Mosby's
Emergency
Nursing
Reference

Mosby's Emergency Nursing Reference

PAMELA STINSON KIDD, RN, PhD, CEN
Associate Professor
University of Kentucky College of Nursing
University of Kentucky Hospital
Lexington, Kentucky

PATTY STURT, RN, MSN, CEN
Staff Development Specialist
Emergency Department
University of Kentucky Hospital
Lexington, Kentucky

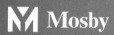 Mosby

St. Louis   Baltimore   Boston
Carlsbad   Chicago   Naples   New York   Philadelphia   Portland
London   Madrid   Mexico City   Singapore   Sydney   Tokyo   Toronto   Wiesbaden

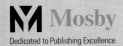

Mosby

Dedicated to Publishing Excellence

A Times Mirror
Company

Editor: Robin Carter
Developmental Editor: Jeanne Allison
Project Manager: Carol Sullivan Weis
Production Editor: Marie Doss
Designer: Sheilah Barrett
Illustrator: Jack Reuter

Printed in the United States of America
Composition by Shepherd, Inc.
Printing/binding by R.R. Donnelley

Mosby-Year Book, Inc.
11830 Westline Industrial Drive, St. Louis, Missouri 63146

Library of Congress Cataloging-in-Publication Data
Mosby's emergency nursing reference / [edited by] Pamela Stinson Kidd,
 Patty Sturt.
    p.   cm.
   Includes bibliographical references.
   ISBN 0–8151–5226–4
   1. Emergency nursing—Handbooks, manuals, etc.   I. Kidd, Pamela
Stinson.   II. Sturt, Patty.
   [DNLM: 1. Emergency Nursing—handbooks.   WY 49 M8935 1996]
RT120.E4M69 1996
610.73'61–dc20
DNLM/DLC
for Library of Congress   95–24351
                                                                          CIP

International Standard Book Number ISBN 0-8151-5226-4

95   96   97   98   99   /   9   8   7   6   5   4   3   2   1

Contributors

MARY ROSE BAUER, RN, BSN
Staff Nurse
Emergency Department
University of Kentucky Hospital
Lexington, Kentucky

BARBARA BLAKE, RN, BSN
Staff Nurse
Emergency Department
University of Kentucky Hospital
Lexington, Kentucky

PATRICIA L. BRISKY, RN, BSN, CEN
Staff Nurse
Emergency Department
University of Kentucky Hospital
Lexington, Kentucky

LISA L. CREECH, RN, BSN
Staff Nurse
Emergency Department
University of Kentucky Hospital
Lexington, Kentucky

JULIA H. FULTZ, RN, BSN
Flight Nurse
Aeromedical Services
University of Kentucky Hospital
Lexington, Kentucky

LEE GARNER, RN, ADN, CEN
Divisional Charge Nurse
Emergency Department
University of Kentucky Hospital
Lexington, Kentucky

GEORGE P. GLESSNER III, EMT-P
Flight Paramedic
Aeromedical Services
University of Kentucky Hospital
Lexington, Kentucky

THERESA M. GLESSNER, RN, BSN, CCRN, CEN
Staff Nurse
Emergency Department/Cardiothoracic Intensive Care Unit
University of Kentucky Hospital
Lexington, Kentucky

REGINA M. HEISER, RN, MSN
Operating Room Services
Emergency Department Case Manager
University of Kentucky Hospital
Lexington, Kentucky

CHRISTINE E. LINDSEY, RN
Divisional Charge Nurse
Emergency Department
University of Kentucky Hospital
Lexington, Kentucky

MARCIA G. MESSER, RN, BSN
Outpatient Case Manager
Flight Nurse
Clark Regional Medical Center
Winchester, Kentucky

ELIZABETH GAUDET NOLAN, RN, BSN, CEN
Clinical Staff Nurse
Emergency Department
University of Kentucky Hospital
Lexington, Kentucky

MICHELE NYPAVER, MD
Pediatric Emergency Medicine
University of Kentucky Hospital
Lexington, Kentucky

MARK B. PARSHALL, RN, BSN, CEN
Clinical Nurse III
St. Vincent Hospital
Santa Fe, New Mexico
Doctoral Student
University of Kentucky College of Nursing

MARY PHILLIPS, RN, BSN, CEN
Weekend Divisional Charge Nurse
Emergency Department
University of Kentucky Hospital
Lexington, Kentucky

JANET RODGERS, RN, CFRN
Aeromedical Services
University of Kentucky Hospital
Lexington, Kentucky

CELESTE SHAWLER, MSN, RN, CS
Psychiatric Clinical Nurse Specialist
University of Kentucky Hospital
Lexington, Kentucky

KIMBERLY SHORT, RN, BSN, CEN
Staff Nurse
Emergency Department
University of Kentucky Hospital
Lexington, Kentucky

KIM SPARKS, RN, CEN, EMT-P
Staff Nurse
Emergency Department
University of Kentucky Hospital
Lexington, Kentucky

COLLEEN H. SWARTZ, RN, MSN, CCRN
Trauma Nurse Coordinator
Chief Flight Nurse, Aeromedical Services
University of Kentucky Hospital
Lexington, Kentucky

STEVEN R. TALBERT, RN, MSN, CEN, EMT
Flight Nurse
Aeromedical Services
University of Kentucky Hospital
Lexington, Kentucky

DARLENE WELSH, RN, MSN
Nursing Instructor
College of Nursing
Critical Care Clinical Nurse Specialist
University of Kentucky Hospital
Lexington, Kentucky

JUDITH E. LOMBARDI, RN, MSN, ENP
Emergency Department
Dartmouth Hitchcock Medical Center
Lebanon, New Hampshire

KATHLEEN B. MCLEOD, RN, MA, CEN
Tucson Medical Center
Tucson, Arizona

WAYNE C. MCLEOD, BA, CFRN, REMTP
Snell & Wilmer
Tucson, Arizona

DARLENE T. SCHELPER, MSN, RN, CEN
Emergency Services
Milton S. Hershey Medical Center
Pennsylvania State University
Hershey, Pennsylvania

JUNE THOMPSON, RN
New Mexico Department of Health
Division of Epidemiology
Reynoldsburg, Ohio

To the greatest son in the world, Richard, and to Pam for constantly motivating and encouraging me. PS

To Elliot who patiently waited to arrive until the manuscript was done. To Baby and Pa Bog who kept the home fires burning. Can we go camping now? PK

This book is written by emergency nurses for emergency nurses. After years of carrying index cards in our labcoats, the nurses in the ED decided it was time to organize our knowledge in a manner that all emergency nurses could use and appreciate. This handbook is designed to fit in the pocket, be there when needed, and provide the essentials to manage the variety of situations that are seen every day in an emergency department. Unless detailed information is needed on a particular topic, this book should eliminate the need to "track down" other reference books when time is of the essence.

Emergency nurses must constantly prioritize because patient acuity and census prevent the provision of comprehensive care to everyone. The chapters are organized in the same manner as care evolves in the ED. They start with triage priorities, followed by assessment, diagnostic, and intervention priorities. Pertinent cues to address are presented throughout each chapter, since emergency nurses use cues to prioritize care demands. Independent interventions initiated by the nurse before physician examination are included, since emergency nurses "get the treatment process going" while tracking down the emergency physician to inform him/her of patient needs. Each chapter ends with discharge implications and includes expected patient outcomes (EPOs) realistic for patient progress and stabilization while in the ED. These EPOs can be used as concrete measures of the effectiveness of the ED visit. Nursing Alert boxes are included to remind us even in the midst of a chaotic shift of how to prevent errors or to address circumstances that may impact patient outcomes.

The book includes a section on frequently performed ED procedures so that the reader can anticipate needed equipment and review the "how-to" steps just before approaching the patient. Diagnostic tests are discussed to explain why they are ordered and what results indicate to enhance patient preparation and teaching. The Reference Guide section provides easy access to frequently used scales and guides. Tables and figures are used to package information in a concise, easy-to-find manner. Life Span issues, including pediatrics, pregnancy, and geriatrics, are integrated preventing the need for additional books. Drug summary tables are listed at the end of most chapters so that you don't have to wait for the drug insert to be sent from pharmacy. These summaries are just that. Enough information to be safe in administration but not too much to confuse the situation.

Because the editors and contributors are practitioners, they are acutely aware of the changing ED patient population and the need to prioritize care as a result of limited hospital resources (such as hospital beds and ancillary services). In anticipation of decreased laboratory resources, the Reference Guide includes how much blood is needed and the type of specimen tube for each test. It also includes information on ventilator settings and alarms in anticipation of decreased respiratory therapy services.

So throw away those old tattered cards and pieces of paper in your labcoat pocket that contain the pearls of wisdom you have collected over the years! Finally there is a handbook available that has our collective pearls of wisdom that should last us a couple of more years.

Pamela Stinson Kidd

Patty Stuart

Acknowledgments

We want to express our deepest appreciation to Elitha Farmer and Wanda Gabbard for their assistance in producing a beautifully typed manuscript.

Contents

UNIT III: PROCEDURES

UNIT ONE

**Reference
Guide**

REFERENCE GUIDE 1

ACLS Algorithms: Adults

Ventricular Fibrillation/Pulseless Ventricular Tachycardia (VF/VT) Algorithms

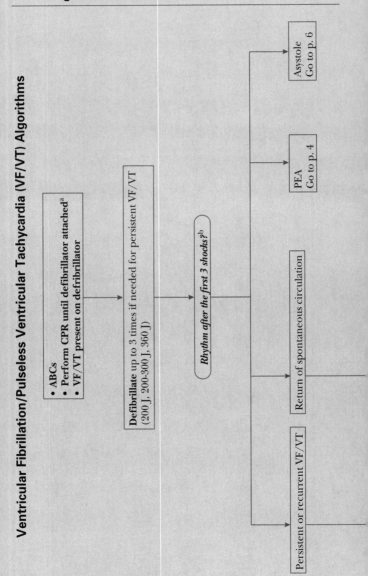

- ABCs
- Perform CPR until defibrillator attached[a]
- VF/VT present on defibrillator

Defibrillate up to 3 times if needed for persistent VF/VT
(200 J, 200-300 J, 360 J)

Rhythm after the first 3 shocks?[b]

Persistent or recurrent VF/VT

Return of spontaneous circulation

PEA
Go to p. 4

Asystole
Go to p. 6

Class I: definitely helpful
Class IIa: acceptable, probably helpful
Class IIb: acceptable, possibly helpful
Class III: not indicated, may be harmful

a. Precordial thump is a Class IIb action in witnessed arrest, no pulse, and no defibrillator immediately available.

b. Hypothermic cardiac arrest is treated differently after this point.

c. The recommended dose of *epinephrine* is 1 mg IV push every 3-5 min. If this approach fails, several Class IIb dosing regimens can be considered:
- Intermediate: *epinephrine* 2-5 mg IV push, every 3-5 min
- Escalating: *epinephrine* 1 mg, 3 mg, 5 mg IV push, 3 min apart
- High: *epinephrine* 0.1 mg/kg IV push, every 3-5 min

d. *Sodium bicarbonate* 1mEq/kg is Class I if patient has known preexisting hyperkalemia.

e. Multiple sequenced shocks are acceptable here (Class 1), especially when medications are delayed.

f. Medication sequence:
- *Lidocaine* 1.0-1.5 mg/kg IV push. Consider repeat in 3-5 min to maximum dose of 3 mg/kg. A single dose of 1.5 mg/kg in cardiac arrest is acceptable.
- *Bretylium* 5 mg/kg IV push. Repeat in 5 min at 10 mg/kg.
- *Magnesium sulfate* 1-2g IV in torsades de pointes or suspected hypomagnesemic state or refractory VF.
- *Procainamide* 30 mg/min in refractory VF (maximum total 17 mg/kg).

g. *Sodium bicarbonate* 1 mEq/kg IV:
  Class IIa
  - If known preexisting bicarbonate-responsive acidosis
  - If overdose with tricyclic antidepressants
  - To alkalinize the urine in drug overdoses
  Class IIb
  - If intubated and continued long arrest interval
  - Upon return of spontaneous circulation after long arrest interval
  Class III
  - Hypoxic lactic acidosis

Continued.

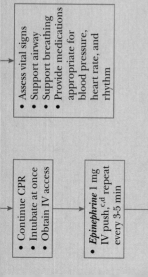

- Assess vital signs
- Support airway
- Support breathing
- Provide medications appropriate for blood pressure, heart rate, and rhythm

- Continue CPR
- Intubate at once
- Obtain IV access

- *Epinephrine* 1 mg IV push,[c,d] repeat every 3-5 min

- **Defibrillate** 360 J within 30-60 sec[e]

- Administer medications of probable benefit (Class IIa) in persistent or recurrent VF/VT[f,g]

- **Defibrillate** 360 J, 30-60 sec after each dose of medication[e]
- Pattern should be drug-shock, drug-shock

Pulseless Electrical Activity (PEA)

Includes
- Electromechanical dissociation (EMD)
- Pseudo-EMD
- Idioventricular rhythms
- Ventricular escape rhythms
- Bradyasystolic rhythms
- Postdefibrillation idioventricular rhythms

- Continue CPR
- Intubate at once
- Obtain IV access

- Assess blood flow using Doppler ultrasound, end-tidal CO_2, echocardiography, or arterial line

Consider possible causes
(Parentheses = possible therapies and treatments)

- Hypovolemia (volume infusion)
- Hypoxia (ventilation)
- Cardiac tamponade (pericardiocentesis)
- Tension pneumothorax (needle decompression)
- Hypothermia
- Massive pulmonary embolism (surgery, *thrombolytics*)

- Drug overdoses such as tricyclics, digitalis, β-blockers, calcium channel blockers
- Hyperkalemia[a]
- Acidosis[b]
- Massive acute myocardial infarction

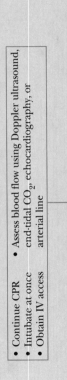

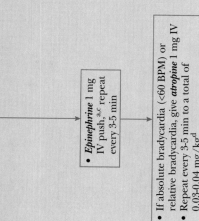

* *Epinephrine* 1 mg IV push,[a,c] repeat every 3-5 min

* If absolute bradycardia (<60 BPM) or relative bradycardia, give *atropine* 1 mg IV
* Repeat every 3-5 min to a total of 0.03-0.04 mg/kg[d]

Class I: definitely helpful
Class IIa: acceptable, probably helpful
Class IIb: acceptable, possibly helpful
Class III: not indicated, may be harmful

a. *Sodium bicarbonate* 1 mEq/kg is Class I if patient has known preexisting hyperkalemia.
b. *Sodium bicarbonate* 1 mEq/kg:
   Class IIa
   • If known preexisting bicarbonate-responsive acidosis
   • If overdose with tricyclic antidepressants
   • To alkalinize the urine in drug overdoses
   Class IIb
   • If intubated and continued long arrest interval
   • Upon return of spontaneous circulation after long arrest interval
   Class III
   • Hypoxic lactic acidosis
c. The recommended dose of *epinephrine* is 1 mg IV push every 3-5 min. If this approach fails, several Class IIb dosing regimens can be considered:
   • Intermediate: *epinephrine* 2-5 mg IV push, every 3-5 min
   • Escalating: *epinephrine* 1 mg, 3 mg, 5 mg IV push, 3 min apart
   • High: *epinephrine* 0.1 mg/kg IV push, every 3-5 min
d. The shorter *atropine* dosing interval (3 min) is possibly helpful in cardiac arrest (Class IIb).

Continued.

Asystole Treatment Algorithm

- Continue CPR
- Intubate at once
- Obtain IV access
- Confirm asystole in more than one lead

↓

Consider possible causes
- Hypoxia
- Hyperkalemia
- Hypokalemia
- Preexisting acidosis
- Drug overdose
- Hypothermia

↓

Consider immediate transcutaneous pacing (TCP)[a]

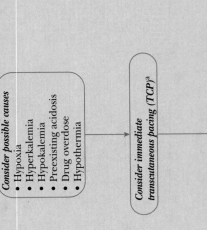

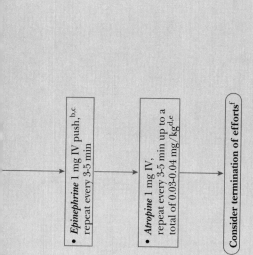

- *Epinephrine* 1 mg IV push,[b,c] repeat every 3-5 min

- *Atropine* 1 mg IV, repeat every 3-5 min up to a total of 0.03-0.04 mg/kg[d,e]

Consider termination of efforts[f]

Class I: definitely helpful
Class IIa: acceptable, probably helpful
Class IIb: acceptable, possibly helpful
Class III: not indicated, may be harmful

a. TCP is a Class IIb intervention. Lack of success may be due to delays in pacing. To be effective TCP must be performed early, simultaneously with drugs. Evidence does not support routine use of TCP for asystole.

b. The recommended dose of *epinephrine* is 1 mg IV push every 3-5 min. If this approach fails, several Class IIb dosing regimens can be considered:
   - Intermediate: *epinephrine* 2-5 mg IV push, every 3-5 min
   - Escalating: *epinephrine* 1 mg-3 mg-5 mg IV push, 3 min apart
   - High: *epinephrine* 0.1 mg/kg IV push, every 3-5 min

c. *Sodium bicarbonate* 1 mEq/kg is Class I if patient has known preexisting hyperkalemia.

d. The shorter *atropine* dosing interval (3 min) is Class IIb in asystolic arrest.

e. *Sodium bicarbonate* 1 mEq/kg:
   Class IIa
   - If known preexisting bicarbonate-responsive acidosis
   - If overdose with tricyclic antidepressants
   - To alkalinize the urine in drug overdoses
   Class IIb
   - If intubated and continued long arrest interval
   - Upon return of spontaneous circulation after long arrest interval
   Class III
   - Hypoxic lactic acidosis

f. If patient remains in asystole or other agonal rhythm after successful intubation and initial medications and no reversible causes are identified, consider termination of resuscitative efforts by a physician. Consider interval since arrest.

Continued.

Bradycardia Algorithm (Patient is not in cardiac arrest)

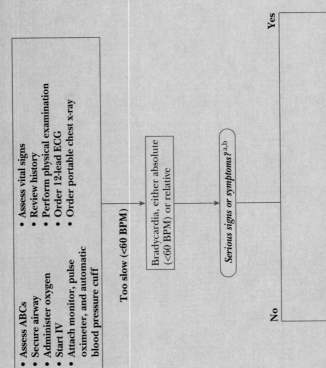

- Assess ABCs
- Secure airway
- Administer oxygen
- Start IV
- Attach monitor, pulse oximeter, and automatic blood pressure cuff

- Assess vital signs
- Review history
- Perform physical examination
- Order 12-lead ECG
- Order portable chest x-ray

Too slow (<60 BPM)

Bradycardia, either absolute (<60 BPM) or relative

Serious signs or symptoms?[a,b]

No   Yes

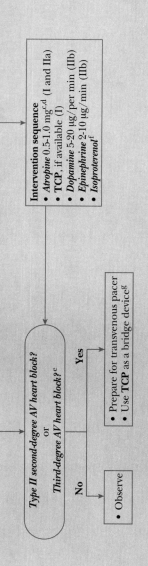

Intervention sequence
- *Atropine* 0.5-1.0 mg[c,d] (I and IIa)
- **TCP**, if available (I)
- *Dopamine* 5-20 µg/per min (IIb)
- *Epinephrine* 2-10 µg/min (IIb)
- *Isoproterenol*[f]

Type II second-degree AV heart block?
or
Third-degree AV heart block?[e]

No → • Observe

Yes →
- Prepare for transvenous pacer
- Use **TCP** as a bridge device[g]

a. Serious signs or symptoms must be related to the slow rate. Clinical manifestations include:
  - Symptoms (chest pain, shortness of breath, decreased level of consciousness)
  - Signs (low BP, shock, pulmonary congestion, CHF, acute MI)

b. Do not delay TCP while awaiting IV access or for *atropine* to take effect if patient is symptomatic.

c. Denervated transplanted hearts will not respond to *atropine*. Go at once to pacing, *catecholamine* infusion, or both.

d. *Atropine* should be given in repeat doses every 3-5 min up to a total of 0.03-0.04 mg/kg. Use the shorter dosing interval (3 min) in severe clinical conditions. It has been suggested that *atropine* should be used with caution in atrioventricular (AV) block at the His-Purkinje level (type II AV block and new third-degree block with wide QRS complexes) (Class IIb).

e. Never treat third-degree heart block plus ventricular escape beats with *lidocaine.*

f. *Isoproterenol* should be used, if at all, with extreme caution. At low doses it is a Class IIb (possibly helpful); at higher doses it is Class III (harmful).

g. Verify patient tolerance and mechanical capture. Use analgesia and sedation as needed.

TCP, Transcutaneous pacing.

Continued.

REFERENCE GUIDE 1 (cont'd)

Tachycardia Algorithm

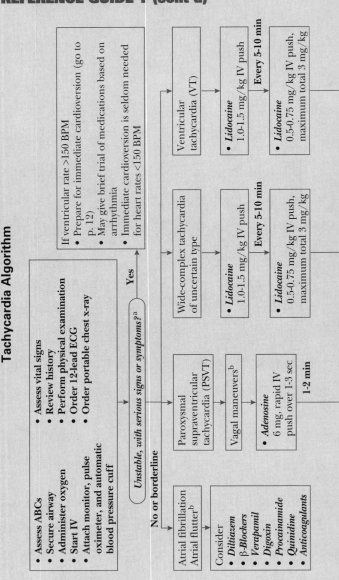

- Assess ABCs
- Secure airway
- Administer oxygen
- Start IV
- Attach monitor, pulse oximeter, and automatic blood pressure cuff
- Assess vital signs
- Review history
- Perform physical examination
- Order 12-lead ECG
- Order portable chest x-ray

Unstable, with serious signs or symptoms?[a]

No or borderline

Yes

If ventricular rate >150 BPM
- Prepare for immediate cardioversion (go to p. 12)
- May give brief trial of medications based on arrhythmia
- Immediate cardioversion is seldom needed for heart rates <150 BPM

Atrial fibrillation
Atrial flutter[b]

Consider
- *Diltiazem*
- *β-Blockers*
- *Verapamil*
- *Digoxin*
- *Procainamide*
- *Quinidine*
- *Anticoagulants*

Paroxysmal supraventricular tachycardia (PSVT)

Vagal maneuvers[b]

- *Adenosine*
6 mg, rapid IV push over 1-3 sec

1-2 min

Wide-complex tachycardia of uncertain type

- *Lidocaine*
1.0-1.5 mg/kg IV push

Every 5-10 min

- *Lidocaine*
0.5-0.75 mg/kg IV push, maximum total 3 mg/kg

Ventricular tachycardia (VT)

- *Lidocaine*
1.0-1.5 mg/kg IV push

Every 5-10 min

- *Lidocaine*
0.5-0.75 mg/kg IV push, maximum total 3 mg/kg

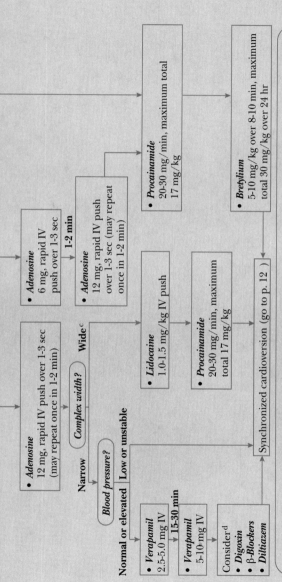

- *Adenosine*
12 mg, rapid IV push over 1-3 sec
(may repeat once in 1-2 min)

Narrow ← **Complex width?** → **Wide**ᶜ

- *Adenosine*
6 mg, rapid IV
push over 1-3 sec

1-2 min

- *Adenosine*
12 mg, rapid IV push
over 1-3 sec (may repeat
once in 1-2 min)

- *Procainamide*
20-30 mg/min, maximum total
17 mg/kg

- *Bretylium*
5-10 mg/kg over 8-10 min, maximum
total 30 mg/kg over 24 hr

- *Lidocaine*
1.0-1.5 mg/kg IV push

- *Procainamide*
20-30 mg/min, maximum
total 17 mg/kg

Blood pressure?

Normal or elevated | **Low or unstable**

- *Verapamil*
2.5-5.0 mg IV

15-30 min

- *Verapamil*
5-10 mg IV

Considerᵈ
- *Digoxin*
- *β-Blockers*
- *Diltiazem*

Synchronized cardioversion (go to p. 12)

a. Unstable condition must be related to the tachycardia. Signs and symptoms may include chest pain, shortness of breath, decreased level of consciousness, low blood pressure (BP), shock, pulmonary congestion, congestive heart failure, acute myocardial infarction.
b. Carotid sinus pressure is contraindicated in patients with carotid bruits; avoid ice water immersion in patients with ischemic heart disease.
c. If the wide-complex tachycardia is known with certainty to be PSVT and BP is normal/elevated, sequence can include *verapamil*.
d. Use extreme caution with β-blockers after *verapamil*.

Continued.

Electrical Cardioversion Algorithm (Patient is not in cardiac arrest)

Tachycardia
With serious signs and symptoms related to the tachycardia

If ventricular rate is >150 BPM, prepare for **immediate cardioversion**. May give brief trial of medications based on specific arrhythmias. Immediate cardioversion is generally not needed for rates <150 BPM.

Check
- Oxygen saturation
- Suction device
- IV line
- Intubation equipment

Premedicate whenever possible[a]

Synchronized cardioversion[b,c]

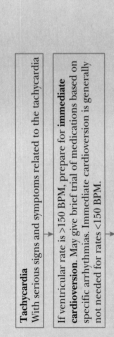

VT[d]	100 J, 200 J
PSVT[e]	300 J, 360 J
Atrial fibrillation	
Atrial flutter[e]	

a. Effective regimens have included a sedative (e.g., *diazepam, midazolam, barbiturates, etomidate, ketamine, methohexital*) with or without an analgesic agent (e.g., *fentanyl, morphine, meperidine*). Many experts recommend anesthesia if service is readily available.

b. Note possible need to resynchronize after each cardioversion.

c. If delays in synchronization occur and clinical conditions are critical, go to immediate unsynchronized shocks.

d. Treat polymorphic VT (irregular form and rate) like VF: 200 J, 200-300 J, 360 J.

e. PSVT and atrial flutter often respond to lower energy levels (start with 50 J).

Modified from *Textbook of advanced cardiac life support*, Dallas, 1994, American Heart Association.

REFERENCE GUIDE 2
Arterial Blood Gas Interpretation

Blood gases: normal values

Arterial	Value	Venous
7.35-7.45	pH	7.31-7.41
80-100 mm Hg	Po_2*	30-40 mm Hg
35-45 mm Hg	Pco_2	41-51 mm Hg
21-25 mEq/L	HCO_3^-	22-29 mEq/L
95%-99%	O_2 sat	60%-85%
−2 to +2	BE	0 to +4

Interpretation of arterial blood gas values

	pH	Pco_2	HCO_3^-
Respiratory acidosis	↓	↑	Normal
Respiratory acidosis with ↓ metabolic compensation	↓	↑	↑
Metabolic acidosis	↓	Normal	↓
Metabolic and respiratory acidosis	↓	↑	↓
Metabolic alkalosis	↑	Normal	↑
Metabolic alkalosis with ↓ respiratory compensation	↑	↑	↑
Respiratory alkalosis	↑	↓	Normal
Metabolic and respiratory alkalosis	↑	↓	↑

Modified from Lee G: *Quick emergency care reference*, St Louis, 1992, Mosby.
*In a patient over 60 years old, Pao_2 is equal to 80 mm Hg minus 1 mm Hg for every year over 60. Expected Pao_2 can be determined by multiplying the Fio_2 by 5.

REFERENCE GUIDE 3
Calculations and Conversions

Conversions

Volume

5 ml = 1 teaspoon (tsp)
15 ml = 1 tablespoon (T)
30 ml = 1 ounce (oz) = 2 T
500 ml = 1 pint (pt)
1000 ml = 1 quart (qt)

Weight

1 kilogram (kg) = 2.2 pounds (lb)
1 gram (g) = 1000 milligrams (mg)
1 mg = 1000 micrograms (µg)
1 grain (gr) = 60 mg
$\frac{1}{100}$ gr = 0.6 mg
$\frac{1}{150}$ gr = 0.4 mg

Length

2.5 centimeters (cm) = 1 inch

Centigrade (C)/Fahrenheit (F)

$°C = (F - 32) \times \frac{5}{9}$
$°F = (C \times \frac{9}{5}) + 32$

Pressure

1 mm Hg = 1.36 cm H_2O

Critical care calculations

Drug concentration

mg/ml = Drug in solution (mg)/Volume of solution (ml)
µg/ml = mg/ml × 1000

Delivery rate

ml/min = ml/hr ÷ 60

$$µg/kg/min = \frac{µg/ml \times ml/min}{Weight\ (kg)}$$

$$ml/hr = \frac{µg/kg/min\ prescribed \times kg \times 60\ min}{µg/ml}$$

From Keen J, Baird M, Allen J: *Mosby's critical care and emergency drug reference*, St Louis, 1994, Mosby.

REFERENCE GUIDE 4
Diabetic Ketoacidosis (DKA): Adult

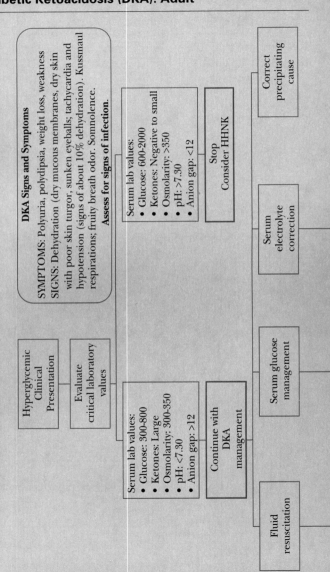

DKA Signs and Symptoms

SYMPTOMS: Polyuria, polydipsia, weight loss, weakness

SIGNS: Dehydration (dry mucous membranes, dry skin with poor skin turgor, sunken eyeballs; tachycardia and hypotension (signs of about 10% dehydration). Kussmaul respirations; fruity breath odor. Somnolence.

Assess for signs of infection.

Hyperglycemic Clinical Presentation

Evaluate critical laboratory values

Serum lab values:
- Glucose: 300–800
- Ketones: Large
- Osmolarity: 300–350
- pH: <7.30
- Anion gap: >12

Serum lab values:
- Glucose: 600–2000
- Ketones: Negative to small
- Osmolarity: >350
- pH: >7.30
- Anion gap: <12

Continue with DKA management

Stop
Consider HHNK

Fluid resuscitation

Serum glucose management

Serum electrolyte correction

Correct precipitating cause

Goal: Attain normovolemia
Initial 1-2 hr: 0.9% NS at 1000 ml/hr
Maintenance: 0.9% NS at 250-400 ml/hr

When glucose ≤250, begin 5% dextrose/0.45% NS solution (See Glucose Correction)

IF

Glucose = 100-250 with ketones of moderate to large, consider starting 10% dextrose

Regular insulin (IV) bolus: 0.3 U/kg or 10 U IV push (optional)
followed by:
Continuous IV regular insulin drip at 0.1 U/kg/hr (6-10 U/hr)
Increase insulin 2-10 fold if no response by 4 hr

Monitor serum:
Glucose: q 1-2 hr
Acetone: q 4 hr
Arterial pH: q 4-12 hr
[Blood glucose should drop approx. 10%/hr]

Evaluate serum electrolytes:
K^+ = q 1-2 hr
Na^+Cl = q 4 hr
PO_4 = q 12-24 hr
12-lead ECG; Continuous cardiac monitoring;
Phosphate therapy if hypophosphatemia:
Sodium or potassium phosphate at ≤10 mmol/hr
Cautious use of bicarbonate for correction of severe acidosis
K^+ replacement: Initiate with second liter of IV fluid

Patient Level/	Replacement
3.5	40 mEq
3.5-5.5	20 mEq
>5.5	Hold replacement

Glucose: 200-300
Ketones: Negative to moderate
pH: 7.30-7.45
Initiate clear liquid diet and advance as tolerated
Initiate SQ insulin 30-60 min before DC of IV insulin
Placed on maintenance regular insulin q 6 hr or NPH with supplemental regular insulin SQ

Patient stable: Continue current therapy

Glucose: >300
Ketones: Moderate to large
pH: <7.30
Continue current therapy

Patient unstable: Consider pulmonary artery catheter or CVP
If circulatory collapse, may administer plasma expanders

Developed by Kathleen Wagner RN, MSN, Critical Care CNS, University Hospital/University of Kentucky College of Nursing.

REFERENCE GUIDE 5

Electrocardiogram Changes in Myocardial Infarction

Type of infarction	Anatomical location	ECG patterns
Lateral		I, a V_L, V_5, V_6: abnormal Q wave, ST elevation, T wave inversion
Inferior		II, III, a V_F: abnormal Q wave, ST elevation, T wave inversion
Anterior		V_1-V_4: abnormal Q wave, loss of R wave progression, ST elevation, T wave inversion
Posterior		V_1, V_9: tall R wave, ST depression, tall symmetrical T wave
Note: RV infarction		V_{4R}: ST elevation >1 mm

From Lee G: *Quick emergency care reference*, St Louis, 1992, Mosby.

REFERENCE GUIDE 6

Glasgow Coma Scale*: Adult and Infant

| Activity | Adult | | Infant |
	Best response	Points	Best response
Eye opening	Spontaneous	4	Spontaneous
	To verbal stimuli	3	To speech
	To pain	2	To pain
	No response to pain	1	No response to pain
Motor	Follows commands	6	Normal spontaneous movements
	Localizes pain	5	Localizes pain
	Withdrawal in response to pain	4	Withdrawal in response to pain
	Flexion in response to pain	3	Flexion in response to pain
	Extension in response to pain	2	Extension in response to pain
	No response to pain	1	No response to pain
Verbal	Oriented	5	Coos, babbles
	Confused	4	Irritable, crying
	Inappropriate words	3	Cries to pain
	Incomprehensible sounds	2	Moans to pain
	No verbal response	1	No verbal response

From Stillwell SB: *Mosby's critical care nursing reference,* St Louis, 1992, Mosby.
*Possible points of 3-15; score of <8 = coma.

Hemodynamic Values

Parameter	Formula	Normal range
Cardiac output (CO)	$HR \times SV$	4-8 L/min
Cardiac index (CI)	$\dfrac{CO}{BSA}$	2.5-4.0 L/min/m^2
Stroke volume (SV)	$\dfrac{CO \times 1000}{HR}$	55-100 ml/beat
Stroke volume index (SVI)	$\dfrac{SV}{BSA}$	33-75 ml/m^2/beat
Stroke index (SI)	$\dfrac{CI \times 1000}{HR}$	30-65 ml/m^2/beat
Mean arterial pressure (MAP)	$\dfrac{2(DBP) + SBP}{3}$	70-105 mm Hg
Systemic vascular resistance (SVR)	$\dfrac{MAP - CVP \times 80}{CO}$	700-1600 dynes/sec/cm^{-5}
Pulmonary vascular resistance (PVR)	$\dfrac{PAM - PAWP \times 80}{CO}$	20-130 dynes/sec/cm^{-5}
Arterial oxygen content (CaO_2)	$SaO_2 \times Hgb \times 1.38 + (PaO_2 \times .0031)$	18-20 ml/100 ml or 20 vol %
Venous oxygen content (CvO_2)	$SvO_2 \times Hgb \times 1.38 + (PvO_2 \times .0031)$	15.5 ml/100 ml or 20 vol %
Arterial venous oxygen content difference ($CO_{2(a-v)}$)	$CaO_2 - CvO_2$	4-6 ml/100 ml or vol %
Arterial oxygen delivery (DaO_2)	$CO \times 10 \times CaO_2$	900-1200 ml/min
Venous oxygen delivery (DaO_2)	$CO \times 10 \times CvO_2$	775 ml/min
Oxygen consumption (VO_2)	$CO \times 10 \times CO_{2(a-v)}$	200-250 ml/min
Mixed venous oxygen saturation (SvO_2)	$1 - VO_2/DO_2$	60-80%
Alveolar-arterial oxygen gradient ($DO_2)_{(A-a)}$	$PAO_2 - PaO_2$	<15 mm Hg
Respiratory quotient (RQ)	$\dfrac{O_2 \text{ consumption}}{CO_2 \text{ consumption}}$	0.8-1
Cerebral perfusion pressure (CPP)	$MAP - ICP$	80-100 mm Hg

Modified from Keen J, Baird M, Allen J: *Mosby's Critical care and emergency drug reference,* St Louis, 1994, Mosby.

BSA, Body surface area; *PAM,* pulmonary artery mean (pressure).

REFERENCE GUIDE 8
Immunization Schedule

Age(s)	Vaccine(s)
Birth	HBV*$_1$
2 months	HBV$_{1,2}$, DTP†, OPV‡, HbCV§$_{1,2}$
4 months	HBV$_2$, DTP, OPV, HbCV$_{1,2}$
6 months	HBV$_1$, DTP, HbCV$_1$, OPV (optional)
12 months	HbCV$_2$
15 months	DTaP or DTP‖, OPV, MMR¶, HbCV$_1$, HBV$_{1,2}$ (depending on schedule)
4-6 years	DTaP or DTP‖, OPV, MMR
14-16 years (and every 10 years throughout life)	Td#

From Centers For Disease Control and Prevention: *ACIP recommended immunization schedule,* Atlanta, 1992, The Center.

* Hepatitis B vaccine. May be given in either of 2 schedules:
  1. Birth, 1-2 months, 6-18 months (Note: The third dose of HBV should be given 6 months after the second dose.)
  2. 2 months, 4 months, 12-16 months
† Diphtheria, tetanus, and pertussis.
‡ Oral polio vaccine.
§ *Haemophyllus* b conjugate vaccine:
  1. HbOC is given at 2, 4, 6, and 15 months
  2. PRP-OMP is given at 2, 4, and 12 months
‖ DTP preparation containing acellular pertussis vaccine (DTaP) is recommended for this dose, but whole-cell DTP may still be used if TaP is not available.
¶ Measles, mumps, and rubella.
# Tetanus and diphtheria.

REFERENCE GUIDE 9

Intracranial Pressure Monitoring Checklist

Problem	Action
No waveform	Check power to monitor and to trace
	Check gain setting
	Check all connections
	Check for air bubbles in system*
High pressure reading	Check transducer level placement
	Check calibration and rezero
	Evaluate patient:
	Check airway
	Check ventilator settings
	Check ABGs for hypoxemia, hypercarbia
	Check HOB (15-30°)
	Check position of head (do not rotate head)
	Check extremities (limit flexion in lower extremities and hips)
	Check excessive muscle activity (administer muscle relaxants, paralyzing agents as ordered)
	Check abdominal distention
	Check noxious stimuli and remove
	Check temperature
	Check PAP, CO, Svo_2, BP
	Check electrolytes
Low pressure reading	Check transducer level placement
	Check for otorrhea and rhinorrhea
	Check for dislodged catheter—notify physician
	Check if 15-20 mm Hg positive pressure exists (with use of external ventriculostomy)

From Stillwell SB: *Quick critical care reference guide,* ed 2, St Louis, 1994, Mosby.
*Only flush intraventricular catheter or screw under direction of physician.

REFERENCE GUIDE 10

Intracranial Pressure Transducer Placement

The foramen of Monro is the reference point. The outer canthus of the eye or top of ear or external auditory meatus can also be used.

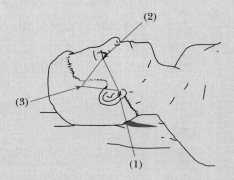

Location of foramen of Monro for transducer placement. Map an imaginary equilateral triangle from *(1)* the external auditory meatus to *(2)* the outer canthus of the eye to *(3)* behind the hairline. Point *3* is the location of the foramen of Monro.

From Stillwell SB: *Quick critical care reference guide,* ed 2, St Louis, 1994, Mosby.

REFERENCE GUIDE 11
Intracranial Pressure Waveforms

A. Pressure
Normal ICP: 0-15 mm Hg
Severe ICP increase: >20 mm Hg
Normal cerebral perfusion pressure: 70-90 mm Hg

B. Waveform
The waveform consists of at least 3 peaks. All components will increase initially if ICP is increased. As ICP progresses, P_2 becomes elevated. If P_2 is equal to or higher than P_1, suspect decreased compliance.

Waveform Types

A waves (plateau waves)
Occur with ICP >20 mm Hg
Sudden transient elevations of 50-100 mm Hg that last 5-20 min, notify physician

B waves (sawtooth waves)
Occur every 30 sec to 2 min
Raise ICP to 50 mm Hg
Signify unstable ICP; precursor to A waves

C waves (small, rhythmic waves)
Occur every 4-8 min
Correlate to normal fluctuations in respirations and blood pressure

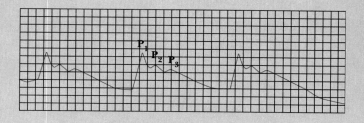

From Stillwell SB: *Quick critical care reference guide,* ed 2, St Louis, 1994, Mosby.

REFERENCE GUIDE 12

Laboratory Values

Test	Normal value	Minimal amount of blood needed for test	Type of specimen tube*
Blood studies			
RBC	4.25-$5.5 \times 10^6 \mu l$ (males)	2 cc (adults)	purple top
	3.6-$5.0 \times 10^6 \mu l$	0.5 cc (pediatrics)	
	(females; *pregnancy:* 4.5-5.5)		
WBC	5-$10^3 \mu l$ (*pregnancy:* 5-$15^3 \mu l$)	same as above	purple top
Hgb	13.5-17.5 g/dl (males)	same as above	purple top
	12-16 g/dl (females; *pregnancy:* 10-14)		
Hct	40%-54% (males)	same as above	purple top
	37%-47% (females; *pregnancy:* 32-42)		
Platelets	150,000-350,000/μl^3	same as above	purple top
	(*pregnancy:* 200,000-350,000)		
PT	10-14 sec (*pregnancy:* 10% ↓)	4.5 cc (adults)	blue top
		1.5 cc (pediatrics)	
		Tube must be filled	
		to top because of	
		preservative	
PTT	30-45 sec (*pregnancy:* slight ↓)	same as above	blue top
Na	135-148 mEq/L	4 cc	red top
K	3.5-5.0 mEq/L	4 cc	red top
Cl	98-106 mEq/L	4 cc	red top
CO_2	24-32 mEq/L	4 cc	red top

BUN	7-18 mg/dl (*pregnancy*: 4-12)	4 cc	red top
Cr	0.7-1.3 mg/dl (males)	4 cc	red top
	0.6-1.2 mg/dl (females; *pregnancy*: 0.4-0.9)		
Glucose	70-110 mg/dl	4 cc	red top
Ca	8.5-10.5 mg/dl	4 cc	red top
Mg	1.3-2.1 mEq/L	4 cc	red top
Osmolality	275-295 mOsm/kg	4 cc	red top
Bilirubin			
Direct	0-0.2 mg/dl	4 cc	red top
Total	0.2-1.0 mg/dl		
Indirect	total minus direct		
Amylase	50-150 U/L	4 cc	red top
Anion Gap	8-16 mEq/L	4 cc	red top
Lactate	0.5-2.2 mEq/L	7 cc	gray top
AST (SGOT)	6-18 U/L (females)	3-4 cc	red top
	7-21 U/L (males)		
with MI elevations			
Onset:	12-18 hr		
Peak:	24-48 hr		
Duration:	3-4 days		

*Large red tube will hold 10 cc, small red tube will hold 7 cc.

Continued.

Test	Normal value	Minimal amount of blood needed for test	Type of specimen tube*
CK	96-140 U/L (females)	3-4 cc	red top
	38-174 U/L (males)		
with MI elevations			
Onset:	4-6 hr		
Peak:	12-24 hr		
Duration:	3-4 days		
CK-MB	0%	3-4 cc	red top
with MI elevations			
Onset:	4-6 hr		
Peak:	12-24 hr		
Duration:	2-3 days		
LDH	90-200 U/L	3-4 cc	red top
with MI elevations			
Onset:	24-48 hr		
Peak:	3-6 days		
Duration:	7-10 days		

LDH₁	17.5%-28.3% of total LDH	3-4 cc	red top
LDH₂	30.4%-36.4% of total LDH	3-4 cc	red top
with MI			
LDH₁ > LDH₂			
Onset:	12-24 hr		
Peak:	48 hr		
Duration:	variable		
Miscellaneous			
Urine Na	40-220 mEq/L	—	—
Urine K	25-125 mEq/L	—	—
Urine Cl	110-250 mEq/L	—	—
Digoxin level	0.5-2 ng/ml Toxic >2 ng/ml	5-7 cc	red top
Phenytoin level	10-20 μg/ml Toxic >20 μg/ml	5-7 cc	red top
Theophylline level	10-20 μg/ml Toxic >20 μg/ml	5-7 cc	red top
Type and crossmatch		10 cc	red top

Modified from Lee G: *Flight nursing,* St Louis, 1992, Mosby.

REFERENCE GUIDE 13

Organ Procurement Guideline*

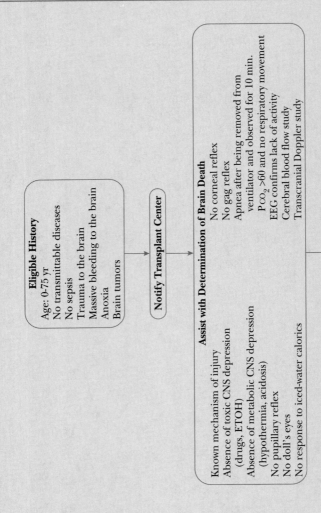

Eligible History
Age: 0-75 yr
No transmittable diseases
No sepsis
Trauma to the brain
Massive bleeding to the brain
Anoxia
Brain tumors

Notify Transplant Center

Assist with Determination of Brain Death
Known mechanism of injury
Absence of toxic CNS depression
  (drugs, ETOH)
Absence of metabolic CNS depression
  (hypothermia, acidosis)
No pupillary reflex
No doll's eyes
No response to iced-water calorics
No corneal reflex
No gag reflex
Apnea after being removed from
  ventilator and observed for 10 min.
$PCO_2 > 60$ and no respiratory movement
EEG confirms lack of activity
Cerebral blood flow study
Transcranial Doppler study

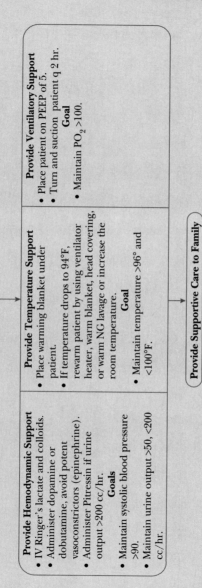

Provide Hemodynamic Support
- IV Ringer's lactate and colloids.
- Administer dopamine or dobutamine, avoid potent vasoconstrictors (epinephrine).
- Administer Pitressin if urine output >200 cc/hr.

Goals
- Maintain systolic blood pressure >90.
- Maintain urine output >50, <200 cc/hr.

Provide Temperature Support
- Place warming blanket under patient.
- If temperature drops to 94°F, rewarm patient by using ventilator heater, warm blanket, head covering, or warm NG lavage or increase the room temperature.

Goal
- Maintain temperature >96° and <100°F.

Provide Ventilatory Support
- Place patient on PEEP of 5.
- Turn and suction patient q 2 hr.

Goal
- Maintain PO_2 >100.

Provide Supportive Care to Family

PEEP, positive end expiratory pressure; *CNS*, central nervous system; *NG*, nasogastric.
*Laboratory and radiographic tests may be ordered at any time throughout this process as required for tissue and organ donation.
Modified from Thacker D: *Organ and tissue donation*, Lexington, KY, 1994, Kentucky Organ Donation Association.

REFERENCE GUIDE 14

Oxygen Delivery Devices: Adults

Flow rate	Oxygen concentrations	Advantages	Disadvantages
Nasal cannula 2–6 L/min	25%–40%	No rebreathing of expired air	Can be used only on patients who are breathing spontaneously
Face mask 10 L/min	50%–60%	Higher O_2 concentration than nasal cannula	Not tolerated well by severely dyspneic patients; can be used only on patients who are breathing spontaneously
Oxygen reservoir mask 10–12 L/min	90%	Higher O_2 concentration than nasal cannula or face mask	Must have tight seal on mask; can be used only on patients who are breathing spontaneously
Venturi mask 4 L/min 8 L/min	24%–28% 35%–40%	Fixed O_2 concentration	Can be used only on patients who are breathing spontaneously
Pocket mask Expired air to 10 L/min	18%–50%	Avoids direct contact with patient's mouth; may add O_2 source; may be used on apneic patient; may be used on child	Rescuer fatigue

Bag-valve-mask			
Room air	21%	Quick; O₂ concentration may be increased; rescuer can sense lung compliance; may be used on both apneic and spontaneously breathing patients	Air in stomach; low tidal volume
12 L/min part	40%-90%		
O₂-powered breathing device			
100 L/min	100%	High O₂ flow; positive pressure	Gastric distension; overinflation; standard device cannot be used for children without special adapter

Modified from Lee G: *Quick emergency care reference*, St Louis, 1992, Mosby.

REFERENCE GUIDE 15

Pain Scales: Children

Pain scale/Description	Instructions	Recommended age
Faces Scale (Wong and Baker, 1988) Consists of six cartoon faces ranging from very happy, smiling face for "no pain" to increasingly less happy faces to final sad, tearful face for "worst pain"	Explain to child that each face is for a person who feels happy because there is no pain (hurt) or sad because there is some or a lot of pain. Face 0 is very happy because there is no hurt. Face 1 hurts just a little bit. Face 2 hurts a little more. Face 3 hurts even more. Face 4 hurts a whole lot, but Face 5 hurts as much as you can imagine, although you don't have to be crying to feel this bad. Ask child to choose the face that best describes own pain. 	Children as young as 3 yr
Oucher (Beyer, 1988) Consists of six photographs of child's face representing "no hurt" to "biggest hurt you could ever have;" also includes a vertical scale with numbers from 0 to 100	*Photographs:* Explain to child that face at bottom has "no hurt, no hurt at all;" second picture, "just a little bit of hurt;" third picture, "a little bit more;" fourth picture, "even more hurt;" fifth picture, *"pretty* much hurt;" and the last picture, "biggest hurt you could ever have." Ask child to choose face that best describes own pain.	Children as young as 3 yr; use numeric scale if child can count to 100; otherwise use photographic scale

Numeric Scale
Uses straight line with end points identified as "no pain" and "worst pain;" divisions along line are marked in units from 0 to 10 (high number may vary)

Numbers: Explain to child that 0 means you have "no hurt;" 0 to 29, "little hurts;" 30 to 69, "middle hurts;" 70 to 99, "big hurts;" and 100, "biggest hurt you could ever have." Ask child to choose any number between 0 and 100, not just numbers pictured on Oucher, that best describes own pain.

Explain to child that at one end of the line is a 0, which means that a person feels no pain (hurt). At the other end is a 10, which means the person feels the worst pain imaginable. The numbers 1 to 9 are for a very little pain to a whole lot of pain. Ask child to choose number that best describes own pain.

Children as young as 5 yr, provided they can count and have some concept of numbers

```
No pain                                            Worst pain
   |____|____|____|____|____|____|____|____|____|____|
   0    1    2    3    4    5    6    7    8    9    10
```

Poker Chip (Hester, 1979, 1989)
Uses plastic (poker) chips; several variations in color and number of chips have been described; original used four white chips

Explain to child that these are "pieces of hurt." One piece is a "little bit of hurt," and four pieces is the "most hurt." Ask child to choose number of pieces that describes own pain. If child replies "no pain," record a 0.

Children as young as 4 to 4½ yr, provided they can count and have some concept of numbers

Continued.

Pain Scales: Children (cont'd)

Pain scale/Description	Instructions	Recommended age
Color Tool (Eland, 1985) Uses crayons or markers for child to construct own scale	Ask child to identify things that have hurt in the past and what has hurt the worst. Give child eight crayons or markers (yellow, orange, red, green, blue, purple, brown, and black) in a random order. Ask child which color is like the worst pain experienced. Place that crayon or marker aside and ask child to identify crayon that is like a hurt not quite as bad as the worst hurt. Place that crayon aside and ask which other crayon is like something that hurts just a little. Place that crayon with the others and ask child which crayon is like no hurt at all. Show four crayon choices to child in order from worst-hurt color to no-hurt color. Ask child to show on body outline where it hurts using crayon of color that most nearly is like own pain. When colors are ranked, assign them a numeric value of 0 to 3.	Children as young as 4 yr, provided they know their colors and are not color blind
Simple Descriptive Scale Uses descriptive words (may vary according to scale) to denote varying intensities of pain.	Explain to child that at one end of line is *no pain* because person feels no hurt. At the other end is *worst pain* because person feels the worst pain imaginable. The words in between are *mild* for just a little pain, *moderate* for a little more, *quite a lot* for even more, and *very bad* for a whole lot of pain. Ask child to choose word that best describes own pain.	Children as young as 5 yr, although words may need explanation

No pain	Mild	Moderate	Quite a lot	Very bad	Worst pain
0	1	2	3	4	5

Visual Analogue Scale
Uses 10 cm horizontal line with end points marked "no pain" and "worst pain"

Ask child to place a mark on line that best describes amount of own pain. With a centimeter ruler, measure from the "no pain" end to the mark and record this measurement as the pain score.

Young school-age children: may understand concept better if presented as vertical line with anchor phrases such as "no hurt" and "biggest hurt you could ever have" (Beyer and Aradine, 1987) and described as thermometer

From Whaley LF, Wong DL: *Whaley & Wong's essentials of pediatric nursing,* ed 4, St Louis, 1993, Mosby.

REFERENCE GUIDE 16

Pain Treatment: Pediatrics and Adults

Drug	Usual adult dose	Usual pediatric dose*	Comments
Oral NSAIDs			
Acetaminophen	650-975 mg q 4 hr	10-15 mg/kg q 4 hr	Acetaminophen lacks the peripheral anti-inflammatory activity of other NSAIDs
Aspirin	650-975 mg q 4 hr	10-15 mg/kg q 4 hr†	The standard against which other NSAIDs are compared; inhibits platelet aggregation; may cause postoperative bleeding
Choline magnesium trisalicylate (Trilisate)	1000-1500 mg bid	25 mg/kg bid	May have minimal antiplatelet activity; also available as oral liquid
Diflunisal (Dolobid)	1000 mg initial dose followed by 500 mg q 12 hr		
Etodolac (Lodine)	200-400 mg q 6-8 hr		
Fenoprofen calcium (Nalfon)	200 mg q 4-6 hr		
Ibuprofen (Motrin, others)	400 mg q 4-6 hr	10 mg/kg q 6-8 hr	Available as several brand names and as generic; also available as oral suspension
Ketoprofen (Orudis)	25-75 mg q 6-8 hr		
Magnesium salicylate	650 mg q 4 hr		Many brands and generic forms available
Meclofenamate sodium (Meclomen)	50 mg q 4-6 hr		

Mefenamic acid (Ponstel)	250 mg q 6 hr		
Naproxen (Naprosyn)	500 mg initial dose followed by 250 mg q 6-8 hr	5 mg/kg q 12 hr	Also available as oral liquid
Naproxen sodium (Anaprox)	550 mg initial dose followed by 275 mg q 6-8 hr		
Salsalate (Disalcid, others)	500 mg q 4 hr		May have minimal antiplatelet activity Available in generic form from several distributors
Sodium salicylate	325-650 mg q 3-4 hr		
Parenteral NSAID			
Ketorolac (Toradol)	IV: Begin with 30-60 mg IV undiluted form through a Y-tube or three-way stopcock of infusion set administered over 5 minutes. All succeeding doses are reduced by half (15-30 mg). IV dosage is considered investigational. 30 or 60 mg IM initial dose followed by 15 or 30 mg q 6 hr		Intramuscular dose not to exceed 5 days
	Oral dose following IM dosage: 10 mg q 6-8 hr		

Continued.

Note: Only the above NSAIDs have FDA approval for use as simple analgesics, but clinical experience has been gained with other drugs as well.

*Drug recommendations are limited to NSAIDs where pediatric dosing experience is available.

†Contraindicated in presence of fever or other evidence of viral illness.

Pain Treatment: Pediatrics and Adults (cont'd)

Drug	Approximate equianalgesic oral dose	Approximate equianalgesic parenteral dose	Recommended starting dose (adults >50 kg body weight)		Recommended starting dose (children and adults <50 kg body weight)‡	
			oral	parenteral	oral	parenteral
Opioid Agonist						
Morphine§	30 mg q 3-4 hr (around-the-clock dosing) 60 mg q 3-4 hr single dose or intermittent dosing	10 mg q 3-4 hr	30 mg q 3-4 hr	10 mg q 3-4 hr	0.3 mg/kg q 3-4 hr	0.1 mg/kg q 3-4 hr
Codeine‖	130 mg q 3-4 hr	75 mg q 3-4 hr	60 mg q 3-4 hr	60 mg q 2 hr (IM, SC)	1 mg q 3-4 hr¶	Not recommended
Hydromorphone§ (Dilaudid)	7.5 mg q 3-4 hr	1.5 mg q 3-4 hr	6 mg q 3-4 hr	1.5 mg q 3-4 hr	0.06 mg q 3-4 hr	0.015 mg/kg q 3-4 hr
Hydrocodone (in Lorcet, Lortab, Vicodin, others)	30 mg q 3-4 hr	Not available	10 mg q 3-4 hr	Not available	0.2 mg q 3-4 hr	Not available
Levorphanol (Levo-Dromoran)	4 mg q 6-8 hr	2 mg q 6-8 hr	4 mg q 6-7 hr	2 mg q 6-8 hr	0.04 mg q 3-4 hr	0.02 mg/kg q 6-8 hr
Meperidine (Demerol)	300 mg q 2-3 hr	100 mg q 3 hr	Not recommended	100 mg q 3 hr	Not recommended	0.75 mg/kg q 2-3 hr

Methadone (Dolophine, others)	20 mg q 6-8 hr	10 mg q 6-8 hr	20 mg q 6-8 hr	10 mg q 6-8 hr	0.2 mg q 6-8 hr	0.1 mg/kg q 6-8 hr
Oxycodone (Roxicodone, also in Percocet, Percodan, Tylox, others)	30 mg q 3-4 hr	Not available	10 mg q 3-4 hr	Not available	0.2 mg q 3-4 hr[¶]	Not available
Oxymorphone[§] (Numorphan)	Not available	1 mg q 3-4 hr	Not available	1 mg q 3-4 hr[¶]	Not recommended	Not recommended

From Acute Pain Management Guideline Panel: *Acute pain management operative or medical procedures and training: clinical practice guidelines,* Rockland, Md, 1992, Aging for Health Care Policy and Research, Public Health Service, U.S. Department of Health and Human Services.

Note: Published tables vary in the suggested doses that are equianalgesic to morphine. Clinical response is the criterion that must be applied for each patient; titration to clinical response is necessary. Because there is not complete cross tolerance among these drugs, it is usually necessary to use a lower equianalgesic dose when changing drugs and to retitrate to response. Caution: Recommended doses do not apply to patients with renal or hepatic insufficiency or other conditions affecting drug metabolism and kinetics.

[‡]**Caution:** Doses listed for patients with body weight less than 50 kg cannot be used as initial starting doses in babies younger than 6 months of age.

[§]For morphine, hydromorphone, and oxymorphone, rectal administration is an alternative route for patients unable to take oral medications, but equianalgesic doses may differ from oral and parenteral doses because of pharmacokinetic differences.

[ǁ]**Caution:** Codeine doses above 65 mg often are not appropriate because of diminishing incremental analgesia with increasing doses but continually increasing constipation and other side effects.

[¶]**Caution:** Doses of aspirin and acetaminophen in combination opioid/NSAID preparations must also be adjusted to the patient's body weight.

Continued.

Drug	Approximate equianalgesic oral dose	Approximate equianalgesic parenteral dose	Recommended starting dose (adult <50 kg body weight)		Recommended starting dose (children and adults >50 kg body weight)‡	
			oral	parenteral	oral	parenteral
Opioid Agonist-Antagonist and Partial Agonist						
Buprenorphine (Buprenex)	Not available	0.3-0.4 mg q 6-8 hr	Not available	0.4 mg q 6-8 hr	Not available	0.004 mg/kg q 6-8 hr
Butorphanol (Stadol)	Not available	2 mg q 3-4 hr	Not available	2 mg q 3-4 hr	Not available	Not recommended
Nalbuphine (Nubain)	Not available	10 mg q 3-4 hr	Not available	10 mg q 3-4 hr	Not available	0.1 mg/kg q 3-4 hr
Pentazocine (Talwin others)	150 mg q 3-4 hr	60 mg q 3-4 hr	50 mg q 4-6 hr	Not recommended	Not recommended	Not recommended

REFERENCE GUIDE 16
Pediatric Pain Medications

Mild pain

Acetaminophen	10-15 mg/kg PO q 4 hr
Ibuprofen (Motrin, others)	5-10 mg/kg PO 6-8 hr

Moderate pain

Acetaminophen with codeine	1 mg/kg codeine PO q 3-4 hr

Severe pain

Morphine[†]	0.1 mg/kg IV/IM 3-4 hr
or Meperidine	0.75 mg/kg IV/IM 2-3 hr
or Hydromorphone (Dilaudid)	0.015 mg/kg 3-4 hr

From Acute Pain Management Guideline Panel: *Acute pain management, operative or medical procedures and trauma: clinical practice guidelines.* Rockland, Md, 1992, Agency for Health Care Policy and Research, Public Health Service, U.S. Department of Health and Human Services.
[†]Fentanyl may be preferable when cardiovascular stability is an issue and patients are closely monitored and/or intubated. Meperidine should be used in exceptional circumstances.

REFERENCE GUIDE 17

Pediatric Emergency Drugs Used in Advanced Life Support

Drug	Dose	Remarks
Adenosine	0.1-0.2 mg/kg Maximum single dose: 12 mg	Rapid IV bolus
Atropine sulfate	0.02 mg/kg per dose	Minimum dose: 0.1 mg Maximum single dose: 0.5 mg in child, 1.0 mg in adolescent
Bretylium	5 mg/kg; may be increased to 10 mg/kg	Rapid IV
Calcium chloride 10%	20 mg/kg per dose	Give slowly

Continued.

REFERENCE GUIDE 17

Pediatric Emergency Drugs Used in Advanced Life Support (cont'd)

Drug	Dose	Remarks
Dopamine hydrochloride	2-20 µg/kg/min	α-Adrenergic action dominates at ≥ 15-20 µg/kg/min
Dobutamine hydrochloride	2-20 µg/kg/min	Titrate to desired effect
Epinephrine* For bradycardia	IV/IO: 0.01 mg/kg (1:10,000) ET: 0.1 mg/kg (1:1000)	—
For asystolic or pulseless arrest	*First dose:* IV/IO 0.01 mg/kg (1:10,000) ET: 0.1 mg/kg (1:1000) Doses as high as 0.2 mg/kg may be effective *Subsequent doses:* IV/IO/ET: 0.1 mg/kg (1:1000) Doses as high as 0.2 mg/kg may be effective	—
Epinephrine infusion	Initial at 0.1 µg/kg/min Higher infusion dose used if asystole present	Titrate to desired effect (0.1-1.0 µg/kg/min)
Lidocaine	1 mg/kg per dose	
Lidocaine infusion	20-50 µg/kg per minute	
Sodium bicarbonate	1 mEq/kg per dose or 0.3 × kg × base deficit	Infuse slowly and only if ventilation is adequate

From AHA Committee: *Guidelines for cardiopulmonary resuscitation and emergency care,* Part IV, pediatric advanced life support, *JAMA,* 1992, American Heart Association.
*Be aware of effective dose of preservative administered (if preservatives present in epinephrine preparation) when high doses are used.
IV, intravenous route; *IO,* intraosseous route; *ET,* endotracheal route.

REFERENCE GUIDE 18

ACLS Algorithms: Pediatrics

Bradycardia Decision Tree

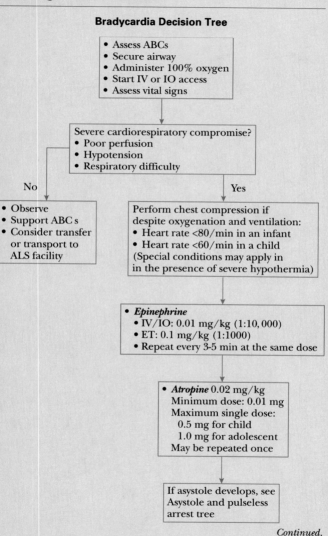

- Assess ABCs
- Secure airway
- Administer 100% oxygen
- Start IV or IO access
- Assess vital signs

Severe cardiorespiratory compromise?
- Poor perfusion
- Hypotension
- Respiratory difficulty

No

Yes

- Observe
- Support ABCs
- Consider transfer or transport to ALS facility

Perform chest compression if despite oxygenation and ventilation:
- Heart rate <80/min in an infant
- Heart rate <60/min in a child
(Special conditions may apply in in the presence of severe hypothermia)

- *Epinephrine*
  - IV/IO: 0.01 mg/kg (1:10,000)
  - ET: 0.1 mg/kg (1:1000)
  - Repeat every 3-5 min at the same dose

- *Atropine* 0.02 mg/kg
  Minimum dose: 0.01 mg
  Maximum single dose:
  0.5 mg for child
  1.0 mg for adolescent
  May be repeated once

If asystole develops, see Asystole and pulseless arrest tree

Continued.

REFERENCE GUIDE 18

ACLS Algorithms: Pediatrics (cont'd)

Asystole and Pulseless Arrest Decision Tree

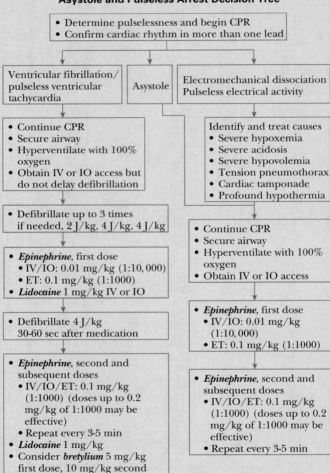

- Determine pulselessness and begin CPR
- Confirm cardiac rhythm in more than one lead

Ventricular fibrillation/ pulseless ventricular tachycardia

Asystole

Electromechanical dissociation Pulseless electrical activity

- Continue CPR
- Secure airway
- Hyperventilate with 100% oxygen
- Obtain IV or IO access but do not delay defibrillation

Identify and treat causes
- Severe hypoxemia
- Severe acidosis
- Severe hypovolemia
- Tension pneumothorax
- Cardiac tamponade
- Profound hypothermia

- Defibrillate up to 3 times if needed, 2 J/kg, 4 J/kg, 4 J/kg

- Continue CPR
- Secure airway
- Hyperventilate with 100% oxygen
- Obtain IV or IO access

- *Epinephrine*, first dose
  - IV/IO: 0.01 mg/kg (1:10,000)
  - ET: 0.1 mg/kg (1:1000)
- *Lidocaine* 1 mg/kg IV or IO

- Defibrillate 4 J/kg 30-60 sec after medication

- *Epinephrine*, first dose
  - IV/IO: 0.01 mg/kg (1:10,000)
  - ET: 0.1 mg/kg (1:1000)

- *Epinephrine*, second and subsequent doses
  - IV/IO/ET: 0.1 mg/kg (1:1000) (doses up to 0.2 mg/kg of 1:1000 may be effective)
  - Repeat every 3-5 min
- *Lidocaine* 1 mg/kg
- Consider *bretylium* 5 mg/kg first dose, 10 mg/kg second dose IV

- *Epinephrine*, second and subsequent doses
  - IV/IO/ET: 0.1 mg/kg (1:1000) (doses up to 0.2 mg/kg of 1:1000 may be effective)
  - Repeat every 3-5 min

- Defibrillate 4 J/kg 30-60 sec after medication

REFERENCE GUIDE 19

Adult Emergency Drugs

Drug/Actions	Indications for use	Side effects	Normal dosage and rate of administration
Lidocaine Antiarrhythmic agent that decreases automaticity	Suppression of ventricular ectopy PVCs Ventricular tachycardia Ventricular fibrillation	Drowsiness Disorientation Decreased hearing ability Paresthesias Muscle twitching Agitation Seizures	PVCs and ventricular tachycardia 1 mg/kg —additional bolus of 0.5 mg/kg every 2-10 min to a total dose of 3 mg/kg Primary prophylaxis for ventricular fibrillation 1.5 mg/kg continuous IV infusion Patient with impaired hepatic flow or age over 70, reduce dosage by 50%
Epinephrine Catecholamine with both α- and β-adrenergic activity Increased SVR, arterial BP, HR, coronary and cerebral blood flow, myocardial contraction; myocardial oxygen requirements; automaticity	Acute bronchospasm Cardiac arrest Anaphylactic reactions Severe hypotension	Ventricular arrhythmias Myocardial ischemia Hypertension	1.0 mg IV push of 1:10,000 solution repeated at 3-5 min intervals Escalating: 1 mg, 3 mg, 5 mg IV of 1:10,000 solution q 3 min 0.1 mg/kg of 1:10,000 solution IV push every 3-5 min Give slow IV push

Continued.

Drug/Actions	Indications for use	Side effects	Normal dosage and rate of administraton
Atropine Parasympatholytic drug that enhances SA node automaticity and AV conduction	Symptomatic bradycardia Asystole Should be used with caution in presence of myocardial ischemia	Tachycardia Delirium Coma Ataxia Flushed, hot skin Dilated pupils	0.5-1.0 mg repeated up to 3.0 mg or 0.04 mg/kg
Adenosine Slows AV nodal conduction; interrupts reentrant pathway	Paroxysmal supraventricular tachycardia	Facial flushing Shortness of breath Chest pressure Light-headedness Nausea Asystole Effect inhibited by theophylline Effect enhanced by dipyridamole	Initial dose: 6 mg over 1-2 sec, if no response in 1-3 min, administer 12 mg over 1-2 sec
Narcan Antagonizes the actions of narcotic and some non-narcotic analgesics	Reverses the analgesic effects and the respiratory depression of narcotics	Side effects are rare Closely monitor HR, BP, respirations, and pupillary response Pulmonary edema	0.4-0.8 mg IV push

Skin Rash Diseases

Disease	Type of rash	Incubation	Duration	Cause
Maculopapular rashes				
Rubella (German measles, 3-day measles)	Macular, pink to red. First appears on head and spreads downward.	14-21 days; contagious from 7 days before to 5 days after rash appears	3-4 days	Viral; can cause joint pain; fever is uncommon
Rubeola (measles, red measles)	Preceded for 2-3 days by cough, coryza, and conjunctivitis. Koplik's spots appear on buccal mucosa (pinpoint white lesions on a red base) 12-24 hrs before rash. Rash consists of reddish macules and begins on face and spreads downward. Within 1-2 days, rash is confluent.	10-20 days; contagious from 4 days before to 5 days after rash appears	10-15 days	Viral
Roseola	Maculopapular, small, pink, widely disseminated, and nonpruritic. Onset follows 3-4 days of fever.	Unknown	1-2 days	Probably viral
Erythema infectiosum (fifth disease)	Macular; facial distribution ("slapped cheeks" appearance). Lacy rash is found on flexor surfaces of arms and legs.	6-14 days	Acute phase, 3-4 days; may recur for several weeks if exposed to strong sunlight	Viral (parvovirus B19)
Scarlet fever	Fine, raised generalized maculopapular rash ("sandpaper rash"). May be absent around mouth and face. Red "strawberry" tongue. Bright red lines found in axilla and antecubital fossae (Pastia's lines). May peel after 5 days.	1-7 days; contagious during incubation period	Up to 3 weeks, until treated	Bacterial: group A strep toxin

Continued.

Skin Rash Diseases (cont'd)

Disease	Type of Rash	Incubation	Duration	Cause
Rocky Mountain spotted fever	Systemic signs for 1-3 days, consists of fever, headache, vomiting, and myalgias. Rash consists of pink macules on peripheral extremities that become papular after 1-2 days.	2-10 days	Until treated	Tick-introduced *Rickettsia*
Scabies	Initial: linear, threadlike gray to brown lesions between fingers and toes, and on ankles and axillae. Advanced: pruritic red papules.	Up to 30-60 days	Until treated	Parasitic mite that burrows under the skin
Contact dermatitis	Red maculopapular lesions; sharp demarcation exists between involved and uninvolved areas of skin. May develop into a secondary lesion (e.g., vesicles or wheals).	Lesions developing within a few minutes to a few hours after contact with allergen	Until treated; may gradually disappear without treatment	Irritating agents such as soaps, detergents, and rough sheets
Varicella (chickenpox)	Rash begins as small red macules and then progresses to papules and then vesicles. After the vesicles rupture, a dry crust forms over the lesion. May have all types of lesions present at the same time.	14-21 days; contagious from 1 day before eruption of lesions until 6-7 days after all lesions are crusted over	5-20 days	Viral; scratching may cause a secondary bacterial infection
Tinea corporis (ringworm)	Round or oval, red scaly patch that spreads peripherally and clears centrally.	N/A	Until treated	Fungus acquired through direct or indirect contact

Impetigo	Rash begins as vesicular lesions, advances to yellow crusts on a red base. Usually seen on feet, hands, and around the mouth. May cause cellulitis.	N/A	Until treated	Bacterial (staphylococcal or streptococcal)
Candida (Monilia)	Oral: white patches on mucous membranes; will not scrape off. Skin: red lesions with serous drainage, white crust (usually in diaper area).	N/A	Until treated	Yeast infection, which proliferates in warm, moist environments
Kawasaki syndrome	Rash begins as red maculopapular lesions, commonly in the perineum area. Progresses to confluent pruritic wheals. Desquamation of lesions occurs within 2-7 days	Unknown	6-8 weeks	Unknown

Rash type	Appearance	Disease(s)
Associated with hemorrhagic lesions		
Petechiae	Small (1-2 mm) pinpoint reddish purple macular lesions that do not blanch with pressure	Platelet disorders, leukemia, meningococcemia, bacterial meningitis
Purpura (ecchymoses)	Larger ecchymotic lesions that are macular and do not blanch with pressure	Henoch-Schönlein purpura, idiopathic thrombocytic purpura, hemophilia, trauma, viral infections

From Thomas DO: *Quick reference to pediatric emergency nursing*, Gaithersburg, MD, 1991, Aspen Publishers.

REFERENCE GUIDE 21

Tetanus Guidelines

History of adsorbed tetanus toxoid (doses)	Clean, minor wounds		All other wounds*	
	Td[†]	TIG	Td[†]	TIG
Unknown or < three	Yes	No	Yes	Yes
≥ three[‡]	No[§]	No	No[‖]	No

Adapted from Centers for Disease Control: MMWR 34(27):422, 1985.

*Such as, but not limited to, wounds resulting from missiles, crushing, burns, frostbite.

[†]For children <7 yr; DPT (DT, if pertussis vaccine contraindicated) preferred to tetanus toxoid alone. For persons ≥7 yr, Td preferred to tetanus toxoid alone.

[‡]If only 3 doses of *fluid* toxoid received, fourth dose of toxoid, preferably adsorbed toxoid, should be given.

[§]Yes, if >10 yr since last dose.

[‖]Yes, if >5 yr since last dose. (More frequent boosters not needed, can accentuate side effects.)

From: Keen J, Baird M, Allen J: *Mosby's critical care and emergency drug reference,* St Louis, 1994, Mosby.

REFERENCE GUIDE 22

Trauma Score (Revised): Adults

Glasgow Coma Scale

Find a subtotal for GCS. Use this subtotal to obtain a corresponding
revised trauma score (RTS). Add this value to the score of the
two other categories.

Eye opening	Spontaneous	4
	To voice	3
	To pain	2
	None	1
Verbal response	Oriented	5
	Confused	4
	Inappropriate words	3
	Incomprehensible sounds	2
	None	1
Motor response	Obeys commands	6
	Purposeful movement (pain)	5
	Withdrawal (pain)	4
	Flexion (pain)	3
	Extension (pain)	2
	None	1
GCS subtotal		3-15

Revised Trauma Score (RTS)

Glasgow coma scale

Find a subtotal for GCS. Use this subtotal to	13-15	4
obtain a corresponding RTS. Add this value	9-12	3
to the scores of the two other categories.	6-8	2
	4-5	1
	3	0

Respiratory rate

Number of respirations in 15 seconds;	10-29	4
multiply by four	>29	3
	6-9	2
	1-5	1
	0	0

Systolic blood pressure

Systolic cuff pressure obtained from	>89	4
either arm palpitation or	76-89	3
auscultation	50-75	2
	1-49	1
	No pulse	0
Total RTS		1-12

From Lee G: *Quick emergency care reference,* St Louis, 1992, Mosby.

REFERENCE GUIDE 23

Tube Sizes: Pediatric

Equipment	Premature	Neonate	6 mo	1 Yr	2 Yr
Airway					
Oral airway† (size)	Infant	Infant/ Small	Small	Small	Small
Endotracheal tube‡ (mm) *=cuffed	2.5-3.0	3.0-3.5	3.5-4.0	4.0-4.5	4.0-4.5
Laryngoscope blade† s = straight c = curved	0 s	1 s	1 s	1 s	1 s
Suction catheter‡ (French)	5	6	6	8	8
Breathing					
Face mask† (size)	Premie NB	NB	NB	Ped	Ped
Bag-valve device† (size)	Inf	Inf	Inf	Ped	Ped
Chest tube† (French)	10-14	12-18	14-20	14-24	14-24
Circulation					
Over-the-needle catheter§ (gauge)	22-24	22-24	22-24	20-22	20-22
Intraosseous device (gauge)	18	15	15	15	15
Gastrointestinal/ Genitourinary					
Nasogastric tube‖ (French)	5	5	8	8	10
Urinary catheter† (French)	5 feeding tube	5-8 feeding tube	8	10	10

From Bernardo L: *Pediatric emergency nursing procedures,* Boston, 1993, Jones & Bartlett.
*This reference demonstrates suggested sizes only. Always consider each child's size and health condition when selecting appropriate equipment for procedures.
†Committee on Trauma: *Advanced trauma life support student manual,* Chicago, 1989, American College of Surgeons.
‡Motoyama E: "Endotracheal intubation". In Motoyama E, Davis P, editors, *Smith's anesthesia for infants and children,* St. Louis, 1990, Mosby.
§Chameides L, editor: *Textbook of pediatric advanced life support,* Dallas, 1988, American Heart Association and American Academy of Pediatrics.
‖Skale N: *Manual of Pediatric nursing procedures,* Philadelphia, 1992, JB Lippincott.
NB, Newborn; *INF,* Infant; *Ped,* Pediatric; *Ad,* Adult.

3 Yr	4 Yr	5 Yr	6 Yr	7 Yr	8 Yr	9 Yr	10 Yr	11-18 Yr
Small	Med	Med	Med	Med	Med/Lg	Med/Lg	Med/Lg	Large
4.0-4.5	5.0-5,5	5,0-5.5	5.5-6.0	5.5-6.0	6.0†-6.5†	6.0†-6.5†	6.0†-6.5†	7.0†-8.0†
1 s	2 s/c	2 s/c	2 s/c	2 s/c	2-3 s/c	2-3 s/c	2-3 s/c	3 s/c
8	10	10	10	10	10	10	10	12
Ped	Ped	Ped	Ped	Ped	Ad	Ad	Ad	Ad
Ped	Ped	Ped	Ped	Ped/Ad	Ad	Ad	Ad	Ad
14-24	20-32	20-32	20-32	20-32	28-38	28-38	28-38	28-38
20-22	20-22	18-22	18-20	18-20	16-20	16-20	16-20	14-18
15	15	15	—	—	—	—	—	—
10	10	10	10	12	12	12	12	14-16
10	10-12	10-12	10-12	10-12	12	12	12	12-18

REFERENCE GUIDE 24
Ventilator Alarms Troubleshooting

Alarm	Possible causes
High pressure	Secretion build-up, kinked airway tubing, bronchospasm, coughing, fighting the ventilator, decreased lung compliance
Low exhaled volume	Disconnection from ventilator, loose ventilator fittings, leaking airway cuff
Low inspiratory pressure	Disconnection from ventilator, loose connections, low ventilating pressure
High respiratory rate	Anxiety, pain, hypoxia, fever
Apnea alarm	No spontaneous breath within preset time interval

From Stillwell SB: *Mosby's critical care nursing reference,* St Louis, 1992, Mosby.

REFERENCE GUIDE 25
Ventilator Modes: High-Frequency Ventilation

Type	Description
HF positive pressure ventilation (HFPPV)	Extremely short inspiratory times with V_T equivalent to deadspace at a rate of 60-100 cycles/min
HF jet ventilation (HFJV)	Small volumes, $\leq$ anatomical deadspace, are pulsed through a jet injector catheter at rates of 60-600 cycles/min
HF oscillation (HFO)	Small volume of gas is continually vibrated in the airways at rates of 900-3000 cycles/min
Assist-controlled mode ventilation (ACV)	Patient triggers a breath and the ventilator delivers a preset volume; the control mode takes over at a preset backup rate if patient becomes apneic
Bilevel CPAP (BiPAP)	Positive pressure applied during spontaneous breathing that allows the inspiratory positive airway pressure (IPAP) and expiratory positive airway pressure (EPAP) to be independently adjusted

REFERENCE GUIDE 25

Ventilator Modes: High-Frequency Ventilation (cont'd)

Type	Description
Continuous positive - airway pressure (CPAP)	Positive pressure applied during spontaneous breathing and maintained throughout the entire respiratory cycle; decreases intrapulmonary shunting
Controlled mandatory ventilation (CMV)	Ventilator delivers a preset tidal volume at a fixed rate regardless of the patient's efforts to breathe
Intermittent mandatory ventilation (IMV)	Patient may be able to breathe spontaneously but receives intermittent ventilator breaths at a preset rate and tidal volume; tidal volume stacking can occur
Inverse-ratio ventilation	Provides inspiratory time greater than expiratory time, thereby improving distribution of ventilation and preventing collapse of stiffer alveolar units
Positive end-expiratory pressure (PEEP)	Positive pressure applied during machine breathing and maintained at end-expiration; decreases intrapulmonary shunting
Pressure support ventilation (PSV)	Clinician-selected amount of positive pressure applied to airway during patient's spontaneous inspiratory efforts; PSV decreases work of breathing caused by demand flow valve, IMV circuit, and narrow inner diameter of ETT
Synchronized IMV (SIMV)	Intermittent ventilator breaths synchronized to spontaneous breaths to reduce competition between ventilator and patient

From Stillwell SB: *Mosby's critical care nursing reference,* St Louis, 1992, Mosby.

REFERENCE GUIDE 26

Vital Sign Norms: Pediatric

	6 mo	1 yr	3 yr	6 yr	10 yr
Heart rate (beats/min)	90-120	90-120	80-120	70-110	60-90
Respirations (breaths/min)	25-40	20-30	20-30	18-25	15-20
Systolic blood pressure (mm Hg)	80-100	80-100	80-110	80-110	90-120

From Stillwell SB: *Quick critical care reference guide,* ed 2, St Louis, 1994, Mosby.

UNIT TWO

Clinical
Conditions

Chapter I

Abdominal Conditions

Regina Heiser

CLINICAL CONDITIONS
Appendicitis
Bowel Obstruction
Cholecystitis
Crohn's Disease
Dehydration
Esophageal Varices
Gastric/Gastroenteritis
Fulminant Hepatic Failure
Acute Pancreatitis

TRIAGE ASSESSMENT

One of the most common reasons patients seek treatment in the emergency department is abdominal pain or abdominal complaints. Pain may indicate an acute or chronic problem and may be accompanied by other associated symptoms such as nausea, vomiting, fever, or diarrhea.

Women of childbearing age who complain of abdominal pain present an additional challenge. Pelvic inflammatory disease, ectopic pregnancy, and ovarian cysts and abscesses are conditions that mimic other abdominal conditions. Classic symptoms of pelvic inflammatory disease include lower abdominal pain that increases with ambulation, pain on manual palpation of the cervix, and foul-smelling vaginal discharge. Right-sided ectopic pregnancy mimics the pain patterns of appendicitis. Pain may radiate to one or both shoulders with a ruptured ovarian cyst or ruptured ectopic pregnancy. In addition, the patient may complain of vaginal bleeding that may be intermittent or significant. Identification of sexually active patients with missed or abnormal menses are key indications of ectopic pregnancy. Ruptured ectopic pregnancy can produce hemorrhagic shock.

A

Patients with ovarian cysts complain of the same symptoms as ectopic pregnancy except laboratory pregnancy tests are negative. Patients with ruptured ovarian cysts may also present in hemorrhagic shock. Ovarian abscesses may also rupture resulting in septic shock (see Chapter 16).

The initial triage assessment should focus on some general observations of the patient. The primary survey focuses on assessing airway, breathing, and circulation. Any condition that causes an alteration in the patient's ability to maintain a patent airway, breathe normally, or maintain adequate circulation must be corrected before a focused or secondary survey begins. Symptoms at triage that warrant the need for immediate treatment include severe, debilitating pain (the patient is unable to sit or stand); protractive vomiting or diarrhea; and vital signs indicative of early shock (tachycardia, tachypnea, and hypotension).

The triage history and assessment are invaluable tools that can direct an accurate work-up and diagnosis in this population. A brief history should include the following:

Chief complaint
Nausea and vomiting—suspect appendicitis, bowel obstruction; colicky, epigastric pain—suspect gastritis, gastroenteritis; anorexia with diarrhea—suspect Crohn's disease.

Social and medical history
History of alcohol use and abuse—suspect liver disease; intravenous drug use—suspect withdrawal; previous abdominal surgeries—suspect bowel obstruction; prolonged salicylate or ibuprofen use—suspect liver disease, gastritis; antibiotic use—suspect dehydration, gastroenteritis.

Reason for seeking treatment
Identify changes in symptoms; identify contact with other health care providers with this illness.

Treatment before arrival
Identify use of home remedies, alteration in diet, use of over-the-counter medicines.

Pain
History and duration of pain; use the **PQRST** mnemonic as a systematic way to obtain information about pain:
  P—provoke. What provokes the pain? Makes it better or worse? Position of comfort/discomfort?

Q—quality or character. What type of pain is it? Burning, tight, crushing, tearing, pressure?

R—radiation. Where does the pain go? Where does it start? Have patient point with one finger where pain is the most uncomfortable.

S—severity. How severe is the pain on a scale of 0 to 10? (0 is equivalent to no pain, 10 is the worst pain.)

T—time. When did the pain start? How long did it last? What time did the intensity change?

CHARACTERISTICS AND TYPES OF PAIN

There are three types of abdominal pain: primary, somatic, and referred. *Primary,* or visceral, pain originates in the organ itself. It is cramping, gaslike, and intensifies, then decreases. The pain is usually periumbilical (e.g., appendicitis, pancreatitis, bowel obstruction).

Somatic, or secondary, pain results from irritation of surrounding structures and nerve fibers resulting from bacterial or chemical causes. Somatic pain is described as sharp and localized, and patients frequently assume a knee-chest position for comfort (e.g., peritonitis, gastroenteritis).

Referred pain is located distant from the affected organ and results from irritation of the same dermatome of the effected organ (e.g., cholecystitis, renal colic).

FOCUSED NURSING ASSESSMENT

A focused assessment should briefly reassess the ABCs for changes and necessary interventions. Ruptured esophageal varices, aortic aneurysm, hemorrhagic pancreatitis, and severe gastroenteritis may produce sudden and severe hypotension with resultant shock. Nursing assessment should focus on ventilation, perfusion, cognition, elimination patterns, and associated signs and symptoms.

Ventilation
Breath sounds and breathing patterns

Atelectasis, pleural effusions, and crackles are common in pancreatitis and hepatic failure. In pancreatitis, left-sided effusions are most common. While the exact cause is unknown, effusions are believed to be a result of diaphragmatic inflammation that occurs when enzymes are released from the ascitic abdomen (9). The respiratory problems associated with liver failure are due to arterial hypoxemia secondary to intrapulmonary dilatation and noncardiogenic pulmonary edema (10). Acute pain may cause an increased respiratory rate or splinting respirations in an effort to decrease pressure on the abdomen. Patients who receive narcotics for pain management are at risk for respiratory depression with inappropriate dosing.

Perfusion
Apical heart rate
Obtain an apical heart rate and compare to all peripheral pulses. Moderate-to-severe dehydration that results from gastroenteritis or shock states cause weak, thready, and rapid pulse rates. Tachycardia is the most common dysrhythmia in pancreatitis and fulminate hepatic failure (9,10).
Blood pressure
As dehydration or shock progresses from fluid volume loss, peripheral vasoconstriction increases and blood pressure decreases. Fifty percent of patients with fulminant hepatic failure present with a systolic blood pressure less than 90 mm Hg (10).
Skin
Assess skin color, temperature, and capillary refill. Nausea, vomiting, and severe pain may produce diaphoresis. Pancreatitis and appendicitis are associated with fever.

Cognition
Neurologic status
Severe hepatic failure causes decreased carbohydrate metabolism and increased circulating ammonia and bilirubin producing encephalopathic changes. Within hours, hepatic encephalopathy may progress from mild confusion to coma. Level of consciousness is regarded as the most critical indicator of encephalopathic changes (10). Decreased level of consciousness is also a warning sign of early shock from hypovolemia resulting from gastrointestinal bleeding, dehydration from vomiting and diarrhea, or sepsis secondary to peritonitis.

Elimination Patterns
Inspection
Inspection is best done from the patient's right side. Note symmetry, presence or absence of movement, distention,

dilated veins, ascites, and bruises. Coughing may elicit bulges or pain. Hemorrhagic pancreatitis has signs and symptoms consistent with abdominal trauma (blood and bruising periumbically or on the left lower flank). An asymmetric abdominal wall may indicate the presence of masses, air, or fluid. A palpable, visible mass may indicate an abdominal aneurysm.

Auscultation

Auscultation should be documented in all four quadrants. Frequency, quality, and pitch should be noted. Most bowel sounds originate in the small intestine located in the right lower quadrant. Bowel sounds may be hyperactive with gastroenteritis and accompanied by nausea, vomiting, and diarrhea. Abdominal bruits may be noted with dissecting aneurysms and renal artery stenosis. Friction rubs may indicate inflammation of an organ surface or presence of fluid. Early bowel obstruction and complete obstruction produce high-pitched, frequent, peristaltic bowel sounds. Absence of bowel sounds may indicate paralytic ileus or peritonitis.

Percussion

Tympanic sounds occur when air masses are percussed. Dull sounds are noted over solid structures such as tumors or organs. The liver should be percussed separately and its size noted. Borders of the liver can be obscured by right-sided pleural effusions, commonly a result of fulminant hepatic failure, and less commonly secondary to acute pancreatitis.

Palpation

Note tenderness, masses, guarding, rigidity, or rebound. Ask the patient to cough and note where pain occurs. Gentle palpation is recommended with suspected appendicitis because frequent deep palpation can result in perforation.

Bowel patterns

Stool initially passes in small bowel obstruction then stops. Dehydration and large bowel obstruction cause constipation. Pancreatitis produces steatorrheic (fatty, frothy, foul-smelling) stools. Diarrhea is associated with gastroenteritis, gastritis, and appendicitis. Tarry stools or occult blood in the stool may be found in diverticulitis, ulcerative colitis, and dysentery. Clay-colored stools are common with biliary tract obstruction.

Emesis

Vomiting is one of the major gastrointestinal symptoms. If vomiting is significant, gastritis, gastroenteritis, diverticulitis, pancreatitis, and small bowel obstruction are likely. Cholecystitis is associated with anorexia.

Risk Factors

1. Ingestion of noxious substances such as alcohol or caffeine: risk for acute gastritis.
2. Overeating, rapid food intake, high fat diet: risk for gastritis, pancreatitis, cholecystitis.
3. Improperly prepared foods and water: risk for gastroenteritis.
4. Over-the-counter medication (antacids, aspirin, ibuprofen) abuse: risk for gastrointestinal bleeding, gastritis.
5. Pregnancy: risk for gastritis.
6. Chronic bowel problems, laxative abuse, multiple abdominal surgeries with adhesions: risk for bowel obstruction, Crohn's disease.
7. Parous females (smokers): risk for cholecystitis (12).

Life Span Issues

1. Pain assessment in pediatric and geriatric patients can be problematic.
2. Pain assessment in pediatric patients may require use of more than one method (e.g., smiley faces, numerical scales, color-intensity scales may work with children of various ages).
3. The geriatric patient has pain from multiple causes and is high risk for drug-drug and drug-disease interactions (6). Drug absorption is least affected by age. Drug distribution, however, is affected by changes in serum albumin that decreases with age. In addition, total body water and lean muscle mass decrease with age, while fat increases. Drugs that distribute to lean mass compartments will have less absorption and may result in toxicity (e.g., antimicrobials, digoxin, lithium, alcohol). Drugs that distribute to fatty mass compartments may have a prolonged effect and take more drug to obtain therapeutic levels (e.g., psychotropic drugs). Finally, metabolism and excretion are factors that affect drug-drug interactions and drug-disease interactions in the geriatric patient (6).

4. The geriatric patient is at risk for undertreatment and overtreatment. Intraabdominal infections are clinically worse in the geriatric patient. This is attributed to delayed recognition and surgical intervention. Cholecystitis, appendicitis, and intraabdominal sepsis, which result from diverticular leaks and cancers, are the most common infections and cause greater morbidity and mortality in geriatric patients because of delays in recognition and treatment (11).

5. Both the geriatric and pediatric populations are at risk for infection because of their immune systems. Changes in the geriatric population include a reduction of polymorphonuclear leukocytes with a resultant decrease in phagocytosis (11). In the pediatric population an immature immune system and gut can result in infection (4).

6. Pain management in the geriatric population is difficult because of cognitive impairment, the inability to express pain, and problems with chronic pain (1).

7. Both the pediatric and geriatric populations are more susceptible to hypothermia. In the pediatric population, less body fat and a larger surface area result in a higher basal metabolic rate to maintain normal body temperature (4). The geriatric population has diminished sensation to cold, impaired sensation to temperature changes, impaired shiver, abnormal autonomic vasoconstriction in response to cold, and diminished thermogenesis (6). Rapid rehydration with room temperature fluids and repeated abdominal examinations can cause hypothermia and acidosis in these groups.

8. Both populations are more susceptible to dehydration. Infants have greater surface areas related to mass with a greater proportion of extracellular fluid. The geriatric population has decreased thirst perception and diminished urine concentrating capabilities (decreased renal blood flow and decreased glomerular filtration rates) (3).

INITIAL INTERVENTIONS

Most abdominal conditions in the emergency department will require similar treatment. *REMEMBER:* interventions are based on acuity and many abdominal conditions may be life threatening.

1. Maintain NPO status. Document time and type of last oral intake.
2. Anticipate diagnostic work-up: laboratory tests and radiography.
3. Anticipate and prepare for intravenous rehydration (see Chapter 11).
4. Provide comfort measures (positioning, access to bathroom, emesis basin).
5. Provide for and monitor pain needs.

PRIORITY NURSING DIAGNOSES

Risk for fluid volume deficit
Risk for pain
Risk for anxiety
Risk for impaired gas exchange
Risk for knowledge deficit

♦ **Fluid volume deficit** related to anorexia, nausea, vomiting, and diarrhea.
INTERVENTIONS
- Monitor vital signs
- Monitor intake and output
- Check urine specific gravity and color
- Hemoccult all vomitus and stool
- Assess for signs and symptoms of dehydration: mucous membranes (dry), tongue (furrowed), skin turgor (decreased), capillary refill (delayed), color (pale, flushed), and fontanel in infants (depressed)
- Assess neck veins (collapsed when lying flat)

♦ **Pain** related to cramping, burning, vomiting, diarrhea, and distention.
INTERVENTIONS
- Provide pain medications as ordered, preferably intravenously
- Monitor oxygen saturation with pulse oximetry (maintain saturation above 94%)
- Monitor vital signs after pain medication administration
- Reassess pain with pain scale
- Insert nasogastric tube as ordered

♦ **Anxiety** related to potential surgery, hospitalization, and invasive procedures.
INTERVENTIONS
- Explain all procedures, answer questions
- Provide reassurance and comfort

TABLE 1-1 Electrolyte and Acid-base Imbalances and Associated Abdominal Conditions

Laboratory	Condition
Elevated glucose	Pancreatitis
Decreased glucose	Fulminant hepatic failure
Decreased calcium	Pancreatitis, fulminant hepatic failure
Elevated ammonia	Fulminant hepatic failure
Decreased magnesium	Pancreatitis, fulminant hepatic failure
Decreased phosphorus	Fulminant hepatic failure
Elevated potassium	Pancreatitis with acute renal failure
Decreased potassium	Pancreatitis with vomiting, fulminant hepatic failure, bowel obstruction, cholecystitis with vomiting, gastritis with vomiting and dehydration
Decreased sodium	Fulminant hepatic failure, hyponatremic dehydration
Elevated sodium	Dehydration
Acidosis—metabolic	Fulminant hepatic failure secondary to lactic acid from necrosis
	Bowel obstruction (lower small intestine)
Alkalosis—respiratory	Pancreatitis
Alkalosis—metabolic	Fulminant hepatic failure with hypokalemia
Elevated BUN	Dehydration
	Esophageal varices with hypovolemia
Elevated creatinine	Dehydration, fulminant hepatic failure

- Provide calm, quiet environment
- Involve family in patient teaching
- **Impaired gas exchange** related to electrolyte imbalance, acid-base imbalance, and altered respiratory pattern due to pain and distention (Table 1-1).
  INTERVENTIONS
  - Monitor oxygen saturation
  - Administer oxygen as needed
  - Assess respiratory effort and pain relief methods
  - Replace electrolytes as ordered
- **Knowledge deficit** related to diet, fluid intake, and medication use.
  INTERVENTIONS
  - Initiate patient teaching

- Utilize family to reinforce teaching whenever possible
- Dietary consult or nutritionist visit

PRIORITY DIAGNOSTIC TESTS

Laboratory

Serum electrolytes (including BUN and creatinine):

BUN will be abnormal in moderate-to-severe dehydration states and with fluid shifts that accompany bowel obstruction, hepatic failure, and pancreatitis. Severe vomiting and diarrhea accompanying fulminant hepatic failure, pancreatitis, and severe gastroenteritis can cause hypokalemia.

Complete blood count with differential: The white count may be elevated due to the stress response secondary to infection.

Platelets: Will have immature platelets and decreased patient count in fulminant hepatic failure.

PT/PTT and fibrinogen: Abnormal values in hepatic failure and disease.

Serum amylase and lipase: Elevated in pancreatitis.

Serum bilirubin, aspartate aminotransferase (AST), alanine aminotransferase (ALT), and alkaline phosphatase (ALP): Mildly elevated in acute cholecystitis.

Serum ammonia: Elevated in fulminant hepatic failure and states of severe hypokalemia

Urinalysis: Baseline urinalysis should be done to rule out any genitourinary problems, especially in patients who complain of lower abdominal pain.

Type and crossmatch: Blood and blood products may be needed in patients who do not respond to fluid resuscitation.

Radiographic

Flat and upright abdominal film: Done to detect air, dilation, looped bowel, thickening of bowel wall, and foreign bodies. No preparation needed.

Upright chest film: Helpful in diagnosing pleural effusions. No preparation needed.

Abdominal ultrasound and abdominal CT scan: Useful in pancreatitis and identifying gallstones in acute cholecystitis. May need oral or intravenous contrast before study.

Upper GI series: Used to identify patency and motility of esophagus, stomach, and small intestine through serial radiogaphs over 4 to 6 hours after barium is ingested. *Preparation*: The patient is placed on a low residue diet 2 days before the test, NPO after midnight the night before the examination. There is no need for a laxative or enema.

Lower GI series: Barium enema is used to reveal the contour and motility of the colon, cecum, and appendix. *Preparation*: Minimal residue diet 2 days before the examination: 24 hours before the examination the patient is given a cathartic (mineral oil). A cleansing enema is given the night before and the morning of the examination. The patient is NPO after midnight the night before the test.

Cholecystography: Detects gallstones and estimates the ability of the gallbladder to fill and empty. *Preparation*: Patient receives an iodine-containing contrast (e.g., Telepaque) 3.6 g orally 12 hours before the radiograph and then nothing else by mouth. The patient must NOT be allergic to iodine/iodine products.

COLLABORATIVE INTERVENTIONS

Overview

1. Initiate intravenous access with large bore catheter, usually Ringer's lactate, except in cases of liver disease (include variceal bleeding). Isotonic solutions are the fluids of choice in these cases due to the inability of the liver to break down lactate to sodium bicarbonate. Fluid resuscitation, antibiotics, antiemetics, and pain medications may all be required intravenously (Table 1-2). Draw the appropriate laboratory tests with initiation of intravenous access (2 large red top tubes, purple top tube, blue top tube).
2. Initiate continuous cardiac monitoring, pulse oximetry, and frequent hemodynamic monitoring in patients with severe fluid volume loss, active bleeding, or decreased level of consciousness. Anticipate the need for blood and blood product replacement.
3. Initiate replacement of electrolytes.
4. Place nasogastric tube and indwelling urinary catheter.
5. Anticipate and prepare to place esophagogastric tamponade tube with ruptured esophageal varices.

TABLE 1-2 Drug Summary

Drug	Dose/Route	Special considerations
Phenergan	12.5-25 mg IV every 4 hours	Should not be ambulatory; Rate not to exceed 25 mg/min
Morphine sulphate	0.1 mg/kg pediatric patient IV 1 mg/min to 10 mg/min IV	Respiratory depression
Meperidine	1 mg/cc up to 10 mg IV 50-100 mg IM pediatric patient 1.1-1.8 mg/kg IV	Not to be used in patients with glaucoma, closed head injury, liver disease
Fentanyl	0.025-0.1 mg/kg	Shorter acting respiratory depression
Vasopressin	Bolus—20 U over 20 min IV infusion; 0.2–0.8 U/min	Reduction in coronary blood flow; monitor for dysrhythmia and ST segment changes
Nitroglycerin	5-20 mcg/min to counteract vasopressin	Monitor for hypotension
Neomycin	4-12 g/day in divided doses over 5-6 days	Ototoxicity, nephrotoxity
Lactulose	20-30 g tid po	—
Mannitol	12.5 g of 15%-20% over 3-5 min	Not to be used in anuric or dehydrated patients; monitor electrolytes

Clinical Conditions
Appendicitis
Appendicitis is one of the most common abdominal emergencies.

SYMPTOMS

- Classic progression of nausea and vomiting, followed by pain, and finally, fever
- Pain starts periumbilically, then localizes at McBurney's point (midway between the anterior iliac crest and umbilicus).
- Pain is steady, severe, and increases with movement and perforation.

DIAGNOSIS

- The white count is usually elevated but may not be in geriatric patients who are immunocompromised.
- Radiography is not always diagnostic but is useful in ruling out other conditions.
- Ultrasound shows a thickened cecum (14).
- Diagnosis is usually made by physical examination.

TREATMENT

- The treatment for a patient who does not "rule in" for appendicitis consists of observation with serial examinations (physical and white count) and intravenous rehydration.
- With classic symptoms, treatment involves intravenous hydration (IVFs), broad-spectrum antibiotics, and laparoscopic surgery with removal of the appendix.

Bowel obstruction

One of the two most common causes of abdominal pain is bowel obstructions that result from many causes: ileus, impaction, stricture, volvulus, worms, or malignancy. These obstructions may be partial or complete and are most commonly located in the area of the duodenum, small, or large bowel. Bowel obstruction is an extremely dangerous condition resulting in a high incidence of infection and perforation with resultant peritonitis, especially in the geriatric patient.

SYMPTOMS

- Include nausea and vomiting (frequently fecal-smelling emesis), abdominal pain that is localized and colicky, constipation, and abdominal distention.

DIAGNOSIS

- Radiography shows dilated, fluid-filled loops of bowel proximal to the obstruction.
- Serum electrolytes are abnormal due to the massive loss of fluid and electrolytes from accumulated abdominal contents.

TREATMENT

- Includes rehydration with Ringer's lactate solution, electrolyte replacement, insertion of a nasogastric tube and indwelling urinary catheter, antibiotics, and hospital admission.
- Patients may require intensive care based on the degree of dehydration and electrolyte abnormality.
- Surgical intervention is considered in cases of perforation and ischemic bowel.

Cholecystitis

Cholecystitis is the second most common cause of abdominal pain. Pain is produced primarily from obstruction of the cystic duct in the gallbladder or secondarily, from staphylococcal or streptococcal infection.

SYMPTOMS

- Acute onset of steady, noncrampy right upper quadrant pain and tenderness, with nausea, anorexia, vomiting, and fever.

DIAGNOSIS

- Ultrasound of the right upper quadrant will usually identify gallstones.
- Laboratory is positive for leukocytosis with increased polymorphonuclear cells (basophils, eosinophils, granulocytes, and neutrophils) and bands, and elevated bilirubin and liver function studies.
- Imaging studies (cholescintigraphy) while highly accurate, remain controversial due to cost, availability, and specificity to cystic duct obstruction (5).

TREATMENT

- Treatment for the first 24 to 48 hours is usually conservative, consisting of intravenous fluid therapy, pain control, and antibiotic therapy.
- Nasogastric tube insertion may be indicated in the patient with vomiting, gastric distention, or ileus.
- Early surgery can be anticipated for patients for whom medical management is not successful.
- Laparoscopic cholecystectomy, as opposed to open laparotomy, has become the procedure of choice for this condition.
- Laparoscopic cholecystectomy has been shown to be successful in decreasing hospital stay and expediting recovery resulting in earlier return to work and ability to perform activities of daily living (7).

Crohn's disease

Crohn's disease is an inflammatory process of the bowel
that produces thickened, incompressible bowel wall.
This disease tends to occur in families, frequently among
Eastern-European Jews between the ages of 15 and 35
years.

SYMPTOMS

- Symptoms and onset are varied.
- Patients may complain of localized pain; typically, pain is
  worse after eating, especially after ingestion of milk
  products or mechanically or chemically irritating foods.
- The patient is usually anorexic, febrile, and has frequent
  loose stools.
- Symptoms are insidious and sporadic but episodes
  gradually become more severe and more frequent.

DIAGNOSIS

- Barium enema is diagnostic for thickened bowel walls
  with a narrowed passage through which a thin trickle of
  barium is able to pass.

TREATMENT

- Treatment is aimed at palliation, not cure. Therapy is
  directed toward pain control, reduction of inflammation
  through steroid treatment, hydration, antibiotic therapy,
  replacement of electrolytes, and dietary changes.

Dehydration

Many patients with abdominal conditions may exhibit some
degree of dehydration and electrolyte imbalance based
on the severity of the illness. The most susceptible
groups are the geriatric and pediatric patient.

SYMPTOMS

- Symptoms vary with the degree of dehydration.
- Mild (5%)—skin is pale, cool, skin turgor decreases,
  mucous membranes are normal to slightly dry, and
  urinary output is diminished.
- As the degree of dehydration increases, signs and
  symptoms of shock are more marked.
- The patient becomes anuric, pulse becomes increasingly
  rapid, weak, and thready, skin color changes and
  becomes gray and mottled with loss of elasticity (positive
  "tenting" sign), and level of consciousness decreases.
- In the pediatric patient, dehydration is based on the
  percent of body weight loss and is most often due to
  gastroenteritis.

- Additional causes include antibiotic intolerance, ingestion, food or formula allergies, and improper handling of formula.
- The most common form of dehydration in the pediatric population is isotonic (defined as a serum sodium of 130 to 150 mEq/L).
- Hyponatremic dehydration (serum sodium <130 mEq/L) and hyponatremic dehydration (serum sodium >150 mEq/L) are both less common.

DIAGNOSIS

- Diagnosis (in adults) is confirmed by a change in baseline weight, increased hematocrit, serum sodium >148 mm/L, and serum BUN/creatinine ratio >25 (3).
- In pediatrics, diagnosis is confirmed by change in weight, serum sodium level, diaper use number and percent saturation in the past 6 hours, and fluid intake.

TREATMENT

- Varies with the degree of dehydration and electrolyte imbalance.
- Mild dehydration is treated with fluids and observation. Severe dehydration requires rapid intravenous rehydration, cardiac monitoring, hospitalization, electrolyte replacement over 2 to 3 days, accurate intake and output, and supportive care.
- In mild to moderate cases of dehydration in the pediatric population, the American Academy of Pediatrics recommends oral rehydration with an oral glucose-electrolyte solution in the first 4 to 6 hours, followed by diluted formula or milk (2).
- In older children, after oral rehydration, a BRAT (Bananas, Rice, Applesauce, Tea, Toast) diet is recommended (Table 1-3).
- In cases of severe dehydration, boluses of warm Ringer's lactate are given at a rate of 20 cc/kg and repeated until the heart rate is within normal range.
- Maintenance fluids are based on weight at a cc/kg/hr dose.

Esophageal varices

Esophageal varices are dilated lower esophageal veins that result from portal hypertension. Ninety percent of cases of portal hypertension are due to cirrhotic changes (8). It is the rupture and subsequent bleeding of these vessels that constitutes a life-threatening emergency. Within

TABLE 1-3 Special Diets for Abdominal Conditions

Condition	Diet	Special considerations
Crohn's disease Prep for upper and lower gastrointestinal series	Low residue Low fiber Low fat High calorie High carbohydrate High protein	Avoid milk, milk products, vegetable fiber (salads, fruit peels), nuts
Chronic pancreatitis	Bland, low fat with six meals per day	Avoid alcohol Use antacid with meals
Dehydration in older pediatric patients	*BRAT: B*ananas, *R*ice, *A*pplesauce, *T*ea, *T*oast	—
Mild to medium dehydration, gastritis, gastroenteritis	Clear liquids: broth, gelatin, Jell-o water, Pedialyte	Avoid orange juice

1 year of their first episode of hemorrhage, 70% of patients die (13), and 50% die within the first 6 weeks (8).

SYMPTOMS

- Patients present with sudden painless hemorrhage associated with nausea.
- The hematocrit is low, which usually requires transfusion.
- On physical examination, the spleen is enlarged.
- In serious cases of active bleeding, the patient presents in shock.

DIAGNOSIS

- Diagnosis is made on history, laboratory values (decreased hematocrit, abnormal liver function studies), angiography, and/or esophagoscopy.

TREATMENT

Treatment ranges from conservative management to aggressive resuscitation. Patients are hospitalized for fluid resuscitation with isotonic fluids and blood. The goal of blood administration is to maintain the hematocrit near

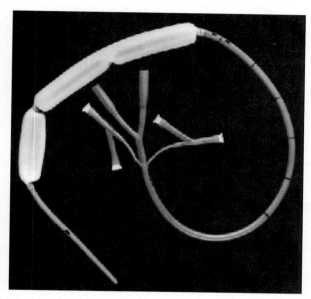

Figure 1-1 Minnesota Four Lumen Tube. (Courtesy Davol, Inc.)

30. Overtransfusion can increase portal hypertension and cause rebleeding (8). Ringer's lactate is not recommended for volume replacement in these patients because of the inability of the diseased liver to convert lactate to sodium bicarbonate for excretion (causes metabolic alkalosis). Procedures that have been effective in the emergency department include insertion of an esophagogastric balloon tamponade tube (Figure 1-1). Ice water lavage with or without epinephrine is no longer recommended in the acute bleed. Emergent endoscopy with scleraltherapy is the most effective treatment and is effective in up to 95% of cases (8). Temporizing measures also include vasopressin infusion with concomitant nitroglycerin infusion to lower portal pressure by reducing blood flow in the arterial bed (8). Surgical intervention may include placement of a portal-systemic shunt or devascularization procedure to arrest bleeding.

Gastritis/gastroenteritis

Gastritis occurs when food is ingested too quickly or with the ingestion of noxious agents (e.g., coffee, alcohol). Gastroenteritis is an infection which may be bacterial (e.g., food poisoning-causative agents: *Campylobacter, Salmonella, Shigella*), viral, protozoan (e.g., *Giardia lamblia*, "amoebic dysentery"), or parasitic (e.g., worms) in origin.

SYMPTOMS

- Symptoms are similar for both conditions.
- Pain is colicky and epigastric in origin.
- Patients complain of nausea, vomiting, and diarrhea frequently within 6 to 8 hours after eating.

DIAGNOSIS

- Diagnosis is based on history and stool culture results.

TREATMENT

- Treatment is related to the severity of the incident.
- Patients with gastritis should alter frequency and composition of meals.
- Gastroenteritis is treated by identifying and correcting the causative agent, intravenous rehydration, and electrolyte replacement.
- Severe episodes require hospitalization for observation and monitoring.

Fulminant hepatic failure

Most cases of hepatic failure result from an acute episode of viral hepatitis, although common drug use such as acetaminophen, valproate, methyldopa, tetracycline, and nonsteroidal antiinflammatory medications can cause failure. Massive cellular liver necrosis and disruption of all metabolic functions of the liver occur producing neurologic, cardiopulmonary, renal, hematologic, and metabolic deficiencies.

SYMPTOMS

- Symptoms include encephalopathy (mild confusion to coma), jaundice, edema, dehydration, bleeding and bruising, acute tubular necrosis (ATN) and renal failure, fever, and anorexia.

DIAGNOSIS

- Diagnosis is made on history, physical examination, and laboratory values (abnormal coagulation studies, liver function studies).

TREATMENT

* Acetaminophen toxicity is the only cause of fulminant hepatic failure that is treatable (see Chapter 20). Treatment of hepatic failure involves supportive care with admission to intensive care, monitoring, strict intake and output, fluid and electrolyte replacement, treatment of coagulopathy, routine culture and sensitivity of body secretions to determine sepsis (fever and leukocytosis occur with liver failure and cannot be used as a sign of sepsis), routine chest radiography, and restriction of dietary protein (to decrease nitrogen load). Hypotension is treated with blood, blood products, albumin, and isotonic fluids.

Acute pancreatitis

The pancreas becomes inflamed as a result of alcohol intake or blockage of the ampulla of Vater from gallstones resulting in pancreatic autodigestion.

SYMPTOMS

* Onset of excruciating sharp, upper abdominal pain that increases with supination and radiates to the back, chest, and epigastric area.
* Pain is knifelike, severe, and twisting.
* Pain usually occurs after drinking large quantities of alcohol or ingestion of high fat meal.
* Other symptoms include fever, signs of shock, vomiting, abdominal distention, ascites, and diminished-to-absent bowel sounds.

DIAGNOSIS

* Pancreatitis mimics other conditions.
* Diagnosis is based on laboratory and radiographic studies.
* The chest film is positive for pleural effusions.
* Increased lipase and amylase levels are present.
* Ultrasound, in combination with laboratory studies, has the best specificity and sensitivity for diagnosis (5).
* Abdominal CT with contrast may also be done.

TREATMENT

Treatment is supportive, including admission to intensive care, invasive monitoring, and aggressive fluid replacement with Ringer's lactate and colloids. High doses of fresh frozen plasma, in theory, may be of value by inhibiting further proteolytic activity (9). Pain management with intravenous narcotics is preferred, however, controversy exists over the narcotic of preference. Nonopioid-containing analgesics have been preferred (meperidine, fentanyl) because they do not produce spasm at the sphincter of Oddi, which is thought to be the pain source. Morphine, initially avoided, is currently thought to have minimal effect on the sphincter (9). Strict NPO maintenance is critical until serum amylase returns to normal to prevent recurrence of autodigestion. Eighty-five to ninety percent of patients respond to medical management. There is considerable debate about delayed versus early surgical intervention for removal of gallstones (5). Surgical intervention is based on clinical and morphologic criteria such as renal failure, sepsis, persistent acute abdomen, or intestinal perforation (9). In these cases, surgery is necessary. Severity of the disease is related to the amount of tissue necrosis, and treatment is based on severity. Hemorrhagic pancreatitis requires immediate surgical intervention.

NURSING SURVEILLANCE

1. Monitor severity of condition based upon changes in airway, breathing, and circulation.
2. Monitor level and type of pain and response to pain management strategies.
3. Monitor intake and output, check gastric and rectal secretions for occult and/or gross bleeding.
4. Monitor for cardiac dysrhythmia.
5. Monitor for signs and symptoms of decreased perfusion.
6. Assess changes in level of consciousness (as appropriate).

EXPECTED PATIENT OUTCOMES

1. Rehydration and volume replacement will support mean arterial pressure between 90 and 105 mm Hg.
2. Antibiotic therapy will be initiated (as appropriate).
3. Pain management will be initiated (as appropriate).

DISCHARGE IMPLICATIONS

1. Check orthostatic vital signs before discharge (pulse within normal limits 50 to 100 beats/min, no hypotension when transfer from lying to standing).

2. Dietary instructions given to family and patient (e.g., clear liquids, bland diet, small frequent meals, BRAT diet) (see Table 1-3).
3. Teach family and patient signs/symptoms of dehydration. Pediatric and geriatric patients may need teaching about potential for aspiration with recurrent vomiting.
4. Instruct patient/family about need for follow-up (e.g., fever over 101°F, vomiting greater than 6 times in 24 hours, diarrheal stools greater than 8 in 24 hours, cultures/sensitivities pending from emergency department laboratory work).

References

1. Agency for Health Care Policy and Research: *Acute pain management: operative or medical procedures and trauma*, 1992, Rockville, MD US Department of Health and Human Services.
2. Bezerra JA, Stathos TH, Duncan B, Gaines JA, and Udall JN: Treatment of infants with acute diarrhea: what's recommended and what's practiced, *Pediatr* 90(1):1-4, 1992.
3. Hoffman NB: Dehydration in the elderly: insidious and manageable, *Geriatr* 46(6):35-38, 1991.
4. Huddleston KC, Ferraro-McDuffie A, and Wolff-Small T: Nutritional support of the critically ill child, *Crit Care Nur Clin North Am* 5(1):65-77, 1993.
5. Kadakia SC: Biliary track emergencies: acute cholecystitis, acute cholangitis, and acute pancreatitis, *Med Clin North Am* 77(5):1015-1030, 1993.
6. Kane RL, Ouslander JG, and Abrass IB: *Essentials of clinical geriatrics*, ed 3, New York, 1994, McGraw-Hill.
7. Kelley JE, Burrus RG, Burns RP, Graham LD, and Chandler KE: Safety, efficacy, cost and morbidity of laparoscopic versus open cholecystomy: a prospective analysis of 228 consecutive patients, *Am Surg* 59(1):23-27, 1993.
8. Kerber K: The adult with bleeding esophageal varices, *Crit Care Nurs Clin North Am* 5(1):153-161, 1993.
9. Krumberger JM: Acute pancreatitis, *Crit Care Nurs Clin North Am.* 5(1):185-201, 1993.
10. Kucharski SA: Fulminant hepatic failure, *Crit Care Nurs Clin North Am* 5(1):141-149, 1993.
11. Louria DB, Sen P, Sherer CB and Farrer WE: Infections in older patients: a systematic clinical approach, *Geriatr* 48(1): 28-34, 1993.
12. Murray FE, Logan RF, Hannaford PC and Kay CR: Cigarette smoking and parity as risk factors for the development of symptomatic gall bladder disease in women: results of the

Royal College of General Practitioner's oral contraception study, *Gut* 35:107-111, 1994.

13. Schwartz SI, Shires GT, Spencer FC, and Storer EH: *Principles of surgery*, ed 4, New York, 1984, McGraw-Hill.

14. Spiro HM: An internist's approach to acute abdominal pain, *Med Clin North Am* 77(5):963-971, 1993.

Bibliography

Brunner LS and Suddarth DS: *Lippincott manual of nursing practice*, ed 4, Philadelphia 1986, JB Lippincott.

Dossey BM, Guzetta CE, and Kenner CV: *Essentials of critical care nursing: body, mind, spirit*, Philadelphia, 1990, JB Lippincott.

Guyton AC: *Textbook of medical physiology*, ed 8, Philadelphia, 1991, WB Saunders.

Kidd PS and Wagner KD: *High acuity nursing: preparing for practice in today's health care settings*, Norwalk, Conn., 1992, Appleton & Lange.

Shaffer H: Perforation and obstruction of the gastrointestinal tract: assessment by conventional radiology, *Radiol Clin North Am* 30(2):405-414, 1992.

Sheehy SB: *Emergency nursing: principles and practice*, ed 3, St. Louis, 1992, Mosby.

Abuse

Patty Sturt

CLINICAL CONDITIONS

Physical Abuse in Children
    Injuries to Skin and Subcutaneous Tissues
    Burns
    Head Injuries
    Shaken Impact (or baby) Syndrome
    Abdominal Injuries
    Münchausen's Syndrome by Proxy
Sexual Abuse (in children)
Battered Women
Elder Abuse
    Physical Abuse
    Psychologic/Emotional Abuse
    Neglect
    Exploitation

TRIAGE ASSESSMENT

Abuse occurs among people of all ages, races, religions, socioeconomic and educational levels, and religious backgrounds. The most vulnerable individuals of abuse are children, women, and the elderly. However, abuse can also occur in men.

The emergency department nurse may be the first health care professional to interact with the patient. Individuals reporting rape, sexual assault, or abuse should not be questioned at triage. This may increase the emotional trauma (guilt, embarrassment) the person may be experiencing. If no life-threatening injuries are present, escort the patient immediately to a private treatment area to obtain the triage assessment data.

Abuse is not always apparent. The triage nurse must have a high index of suspicion any time an injury is not congruent with the history. If life-threatening injuries are absent, the following data should be obtained.

Children
Deficits

Determine if there is a history of physical, mental, or psychosocial deficits.

Increased stress within the family may be associated with children who have a variety of problems or who are perceived as "different" or difficult by their parents. These problems may be physical, such as cerebral palsy, mental (retardation), temperamental (moody, difficult), or behavioral (hyperactive).

Stressors

Ask about recent or multiple stressors in the family unit.

Factors such as unemployment, poverty, parental discord, and family crisis can create a stressful environment where abuse can occur.

Caregiver

Determine who is the primary caregiver. Who does the child live with? Where do they live?

Single parents are more likely to experience social isolation and poverty, which may place the child at greater risk of being abused. Parents may drive great distances and bypass hospitals closer to home for fear of detection. See box for summary of risk factors for child abuse.

Injury

If an injury (or injuries) is present, determine the following:
1. Where is the child complaining of pain?
2. How did the injury occur?
3. Where did the injury occur?
4. Who was present or witnessed the injury?
5. When did the injury occur?

This information is important to determine if the injury is consistent or possible with the history. The following are cues of possible abuse:

- Inconsistencies in the history obtained from the parents or child.
- Parent is reluctant to describe the circumstances around the injury.
- Parent denies any knowledge of how injury occurred.
- Sibling, another child, or babysitter is blamed for the injury.
- Child is developmentally incapable of causing injury (e.g., 6-month-old pulls down a pan of hot water from the stove).
- Delay in seeking medical treatment.

RISK FACTORS FOR CHILD ABUSE

Child risk factors

Physical disability

Mental or psychosocial deficits
(e.g., mental retardation)

Parents' perceptions of the
child as "different" or difficult

Prematurity

Product of a multiple birth

Chronic illness

Parental risk factors

Childhood history of
abuse

Drug and/or alcohol
dependency

Unmet emotional needs

Single parent

Social isolation

Low self-esteem

Inadequate social supports
or role models

Belief in use of corporal
punishment

Unemployment and/or
poverty

Parental discord

Unrealistic expectations
of child

Immunizations

Determine if childhood immunizations are up-to-date.
If not, this may indicate lack of appropriate health
care.

History

1. History of repeated injuries or hospitalizations.
2. History of failure to gain weight at home. Failure to gain
   weight, particularly in infants, may be due to
   underfeeding.
3. History of genital or rectal discharge, bleeding, and/or
   pain (suspect sexual abuse).
4. History of dysuria or frequency (suspect sexual abuse).

Vital Signs

- *Tachycardia and hypotension:* May result from blood loss
  secondary to vaginal-cervical tears from sexual abuse,
  internal injuries from physical abuse, or dehydration
  secondary to malnourishment.
- *Fever:* May be noted in children with genital-pelvic or
  urinary tract infections secondary to sexual abuse.

General Observations

The following should increase the nurse's suspicion of possible abuse:

- Appears frightened of parent or caregiver.
- Goes easily to strangers.
- Extreme apprehension when hearing other children cry.
- Human bite marks.
- Bruises in various stages of healing.
- Bruises suggestive of being struck by an object, such as a looped cord, belt buckle, or hand imprint.
- Cigarette burns.
- Burns in the configuration of the object used to cause the harm.
- Rectal burns and burns with a clear line of demarcation (dunking burns).
- Inappropriate clothing.

Women

Privacy is a must when interviewing a suspected battered woman. Escort the woman to a private treatment room to obtain the needed history. The husband, friend, or family member should remain in the lobby. The following information should be elicited.

Anxiety

Anxiety, nervousness, difficulty sleeping, and depression are common complications associated with battering.

Vague complaints

Frequent visits to the emergency department (ED) with vague complaints and/or chronic pain is suggestive of battering. Women who are beaten at regular intervals may come to the ED with psychosomatic or emotional complaints just before they expect another beating.

History of suicide attempt

Attempted suicide has been associated with battering.

Past injuries

Determine if there is history of previous ED visits as a result of injuries. Repeated ED visits with injuries becoming more severe is highly suggestive of battering.

Present injuries

If an injury is present, determine the following:

1. Location of the injury and pain
2. How the injury occurred
3. Time the injury occurred

Many times the extent or type of injury will be inconsistent with the explanation the patient gives. There may be a substantial delay between time of injury and presentation for treatment. Common sites of injury are the face, head, neck, chest, breasts, abdomen, and genitals.

Menstruation

Determine last menstrual period and ask about possibility of pregnancy. A significant number of pregnant women are beaten, often in the breasts and abdomen.

NURSING ALERT

When a woman has one injury from abuse, there may be multiple old and new injuries that may be overlooked, especially if the presenting problem is a painful, obvious facial injury. The more subtle injury, such as in the abdomen, may be hidden by clothing and may be life threatening.

Vital Signs

- *Tachycardia:* Often present as a result of pain, anxiety, and fear secondary to abusive episodes from husband or male partner.
- *Tachycardia and hypotension:* May result from blood loss secondary to inflicted blunt or penetrating trauma (see Chapter 21).

General Observations

The following observations should increase the nurse's index of suspicion for possible battering:

- Unexplained lacerations, abrasions, burns, or bruises in various stages of healing.
- The patient minimizes the frequency or seriousness of the injuries.
- The patient describes in a hesitant, embarrassed, or evasive manner the circumstances around the alleged accident.
- The husband or male partner that accompanies the patient insists on staying with her, makes hostile or threatening statements to the patient, answers the triage nurse's questions, makes defensive or derogatory comments to the triage nurse, and/or appears to be under the influence of alcohol or drugs.

NURSING ALERT

Any trauma in a female patient without clear indication of cause needs to be considered battering until it is ruled out (1).

Elderly
Age and gender
Note the patient's age and gender; the typical abused elder is female and more than 70 years of age (9).
Caregiver
Determine with whom the patient lives. Does the patient have a history of any mental and/or physical impairments? Often the abused elder will have a physical impairment such as difficulty walking, hearing and/or vision deficits, and incontinence. Mental impairments may include confusion and senility secondary to Alzheimer's disease, previous strokes or head injuries, and organic brain syndrome. Daughters and daughters-in-law frequently have the responsibility of caring for aged parents. The abuser is often a middle-aged female (7).
Transportation to the ED
Determine who brought the patient to the ED. The abused elder is often brought to the ED by someone other than the caregiver.
Medications
Determine current medications. Ask to look at the bottles. Try to determine if medications are being given as prescribed.
Past injuries
Frequent hospitalizations from injuries is suggestive of abuse.
Time of injury/illness
Determine the interval between the injury or illness and presentation to the ED. Often this interval will be prolonged.
Chief complaint
Determine chief complaint or reason for transfer to the ED. Although hip and proximal femoral fractures are common after accidental falls, identical injuries can occur if the patient has been pushed or tripped. The presence of multiple, untreated, or poorly treated decubiti is an important physical indicator of elder neglect (8).

Weight loss

Excessive weight loss can result from malnourishment.

Vital Signs

- *Tachycardia and hypotension:* May result from blood loss secondary to inflicted trauma (usually chest, abdominal, or femur) or severe dehydration secondary to malnourishment.
- *Fever:* May occur in patients with untreated decubiti.

NURSING ALERT

Hypovolemic elderly may not experience tachycardia if taking beta-blockers such as Inderal.

General Observations

The following observations should increase the triage nurse's index of suspicion for abuse:

- Symptoms of severe dehydration such as pallor, poor skin turgor, sunken eyes and cheeks, and dry lips.
- The elder appears very nervous or fearful.
- The elder is notably passive and withdrawn.
- The caregiver verbalizes and/or demonstrates overt hostility, frustration, defensiveness, denial, or concern over the elder's "behavior."
- The caregiver demonstrates lack of eye contact with the elder.

FOCUSED NURSING ASSESSMENT

Nursing assessment for all individuals of suspected abuse should focus on oxygenation/ventilation, perfusion, cognition, sexuality, and safety and security.

Oxygenation/Ventilation
Airway

Stridor and respiratory distress may be present in cases where the victim was strangulated by hands, rope, or other objects. Patients with a decreased level of consciousness, such as infants with shaken impact syndrome (shaken baby syndrome), are at high risk for airway compromise.

Breath sounds

Absent or decreased breath sounds may occur with inflicted blunt or penetrating injuries to the chest. Suspect a pneumothorax or hemothorax. Breath sounds may be decreased if the patient is hypoventilating secondary to increased intracranial pressure from a head injury.

Perfusion

Assess skin color and temperature, capillary refill, and peripheral pulses. Pale, cool skin may indicate hemorrhage from inflicted blunt or penetrating abdominal trauma to the spleen and/or liver. Delayed capillary refill is a reliable indicator of hypovolemia/hemorrhage in infants and children. Weak or absent pulses distal to an injured extremity is indicative of impingement on vascular structures.

Cognition

Perform a neurologic assessment. An alternation in level of consciousness may be seen with head injuries resulting from abuse. Some examples would include shaken impact syndrome in infants, children repeatedly hit across the head, and women forcibly thrown against an object and striking their head. Obtain a Glasgow Coma Scale score (see Reference Guide 6) and assess pupil size and reaction (see Chapter 15).

Sexuality

Sexual abuse can occur in both sexes and at any age. Assess for any trauma, discharge, or drainage from the genitals or rectum. Determine last menstrual period. Ask about use of birth control and the possibility of pregnancy (see Sexual Assault Evidence Collection Procedure 26, and Child Sexual Abuse Under Collaborative Interventions in this chapter).

NURSING ALERT

Any patient with suspected sexual abuse should be interviewed and examined in a private area.

Safety/Security

- Assess suicide potential. Approximately 25% of battered women attempt suicide (see Chapter 14).
- Assess homicide potential. Battering is considered the most important precipitant for women killed by men

and men killed by women. Determine if partner has threatened to kill the victim. Risk factors for homicide include sexual abuse; guns in the home; partner is addicted to cocaine and/or is intoxicated daily; the woman is making plans to leave; and either partner has threatened or attempted suicide.

Risk Factors
Child abuse
See the box on p. 85 for the risk factors for child abuse.
Battering
- *Characteristics of the batterer*
  1. Heavy drinking. Experts report that 40% to 95% of wife beating involves drinking.
  2. Physical abuse during dating and courtship.
  3. Cruelty to animals. Any man who savagely beats a dog or other pet should be considered a potential abuser.
  4. Violent home environment. If a man was abused as a child or grows up seeing his mother beaten by his father, he is apt to think of family violence as normal behavior.
  5. Poor self-image. Men often attack their wives when they feel that their masculinity has been threatened.
  6. Excessive jealousy. Battered women often report that husbands isolate them from social contacts (e.g., friends, neighbors, and relatives) and sources of transportation (e.g., take away the car keys).
  7. Inability to differentiate feelings. Emotions such as fear and loneliness are expressed as anger.
  8. Rigid expectations of wife. The mate must conform to *his* definitions of her role.
  9. Negative and derogatory opinion of women in general.
- *Characteristics of the battered mate*
  1. Engages in excessive minimization and denial.
  2. High economic and emotional dependency.
  3. Unsure of own ego needs. Defines self only in terms of her roles as wife and mother.
  4. Unlimited patience in hopes for discovery of a magic combination in solving marital problems.
  5. Family history of abuse. Witnessed mother being abused by the father.
  6. Approval seekers. Constantly seeking approval from spouse.

Elder abuse

Victims of elder abuse are likely to be individuals with characteristics that render them vulnerable—more than 70 years of age, female, limited economic resources, lack of alternative living arrangements, physically and/or mentally impaired (unable to walk or requires assistance to walk, hearing and/or visual impairments, partially or totally confused, and incontinent) and living in the community with an adult child or other family member.

- *Characteristics of the elder abuser*
  1. Violent background—grew up being abused by the parent or witnessing abuse.
  2. History of alcohol and/or drug addiction.
  3. Long-term financial problems.
  4. Displaces anger. Often displaces anger meant for some authority figure onto a family member.
  5. Confuses roles. Expects the victim to meet a wide range of their needs.
- *Characteristics of the elderly victim*
  1. Have a tendency to internalize blame. Believe they cause the "assaults."
  2. Passive and compliant. Do not usually fight back.
  3. Loyal—despite pain and anger, they defend the abuser.

Life Span Issues

1. Approximately 25% of obstetric patients, 45% of mothers of abused children, 25% of women who attempt suicide, and 30% to 50% of female psychiatric patients are abused women (3).
2. Domestic assaults account for approximately 99,800 hospital days and 28,700 ED visits.
3. Violence occurs even after a relationship has ended. Approximately one fifth of both fatal and nonfatal incidents involve relationships that have been terminated or estranged.
4. Studies indicate that 2% to 5% of people over the age of 65 have been abused.

INITIAL INTERVENTIONS

Regardless of the victim's age or the type of suspected abuse, the following interventions must be considered:

1. Perform a primary survey to identify all life-threatening injuries.

2. Implement measures to maintain a patent airway (see Chapter 17). Always consider the possibility of spine injury in patients with inflicted trauma to the head and upper torso.
3. If the patient exhibits signs and symptoms of hypovolemic shock, initiate 100% oxygen per nonrebreather mask and two large bore IVs of Ringer's lactate or normal saline.
4. Perform a secondary survey (see Chapter 21) to identify all injuries.
5. Splint and immobilize all extremities as indicated.
6. Implement measures to decrease and control increased intracranial pressure in patients with a head injury sustained from physical abuse (see Chapter 15).
7. Maintain confidentiality and privacy for any patient with suspected abuse.
8. Use words appropriate to the developmental level of the patient. For example, a four-year-old may not understand the word "urine" but will understand "pee."
9. Treat the abused individual with respect and empathy. Many abused victims experience embarrassment, guilt, and shame.
10. Determine the tetanus/diphtheria immunization status on any patient with altered skin integrity as a result of suspected abuse.

PRIORITY NURSING DIAGNOSES

Risk for ineffective airway clearance
Risk for impaired gas exchange
Risk for fluid volume deficit
Risk for potential for injury
Risk for rape trauma syndrome
Risk for potential for violence
Risk for knowledge deficit (caregiver)

◆ **Ineffective airway clearance** related to decreased level of consciousness secondary to inflicted head trauma.
   INTERVENTIONS
   • Maintain patent airway (see Chapter 17).
◆ **Impaired gas exchange** related to injury of the airway structures or lungs secondary to strangulation, or inflicted penetrating or blunt trauma to the chest.
   INTERVENTIONS
   • Provide 100% oxygen per nonrebreather mask.

- Anticipate need for stat chest x-ray.
- Prepare for chest tube insertion if pneumothorax or hemothorax present (see Chapter 21).

◆ **Fluid volume deficit** related to severe malnutrition or hemorrhage from chest, abdominal, or genital trauma secondary to neglect, physical abuse or sexual abuse (large vaginal tears with vascular involvement in children).

INTERVENTIONS

- Initiate two large bore IVs with Ringer's lactate or normal saline.
- Obtain type and crossmatch for blood.
- Administer blood products as ordered.
- Prepare the patient for surgery.

◆ **Potential for injury** related to abusive home environment.

INTERVENTIONS

- Report abuse to the appropriate authorities as based on hospital policy and state laws.
- Provide written and verbal information to abused women about a safety plan and community resources.
- Provide information on spouse abuse shelters.
- Give parents information on support services for children with physical, developmental, or mental impairments (e.g., support groups for parents with children with cerebral palsy).
- Provide telephone numbers of community agencies that assist with child care and elder care.
- Provide information on coping techniques to deal with stressful situations.

◆ **Rape trauma syndrome** related to child sexual abuse, marital rape, or sexual assault (see Procedure 26).

◆ **Potential for violence** self-directed or directed at others related to suicide or homicide potential secondary to history of battering.

INTERVENTIONS

- Discuss removing gun or disarming gun in the home.
- Assess if victim has a plan to harm self or mate.
- Utilize suicide precautions (see Chapter 14).

◆ **Knowledge deficit (caregiver)** related to normal child development, parental skills, constructive stress management, and nonphysical methods of discipline.

INTERVENTIONS

- Provide parent (caregiver) with information regarding child development, social and community agencies for support and therapy, and alternatives to corporal punishment.

PRIORITY DIAGNOSTIC TESTS

Laboratory

Complete blood count: Obtain to assess hemoglobin and hematocrit in patients when symptoms of hemorrhage (hypovolemic shock) are present. Also use to assess the white blood count (WBC) in children and elderly to determine if weight loss is related to an infectious process or malnutrition. However, malnutrition increases the individual's susceptibility to an infection.

Type and crossmatch: Obtain when symptoms of hypovolemic shock are present.

Electrolytes and glucose: Hypokalemia and hypoglycemia, as well as other electrolyte abnormalities, may be present in malnourished children and elderly.

Coagulation profile: Obtain to determine if multiple unexplained bruises are from a bleeding disorder (7).

Radiographic

Radiographs: A complete skeletal survey is usually indicated in all infants less than 2 years of age who have clinical evidence of abuse or in infants less than 1 year of age who show evidence of significant neglect (2). Fractures in infants under 1 year of age are rare and suggest the possibility of abuse. Bone injuries are more common in abused children under 4 years of age, whereas accidental fractures occur more commonly in school-age children (6). In the absence of major identifiable trauma or intrinsic bone disease, unexplained fractures of the ribs, sternum, skull, humerus, and femur may indicate abuse. Other skeletal radiologic findings suggestive of abuse include multiple and often symmetric fractures of the limbs, and multiple fractures at different stages of healing. In the elderly, unexplained fractures of the skull, nose, facial bones; multiple fractures in various stages of healing; or spinal fractures are suggestive of abuse.

CT Scan: May reveal skull fractures. Bilateral skull fractures or skull fractures in an infant are suggestive of abuse. Cerebral edema may occur in shaken baby syndrome. CT scans in adults may reveal skull fractures, contusions, or intracranial bleeds from inflicted head trauma.

Sexual Abuse or Assault (Laboratory)

Venereal disease research laboratory test (VDRL).

Serum pregnancy test.

Gonococcal and chlamydia cultures of the oropharynx, rectum, and/or vagina depending on the history. In young children, all three should be obtained.

Vaginal swabs to test for spermatozoa and seminal plasma contents.

Saliva swabs to test for ABO-antigen typing. The swabs determine if the patient secretes properties of his/her blood type in body fluids (4).

Head and vaginal hair for forensic analysis under a microscope to compare with suspected abuser's hair. Head hair should be pulled from different areas. Vaginal hair should be combed and then pulled.

HIV antibody testing of adult abuse victims in the ED is controversial, since most EDs do not provide private counseling to individuals with a positive test. Patients can be referred to health departments or clinics that specialize in sexually transmitted diseases.

COLLABORATIVE INTERVENTIONS

Child Abuse

Child abuse can entail one or more of the following:

1. Physical abuse: Any intentionally inflicted injury to a child by a caregiver.
2. Sexual abuse: Any sexual activity or contact between a child and adult (or older child) whether by physical force, persuasion, or coercion.
3. Emotional abuse: Parental behaviors which are degrading, terrorizing, belittling, isolating, threatening, and/or exposure to spouse abuse.
4. Neglect: Usually involves acts of omission or failure to meet the basic needs of a child. These basic needs include food, clothing, medical care, and a safe environment.

Clinical Conditions
Physical abuse in children

Injuries to skin and subcutaneous tissues are seen in 90% of
abused children (8). Children who fall and injure
themselves accidentally usually have bruises over bony
prominences such as the chin, forehead, elbow, knee,
and shin.

SYMPTOMS

• Often bruises will represent the configuration of the
object used to cause the harm such as outline of
fingers, belt straps or buckles, or circumferential
bruises around the ankles or wrists from cords or rope
(Figures 2-1 to 2-3).

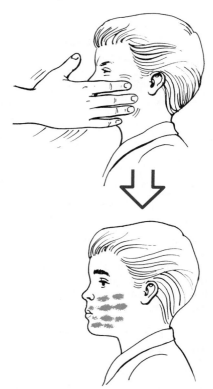

Figure 2-1 Typical slap pattern.

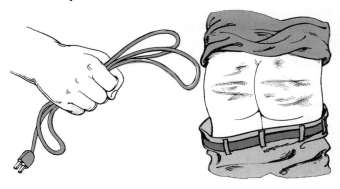

Figure 2-2 Loop or cord marks on buttocks.

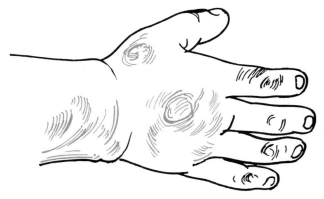

Figure 2-3 Blistering and edema in acute binding injury.

- Stages of bruising include: Purple for 1 to 5 days; green in 5 to 7 days; yellow in 7 to 10 days; and brown in >10 days. Multiple bruises in various stages of healing are suggestive of abuse.

DIAGNOSIS

- Diagnosis is based on an examination and history that do not correlate with the injuries.

TREATMENT

- Apply ice packs and elevate injured extremity. Monitor the amount of swelling.
- Immobilize area for comfort.

Burns: Death rates from abuse related burns are high and children with inflicted burns are likely to be injured again.

SYMPTOMS

- Tap water scalding is a common abusive burn. Splash injuries occur when hot water, liquid, or food is thrown or poured on the victim. The burns will not be uniform in depth and will involve different body areas. The top of the head and the anterior face, chest, and abdomen are most likely to be involved if a child pulls a pot of hot liquid on him or herself.
- In immersion injuries the burn depth is uniform and wound boundaries are distinct. Inflicted immersion injuries from dipping or dunking generally involve the perineum, buttocks, external genitalia, or the face or hands (Figure 2-4).

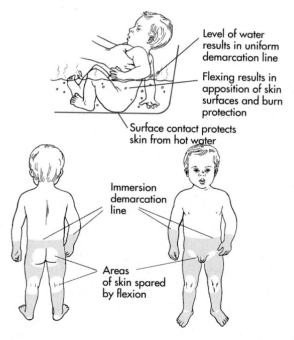

Level of water results in uniform demarcation line

Flexing results in apposition of skin surfaces and burn protection

Surface contact protects skin from hot water

Immersion demarcation line

Areas of skin spared by flexion

Figure 2-4 Typical immersion burn. Uniform degree of injury with interspersed protected areas.

- Circular burns to the soles of the feet and palms of the hands may be seen when cigarettes are intentionally placed on those areas.

DIAGNOSIS
- Diagnosis is based on an examination and history.

TREATMENT
See Chapter 3.

Head injuries are the leading cause of death among children who are physically abused (7).

SYMPTOMS
- Scalp bruises, subgaleal hematomas, and bald patches are common signs of abuse involving the head. The most common intracranial injuries in abuse are subdural and subarachnoid hemorrhages.
- There may be serious intracranial injury without evidence of external injury. Symptoms will include altered level of consciousness, pupillary and respiratory changes, seizures, and other signs of increased ICP.

DIAGNOSIS
- Diagnosis is based on an examination and history that do not correlate with the injury.

TREATMENT
- Monitor for symptoms of increased ICP.
- Initiate nursing interventions to decrease ICP (see Chapter 15).
- Maintain patent airway and cervical spine immobilization.
- Provide 100% oxygen.
- Intubate as necessary.
- Initiate an IV line.
- Prepare patient for surgery.

Shaken impact (or baby) syndrome is a result of vigorous shaking of an infant.

SYMPTOMS
- Symptoms include retinal hemorrhage, altered level of consciousness (usually from increased ICP from an epidural or subdural hematoma), full or bulging anterior fontanel, seizure activity, fixed dilated pupils, decerebrate posturing, abnormal respiratory rate and pattern, and bruising of the upper extremities.

DIAGNOSIS
- Based on examination and history.

TREATMENT

- Initiate nursing interventions to decrease ICP (see Chapter 15).

Abdominal injuries: Bruises over the abdomen are not common in children. Children with abuse-related abdominal injury are usually less than 2 years of age. A blow to the middle abdomen can cause a blow-out rupture of the stomach or intestines. The liver and spleen may be injured due to compressing forces against the abdomen such as kicking (see Chapter 21).

SYMPTOMS

- Symptoms include a distended or rigid abdomen, persistent vomiting and abdominal pain, and symptoms of hypovolemic shock.

DIAGNOSIS

- Diagnosis is based on the CT Scan, CBC, abdominal films, and examination.

TREATMENT

- Administer 100% oxygen per nonrebreather mask.
- Start two large bore IVs of Ringer's lactate or normal saline. In children, large bore IV is 22 gauge or greater.
- Obtain type and crossmatch and administer blood as ordered.
- Insert a nasogastric tube and urinary catheter.
- Prepare patient for surgery.

Münchausen's Syndrome by Proxy is a form of child abuse in which a parent or caregiver (usually the mother) fabricates or induces symptoms of an illness in a child. The mothers involved are usually described as intelligent, knowledgeable, and genuinely concerned for the child (5).

SYMPTOMS

- The fabricated illnesses typically include histories of fever, vomiting, diarrhea, seizures, rash, blackouts, apnea, hematemesis, and hematuria.
- The mother may actually induce symptoms in the child by suffocation, administration of drugs or toxic substances, or placing her own blood in the child's urine, vomitus, or stool specimens.

DIAGNOSIS

- Symptoms are observed only by the caregiver and disappear when the child is separated from the caregiver.

- There is a history of repeated visits to the ED to treat illnesses for which no cause can be determined.
- The child has been treated in numerous medical facilities.
- There are unusual symptoms which make no clinical sense.
- There are discrepancies between the history and physical findings (5).

TREATMENT

- The treatment will be based on the child's actual clinical presentation.
- Do not allow the mother to have access to any laboratory specimens since she may attempt to alter the specimen.
- Document the history given by the mother and all physical findings.

NURSING ALERT

Document all findings thoroughly but in an objective manner. Body diagrams and photographs may be helpful in delineating the location and size of the injuries. This information may be very helpful later in court. Also, do not alienate the parents or caregivers. Keep them informed of the plan of care. Be non-judgmental during your communication and interactions with the parents or caregivers. *REMEMBER:* it is the law in every state to report suspected child abuse to the appropriate child protection agency.

Sexual abuse in children

Explain to the child during the interview that you are there to listen. Convey interest, sincerity, and respect. Never interview the child in front of the possible abuser. Determine and use the child's own terminology for describing body parts. The following questions may help when interviewing the child:

"Sometimes kids are asked to keep secrets. These secrets can be scary. You are safe with me. Has this happened to you? Can you tell me about the secret?" (8)

"Sometimes grown ups do things to kids that hurt and are scary. Has someone hurt you?" (8)

Assessment of the genitals and rectum should only be done once if at all possible to prevent unnecessary psychologic trauma to the child. Thus the nurse and physician should do this together. To examine the genitals, place the child supine in the frog leg position. For anal examination, place the child in the lateral decubitus position. To help the child relax, a family member, social worker, or nurse should be at the head of the examining table to comfort the child. The child should not be restrained for this part of the examination. If the child is very uncooperative, the examination should be stopped and the child sedated if necessary.

SYMPTOMS

- Symptoms include inflammation, redness, drainage, discharge, or bleeding from the genitals; lacerations, abrasions, or ecchymosis of the genitals; and/or tears, abrasions, edema, or discharge of the anus.

NURSING ALERT

Victims of child abuse will often need to be seen in a pediatric or gynecology clinic that is capable of performing a colposcopy. A colposcope allows examination of the external genitalia as well as the vagina and cervix. Vascular changes, scars, and variations are best noted with a colposcope. However, this instrument does not eliminate the need for a gross examination in the ED.

DIAGNOSIS

- Diagnosis is based on an examination and history obtained during interview with child (and parent).

TREATMENT

- Unless life-threatening bleeding is present, definite treatment may not be needed in the ED.
- Document the child's statements from the interview and any abnormal physical findings.
- It may be necessary to refer the child to a play therapist.
- Follow-up of culture results and treatment will be necessary.
- Report the suspected abuse to the appropriate child protection agency.

Battered women

A battered woman is 16 years of age or older and is physically, emotionally, or psychologically abused by a husband or significant other (8). Some characteristics often associated with battered victims include the following:

1. Denial of battering because of fear or shame.
2. Self-blame for what has happened.
3. Feelings of confusion, depression, and low self-esteem.
4. Reluctance to take action because of emotional and/or financial dependence on batterer or lack of emotional and financial resources.
5. Reluctance to take action because of fear of retaliation by the abuser.
6. A tendency to rationalize the "accident" because the batterer was intoxicated.

The batterer will often accompany and stay with the victim to prevent her from reporting the abuse. Ask the accompanying spouse, mate, or friend to wait in the lobby. Interview the woman in a place which affords privacy. Some women will admit that they were beaten by a boyfriend or spouse while others will not. Questioning should be conducted in a supportive, nonjudgmental, and nonassuming manner. The following questions may be helpful in eliciting a history:

"It seems that the injuries you have could have been caused by someone hurting or abusing you. Did someone hurt you?" (8)

"Sometimes when people come to the ED with physical symptoms like yours, we find that they are having some sort of trouble at home. I am concerned that someone is hurting you. Is this happening to you?"

Injuries commonly seen in battered women are listed in the box.

Symptoms
- Symptoms will be based on the injuries.

Diagnosis
- Diagnosis is based on an examination and history obtained from the patient.

Treatment
- Perform a primary survey to identify all life-threatening injuries.
- After intervening for any life-threatening conditions, perform a secondary survey to identify any other injuries.
- Assess homicide potential (see Chapter 14).
- Battered women may stay in an abusive relationship for many understandable reasons. Notify the appropriate adult protection agency based on your hospital policy and state laws.

INJURIES COMMONLY SEEN IN BATTERED WOMEN

Alterations in skin integrity

- Burns resulting from:
  Splashes
  Friction (being dragged on the ground)
  Chemicals
  Cigarettes or cigars
- Knife wounds
- Scalp, facial lacerations
- Oral mucosa lacerations

Alterations in musculoskeletal system

- Facial or nose contusions or fractures
- Skull fractures
- Patterned bruises
- Torso injuries
- Breast contusions
- Fractured ribs
- Abdominal contusions (especially during pregnancy)
- Back or spine injuries

Neurologic impairment

- Altered consciousness from strangulation attempts
- Intracranial hemorrhage
- Postconcussion symptoms
- Visual impairment resulting from corneal abrasion or retinal detachment

Obstetric complications

- Miscarriages
- Abruptio placentae
- Premature uterine contractions
- Intrauterine fetal demise
- Low-birth-weight infant

- Document all injuries. Body maps may be helpful in delineating the location and size of the injury.
- Instruct and assist the woman in developing an emergency safety plan if she needs to leave the home immediately.

- Provide her with the phone number of the closest women's shelter.

Elder abuse

Elder abuse can include any of the following:

1. Physical abuse: The willful infliction of bodily harm onto a person 60 years of age or older by a spouse, child, family member, or primary caregiver. Examples include pushing, kicking, hitting, slapping, and punching. Other examples include rough handling, inappropriate use of physical or chemical restraints and sexual assault/rape.

2. Psychologic/emotional abuse: The infliction of mental anguish caused by actions or verbal assaults against a person's well-being. Examples include name-calling, insults, attacks on person's self-esteem, treating the elder as a child, threats of violence against the elder, and controlling the victim's activities.

3. Neglect: The passive or active withholding of services necessary to maintain the health and welfare of an adult. Such services can include food, clothing, medications, basic hygiene, or health-related services.

4. Exploitation: The improper use of an adult or adult's resources by a caregiver for the purpose of financial or material gains.

Elder abuse rarely occurs in isolation or as a single incident. It is usually a recurring problem that may increase in frequency and severity over time. It will be necessary to interview the caregiver and the elder patient separately. Provide a private, quiet place for the interview. Listen carefully and convey a nonjudgmental, empathetic attitude. Ask open-ended questions. The following questions may be used as a guideline:

"We sometimes see people with injuries like yours. Sometimes they are the result of an argument. Has this happened to you?"

"Can you describe what happens when you and your family member/caregiver argue or have problems? Do these behaviors include hitting or threats to harm you?"

"Have there been threats to abandon or confine you, or to withhold medicine or food from you?"

"Could you describe your routine day to me (e.g., activities, bathing, hygiene)?"

The following questions may be helpful in interviewing the caregiver:

"Caring for someone who is impaired as (the patient) is can be a very difficult task. It must be frustrating at times. How do you handle it?"

"Is it difficult to obtain the medications your (patient) needs?"

"Who is available to help you at home? Do you ever get a break to relax?"

"How do you cope having to care for (the patient) all the time?"

"During the interview we noticed bruises on the patient's face and arms. Do you know how he/she got them?"

SYMPTOMS
* Symptoms depend on the injuries.

DIAGNOSIS
* Diagnosis is based on an examination and information obtained from the history.

TREATMENT
* The treatment will depend on the specific injuries.
* Notify a social worker if possible. The social worker may go into the home to assess the interactions and environment.
* Carefully document information obtained from the interview and any physical findings.
* Provide the caregiver with information regarding community resources and support groups.

EXPECTED PATIENT OUTCOMES

1. Patent airway
2. Bilateral equal breath sounds
3. Heart rate of 60 to 100 beats/min (or age appropriate).
4. Systolic blood pressure of >90 mm Hg (or age appropriate) or at level needed to maintain adequate perfusion. (See Reference Guide 26 for vital signs in children.)
5. Improvement or no further deterioration in neurologic status.
6. Open and effective communication between the patient and nurse.
7. Understanding of abuse/neglect as a crime against the patient.
8. Understanding and verbalization of community resources and support systems.

DISCHARGE IMPLICATIONS

Child Abuse

1. Instruct the parent on alternative coping mechanisms to deal with stress (e.g., leave the room immediately if ready to hit the child or phone a friend or relative).
2. Provide the parent with phone numbers of support groups. These may be listed in local telephone books or under city/county or state information.

Battered Women

If a battered woman decides to return to the home, there are some things she can do to protect herself. Include these with the discharge instructions:

1. Have a room in the house that has a strong lock.
2. Keep a bag or suitcase packed.
3. Hide extra money, car keys, and important documents, such as marriage license, social security card, and family birth certificates, in a safe, secure place so they can be obtained quickly.
4. Teach the children or encourage the neighbors to call the police during an attack.
5. Plan for a place to go in an emergency—a woman's shelter, a social agency, or the home of a trusted friend or relative.
6. When possible, call the police and get names and badge numbers of police officers in case there is need of a record of the attack.
7. Leave the house and take the children if an attack is imminent.
8. Go to a hospital or ask for medical attention when in a safe place. Usually domestic violence shelter programs will provide a staff member to accompany the at risk individual to the hospital or emergency department. Sometimes women are hurt more seriously than they think during a physical assault.
9. Obtain and keep a record of any injuries, including photographs, so that she can have the strongest possible case to press charges.
10. Even if the woman will not admit to being battered or abused, provide her with written information of spouse abuse centers and shelters in the area (when you do suspect battering).

Elder Abuse

1. Community referrals are important in elder abuse. These may include the department for social services, senior citizen centers, community mental health centers, long-term care ombudsman, agencies on aging, and national committees dealing with elder abuse.
2. Instruct caregivers on alternative methods to cope with stress.

References

1. Campbell JC and Sheridan DJ: Emergency nursing interventions with battered women, *J Emerg Nurs* 14(1):12-17, 1989.
2. Emergency Nurses Association: Emergency Nursing Pediatric Course Manual, 1993, Park Ridge, Ill.
3. Fox G: Victims of abuse, *Nurs Times* 87(33):30-31, 1991.
4. Hauber DJ and Stokes JL: Evidence Collection Handbook: Kentucky State Police Laboratory, 1994, Frankfort, Ky.
5. Kelley: Physical abuse of children: recognizing and reporting, *J Emerg Nurs* 14(2), 1988.
6. Kessler DB and Hyden P: Physical, sexual, and emotional abuse of children, *Clin Symp* 43(1):1-32, 1991.
7. Pollick MF: Abuse of the elderly: a review, *Holistic Nursing Practice* 1(2):43-53, 1987.
8. Sheridan D: Family violence. In Kitt S and Kaiser J, editors: *Emergency nursing: a physiologic and clinical perspective*, Philadelphia, 1990, WB Saunders.
9. U.S. Department of Health and Human Services: *Elder abuse*, 1980, Washington, DC.

Burns

Julia Fultz
Marci Messer

CLINICAL CONDITIONS
Thermal Burns
Carbon Monoxide Inhalation
Upper Airway Injury
Pulmonary Inhalation Injury
Electrical Burns
Chemical Burns

TRIAGE ASSESSMENT

The goals of burn management in the emergency department are maintenance of the airway, breathing, and circulation; preservation of viable tissue; and prevention of infection. Eliminating the source of the burning is the first priority of care. Clothing that is producing heat must be removed. Chemical burns must be flushed immediately with copious amounts of water for 20 to 30 minutes until the burning sensation and pain subside. Chemicals in the form of a dry powder should be brushed off the skin before flushing the area.

NURSING ALERT

Certain toxic or hazardous materials may also cause burns (e.g., phosphorus, ammonium, or hydrofluoric acid). Precautions must be taken to prevent injury to the caregiver and to prevent contamination of the emergency department if the patient has been exposed to a hazardous material. Protective gear (gloves, face shield, and clothing) must be donned to prevent accidental contamination of the caregiver. Employer hazardous material policy and procedure must be followed. If the clothing is contaminated, it must be placed in an isolation bag (22).

General Observations

- Ensure the burning has been stopped, and the airway, breathing, and circulation are intact.
- Victims of electrical injury who are in cardiopulmonary arrest can frequently be revived and should receive aggressive resuscitation.
- Assuming life-saving interventions are not necessary, elicit the following data from the patient, family, friends, or emergency medical personnel:
  1. *AMPLE* history (*A*llergies, *M*edications, *P*ast medical history, *L*ast meal, *E*vents of the incident)
  2. Type of burning agent
  3. Length of time of exposure
  4. Whether the patient was in an enclosed area
  5. Concurrent trauma
  6. Any prior treatment
  7. Whether patient used alcohol or drugs before the event
  8. Whether the patient smokes
  9. Voltage, amperage, and current for electrical burns
  10. Advanced directives
  11. Patients with the potential for airway, breathing, or circulation problems should be directly admitted to the treatment area. Patients with what appear to be "minor burns" may also be admitted to the treatment area for pain relief measures.

FOCUSED NURSING ASSESSMENT

After ensuring that the burning process has stopped, attention should be directed toward the patient, not the burn. Nursing assessment should initially be centered on airway, breathing, and perfusion, then evaluation of the extent of the burn. Burn injuries may be associated with concurrent trauma. As with all trauma patients, a high index of suspicion must be maintained to anticipate and treat potentially life-threatening situations.

Airway
Verbal response
Briefly talk to the patient. If an appropriate verbal response can be elicited, it can be momentarily assumed that the airway is patent, ventilation intact, and the brain perfused.

Inspiratory sounds

Monitor for abnormal inspiratory sounds (e.g., crowing, stridor, or hoarseness) that may be associated with partial occlusion of the pharynx or larynx.

History

Inhalation injury should be suspected in patients who have a history of the injury occurring in a confined area or those who present with an altered level of consciousness.

Neck burns

Circumferential burns to the neck may compromise the airway as a result of the tourniquet-type effect of edema.

NURSING ALERT

Many who have inhalation injuries do not exhibit signs and symptoms initially. Significant upper airway edema may not manifest itself for several hours after the injury. The patient may exhibit few early signs of progressive airway compromise. Prepare for prophylactic endotracheal intubation in any patient who exhibits questionable respiratory mechanics.

Breathing
Respiratory rate

Evaluate the respiratory rate, use of accessory muscles, and the symmetry of chest-wall expansion. An increase in respiratory rate is the first sign of hypoxia.

Breath sounds

Auscultate the lungs for bilateral air movement and adventitious sounds.

Level of consciousness

Assess for agitation or change in level of consciousness.

Face/sputum/cough

Physical findings most often associated with inhalation injury include facial burns, singed nasal hairs, carbonaceous sputum, tachypnea, stridor, wheezing, dyspnea, and cough (5,18,19).

NURSING ALERT

Circumferential burns to the chest may impair chest expansion because of eschar formation.

Perfusion
Vital signs
Assess vital signs frequently. Pulse rates >120 beats/min after initial resuscitation may indicate inadequate volume replacement or can be a normal response in patients with large burn areas. Blood pressure is not a reliable measurement for evaluation of fluid resuscitation because of a release of catecholamines caused by hypotension (12). Swelling of a burned limb invalidates the readings from a noninvasive blood pressure cuff placed on that limb. Assess pulses, especially those distal to the burn.

Remove jewelry
Remove rings and other constricting jewelry.

Skin
Assess capillary refill, torso and extremity temperature, and skin color.

Urine
Assess hourly urine output to evaluate the effectiveness of fluid resuscitation in the absence of diuretics (1).

Level of consciousness
Assess cerebral perfusion by evaluating the patient's level of consciousness. As the affinity of hemoglobin for carbon monoxide is over 200 times that for oxygen, signs and symptoms of inadequate perfusion may indicate carbon monoxide poisoning (see box).

SIGNS AND SYMPTOMS OF CARBON MONOXIDE POISONING

0%-10%—Normal, smokers, and those living in urban areas.

10%-20%—Headache, confusion, dyspnea on exertion.

20%-40%—Fatigue, severe headache, visual disturbances, dizziness, nausea and vomiting, chest pains in individuals with coronary artery disease.

40%-60%—Tachycardia, tachypnea, hallucinations, combativeness, respiratory failure, shock, convulsions, coma, cherry red skin color, and death.

>60%—Usually results in death.

From Fitzgerald KA, McLaughlin EG: Inhalation injuries, *ACCN Clin Issues Crit Care Nurs* 1(3):535-542, 1990; and Ruth-Sahd L: Treating carbon monoxide poisoning, *Nurs 92* Jan:33, 1992.

Extent of Burn

The extent of the burn is calculated as a percentage of the total body surface area (TBSA) with partial- or full-thickness burns. First-degree burns are not included in the estimates of TBSA because the skin does not lose its ability to function. The Rule of Nines (Figure 3-1) can be used to estimate the TBSA involved. It must be adapted to accurately assess infants and toddlers as their body proportions are different from adults.

A modified Rule of Nines used for the child proposes that for each year of life after 2 years of age, 1% is subtracted from the head and 0.5% is added to each leg. As in all patients, the palmar surface of the patient's hand equals 1% of the body surface area.

Age-related charts, such as the Lund and Browder chart (Figure 3-2) may provide a more accurate determination of the extent of the injury in children.

Risk Factors

The following risk factors are associated with burn injury:
1. Hot water heaters set too high
2. Work place exposure to chemicals or electricity
3. Complacency in the work place
4. Use of alcohol
5. Carelessness with burning cigarettes
6. Inadequate or faulty electrical wiring
7. Wearing flammable clothing, especially flammable nightwear

Life Span Issues
Pediatrics

1. Airway compromise occurs in the child much more rapidly because of the smaller size of the airway.
2. Ossification of bones in children has not yet occurred; and therefore, bones are more pliable. This results in early exhaustion of a child with constrictive chest burns from the decreased chest wall compliance (19).
3. Children are further compromised by a higher metabolic rate resulting in an increased oxygen consumption (4).
4. Heart rate is a reliable indicator of the degree of shock as cardiac output is maintained in infants by increasing the heart rate rather than the stroke volume (13).

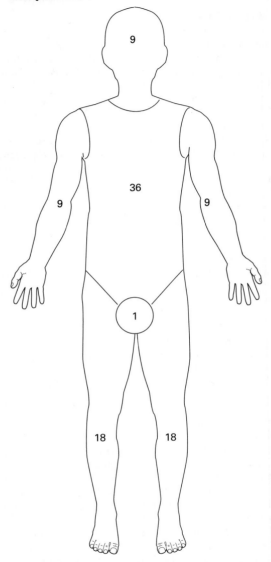

Figure 3-1 Rule of Nines. (From Neff J and Kidd P: *Trauma nursing,* St. Louis, 1993, Mosby.)

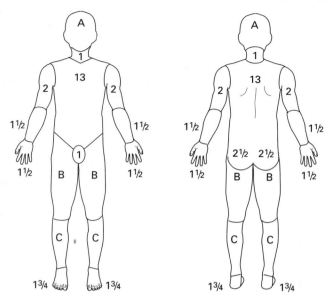

Figure 3-2 Lund and Browder chart. (From Artz C, Moncrief J, and Pruitt B: *Burns: A team approach,* Philadelphia, 1979, WB Saunders.)

5. Blood pressure is not a reliable indicator of shock. Compensation from vasoconstriction will maintain the blood pressure in an acceptable range until cardiovascular decompensation occurs.
6. Young children do not have the motor dexterity to quickly remove themselves from the heat source, and the skin is thinner, producing more severe burns than an adult would sustain given the same exposure (13).
7. Special attention should be given to preserving body heat. Children have a larger body surface area to weight ratio in comparison to an adult and will experience a greater degree of heat and evaporative water loss (13).
8. Children are predisposed to hypoglycemia because of poor glycogen stores. Maintenance fluids (which must be calculated in addition to the burn resuscitation fluids) containing glucose should be used to supplement the Ringer's lactated resuscitation to avoid hypoglycemia (14,20).

Geriatric

1. Preexisting cardiopulmonary disease decreases the ability to tolerate pulmonary stressors such as inhalation burns (10).
2. Increased metabolic need increases the workload of the heart. With a lower attainable maximal heart rate due to diminished beta-adrenergic responsiveness, the geriatric patient's heart is less able to respond effectively to maintain an adequate cardiac output during volume loss (10).
3. Preexisting disease (chronic obstructive pulmonary disease, coronary artery disease, hypertension, renal compromise, and diabetes) results in a reduced reserve capacity of the body system affected by the disease. This affects the body's ability to react to insults such as burns thus predisposing the patient to single- and multiple-organ dysfunction and increased morbidity and mortality (9).
4. Geriatric patients have a diminished sensory capacity and are sometimes cognitively impaired. A reduced reaction time coupled with frequently impaired mobility and declining physical strength increases their potential risk for injury. As in children the skin is thinner, resulting in more severe burns.

Pregnancy

1. Spontaneous termination of pregnancy usually occurs with TBSA burns of 50% or more (16).
2. The fetus totally depends on stable maternal vital signs. Large amounts of supplemental oxygen are required to ensure adequate fetal oxygenation.
3. Patients beyond 20 weeks' gestation (uterus at the level of the umbilicus) need to be placed on either their right or left side to prevent compression of the vena cava by the uterus that results in hypotension.

NURSING ALERT

Plasma volume in pregnancy increases by 40% to 50% with an overall blood volume increase of 48%. As a result of this volume increase, 30% of the blood volume may be displaced before signs of hypovolemia are seen (1). The placenta is very sensitive to catecholamine release and has very little autoregulatory capabilities; thus it cannot compensate for the resulting vasoconstriction and hypoperfusion. Anticipation of shock in the pregnant patient is of the utmost importance in treatment of the fetus.

INITIAL INTERVENTIONS

After the burning has been stopped, attention is directed to management of the airway, breathing, and circulation as in the initial assessment. Once adequacy of the airway, breathing, and circulation has been determined, attention is directed to the areas requiring interventions identified in the focused nursing assessment including the burn.

1. Take precautions to prevent further contamination of burns. (Sterile gloves for all burn wound contact, gowns, masks, and head covers for moderate or major burns.)
2. If the patient is unconscious, use standard cardiopulmonary measures to maintain the airway until it can be secured.
3. Take precautions to prevent aspiration in the unconscious patient by utilizing the rescue position if not contraindicated by concurrent trauma and have functioning suction equipment at hand. Endotracheal intubation and nasogastric tube placement provide definitive protection.
4. Inadequate respiratory effort must be assisted with a bag-valve device attached to a 100% oxygen source.
5. Any patient with potential carbon monoxide poisoning should receive 100% warm humidified oxygen by nonrebreather mask (3).
6. Determine if chemical burns have been flushed adequately. The burns should have been flushed with copious amounts of water at least 20 to 30 minutes, and the patient should voice decreased pain and discomfort.
7. Attach to the patient a cardiac monitor, oxygen saturation monitor, and automatic blood pressure cuff.

NURSING ALERT

Pulse oximetry reading evaluates hemoglobin saturation. It does not differentiate between hemoglobin saturated with carbon monoxide and hemoglobin saturated with oxygen. A high oxygen saturation reading may not indicate adequate oxygenation.

8. Remove any jewelry or clothing that may become constrictive as the damaged tissue swells.
9. Burns may be cooled and exposed nerve endings covered with tepid-to-cool moist compresses.

NURSING ALERT

Care must be taken to avoid hypothermia in cooling burns of >30% TBSA (17). Ice and cold water are contraindicated in cooling burns. After cooling the burns, wet bedding should be removed and patients should be covered with dry, sterile sheets and blankets to maintain body temperature.

10. Eye care involves flushing with copious amounts of water or saline solution after inverting the eyelid and removing any particles (see Chapter 10).
11. Cover burns with dry sterile dressings or sheets until definitive wound care can be initiated.
12. Anticipate fluid resuscitation in patient with burns >10% TBSA in young children and geriatric patients and >20% TBSA in adults (17).

NURSING ALERT

Do not pull tar, asphalt, or melted plastics from the skin unless it is compromising the airway. Cool the substance with water to prevent further tissue damage (7).

PRIORITY NURSING DIAGNOSES

Risk for fluid volume deficit
Risk for impaired gas exchange
Risk for altered peripheral tissue perfusion
Risk for pain
Risk for impaired skin integrity
Risk for infection

◆ **Fluid volume deficit** related to capillary permeability and loss of plasma volume from vascular space (fluid shift) as evidenced by edema, decreased urine output, decreased central venous pressure, decreased pulmonary capillary wedge pressure, hypotension, and/or tachycardia.
INTERVENTIONS
 • Monitor vital signs for tachycardia and hypotension.
 • Place two large bore (14 or 16 gauge) catheters for fluid resuscitation in patients with burns >10% TBSA in young children and geriatric patients and >20% in adults.
 • Place urinary catheter to monitor output.

◆ **Impaired gas exchange** related to alveolar injury, decreased hemoglobin, and a decreased intravascular volume as evidenced by carbonaceous sputum, hoarse voice, singed nasal hairs, burns to the face, a decreased PO_2, and/or an increased PCO_2.

INTERVENTIONS

- Provide 100% oxygen by nonrebreather mask.
- Assist ventilations with bag valve device if inadequate respiratory effort exists.
- Prepare for intubation in patients with signs of potential airway obstruction.
- Elevate the head of the bed for patients with potential inhalation injuries unless concurrent trauma precludes doing so.
- Monitor oxygen saturation by pulse oximetry (pulse oximetry does not differentiate between carbon monoxide and/or oxygen saturated hemoglobin).
- Prepare for escharotomy with circumferential burns of the chest that compromise chest expansion and patient's ability to breathe.
- Monitor hemoglobin.
- Monitor carboxyhemoglobin levels for patients with carbon monoxide poisoning.

◆ **Altered peripheral tissue perfusion** related to generalized edema, avascular tissue, decreased cardiac output, and hypovolemia as evidenced by diminished peripheral pulses, loss of sensory function, and/or cool extremities.

INTERVENTIONS

- Evaluate peripheral pulses, sensory function, skin temperature, and capillary refill.
- Place blood pressure cuff on unaffected limb if possible.
- Remove jewelry and constrictive clothing.
- Prepare to assist with an escharotomy in patients with a circumferential burn of an extremity associated with perfusion deficits.

◆ **Pain** related to stimulation of exposed pain sensors as evidenced by moaning, hostility, crying, clenched teeth, facial grimacing, complaints of pain, irritability, increased heart rate and blood pressure, and/or restlessness.

INTERVENTIONS

- Cool burns with tepid-to-cool moist compresses taking care to avoid hypothermia.
- Administer pain medications as ordered.
- Advise patient of all procedures to be performed and what to expect during the procedure.

◆ **Impaired skin integrity** related to burns, edema, and impaired physical mobility as evidenced by destruction of dermis, epidermis, and underlying structures, fluid-filled blisters, and/or mottled, waxy, white, cherry red, or blackened skin color.

INTERVENTIONS
- Eliminate the source of burning.
- Flush chemical burns with water for 20 to 30 minutes.
- If ears are burned, secure endotracheal and gastric tubes away from ears.
- Tar, asphalt, and plastic that adheres to the skin must be cooled with water.
- Patients who remain in the ED for any length of time must be turned every 2 hours.

◆ **Infection** related to altered integumentary system as evidenced by destruction of dermis and epidermis.

INTERVENTIONS
- Use sterile gloves for all wound contact.
- Use sterile gowns, masks, and shoe and head covers for moderate or major burns.
- Utilize strict aseptic technique.
- Use sterile linens for patients with moderate-to-severe burns.
- Administer antibiotics and tetanus toxoid as ordered.

PRIORITY DIAGNOSTIC TESTS

Laboratory

Blood electrolyte levels: Initially, levels may be normal but will change during the early course of treatment.

BUN and creatinine: Levels may be falsely elevated related to fluid deficits.

Blood glucose: The level may be elevated as a result of the stress response. Hypoglycemia in children may occur because of limited glycogen stores.

Arterial blood gas: The PO_2 may initially be normal with inhalation injuries. It is especially important to document a baseline pH in patients who sustain electrical burns as acidosis is common.

Complete blood count: Initially the hemoglobin and hematocrit may be elevated as a result of the fluid shifting intracellularly.

Blood albumin: The level may be low as a result of plasma proteins, principally albumin, being lost into injured tissue secondary to increased capillary permeability.

Blood drug and alcohol screens and urine drug screen: These are especially important if the patient is unconscious or obtunded.

Carboxyhemoglobin: Signs and symptoms appear if elevated >10% (see Table 3-1).

Myoglobinuria: Myoglobin is released when muscle tissue breaks down. The urine will turn light red or tea colored, but there are no red blood cells present. Myoglobin can cause damage to renal tubules if the kidneys are not well flushed. Urine output needs to be 75 to 100 ml/hr until the color of the urine clears, then reduced to produce urine at 50 ml/hr.

COLLABORATIVE INTERVENTIONS

Overview

1. Provide oxygen. Burn patients should receive 100% oxygen by nonrebreather mask. Patients with a possible inhalation injury should be positioned with the head of the bed elevated to decrease dependent edema of the upper airway unless a potential cervical injury precludes doing so. Prepare to intubate patients with signs of impending airway obstruction (stridor, hoarseness, dyspnea, tachypnea). An endotracheal tube of at least 7.5 mm in diameter is recommended for use in adult patients to facilitate pulmonary toilet or bronchoscopy. Avoid undue pressure against the burned skin and ears when securing an endotracheal tube, particularly during fluid resuscitation when edema formation is greatest.

2. Fluid replacement. Ringer's lactate is the replacement fluid of choice and should be infused through two large bore (14 to 16 gauge) intravenous catheters using the Parkland formula: Administer 4 ml/kg/%BSA burned in the first 24 hours following the time of injury (give one half of the total volume in the first 8 hours, one fourth the second 8 hours, and one fourth the third 8 hours). Use of colloid solutions are controversial during the first 12 to 24 hours of resuscitation as a result of the increased capillary permeability resulting in a loss of plasma proteins interstitially (14,17).

NURSING ALERT

Parkland's formula is a guide to fluid resuscitation. Fluid replacement should be sufficient enough to maintain an hourly urine output of 50 ml/hr in adults, 1 ml/kg/hr in children weighing <30 kg, and 0.5 ml/kg/hr through adolescence.

3. Chest radiograph. Chest radiographic changes are usually seen at approximately 48 hours after inhalation injury. An admission chest x-ray will provide a baseline for comparison with later films.
4. Nasogastric tube. Adynamic ileus usually accompanies most serious burn injuries. These patients should have nasogastric decompression until bowel function returns.
5. Urinary catheter. Output serves as a guide to fluid resuscitation.
6. Escharotomy. Indicated for circumferential burns that constrict chest or extremities and cause circulatory compromise. Preferred sites are medially and/or laterally on the extremities including the joints and bilateral incisions in the anterior axillary lines from the clavicle to the costal margins. Incisions must extend through the entire length of the eschar. This allows separation of the tissue allowing for expansion from edema. Assess extremity pulses after the escharotomy. If pulses are not restored, a fasciotomy is required (1,20).
7. Electrocardiogram. Particularly indicated in electrical burns as cardiac dysrhythmias are common complications.
8. Tetanus toxoid. Necrotic tissue is an ideal medium for *Clostridium tetani* to grow. Administer tetanus toxoid to previously immunized patients. Administer tetanus immunoglobulin for those not previously immunized or where immunization is unknown.

Clinical Conditions
Thermal burns
The extent of the injury is a result of the intensity of the heat and the duration of exposure.
SYMPTOMS
Superficial partial-thickness
(First-degree) burns involve the epidermis and are characterized by erythema that blanches on pressure,

pain, and edema. A patient with extensive superficial burns may exhibit headache, chills, and nausea and vomiting as a result of mild systemic response (7).

Partial-thickness

(Second-degree) burns involve the epidermis and part of the dermis. The skin is hyperemic and moist with thin-walled, fluid-filled blisters. Nerve endings are intact and irritated, causing extreme pain.

Deep partial-thickness

(Second-degree) burns also involve the epidermis and deep layers of the dermis. The skin is pale to waxy-white in color with tissue-paper–like blisters that contain little if any fluid. The wound has a decreased pinprick sensation that can make differentiation from full-thickness burns difficult.

Full-thickness

(Third-degree) burns involve the epidermis, the entire dermis, and extend into the subcutaneous tissues (Figure 3-3). The surface is dry, hard, inelastic, and insensate. The burn appears waxy, white, cherry red, or black in color. Nerve endings have been destroyed, although some sensation may be intact at the edges of the burn and cause discomfort.

DIAGNOSIS

- History and assessment of the skin.

TREATMENT

- Initial treatment is focused on stopping the burning process, airway management, breathing and fluid resuscitation.
- Cool burned areas with tepid-to-cool moist compresses.
- Escharotomy may be indicated if eschar compromises circulation.
- Pieces of clothing, foreign matter, and charred skin should be removed by soaking, rinsing, or gentle cleansing with wet gauze.
- Sloughed or necrotic skin will need to be debrided.
- Tar, asphalt, or plastic burns should be cooled, then covered with a petroleum-based ointment (e.g., mineral oil or bacitracin) to dissolve it (7,19).
- Cover the area with a dressing. The tar will dissolve within 24 to 48 hours (7,14). (Commercially prepared solvents for tar removal will dissolve tar in a shorter period of time.)

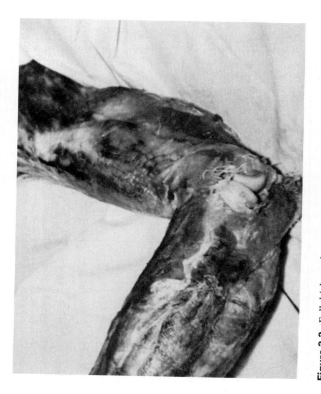

Figure 3-3 Full-thickness burn exposing elbow joint. (From Dressler DP, Hozid JL, and Nathan P: *Thermal injuries*, St. Louis, 1988, Mosby.)

Carbon monoxide inhalation
SYMPTOMS
- Related to the amount of hemoglobin saturated with carbon monoxide (carboxyhemoglobin).
- Mild symptoms include headache and confusion.
- More severe symptoms include vomiting, tachycardia, tachypnea, hallucinations, and eventual coma and death.
- Symptoms result from tissue hypoxia, not from parenchymal injury.

DIAGNOSIS
- History and duration of exposure to products of combustion especially in an enclosed area.
- Carboxyhemoglobin level.

TREATMENT
- Warmed and humidified 100% oxygen by nonrebreather mask if patient can maintain own airway or by intubation if decreased level of consciousness warrants.
- Monitor carboxyhemoglobin levels. In severe cases (carboxyhemoglobin saturations of >50%) hyperbaric oxygen therapy may be suggested (8) or in patients who do not improve with standard oxygen therapy within 2 to 4 hours (11).

Upper airway injury
May result from thermal injury or inhaled chemicals or gases that have a high-water solubility and are rapidly absorbed on the moist surfaces of the mouth, nose, and upper airway (e.g., chlorine, ammonia, sulfur oxides/dioxides) (3,11).

SYMPTOMS
- May be absent initially.
- Erythema, edema, hoarseness, blisters, or ulcerations of oropharynx and larynx.
- Mechanical obstruction of airway secondary to edema (stridor, tachypnea, dyspnea, crowing respirations).

DIAGNOSIS
- History of heat or hot liquids entering airway.
- Visualization of larynx, pharynx, and vocal cords.

TREATMENT
- Elevate the head of the bed.
- Warm, humidified oxygen.
- Early intubation in patients with the potential for airway obstruction.

Pulmonary inhalation injury

Pulmonary inhalation injury results from the chemicals or gases that are inhaled, and severity is related to the amount and composition of the inhaled substances. Substances with low-water solubility (nitrogen oxides, phosgene) dissolve more slowly allowing passage beyond the protective mechanisms of the upper airway (3,11).

SYMPTOMS

- Frequently asymptomatic initially.
- Damage depends on the temperature of the water and chemical content of the inhaled substance.
- May present with sooty sputum (generally reliable), burns to face, singed nasal hairs, inflammation of oropharyngeal mucosa.
- Delayed onset of cough, hoarseness, dyspnea, wheezing.

DIAGNOSIS

- History of exposure to products of combustion.
- Bronchoscopy will reveal parenchymal injuries such as mucosal inflammation, ulcerations, necrosis, soot, foreign particles, and edema (5).
- Xenon ventilation perfusion scan is usually performed within the first 24 to 48 hours after injury. A delay of the clearance of xenon from the lungs is indicative lower airway injury (3).

TREATMENT

Minimal-to-mild injury

- Warm humidified oxygen by nonrebreather mask.
- Incentive spirometry to prevent atelectasis.
- Bronchodilators for bronchospasms and wheezing.
- Monitor arterial blood gases, pulse oximetry, and changes in assessment indicating delayed airway obstruction.
- Those who are asymptomatic but have a history of significant exposure need close observation.

More severe injury

- Early intubation with ventilatory assistance.
- Positive end-expiratory pressure, large tidal volume with as low an oxygen concentration as possible.
- Aggressive pulmonary toilet.
- Bronchodilators for bronchospasms and wheezing.
- Arterial blood gas analysis (nonspecific indicator of inhalation injury, however, with progression of pulmonary dysfunction, arterial oxygen desaturation and retention of carbon dioxide may occur).

Electrical burns

Electrical injuries can cause varying types of injuries depending on the type of electrical contact. Contact with direct current (DC) found in automobile batteries or lightning causes a single violent muscle contraction that frequently throws the victim away from the source. Contact with alternating current (AC) that is found in households and high-tension wires results in tetanic contractions and usually causes more severe damage than DC exposure (2). There are four classes of electrical injuries (2):

- True electrical injuries: The body becomes part of the circuit. The electricity heats up tissues as it travels through the body,
- Flash injuries: Varying degrees of thermal injuries can occur as the current arcs from the source to the victim releasing heat and producing skin temperatures that cause burning or charring.
- Flame injury: burns result from the victim's clothing catching on fire.
- Lightning injuries: Lightning is a direct current causing injuries that are determined by the type of exposure to the lightning. Lightning strikes a victim in one of the following three ways (2,15):

  (1) *Direct strike:* The victim is struck directly and has an obvious entry site and is usually the most serious type;

  (2) *Side flash:* Lightning jumps to the victim from a primary object such as a tree as it continues taking the path of least resistance to the ground and is the most common type of strike; and

  (3) *Ground strike:* The victim is affected by the lightning after it has struck the ground near the victim.

NURSING ALERT

As a result of the implosive and explosive effects of lightning, the victim can be thrown and therefore warrant maintaining a high index of suspicion for life-threatening, blunt, traumatic injury.

SYMPTOMS

- The patient may present in ventricular fibrillation, asystole, and/or respiratory arrest.

NURSING ALERT

Aggressive resuscitation should be performed on patients who are in cardiopulmonary arrest caused by electrical or lightning injuries.

- Internally, nerves and blood vessels have low resistance and are good conductors; whereas, fat and bone have high resistance. Injuries include thrombosis, vascular spasm, peripheral and central neurological injuries, muscle necrosis from cellular damage, and brain injuries (epidural and subdural hematomas, brain parenchymal damage) (2,21).
- Externally, the thermal injuries range in depth from superficial to full-thickness with possible destruction and necrosis of underlying structures and organs. Entrance wounds are usually dry and charred; whereas exit wounds are usually larger with irregular edges (6).

NURSING ALERT

Injuries can be innocuous since damage is difficult to evaluate.

- Lightning strikes frequently result in a flashover phenomenon. The electrical current passes over the body instead of through it. The flashover produces a red-branching pattern on the skin described as featherlike in appearance, which is characteristic of a lightning injury (6).
- Cold extremities with diminished peripheral pulses may occur in the victim of a lightning strike as a result of the vasospasm. This usually resolves spontaneously. If it does not, consider compartmental syndrome or thrombosis of the vessels (21).
- Myoglobinuria may be present.
- Oral burns may be seen in children who have been exposed by chewing on electrical cords.

DIAGNOSIS
- History.
- Assessment of wounds.

TREATMENT
- Manage any airway, breathing, and circulation problems first.

- Spinal immobilization if the potential for fractures from falls is present. Many electrical injuries occur in those who work on elevated electrical wires, cutting trees, or in construction.
- Oxygen administration 100% by nonrebreather mask until an examination has ruled out the need for oxygen.
- Electrocardiographic monitoring. Be prepared to treat dysrhythmias with standard advanced life support measures.
- Massive fluid resuscitation is of the essence to prevent renal failure from myoglobinuria. Fluids should be titrated to maintain a urine output of 0.5-1.0 ml/kg/hr for clear urine or 1.0-1.5 ml/kg/hr for pigmented urine (6).
- The use of traditional burn formulas are not applicable in electrical injuries because of the inability to calculate the TBSA affected.
- An osmotic diuretic such as mannitol may be used initially to promote renal perfusion if myoglobinuria is present. If administered, urine output can no longer be used as the major determinant of adequate fluid resuscitation.
- Tetanus prophylaxis is recommended if appropriate, using the same criteria as used with thermal burns.
- Treat severe acidosis secondary to muscle necrosis by adding 1 ampule of sodium bicarbonate to each liter of intravenous fluids.
- Frequently orient those who are confused.

Chemical burns
SYMPTOMS
- Skin damage resembles that of thermal injury with erythema, blistering, or full-thickness loss.

NURSING ALERT

The extent of tissue injury may be deceptive. Extensive necrosis, fluid loss, and systemic toxicity may occur during the first 24 to 36 hours after the injury.

DIAGNOSIS
- History and assessment of the skin.
- Identification of the chemical agent is appropriate; however, it is secondary to immediate irrigation and removal of contaminated clothing.

TREATMENT

- Emergency caregivers should observe strict universal precaution to avoid contaminating their own eyes, skin, and lungs. The patients contaminated clothing should be removed and disposed of properly.
- Irrigation of the area with water should be done immediately for a minimum of 20 to 30 minutes. Neutralizing solutions have no advantage over water.
- The box provides a list of some chemical burns that require special treatment modalities or antidotes.

Special precautions

Ears: Rupture of the tympanic membrane occurs in 50% of patients struck by lightning (6). Cartilage has a poor blood supply, which means the healing process is slow. With thermal burns, pressure must be kept off the ears; therefore the use of pillows must be avoided. Cloth ties used to secure endotracheal tubes and nasogastric tubes must be kept away from the ears (Figure 3-4).

Lips: Position endotracheal tubes to prevent pressure on the lips. Use bacitracin to prevent drying and cracking.

Eyes: Single most important treatment is copious irrigation with normal saline within seconds of injury. Invert the eyelid and remove any particles before irrigating. Irrigate for 30 minutes. Assess for eyelash inversion that will cause corneal abrasions. The cornea must be kept moist (see Chapter 10).

Hands and Feet: Preserving function is of the utmost importance. Elevate extremity above the heart to prevent dependent edema that will delay healing. Fingers and toes are wrapped individually. Do not mitten them. If the patient cannot maintain the fingers in a position of function independently, the hand needs to be splinted.

Perineum: A Foley catheter must be placed until edema resolves. Massive swelling occurs in the scrotum as a result of dependent edema. If the patient is on bedrest, the area must be cleansed thoroughly and ointment reapplied after voiding or defecation.

Joints: Exposed bone or tendon should be kept moist with saline-soaked sterile gauze.

TREATMENT OF SPECIFIC CHEMICAL BURNS

Hydrofluoric acid—used in manufacturing, research, and in the home as a rust remover.

Action
Penetrates the skin.
Can cause damage to the bones.

Treatment
1. Aggressively lavage with water for 15-20 min immediately after contact.
2. Treat topically with a calcium gluconate gel or a solution of benzalkonium chloride.
3. Eyes must be treated with copious irrigation of water or normal saline.
4. Inhalation injury should be treated with nebulizer treatment of calcium gluconate solution.

Phenols—found in chemical disinfectants.

Action
Causes coagulation necrosis.
May induce fatal systemic toxicity.

Treatment
1. Irrigate with water.
2. Removal and dilution are best accomplished by swabbing with gauze soaked in a 50% solution of Polyethylene glycol for 5-10 min, then flush with water.

Alkalis (potassium, sodium, ammonium, lithium, barium)—commonly found in fertilizers, oven cleaners.

Action
Produces liquefaction necrosis.
Saponifies fats.
Dehydrates cells.

Treatment
1. DO NOT USE WATER.
2. If particulate is on patient, brush off or smother with class D fire extinguisher or sand.
3. Decontaminate the skin with mineral oil or mayonnaise.
4. Immerse sodium and potassium residue in oil so that it will not ignite.

Continued.

TREATMENT OF SPECIFIC CHEMICAL BURNS (cont'd)

Phosphorus

Action   Burns as it becomes phosphorus trioxide. Danger of spontaneous combustion when exposed to air.

Treatment 1. Irrigate with potassium permanganate solution (1:5000).
2. SUBMERGENCE of area in water is necessary to isolate the chemical from air.

Sodium metals

Action   Produces heat in the presence of water. May explode.

Treatment 1. DO NOT USE WATER.
2. Apply oil.

From Doyle CJ and Guzzardi LJ: Chemical burns, *Patient care* 2:232-246, 1992.

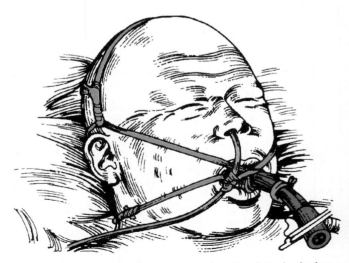

Figure 3-4 Cloth ties used to secure gastric and endotracheal tubes are kept away from the ears.

NURSING SURVEILLANCE

1. Monitor airway patency, anticipate intubation for significant burns of the airway, face, neck, and chest.
2. Monitor for hypoxia.
3. Monitor for hypovolemia.
4. Evaluate tissue perfusion.
5. Monitor urine output.
6. Monitor urine for myoglobin (identified by reddish-brown or tea-colored urine and urinalysis positive for hemoglobin but negative for red cells).
7. Evaluate effectiveness of pain control.
8. Ensure infection control and aseptic techniques.
9. Obtain vital signs and an admission weight.
10. Monitor serum electrolyte levels.

EXPECTED PATIENT OUTCOMES

1. Urine output of 50 ml/hr in an adult, 1 ml/kg/hr for children under 30 kg, 0.5 ml/kg/hr through adolescence, 50-100 ml/hr with electrical burns.
2. Negative urine myoglobin.
3. Adequate pain control evaluated by self-scoring pain scale.
4. Palpable pulses in all extremities.
5. Capillary refill <2 seconds in all extremities.
6. Heart rate <100 beats/min (<120 in patient with extensive burns as a result of hypermetabolic state,[17]), blood pressure, and cardiac rhythm within normal limits for patient's age.
7. Core temperature will remain 37° C or higher.
8. Maintain Glascow coma score of 15.
9. Decreasing carboxyhemoglobin level.
10. Transfer to burn center within 4 hours of injury (see box).

References

1. American College of Surgeons: *Advanced trauma life support,* student manual, ed 5, Chicago, 1993, The College.

BURN CENTER TRANSFER TRIAGE CRITERIA

1. Second- and third-degree burns > 10% of BSA in patients under 10 or over 50 years of age.
2. Second- and third-degree burns > 20% in other age groups.
3. Second- and third-degree burns with serious threat of functional or cosmetic impairment that involve the face, hands, feet, genitalia, perineum, and major joints.
4. Third-degree burns > 5% BSA in any age group.
5. Electrical burns including lightning injury.
6. Chemical burns with serious threat of functional or cosmetic impairment.
7. Inhalation injury with burn injury.
8. Circumferential burns of the extremity and chest.
9. Burn injury in patients with preexisting medical conditions that may complicate management, prolong recovery, or affect mortality.
10. Hospitals without qualified personnel or equipment for the care of children.
11. Any burn patient with concomitant trauma in which the burn injury poses the greatest risk of morbidity or mortality.

From Nebraska Burn Institute: *Advanced burn life support manual*, Lincoln, Neb, 1990, The Institute.
BSA, Body surface areas.

2. Browne BJ, Gaasch WR: Electrical injuries and lightning, *Emerg Med Clin North Am* 10(2):211-229, 1992.
3. Carroucher GJ: Inhalation injury, *AACN Clin Issues Crit Care Nurs* 4(2):367-377, 1993.
4. Chameides L, editor: *Pediatr adv life support*, Dallas, 1990, American Heart Association.
5. Cioffi WG and Rue LW: Diagnosis and treatment of inhalation injuries, *Crit Care Nurs Clin North Am* 3(2):191-199, 1991.
6. Cooper MA and Cantrill SV: Electrical and lightning injuries, *Patient Care* 15:158-175, November 1992.
7. Faldmo L, Kravitz M: Management of acute burns and burn shock resuscitation, *AACN Clin Issues Crit Care Nurs* 4(2):351-366, 1993.
8. Fitzgerald KA, McLaughlin EG: Inhalation injuries, *AACN Clin Issues Crit Care Nurs* 1(3):535-542, 1990.
9. Foyt MM: Does aging magnify the danger of burn injury, Part 1, *J Geront Nurs* 11(11):22-28, 1985.

TABLE 3-1 Drug Summary

Drug	Dose/Route	Special considerations
Tetanus toxoid	0.5 ml IM	For all burn patients. Give in unburned tissue.
Tetanus immuno globulin	250 U-500 U IM	Given if tetanus status is unknown. Give in unburned tissue.
Morphine sulfate	Adult 2-4 mg IV	Do not give morphine IM because poor tissue perfusion results in inadequate absorption. Monitor blood pressure. Repeat every 10 min until pain controlled. Monitor patient for respiratory depression if not intubated.
Mannitol (Osmitrol)	25 g bolus followed by 12.5-25 g/L of Ringer's lactate IV	Administer through a filter. Monitor for hypotension. Evaluate urine for color, amount, and pH.
Mafenide acetate (Sulfamylon)	Spread over burned area topically	Has good eschar penetration capabilities. Choice agent in infected wounds. Painful for 30-40 min when applied. Penetrates cartilage.
Silver sulfadiazine (Silvadene)	Spread over burned area using gloved hand or tongue blade topically	Use sterile technique to apply. Is not painful when applied. Do not apply to face as it may stain the skin.

10. Foyt MM: Does aging magnify the danger of burn injury, Part 2, *J Geront Nurs* 11(12):17-21, 1885.
11. Gough D, Young G: Airway burns and toxic gas inhalation. In Dailey RH et al: *The airway: emergency management*, St. Louis, 1992, Mosby.
12. Griglak MJ: Thermal injury, *Emerg Med Clin North Am* 10(2):369-383, 1992.

13. Helvig E: Pediatric burn injuries, *AACN Clin Issues Crit Care Nurs* 4(2):433-442, 1993.

14. Lasear SE: *Tissue integrity burns.* In Neff JA, Kidd PS, editors: *Trauma nursing*, St. Louis, 1993, Mosby.

15. Lichtenburg R et al: Cardiovascular effects of lightning strikes, *J Am Coll Cardio* 21(2):531-536, 1993.

16. Manley LK: Trauma in pregnancy. In Neff JA, Kidd PS, editors: *Trauma nursing*, St. Louis, 1993, Mosby.

17. Mikhail JN: Acute burn care: an update, *J Emerg Nurs* 14(1):9–17, 1988.

18. Moyan JA: Inhalation injury: a primary determinant of survival following major burns, *J Burn Care Rehabil* 3:78-84, 1981.

19. Nebraska Burn Institute: *Advanced burn life support manual*, Lincoln Neb, 1990.

20. Rue III LW, Cioffi Jr WG: Resuscitation of thermally injured patients, *Crit Care Nurs Clin North Am* 3(2):181-189, 1991.

21. Seward PN: Electrical injuries: trauma with a difference, *Emerg Med* June 15:157-168, 1992.

22. U.S. Department of Health & Human Services: Hospital emergency departments: a planning guide for the management of contaminated patients, *Managing hazardous materials incidents*, vol 2, 1992, U.S. Government Printing Office.

Cardiovascular Conditions

Terri Glessner

CLINICAL CONDITIONS
Myocardial Infarction
Angina
Congestive Heart Failure
Cardiogenic Shock
Sudden Death
Cardiac Arrest
Endocarditis
Pericarditis
Acute Aortic Dissection
Acute Arterial Occlusion
Venous Thrombosis

TRIAGE ASSESSMENT

The most common cardiac conditions encountered in the emergency department are myocardial infarctions (MI), angina, congestive heart failure (CHF), pericarditis, endocarditis, cardiogenic shock, sudden death and cardiac arrest. Common vascular conditions include acute aortic dissection, acute arterial occlusion, and venous thrombosis. At triage it is important to initially assess the patient's airway, breathing, and circulation and to take care of life-threatening conditions first, then determine the exact condition that has presented itself. Many cardiovascular conditions have similar initial presentations, so it is important to do a carefully focused survey. If the patient's cardiovascular system is involved, the patient will need to be closely monitored. Assuming that life-threatening conditions will be cared for per ACLS protocol, the following must be obtained at triage based on the patient's chief complaint.

Pain

Use the **PQRST** mnemonic as a systematic way to obtain information about pain:

P—provoke. What provokes the pain? Does anything change the pain, make it better or worse? Did the pain start suddenly or have a gradual onset?

Q—quality or character. How does the pain feel? Crushing, pressure, tightness, burning, like a brick on the chest?

R—radiation. Where does the pain start and where does the pain go? Can the patient pinpoint the exact area of pain?

S—severity. How severe is the pain on a scale of 1 to 10? (10 being the worst pain ever experienced.)

T—time. When did the pain start? Is the pain intermittent or continuous? How long did the pain last? Has the intensity of the pain ever changed?

If the patient has severe, crushing left-sided chest pain radiating to the left shoulder, arm or jaw, suspect an MI (13).

Shortness of breath

Is the patient short of breath? Is it worse on exertion or with position change? Does the patient experience orthopnea or paroxysmal nocturnal dyspnea (PND)? When did the shortness of breath begin and how long does it last? Is the patient able to function during periods of shortness of breath? If the patient is short of breath on exertion and has chest pain, suspect some type of myocardial ischemia.

Cough

Does the patient have a cough? When did it start? Does it produce any sputum and what does it look like? Is the cough accompanied by pain or shortness of breath? If the patient has a dry, nonproductive cough accompanied by shortness of breath especially on exertion, suspect fluid overload or CHF.

Nausea/vomiting

Has the patient experienced any nausea or vomiting? Was it accompanied by diaphoresis or chest pain? Patients frequently have some vague nausea accompanied by diaphoresis with their chest pain while having an MI or an episode of angina.

Extremity pain

If the complaint involves an extremity, is there pain? What is the color, temperature, capillary refill of the extremity? Is there clubbing or edema? Are the pulses present above and below the involved area of the extremity? What is the size of the involved extremity compared to the uninvolved extremity? If the patient has pain, edema, and cyanosis of one extremity, suspect an arterial or venous occlusion.

Injuries

Has the patient sustained any type of injury that would account for any of the symptoms? What is the location of the injury, time and mechanism of the injury? If the patient was involved in a motor vehicle crash, was the patient restrained? What type of restraint was utilized (lap and/or shoulder)? Was the vehicle equipped with airbags and did they inflate? At what speed did the crash occur? Was there damage to the interior/exterior of the car or steering wheel? What was the extrication time? How many vehicles were involved? Was any object impacted? If the patient has been involved in a motor vehicular crash without impact of the chest area and is having chest pain, suspect angina or MI.

Other symptoms

Other pertinent symptoms would include history of palpitations, syncope or near syncope, numbness, headache and activity intolerance.

Medical history

It is important to determine if the patient has a history of cardiac disease (past myocardial infarctions, angina, congestive heart failure, hypertension, congenital anomalies, angioplasties or cardiac surgery). These patients are at higher risk for developing a recurrence of a problem or developing a related problem. For example, patients who have had an MI are at greater risk for recurrence or for developing angina or congestive heart failure. Also, determine if the patient has a history of pulmonary disease (asthma, chronic bronchitis, emphysema, pulmonary hypertension, pleurisy, congenital pulmonary anomalies or black lung), diabetes (type, how controlled, and history of complications), renal disease (acute or chronic, type of dialysis and access used), vascular disease, hepatic disease, smoking, or alcohol abuse. A history of any of the above puts the patient at higher risk for having cardiac or vascular insufficiency.

Medication history

Determine if the patient is taking any prescribed medications, and determine if the patient is compliant with his/her prescribed medication. Determine if the patient is taking any over-the-counter (OTC) medications or is using any recreational drugs.

FOCUSED NURSING ASSESSMENT

Nursing assessment centers mainly on perfusion.

Perfusion

Heart sounds

Presence of S_3 or S_4 may indicate heart failure; presence of a murmur may indicate valvular or septal insufficiency.

Breath sounds

Presence of rales or crackles that do not clear with coughing may indicate congestive heart failure.

Color

Pale or cyanotic color may indicate poor cardiac output secondary to a myocardial infarction or a great vessel problem.

Peripheral pulses

Weak or absent pulses could indicate an acute arterial or venous occlusion; also weak pulses may indicate low cardiac output secondary to an acute MI, CHF, or a great vessel problem.

Capillary refill

Delayed capillary refill indicates low cardiac output, vessel occlusion, hypothermia, or shock.

Skin temperature

Cool extremities may indicate vessel occlusion or low cardiac output; also check skin for diaphoresis, which may indicate pain, anxiety, or low cardiac output.

Blood pressure and heart rate

Obtain blood pressure and heart rate. A rise in heart rate may indicate anxiety, fluid volume depletion, or low cardiac output. A fall in heart rate may indicate an SA nodal problem or cardiovascular insufficiency. A rise in blood pressure may indicate anxiety, noncompliance with medications, or vasoconstriction. A fall in blood pressure indicates vasodilation or cardiovascular collapse. Also, prescribed medications such as beta-blockers and calcium channel blockers can adversely affect heart rate and blood pressure.

Ventilation
Breathing patterns
Assess the patient's breathing pattern. CHF and low cardiac output produce respiratory distress because of fluid volume overload in the ventricle causing pulmonary congestion. The patient will appear short of breath, have rales on auscultation, and/or exhibit peripheral edema on examination.

Cardiovascular Risk Factors
1. Past medical history: See the box below.

> **NURSING ALERT**
>
> Patients with past cardiac or vascular conditions, diabetes, renal or hepatic disease are at high risk for additional cardiac or vascular conditions because these patients already have some blood vessel compromise and are at risk for additional insult.

2. Congenital conditions: Cardiac or pulmonary anomalies can cause patients to be at risk for an MI or the development of CHF.
3. Smoking history: Patients who smoke or live with smokers have increased risk for cardiac and vascular diseases because cigarette smokers and those inhaling second-hand smoke develop blood vessel changes (2).
4. Medication history: Female patients who use contraceptives and smoke have increased incidence of vascular disease and have been shown to develop blood clots much more readily (2). Cocaine users are at risk for developing tachyarrhythmias and/or myocardial ischemia leading to cardiovascular insufficiency and collapse (15).
5. Gender: Males are at higher risk for heart disease based on research. Hormonal and stress factors have a part in the development of heart disease in men and postmenopausal women (14).
6. Heredity: Patients with a family history of cardiac or vascular disease are at higher risk to develop these conditions (14).
7. Stress and anxiety: Research has shown that stress and anxiety as well as type A personality can lead to MI (14).
8. Age: As the age of a patient increases beyond the third decade, the risk of cardiovascular disease increases because of blood vessel changes associated with aging (3).

9. Hypertension: Those with uncontrolled or undercontrolled hypertension are at increased risk for MI because of increased afterload and increased load on the left side of the heart (2).

10. High cholesterol: Hypercholesterolemia increases risk for MI because of the increased risk for plaque formation leading to occlusions in the coronary arteries (2).

11. Sedentary lifestyle: Lack of exercise and activity increases risk for MI and vascular occlusion that is related to the development of pooled blood leading to blood clots in the small vessels (5,14).

12. Obesity: Because of the increased risk of sedentary lifestyle and increased load on the heart, obese patients are more likely to have vascular occlusions and/or MI (2).

13. Ethnic and racial origin: Non-Caucasians are more likely to develop cardiovascular disease than Caucasians based on research. Blacks are more likely to develop cardiovascular disease at an early age (14).

Life Span Issues
Pediatric

Cardiovascular conditions in pediatric patients may be diagnosed or undiagnosed congenital anomalies and complications related to their treatment. Cardiovascular complications include CHF, acute MI, and/or conduction disturbances. CHF is a result of inadequate pumping and may be related to anomalies such as a ventricular septal defect. An MI is always an ischemic event, not an atherosclerotic event, and may be secondary to an anomaly. Bradycardia can be due to hypoxemia, a conduction disturbance anomaly or may follow surgical correction of a congenital anomaly (10,11).

NURSING ALERT

ALWAYS carefully evaluate chest pain during pregnancy.

Pregnancy

Pregnancy-induced cardiomyopathy and pulmonary embolism are life threatening to the mother and the fetus. Hemodynamic changes during pregnancy include a marked increase in blood volume and cardiac output. Peripheral vascular dilatation causes increased heart rate and decreased blood pressure. During the postpartum period, deep venous thrombosis and pulmonary emboli develop from amniotic emboli. Other conditions that may interfere with the cardiovascular system during pregnancy include pregnancy-induced hypertension, gestational diabetes, vaginal bleeding, spontaneous abortion, placenta previa, abruptio placentae, and postpartum hemorrhage (see Chapter 16) (13).

Geriatric

There is an increased incidence of cardiovascular disease in the geriatric patient because of the development of arteriosclerosis that causes increased peripheral vascular resistance. The heart loses elasticity with age so it is less responsive to demands. It takes the geriatric patient's heart much longer to increase its rate in response to increased activity. There is an increased number of silent myocardial infarctions with increasing age because the nerve innervation to the heart is decreased. Symptoms are not always well described by the geriatric patient because of communication problems, neuropathies, and other physiologic changes associated with aging (3).

INITIAL INTERVENTIONS

Regardless of the cardiovascular condition, the following interventions may be beneficial:

1. Assess breathing and implement measures to facilitate breathing such as elevating the head of the bed, decreasing sensory stimulation, and allowing the patient to assume a position of comfort. Prepare for endotracheal intubation if there is evidence of severe respiratory distress with airway compromise and no evidence of compensation. If the patient is not breathing, open the airway, ventilate the patient, and administer oxygen at 100% per bag/valve/mask, and prepare to intubate.

2. Administer oxygen. If the patient is in no apparent respiratory distress, administer oxygen at 2 L/minute per nasal cannula. If the patient appears to be in respiratory distress, administer oxygen at 100% per nonrebreather mask.

3. Assess circulation. If no pulse is present, administer CPR. If there is a pulse present, assess pulses and capillary refill. Establish peripheral intravenous access, preferably an 18-gauge or larger, and administer D_5W or normal saline at a keep-vein-open rate. If the patient is hypotensive (SBP <90), establish two large bore IVs and administer a bolus of Ringer's lactate or normal saline and then reassess. If hypotension continues, repeat the procedure.

4. Initiate ECG, blood pressure, and pulse oximetry monitoring as soon as possible.

5. Obtain a 12-lead electrocardiogram.

6. Obtain laboratory specimens as ordered by the physician. Anticipate drawing at least an electrolyte panel and a CBC, and possibly a PT/PTT level.

7. If pain is determined to be possibly cardiac in origin, administer nitroglycerin 0.4 mg sublingual as ordered— approximately one every 3 to 5 min as tolerated by the patient's blood pressure (SBP >90 mm Hg) for three doses, then prepare to initiate a nitroglycerin drip as ordered (Table 4-1). The patient may also be started on nitropaste—1 to 2 inches to the chest wall or be given 1 to 3 metered doses of nitrospray to relieve their pain. Continuously monitor the patient's pain, blood pressure, and ECG during nitroglycerin administration and note any changes.

8. If pain is localized to an extremity and possibly related to vascular insufficiency, monitor the color of the extremity, pulses, pain, movement, and edema in the affected extremity.

9. If pain is due to a large vessel problem, the patient's blood pressure should be monitored closely and IV sodium nitroprusside or IV labetalol initiated if hypertension develops. (IV nifedipine is also being used experimentally for control of hypertension.)
Hypotension should be treated with volume resuscitation (Ringer's lactate or normal saline) and dopamine, Levophed, or epinephrine drips and is considered an ominous sign (see Table 4-1).

PRIORITY NURSING DIAGNOSES (4,5)

Risk for decreased cardiac output
Risk for alteration in tissue perfusion

TABLE 4-1 Drug Summary

Drug	Dose/Route	Special considerations
Adenosine	Initial dose: 6 mg rapid IV push (over 1-3 sec). If SVT not resolved in 1-2 min, may administer 12 mg rapid IVP; may repeat × 1 followed by rapid saline flush.	The half-life of adenosine is <5 sec. Side effects are common but resolve quickly; they include flushing, chest pain, and dyspnea. Periods of brady-cardia and ventricular ectopy may be seen after resolution of the SVT. Patients receiving theo-phylline, dipyridamole, and carbamazepine may not be candidates for adenosine therapy.
Bretylium	Load: 5 mg/kg IV push, then increase to 10 mg/kg IV push every 15-30 min up to 30 mg/kg. Maintenance: 1-2 mg/min IV infusion.	Initial bolus may cause hypotension. Continuous infusion causes orthostatic hypotension, nausea, and vomiting. Use with caution in patients who receive digoxin: this drug increases possibility of toxicity.
Digoxin	Load: 0.5-1.0 mg orally or IV in divided doses over 24 hr.	Observe for toxicity (nausea, vomiting, anorexia, irregular pulse); monitor pulse, serum potassium, and renal function closely.
Diltiazem	Bolus: 0.25-0.35 mg/kg IV. Maintenance: initiate infusion at 5mg/hr, titrate to effect.	Monitor for hypotension and bradycardia; regulate infusion accordingly. Use in patients with atrial fibrillation or flutter with rapid ventricular rates. Do not use in patients with AV blocks, WPW, severe hypotension, or shock.

Continued.

TABLE 4-1 Drug Summary (cont'd)

Drug	Dose/Route	Special considerations
Dobutamine	2-10 mcg/kg/min IV infusion.	Monitor blood pressure and ECG closely; these patients are prone to PVCs and tachycardia.
Dopamine	2-20 mcg/kg/min IV infusion.	Monitor urine output, heart rate, and blood pressure closely. DO NOT mix with sodium bicarbonate. Extravasation causes tissue necrosis; can be treated with local Regitine.
Epinephrine	0.1-1.0 mg IV bolus; if no effect may increase to 3-5 mg IV bolus every 5 min. Maintenance: IV infusion 1-4 mcg/min.	DO NOT mix with sodium bicarbonate. Adverse effects include hypertension, tachycardia, and ventricular tachycardia.
Furosemide	20-200 mg at 20 mg/min IV push.	Monitor for alkalosis, nausea, vomiting, diarrhea, hypocalcemia, hyperglycemia, and digoxin toxicity.
Heparin	Bolus: 5000 U IV push. Maintenance: 800-1200 U/hr IV infusion.	Monitor PTT. Initiate bleeding precautions. Can be reversed with protamine.
Hydralazine	10-40 mg IV at 1mg/min or IM.	Monitor for anginal symptoms, tachycardia, hypotension, and palpitations.

Continued.

TABLE 4-1 Drug Summary (cont'd)

Drug	Dose/Route	Special considerations
Lidocaine	Bolus: 1.0-1.5 mg/kg IV; may repeat in 3-5 min at half the initial dose to a total of 3.0 mg/kg. Maintenance: for a 1 mg/kg bolus, infusion rate is 2 mg/min; for a 1.5-2.0 mg/kg bolus, infuse at 3 mg/min, and for a 2.5-3.0 mg/kg bolus, infuse at 4 mg/min.	Maintenance dose may be decreased for geriatric patients or those with poor hepatic function, CNS depression, drowsiness, confusion, or tinnitus.
Metoprolol	5 mg rapid IV push every 2 min for 3 doses.	Monitor heart rate and blood pressure; may precipitate heart failure and angina. Give with caution in patients with COPD. Treat overdose with atropine.
Morphine	1-10 mg every hr IV push or drip. 10-15 mg every 2-4 hr IM.	Titrate dose to effect; may cause respiratory depression and pupil constriction. Use with caution in patients with hypotension or increased intracranial pressure. Give Narcan for overdose.
Nifedipine	10-20 mg PO or SL (may be available IV in the future).	Main side effect is hypotension. Dosage may have to be altered if the patient is receiving concurrent carbamazepine therapy.

TABLE 4-1 Drug Summary (cont'd)

Drug	Dose/Route	Special considerations
Nitroglycerin	Begin IV infusion at 5 mcg/min and titrate to effect. 0.4 mg SL every 3-5 min as tolerated by blood pressure or pain relief.	Closely monitor heart rate and blood pressure. Mix IV nitroglycerin in glass bottle and administer through non-PVC tubing to prevent absorption into plastic.
Nitroprusside	0.5-10 mcg/kg/min IV infusion.	Rapid vasodilator; monitor blood pressure closely; drug may be titrated up every 5 min for effect. Mix in 5% dextrose in water and protect from light. Monitor for toxicity by drawing thiocyanate levels.
Procainamide	Load: 1 g at 20 mg/min IV infusion: 2-5 mg/min.	Stop loading dose for widened QRS or hypotension. Monitor drug levels daily. Signs of toxicity include fever and torsades de pointes.
Streptokinase	1.5 million U IV over 1 hr.	Side effects include bleeding, hypotension, arrhythmias, and allergic reactions. The patient must not have a repeat dose for 6 months because anaphylaxis may develop. Patients that receive streptokinase will be started on heparin therapy after their streptokinase dose.
tPA	100 mg IV over 3 hr (but protocols may vary).	Administer within 6 hr of onset of chest pain. Half-life is 3-5 min. Side effects include bleeding and arrhythmias; screen patient for any history of bleeding

TABLE 4-1 Drug Summary (cont'd)

Drug	Dose/Route	Special considerations
		before drug administration. Patients that receive tPA will also receive heparin therapy following tPA administration.
Urokinase	6000 IU/min for up to 2 hr IA. IV: 4400 U/kg over 10 min followed by 4400 U/kg/hr for 12 hr (16).	Hypotension, bleeding, and arrhythmias are the main side effects. Usually given in conjunction with heparin.
Verapamil	5-10 mg IV bolus over 2 min, then repeat doses of 10 mg after 30 min.	Hypotension and bradycardia followed by asystole are significant adverse effects; bradycardia and asystole usually result from pushing drug too fast. May depress myocardial contractility, so give with caution to patients receiving concurrent beta-blocker therapy. Also, some patients develop reflex tachycardia as result of accessory pathways; if this occurs, administer calcium and choose another drug to slow the heart rate. Also dosage may have to be adjusted if patient is receiving carbamazepine therapy.

From Abrams A: *Clinical drug therapy*, ed 2, New York, 1987, JB Lippincott; American Heart Association: *Textbook of advanced life support*, ed 2, 1987, The Association; Cronin L: Beat the clock: saving the heart with thrombolytic drugs, *Nurs 93* 23(8):34-42, 1993; Lundberg GD, editor: Guidelines for cardiopulmonary resuscitation and emergency cardiac care: recommendations of the 1992 national conference of the american heart association, *JAMA* 268(16):2135-2302, 1992; Newman M, editor: *Curr in Emerg Cardiac Care* 3(4), 1992, American Heart Association (7).

Risk for pain
Risk for anxiety
Risk for impaired gas exchange
Risk for activity intolerance
Risk for fluid volume excess
Risk for impaired skin integrity
Risk for noncompliance, actual or potential

◆ **Decreased cardiac output** related to inability of the damaged myocardial tissue to pump effectively as evidenced by decreased peripheral perfusion, decreased mentation, and poor urinary output.

INTERVENTIONS

- Focus on increasing contractility with medications and decreasing myocardial oxygen demand by decreasing afterload and preload with diuretics, vasodilators, and pain management.

◆ **Alteration in tissue perfusion** related to decreased cardiac contractility, obstruction of blood flow to vital tissues, or decreased blood volume as evidenced by peripheral cyanosis, diminished peripheral pulses, altered mentation, decreased urinary output, chest pain, shortness of breath, decreased cardiac output, cardiac dysrhythmias, increased afterload, increased pulmonary artery pressure, increased central venous and pulmonary capillary wedge pressure.

INTERVENTIONS

- Focus on increasing contractility with medications and increasing circulating blood volume with fluid.
- Vessel obstruction should be relieved with vasodilators, anticoagulants, or thrombolytic therapy.

◆ **Pain** related to poor tissue perfusion because of obstruction in blood flow as evidenced by verbal complaints of crushing chest pain and extremity pain.

INTERVENTIONS

- Focus on pain relief with medications or positioning.

◆ **Anxiety** related to pain and poor mentation as evidenced by behavior, restlessness, and repetitive questioning about condition.

INTERVENTIONS

- Focus on relieving anxiety with medication or by offering reassurance.

◆ **Impaired gas exchange** related to diminished cardiac contractility and increased afterload as evidenced by poor arterial blood gases, increasing shortness of breath, and decreased pulse oximetry readings.

INTERVENTIONS
- Administer oxygen to the patient.
- Possible diuresis to relieve some of the volume overload.

◆ **Activity intolerance** related to decreased functional capacity of the heart as evidenced by shortness of breath, fatigue, chest pain, and vital sign changes with activity.

INTERVENTIONS
- Keep the patient on bedrest during the acute phase of the illness.

◆ **Fluid volume excess** related to decreased contractility, increased afterload, and decreased renal perfusion as evidenced by decreased urinary output, increased peripheral edema, increased pulmonary secretions, decreased cardiac output, and increased pulmonary capillary wedge pressure.

INTERVENTIONS
- Relieve the fluid overload with diuretics and afterload reduction.

◆ **Impaired skin integrity** related to decreased peripheral perfusion as evidenced by skin breakdown in the affected areas.

INTERVENTIONS
- Turn the patient frequently.
- Provide pressure relief with pillows and pressure reduction mattresses.

◆ **Noncompliance, actual or potential** related to denial of the severity of the condition as evidenced by repeated admissions, low blood levels of measurable cardiac drugs, and verbalization that medication and activity regimen are not being followed.

INTERVENTIONS
- Includes good discharge teaching with the patient and family.
- Follow-up needs to be stressed.

PRIORITY DIAGNOSTIC TESTS
Cardiac Conditions
ECG: Determines areas of cardiac injury, myocardial infarction, or conduction disturbance (Table 4-2).

Laboratory tests
Cardiac isoenzymes: CK and CKMB elevate after an MI. CK first appears in the blood 4 to 6 hours after the onset of

TABLE 4-2 Location of Infarct and ECG Changes

Location	Changes
Anterior MI	ST elevation in V_1-V_4
Septal infarct	ST elevation in V_1 and V_2
Inferior MI	ST evelation in lead 2, 3 and aV_F
Lateral MI	ST elevation in lead 1, aV_L, V_5 and V_6
Posterior MI	Reciprocal changes in V_1 and V_2—tall R wave, ST depression and upright T wave
Right Ventricular MI	Significant ST elevation in aV_R in patients with an inferior wall MI
Apical infarct	ST elevation in V_5 and V_6

From Dubin D: Rapid interpretation of EKG's, ed 3, Tampa, 1978, Cover Publishing; Lewis V: Monitoring the patient with an acute myocardial infarction, *Nurs Clin of North Am* 22(1):15-32, 1987; Marriott HJ: *Practical electrocardiography*, ed 7, Baltimore 1983, Williams & Wilkins (1).

pain and peaks at 16 to 36 hours. CKMB is cardiac specific. Also, there is inversion of LDH_1 and LDH_2 isoenzymes that occurs approximately 24 hours after the onset of pain (9).

Complete blood count: WBC count is elevated with any type of infectious process, and this can be a cause for chest or cardiac pain. Decreased hematocrit would indicate bleeding.

Serum electrolytes: Electrolyte abnormalities can cause a variety of symptoms that are similar to those caused by decreased cardiac output. If diuretics are administered to decrease preload, potassium, sodium, and chloride levels could be altered.

Serum magnesium, phosphorous and calcium: Low levels of any of the above could diminish the ability of the heart to pump even further.

PT/PTT: Initially a baseline is helpful. It is nice to know if the patient has an underlying clotting problem especially if thrombolytic therapy needs to be administered.

Liver function tests: Many of the cardiac drugs administered are metabolized by the liver and a baseline is helpful.

Arterial blood gases: Deterioration in the respiratory status can be monitored and an initial baseline is helpful.

Serum creatinine and BUN: Gives an indication of renal function. One or both of these values will be elevated in renal failure and will continue to increase in the presence of renal insufficiency or hypoperfusion.

Radiographic
Chest x-ray: Rules out any radiographic cause of chest pain and gives an indication of presence of pulmonary disease and edema.

Other
Echocardiogram: Gives an indication of myocardial damage by looking at wall motion and giving an indication of ejection fraction. Echocardiography is helpful in assessing valve function utilizing the transthoracic approach (14).

Pericardiocentesis: Done in the event of ventricular asystole or pulseless electrical activity. If fluid is present and can be evacuated, cardiac function will increase because the heart will be able to contract better.

Diagnostic cardiac catheterization: Visualizes patency of the coronary arteries and valves and measures ventricular ejection fraction. Coronary angioplasty can be done at the same time as the catheterization if the lesions are such that the patient will benefit from the procedure.

Exercise tolerance test: Dramatic increase in heart rate with little work indicative of the heart's inability to pump effectively. ST depression (>1 mm) during exercise indicates ischemia. This is a test that may be ordered on an outpatient basis and may be part of the discharge instructions (14).

Vascular Conditions
Angiography: Directly images an artery in order to visualize any narrowing, occlusion, or rupture (12).

Laboratory tests
Serum electrolytes: Assess for any electrolyte imbalance and give a baseline prior to any drug administration.

Serum creatinine and BUN: Indication of renal function.

Complete blood count: Indicates any blood loss or infectious process.

Liver function tests: Indicates any liver damage that could interfere with drug administration or blood clotting.

Type and crossmatch: Important to have blood available if bleeding starts or if operative management of the condition will occur.

Arterial blood gases: Baseline acid-base status is important and oxygenation to poorly perfused areas should be optimal. Also gives an indication of pulmonary function that would be important if operative management was necessary.

PT/PTT: Baseline and continuous monitoring are necessary especially if anticoagulants are administered.

Radiographic

Chest x-ray: Will detect any widening of the mediastinum indicating aortic dissection. Also done preoperatively for patients who have occlusions that need to be managed surgically.

Acute abdominal series: Indicates any problem or disruption of the abdominal aorta—will occasionally see aneurysm on x-ray (12).

CT scan of the abdomen: Will give a transverse view that will show an abdominal aortic aneurysm and give a measurement of the aneurysm (12).

Other

Electrocardiogram: Baseline necessary preoperatively. Repeat ECGs may be ordered to monitor for changes in response to treatment.

Doppler flow studies: Noninvasive—gives indication of arterial and venous flow in the extremities; also measures pressures in the extremities. When systolic wave is prolonged, there is a probable occlusion (12).

Venogram: Direct visualization through injected contrast of the vein and any occlusion (12).

COLLABORATIVE INTERVENTIONS

1. Oxygen should be provided to all patients with cardiovascular insufficiency in order to optimize oxygenation to all cells.
2. Initiate intravenous access in order to administer any medications that may be needed and as a precaution if the patient should arrest.
3. Allow patient to assume a comfortable position in bed in order to allow for adequate oxygenation and minimal anxiety.

4. ECG allows for diagnosis of any cardiac problem and gives a basis for treatment.

Clinical Conditions
Myocardial infarction
SYMPTOMS
- Chest pain with or without radiation to the left arm, neck, or jaw, sometimes accompanied by nausea, diaphoresis, pallor, and/or shortness of breath.
- Pain may be described as sharp, heaviness, tightness, crushing, burning or squeezing; it may be severe or vague and may occur at rest or during activity.

DIAGNOSIS
- 12-lead ECG will show changes (see Table 4-2), but changes may not be evident on the initial electrocardiogram so history and risk factors need to be considered.
- Changes in cardiac isoenzymes will occur; the CPK increases 4 to 6 hours after the onset of the infarct and peaks 16 to 36 hours after the infarct (9).
- Presence of the isoenzyme CKMB indicates myocardial damage; it is the most sensitive and reliable test to indicate MI (9).
- LDH also increases within 24 hours of an infarct and peaks 48 to 72 hours postinfarct (9).
- Abnormality in the LDH isoenzymes (LDH_1 and LDH_2), also indicates myocardial necrosis (9).
- Other positive indicators of myocardial damage include an echocardiogram that looks at cardiac wall motion and valvular function; and diagnostic cardiac catheterization that provides direct visualization of the coronary arteries in order to detect spasm or blockage and measures cardiac pressures as well as LV function.

TREATMENT
- Continuous cardiac monitoring.
- Oxygen therapy (2 L/min per nasal cannula if not in respiratory distress).
- Nitroglycerine titrated to pain relief and blood pressure.
- Thrombolytic therapy (tPA or streptokinase) in conjunction with heparin, aspirin, beta-blockers such as Lopressor IV and calcium channel blockers such as diltiazem IV (8).
- If pain continues after the above therapy, morphine sulfate IV may need to be administered.

- Later interventions include PTCA for blocked coronary arteries, coronary artery bypass grafting, and intraaortic balloon pumping for continuing pain.

Angina

SYMPTOMS

- Substernal or epigastric pain that occurs with activity or emotional stress.
- Pain lasts 3 to 5 minutes but may last up to 20 minutes.
- Varies in severity and presents as a heaviness, tightness, fullness, squeezing, or crushing.
- Pain is intermittent in origin and usually presents in those patients who have a history of angina, a previous myocardial infarction, hypertension, or diabetes.

DIAGNOSIS

- If the patient is having pain at the time that the ECG is done, ischemia will be evident on the ECG and will show ST segment depression.
- There will be no elevation in cardiac enzymes.

TREATMENT

- Nitroglycerin for pain relief, beta-blockers, calcium channel blockers, oxygen.
- Anginal symptoms may also be alleviated by decreasing stress, finding a position of comfort, decreasing environmental stimuli, and maintaining a calm manner while caring for the patient.

Congestive heart failure

SYMPTOMS

- Associated with fluid overload.
- Includes peripheral edema, cough, rales, tachypnea, orthopnea, shortness of breath, fatigue, weight gain, S_3 gallop; and later pink, frothy sputum, tachycardia, and cyanosis.

DIAGNOSIS

- Chest x-ray will show infiltrates and an enlarged heart.
- Arterial blood gases will show hypoxemia and acidosis.
- The ECG will show ventricular enlargement.

TREATMENT

- Oxygen (may require higher concentration of oxygen to keep saturation >95%).
- Position of comfort.
- Intravenous access for administration of furosemide; inotropic agents such as digoxin, dobutamine, or morphine to decrease anxiety and decrease the work of breathing.

- Anticipate the use of vasodilators such as nitroglycerin, nitroprusside, or hydralazine to decrease blood pressure as well as afterload.
- Maintaining an anxiety-free environment will also ensure a better outcome for this patient.

Cardiogenic shock
SYMPTOMS

- Most common cause is MI, so symptoms are similar, but much more severe.
- Also can be caused by chest trauma or end-stage cardiomyopathy.
- All symptoms center around decreased cardiac output: confusion; decreased urine output; poor peripheral perfusion; signs of pulmonary congestion including rales, tachypnea, and orthopnea; tachycardia; and usually a feeling of impending doom ("I'm going to die").

DIAGNOSIS

- ECG may show cardiac arrhythmias and usually MI. Arterial blood gases will show hypoxia and metabolic acidosis.

TREATMENT

- Provide oxygen and prepare for endotracheal intubation.
- Establish intravenous access to provide a combination of medications to decrease preload such as furosemide and nitrates; increase contractility such as dopamine and dobutamine; and decrease afterload such as nitroprusside.
- If cardiac output and tissue perfusion continue to be inadequate, consider intraaortic balloon pump therapy (6). Also, be prepared to initiate ACLS protocol; mortality of this state of shock is 80% to 90%.

Sudden death
SYMPTOMS

- Sometimes accompanied by palpitations, dizziness, chest pain, or shortness of breath, but some patients have no warning.
- If the patient has lived through multiple episodes of sudden death, there may be an aura that the patient can relay.
- There is a loss of consciousness with a period of loss of pulse and blood pressure.

DIAGNOSIS
- The electrocardiogram shows ventricular fibrillation or ventricular tachycardia.

TREATMENT
- Per ACLS protocol, establish an airway, begin ventilation, and administer oxygen (see Reference Guide 1).
- Administer CPR.
- Defibrillate.
- Establish IV access and administer antidysrhythmics such as Lidocaine, bretylium and procainamide.
- If the patient survives sudden death, evaluation for an automatic implantable cardioverter-defibrillator should be initiated.
- If the patient presents with an AICD in place, ACLS protocol should be followed. The rescuer will not be shocked by the AICD as long as universal precautions are maintained and the AICD will not be damaged by the defibrillator (10).

Cardiac arrest

SYMPTOMS
- Absence of respiration, absence of pulse and blood pressure.
- Unresponsive, cyanotic, and pupils unreactive to light.

DIAGNOSIS
- ECG shows ventricular fibrillation/tachycardia, pulseless electrical activity or asystole in two leads.
- ABGs show metabolic and respiratory acidosis especially if the patient has been in cardiac arrest for a prolonged period of time.

TREATMENT
- After taking care of the ABCs, try to determine the underlying cause such as cardiac tamponade, hypovolemia, hypoxemia, tension pneumothorax, acidosis, and treat if possible.
- Utilize ACLS protocol to treat cardiac arrest.
- Epinephrine will be the first and most frequently used drug before and after intravenous access has been established; epinephrine may be given through the endotracheal tube if IV access has not been obtained.
- Always assure that the ECG leads are properly applied prior to deciding that the patient is in asystole and ALWAYS check asystole in two leads.

Endocarditis
SYMPTOMS
- Fever, chills, fatigue, weight loss, anorexia, and night sweats.
- The patient usually has a history of cardiac surgery or some other invasive procedure such as IV drug use, congenital heart disease, or rheumatic heart disease.
- The patient is often tachycardic, has a new cardiac murmur, petechiae, and signs of cardiac failure such as peripheral edema.

DIAGNOSIS
- Increased white blood cell count.
- Positive blood cultures.
- Increased serum glucose secondary to the infectious process.
- Chest x-ray will show heart enlargement.
- Definitive diagnosis is made by an echocardiogram that will show valvular incompetence or valvular vegetation.

TREATMENT
- Antibiotics specific to the infectious agent.
- Palliative treatment for fever such as Tylenol.
- Symptomatic treatment of heart failure.

Pericarditis
SYMPTOMS
- Sudden, severe, sharp chest pain that may radiate to the back or shoulders and increases with movement or inspiration; usually after open heart surgery or radiation.
- A pericardial friction rub is audible along the left lower sternal border.
- The patient may experience tachycardia and hypotension that may be the result of decreasing cardiac output associated with cardiac compression from the accumulated fluid in the pericardial sac.

DIAGNOSIS
- Chest x-ray will show cardiomegaly with clear lung fields.
- ECG will show ST elevation in the limb leads and in the precordial leads, but there are no QRS changes.
- An echocardiogram will be definitive in showing an accumulation of fluid in the pericardial sac.

TREATMENT
- Pericardiocentesis may need to be performed for a large effusion.

- Antiinflammatory drugs or analgesics will help the pain associated with the illness.
- Treatment of the underlying condition such as MI, infection, or rheumatic fever is paramount.
- Surgical interventions such as a pericardial window or pericardiectomy will decrease discomfort and accumulation of fluid.

Acute aortic dissection

SYMPTOMS

- Back pain and pain between the shoulder blades are the most common presenting symptoms.
- Late symptoms include decreasing hematocrit and hypovolemic shock associated with profound blood loss.
- If the dissection involves the thoracic aorta, chest pain may be the presenting symptom. The pain is knifelike and radiates down the back and into the lower extremities.
- There is a blood pressure difference in the right and left extremities and/or in the upper and lower extremities.
- Also peripheral pulses will be diminished or absent.

DIAGNOSIS

- Chest x-ray will show a widening in the area of the aneurysm.
- Definitive diagnosis is an aortogram that will show acute dissection.

TREATMENT

- Controlling the arterial blood pressure to maintain mean arterial pressures between 60 and 80 mm Hg is paramount; use of sodium nitroprusside is indicated acutely.
- If the patient is experiencing shock associated with leaking or rupture, vigorous fluid resuscitation is indicated.
- Replacement of blood loss with packed red blood cells may be necessary.
- If symptoms progress, surgical intervention may be necessary.

Acute arterial occlusion

SYMPTOMS

- Sudden onset of extremity pain and numbness, usually in those patients with a history of peripheral atherosclerotic disease.

- Pale, cool, cyanotic extremity with absence of peripheral pulses associated with paresthesia are common presentations.

DIAGNOSIS

- Doppler flow studies will clearly show arterial occlusion.
- Invasive studies such as arteriograms will also show arterial occlusion (2).

TREATMENT

- Initiation of heparin therapy is common along with intraarterial urokinase infusions.
- If the occlusion is severe, the patient may require an embolectomy or angioplasty.

Venous thrombosis

SYMPTOMS

- Pain, tenderness, swelling, and warmth of the effected extremity along with a positive Homans' sign.
- The patient usually has had a period of bedrest for some reason including acute or chronic illness, or is receiving intravenous injections.

DIAGNOSIS

- Venogram is a definitive indicator of a deep venous thrombosis (2).
- Other diagnostic indicators include measurements of the extremities to show a difference right to left.

TREATMENT

- Heparinization is the definitive treatment for DVT.
- Follow-up treatment includes Coumadin therapy usually for 1 year after deep venous thrombosis.

NURSING SURVEILLANCE

1. Monitor vital signs including oxygen saturation.
2. Monitor for relief of pain.
3. Monitor for increasing pain.
4. Monitor I/0 and continually assess fluid balance.
5. Monitor electrocardiogram for any changes or dysrhythmias.
6. Monitor mentation, an indicator of perfusion.
7. Monitor peripheral perfusion and peripheral pulses.

EXPECTED PATIENT OUTCOMES

1. Pain decreases in severity as documented on the 1 to 10 pain scale.

2. Systolic blood pressure is maintained above 90.
3. Heart rate is maintained above 60 and below 100.
4. Urine output is >30 cc/hr.
5. Mental status is at baseline; patient is awake and alert.
6. Oxygen saturations are >95%.
7. Peripheral perfusion is restored or maintained.

DISCHARGE IMPLICATIONS

Cardiac

1. Teach patient and family the signs of an MI and when medical assistance is needed for symptoms.
2. Teach patient how to use sublingual nitroglycerin or nitropaste.
3. Instruct patient and family about the use of discharge medications, and give medication information sheets to the patient and/or family for reference.
4. Instruct the family on the importance of CPR training in the event of a cardiac arrest.
5. Instruct the patient and family on the importance of follow-up.

Vascular

1. Instruct the patient and family on the importance of getting coagulation studies checked frequently.
2. Instruct the patient on what to look for in the event of reocclusion.
3. For those patients with suspected or documented aortic aneurysms, teach signs of rupture and impending rupture. Stress the importance of follow-up.
4. For patients with peripheral vascular disease, teach palliative measures for their pain such as the use of support hose and elevation of the extremity.

References

1. Caine R: Essentials of monitoring the electrocardiogram, *Nurs Clin of North Am* 22(1):77-87, 1987.
2. Doyle J: Treatment modalities in peripheral vascular disease, *Nurs Clin of North Am* 21(2):241-53, 1986.
3. Ebersole P and Hess P: *Toward healthy aging: human needs and nursing response* ed 3, St. Louis, 1990, Mosby.
4. Gordon M: *Manual of nursing diagnosis*, New York, 1987, McGraw-Hill.
5. Herman J: Nursing assessment and nursing diagnosis in patients with peripheral vascular disease, *Nurs Clin of North Am* 21(2):219-31, 1986.

6. Horvath P, editor: *Care of the adult cardiac surgery patient*, New York, 1984, Wiley.
7. Lamb J and Carlson V: *Handbook of cardiovascular nursing*, Philadelphia, 1986, JB Lippincott.
8. Leach R: A tPA ninety minute protocol, *J of Emerg Nurs* 19: 338-9, 1993.
9. Lewis V: Monitoring the patient with an acute myocardial infarction, *Nurs Clin of North Am* 22(1):15-32, 1987.
10. Lundberg GD, editor: Guidelines for cardiopulmonary resuscitation and emergency cardiac care: recommendations of the 1992 national conference of the american heart association, *JAMA* 268(16):2135-2302, 1992.
11. Majoros K: Comparisons and controversies in clot busting drugs, *Crit Care Nurs Q* 16(2):46-69, 1993.
12. Massey J: Diagnostic testing for peripheral vascular disease, *Nurs Clin of North Am* 21(2):207-18, 1986.
13. Rea R, Bourg P, Parker J and Rushing D, editors: *Emergency nursing core curriculum*, ed 3, Philadelphia, 1987, WB Saunders.
14. Rossi L and Leary E: Evaluating the patient with coronary artery disease, *Nurs Clin of North Am* 27(1):171-88, 1992.
15. Vazquez M, Lazear S and Larson E: *Critical care nursing*, ed 2, Philadelphia, 1992, WB Saunders.
16. Woo M: Clinical management of the patient with an acute myocardial infarction, *Nurs Clin of North Am* 27(1):77-87, 1992.

C

Communicable Diseases

Pamela S. Kidd

CLINICAL CONDITIONS
Acute Rheumatic Fever (ARF)
Acute Streptococcal Infection
Cellulitis/Skin and Soft Tissue Infection
Diphtheria
Food Poisoning
Hepatitis
Human Immunodeficiency Virus
Lyme Disease
Measles
Meningococcal Infection
Mononucleosis
Mumps Parotitis
Pertussis
Rubella (German measles)
Tetanus
Tuberculosis
Varicella (chickenpox)

TRIAGE ASSESSMENT

Many patients will present to the triage area with symptoms of a communicable or infectious disease. This chapter provides an overview of the most frequently encountered communicable and infectious diseases in the emergency department (ED). It is not meant to be a comprehensive review. The reader may need to refer to a communicable disease text for more information. A thorough history at triage is necessary, since many of these patients will need to wait for treatment. The triage nurse must determine if isolation of the patient is necessary before the availability of a treatment bed.

Start with the following questions to help determine if isolation or mask protection may be necessary.

Exposure

Ask if another member of the family and/or work and school contacts has been ill. If so, have them describe symptoms. Table 5-1 includes incubation periods for common communicable diseases.

Travel

Travel to other countries may be associated with a higher incidence of drug-resistant tuberculosis (DR-TB), hepatitis A and E, *E. coli* food poisoning, and Lyme disease (e.g., travel to Asia is associated with higher risk for DR-TB).

Malaise

If the patient complains of malaise, lethargy, anorexia, and frequent colds and cough, ask about the patient's sexual history, history of injection drug use, and hemophilia. Primary HIV infection produces symptoms of fever, myalgia, fatigue, and sore throat.

Communicable disease history

Determine if the patient has or has had a communicable disease. HIV-positive individuals should be considered as tuberculosis positive until proven otherwise (4,5). Determine the date of diagnosis of HIV since progression to acquired immunodeficiency syndrome (AIDS) usually occurs within 10 years after initial infection. Complications such as subacute sclerosing panencephalitis (progressive neurologic deficit) occurs later in childhood after either having a measles infection or from receiving the live measles virus vaccine.

Treatment for previous/current communicable disease

If the patient has had a communicable disease, determine course of treatment. DR-TB generally occurs in people with incomplete treatment for TB or a native of a country with a high rate of DR-TB (e.g., Haiti, Latin America, Southeast Asia). Several factors may activate dormant TB lesions including diabetes, steroid therapy, malnutrition, and alcohol abuse.

Living conditions

Large family size, bedroom overcrowding, inadequate access to clean water and ventilation have been associated with streptococcal infections (e.g., acute rheumatic fever [ARF]), tuberculosis, and hepatitis A.

TABLE 5-1 Comparison of Communicable Diseases

Disease	Adult symptoms	Pediatric symptoms	High risk groups	Diagnosis	Treatment	Incubation period	Transmission route	Peak period	Complications
Pertussis	Persistent cough lasting >7 days	Paroxysmal cough Whoop Cough-induced vomiting Leukocytosis	Infants 1-2 months old Females > males < 3 doses of DPT vaccine	Anti-pertussis toxin 1 g G-antibody measured by enzyme-linked immunosorbent assay Culture of nasopharyngeal secretions	Erythromycin	7-13 days	Respiratory secretions	Every 3-4 yr (1990 last U.S. epidemic)	Pneumonia Seizures Cranial nerve abnormalities
Rubeola (typical)	Fever Macular rash—progressing head to toe Koplik's spots Photophobia	Fever Macular rash progressing head to toe Koplik's spots Photophobia	Persons in late teens and early 20s	Hemoagglutination inhibition and complement-fixation tests	Symptomatic Antipyretics Fluids Dark room Measles vaccine within 72 hours of exposure	10-12 days	Droplets from nasopharyngeal tract	Winter and spring	Encephalitis
Rubeola (atypical)	Headache Arthralgia Abdominal pain Macular rash—starting with extremities moving central	Headache Arthralgia Abdominal pain Macular rash—starting with extremities moving central	Adults born between 1957 and 1967	Hemoagglutination inhibition and complement-fixation tests	Symptomatic	10-14 days	Droplets from nasopharyngeal tract	Winter and spring	Rare

Continued.

C

169

TABLE 5-1 Comparison of Communicable Diseases (cont'd)

Disease	Adult symptoms	Pediatric symptoms	High risk groups	Diagnosis	Treatment	Incubation period	Transmission route	Peak period	Complications
Mumps	Epididymo-orchitis Testicular atrophy Meningitis	Low-grade fever Headache Vomiting Sore throat Unilateral or bilateral parotid swelling	15-19 year old (not vaccinated or infected)	Clinical presentation	Symptomatic Adult males are placed on bed rest Analgesics	2-3 weeks	Droplet, oral contact Contact with articles recently contaminated with saliva	Winter and early spring	Sterility Meningitis
Rubella	Rash Low grade fever Malaise Conjunctivitis Sore throat	Pink papular rash on face and neck that spreads to extremities	7 months to 40 years	Rubella antibody assay tests	Symptomatic Antipyretics (no aspirin)	14-21 days	Droplets from nasopharyngeal tracts	Winter and early spring	Arthralgia Arthritis
Varicella (chicken pox)	Low grade fever Lesions in several stages (macules, papules, vesicles, crusted lesions) Rash appears on trunk then face and scalp Lesions in mouth, throat, conjunctiva	Low-grade fever Lesions in several stages (macules, papules, vesicles, crusted lesions) Rash appears on trunk then face and scalp Lesions in mouth, throat, conjunctiva	Immuno-compromised individuals	By clinical presentation	Antihistamines Varicella immunoglobulin within 96 hours of exposure 125-625 U	10-21 days	Direct contact with vesicle discharge or mucous membranes	Winter and spring	Encephalitis Pneumonia

Disease	Signs and Symptoms		Risk Factors	Diagnosis	Treatment	Incubation	Transmission		Complications
Tetanus	Pain Stiffness in the jaw, abdomen, or back Dysphagia Reflex spasms	Pain Stiffness in the jaw, abdomen, or back Dysphagia Reflex spasms	Occupational groups (wounds obtained in farming, forestry activities) Persons over age 50	By clinical presentation and absence of serum antibody level	500-6,000 U IM of human tetanus immunoglobulin Benzodiazepines to treat spasms Neuromuscular blocking agents (e.g., pancuronium)	2 hours to 7 days	Contact between an open wound and spores in the soil	Variable, based on contact with soil especially where horses are present	Respiratory failure
Multi-drug resistant tuberculosis	Cough Weight loss Diarrhea Abdominal pain Changes in mental status	Cough Weight loss Diarrhea Abdominal pain Changes in mental status	Immunocompromised individuals (HIV positive)	Anergy testing comparing reaction to purified protein derivative with other antigen reactions	Treatment should last for at least 12 months Treatment requires use of at least 3 drugs not used previously	2-10 weeks although can be latent for over 50 years (Immunosuppressed individuals will develop active TB usually within 4-8 weeks)	By droplets from nasopharyngeal tract through coughing, talking, sneezing, singing	Variable	Meningitis Hematologic abnormalities Pleural effusion
Tuberculosis	Weight loss Fever Night sweats Cough Hemoptysis Chest pain (treatment for adults is 6 months)	Children may have more extra-pulmonary symptoms, e.g., abdominal pain (treatment for children is 9 months)	Foreign-born persons from India, China, Philippines, Alcoholics, IV drug abusers Institutionalized individuals (prisons, nursing homes)	Presence of acid-fast bacilli on sputum smear Lesions on chest x-ray Positive tuberculin skin test	Respiratory isolation for 2 weeks Usually treated with isoniazid and rifampin	2-10 weeks although can be latent for over 50 years (Immunosuppressed individuals will develop active TB usually within 4-8 weeks)	By droplets from nasopharyngeal tract through coughing, talking, sneezing, singing	Variable	Meningitis Hematologic abnormalities Pleural effusion

Continued.

171

TABLE 5-1 Comparison of Communicable Diseases (cont'd)

Disease	Adult symptoms	Pediatric symptoms	High risk groups	Diagnosis	Treatment	Incubation period	Transmission route	Peak period	Complications
Hepatitis A	Anorexia Nausea/vomiting Right upper quadrant abdominal pain Jaundice	Same symptoms as adult but less severe	Contact with family member who is infected	Anti-HAV IgM antibody confirms active hepatitis A infection	Immunoglobulin given for anticipated or post-exposure	15-50 days	Fecal-oral transmission spread by saliva, contaminated food and water	Variable	No chronic complications; confers lifelong immunity
Hepatitis B	Anorexia Nausea/vomiting Right upper quadrant abdominal pain Jaundice Rash and arthralgias Jaundice is less severe	Same symptoms as adult but less severe	Health care workers IV drug abusers	HbsAg-presence of hepatitis B surface antigen HbeAg—"e" antigen indicates high infectivity	Hepatitis B immune globulin and hepatitis B vaccine given post exposure	45-160 days	Parenteral or sexual transmission via blood, saliva, semen, and vaginal secretions	Variable	Chronic hepatitis Liver cancer
Non-A, Non-B Hepatitis (Hepatitis C)	Blood dyscrasia Arthritis Hepatomegaly Malaise	Same symptoms as adult but less severe	Health care workers IV drug abusers Hemophiliacs Renal patients	Elevation of alanine aminotransferase Antihepatitis C antibodies in serum	Symptomatic treatment Corticosteroids may be used Acyclovir	2-26 weeks	Percutaneous transmission through blood transfusions, pooled plasma products, IV drug abuse, hemodialysis	Variable	Chronic hepatitis Cirrhosis Liver cancer

Disease	Symptoms	Signs	Population at risk	Diagnostic test	Treatment	Incubation period	Transmission	Season	Complications
Hepatitis D (coinfection with Hepatitis B)	Hepatomegaly Jaundice (more severe symptoms than seen with hepatitis B alone)	—	IV drug abusers Hemophiliacs	Antihepatitis D Antibodies in serum	Hepatitis B immune globulin and hepatitis B vaccine given post exposure	15–64 days	Parenteral or sexual transmission	Variable	Chronic hepatitis
Hepatitis E	Anorexia Nausea/ Vomiting Right upper quadrant abdominal pain Jaundice	Occurs rarely in children	Visitors to Third World developing countries Rare in U.S.	No diagnostic test available	Symptomatic	15–50 days	Fecal-oral spread by contaminated water	Variable	High mortality rate in pregnant women
Human Immunodeficiency Virus (HIV)	Vaginal candidiasis Recurrent shingles Oral candidiasis Skin condition Fatigue Visual changes Fever Sore throat	Vaginal candidiasis Recurrent shingles Oral candidiasis Skin condition Fatigue Visual changes Fever Sore throat	Homosexuals, predominantly male IV drug abusers Hispanics African-Americans Sex workers (prostitutes) Hemophiliacs	Western Blot Test positive for antibodies against HIV	Zidovudine Acyclovir Treatment of opportunistic infections (e.g., pneumocystis, candida)	Unknown	Parenteral or sexual transmission	Variable	May present first with hepatitis B, syphilis, and/or tuberculosis
Lyme disease	Bull's eye rash Fever Headache Neck pain Myalgia	Bull's eye rash Fever Headache Neck pain Myalgia	Children between 5 and 14 years old Hikers in New England, mid-Atlantic, north central U.S. regions	Punch biopsy of rash shows spirochetes with antibodies to B. burgdorferi	Doxycycline, ampicillin or azithromycin	3–30 days	Bite of tick infected with B. burgdorferi	Summer and early fall	Carditis Encephalitis Arthritis

Continued.

c

TABLE 5-1 Comparison of Communicable Diseases (cont'd)

Disease	Adult symptoms	Pediatric symptoms	High risk groups	Diagnosis	Treatment	Incubation period	Transmission route	Peak period	Complications
Acute rheumatic fever (ARF)	Appears rarely as primary disease in adults	Fever Malaise Weight loss Arthralgia Carditis Chorea Subcutaneous nodules	Ethnic groups Children (less likely after puberty)	Presence of streptococcal antibodies Positive throat culture for group A *Streptococcus*	Salicylates Supportive treatment Steroids may be given for carditis	2-3 weeks	Initial infection with group A *Streptococcus* (usually strep throat or scarlet fever)	Variable	Carditis/valve disease Polyarthritis Chorea

Cough

Pertussis should be considered in all persons who have had
a cough lasting more than 7 days (2). Paroxysmal cough
is associated with pertussis in all age groups. Persistent
unrelieved coughing that interrupts sleep is associated
with tuberculosis. When a cough persists for 3 weeks or
more after a cold, TB should be considered (3).
Hemoptysis is also associated with tuberculosis.

Genetic factors

Ask if another member of the family has a positive history
for communicable diseases. ARF has been linked with
genetic factors.

The following information should help in assessing severity
of the condition.

Past medical history

Patients with an earlier diagnosis of streptococcal infection
may have developed ARF. Persons with impaired venous
drainage (e.g., peripheral vascular disease or coronary
bypass graft surgery using the saphenous vein) are at
higher risk for cellulitis. Diabetes associated with
hypertension results in greater number of skin and soft
tissue infections. Latin and Native American diabetic
patients experience diabetic complications earlier.
Hemophiliacs and hemodialysis patients have a higher
incidence of hepatitis B, C, and D.

Speech

Numbness around the mouth and slurred speech with
muscle weakness and malaise are associated with botulism.

Mood/memory changes

Ask about mood and memory changes, headaches, and
neck stiffness, since encephalitis and meningitis are
complications from several communicable diseases (e.g.,
measles, ARF, Lyme disease, chickenpox). Patients may
present with complications and not the initial illness.
These symptoms also suggest the possibility of an
opportunistic infection in an HIV-infected individual.

Injection drug use

Hepatitis B, C, and D, and HIV infection are more
common among injection drug users.

Nausea/vomiting/diarrhea

Gastrointestinal complaints occur in several varieties of
food poisoning. If the patient complains of nausea,
vomiting, diarrhea, and abdominal cramping, get a diet
history for the preceding 24 hours (Table 5-2).

TABLE 5-2 Varieties of Food Poisoning

Organism	Susceptible foods	Symptoms	Incubation period
Staphylococcus aureus	Cream pastries Mayonnaise Mayonnaise-based salads	Vomiting Headache	1-8 hr
Clostridium botulinum	Canned low-acid vegetables Canned fruits Canned fish	Descending weakness Paralysis Ptosis Pupillary abnormalities Dysphagia Dyspnea	18-24 hr
Bacillus cereus	Fried rice	Vomiting Abdominal cramps	1-6 hr
Escherichia coli	Contaminated water Unpeeled vegetables and fruits	Watery diarrhea Abdominal cramps Low-grade fever	24-72 hr
Vibrio cholerae	Contaminated water Unpeeled vegetables and fruits	Severe diarrhea and vomiting Hypovolemic shock	1-3 days

Salmonella	Raw or undercooked poultry, eggs, ground beef	Nausea and vomiting Fever Abdominal pain Watery diarrhea	8-48 hr
Trichinosis	Undercooked pork or wild game	Abdominal pain Nausea Fever Diarrhea	24-48 hr
Ciguatoxin	Barracuda, red snapper, grouper, sea bass	Diarrhea Ataxia, dizziness	1-6 hr

Immunizations

Ask if the patient has had prior immunizations and if so, what vaccine(s), the number of doses, and when received. Underimmunized children are at higher risk for complications from most communicable diseases (see Table 5-1).

Over-the-counter drug use

Ask if over-the-counter medications have relieved their symptoms. The arthritis associated with ARF responds dramatically to aspirin.

Pain

In some communicable diseases, the pain is more severe than associated physical findings would indicate. ARF arthritis pain is very severe, but joint inflammation signs may be minimal.

Insect bite

Ask if the patient was bitten by an insect and if so, what type? Did they bring the insect with them? In Lyme disease, the likelihood of infection increases with the duration of the tick's feeding.

NURSING ALERT

Do not attempt to remove a feeding tick using a lighted match, chemicals, or petroleum jelly. These substances may cause the tick to release more organisms (spirochetes) into the patient's skin. Ticks should be removed using tweezers and gentle traction pulling at the mouth. Squeezing the abdomen may release a greater number of spirochetes. Attach the tick to an index card using clear tape. Label the date of the bite, part of the body bitten, and the locale where the tick came from. The tick can be checked for the presence of spirochetes.

Vital Signs

- *Tachycardia:* Tachycardia out of proportion with fever is a sign of carditis. Carditis is a symptom of ARF. Many times the patient will seek health care for complications from a strep infection but not for the initial infection because the initial infection was mild. Tachycardia with hypotension may be present if the patient is in hypovolemic shock resulting from fluid volume deficit from vomiting and diarrhea associated with food poisoning.
- *Fever:* Temperature elevation is common with communicable diseases. Low-grade fever is present in

chickenpox, measles, and mumps. High-grade fever is associated with atypical measles and *Streptococcus* infection. Very high fever may occur in tetanus because of the overactivity of the autonomic nervous system.

General Observations
Skin rash

- Although it is not possible to have the patient undress at triage, all visible skin should be examined for the presence of a rash or lesion(s). Figure 5-1 illustrates the rash distribution of commonly encountered conditions in the ED. Subcutaneous nodules over bony prominences are associated with ARF. Petechiae or purpura (an indirect indicator of thrombocytopenia) is common in meningococcemia and indicates a very ill patient who needs to be treated immediately.

> **NURSING ALERT**
>
> Do not be fooled by skin and soft tissue infections. Streptococcal skin infection can be life threatening and advances systematically rapidly. When in doubt about the origin of a skin infection, triage immediately to the treatment area.

Skin lesions

- Skin and mucous membrane lesions may appear in histoplasmosis, an opportunistic infection associated with HIV infection. Multiple discrete papules may appear on the extremities, trunk, and face. The lesions will be associated with fever and anorexia.

Wounds

- Examine wounds and lacerations thoroughly. Tetanus-prone wounds include those contaminated with dirt or saliva, puncture wounds, avulsions, gunshot wounds, burns, and frostbite. Closed-fist injuries sustained by hitting knuckles against teeth as well as animal and human bites are particularly prone to cellulitis.
- Examine drainage from wounds, if present. Creamy, yellow pus suggests the presence of staphylococci. Group A beta-hemolytic streptococci produce erythema without drainage. Brownish, foul-smelling drainage suggests anaerobic bacteria.

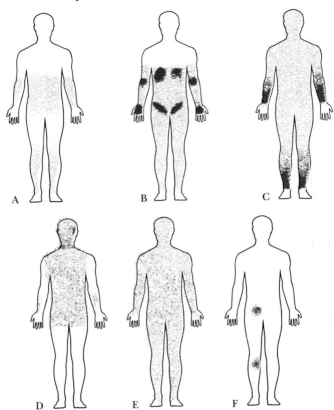

Figure 5-1 **A,** Meningococcemia. Begins as macules, progresses to petechiae, then forms purpura. Located on extremities and trunk. **B,** Atypical measles. Maculopapular rash along skin creases. **C,** Rocky Mountain spotted fever. Diffuse rash with heavier concentration at distal extremities. **D,** Typical measles. Starts behind ears, then moves to face and neck, then downward over rest of body; discrete spots on extremities. **E,** Rubella. Begins on the face, then to neck, trunk, and extremities, respectively. **F,** Lyme disease. Centrifugal rash that varies in diameter with red outer border and clearer center. Higher frequency in popliteal and groin region. May have multiple or singular lesions.

Gland enlargement
- Swelling of the parotid glands may be apparent in cases of mumps.

Throat
- It is helpful to perform a quick inspection of the patient's mouth and throat at triage using a penlight and tongue depressor. A red, irritated pharynx with or without pustules may be present in Streptococcus infection. The patient may be given a mask or asked not to cough without covering his/her mouth while awaiting treatment. A patient with Koplik's spots (bright red macules with a bluish-white spot in the center) on the inner lip buccal mucosa may have measles and is highly contagious requiring immediate isolation. Koplik's spots precedes the measles rash by 48 hours.

Tongue/mouth
- Swelling of the tongue, drooling, dysphagia, and pain in the floor of the mouth are associated with Ludwig's angina. Because of the potential for respiratory compromise resulting from edema, these patients should be triaged immediately to the treatment area.
- Oral mouth lesions may be present in thrush, an opportunistic infection associated with HIV infection.

Height and weight
- Assess height and weight in relation to stature. Weight loss is common in patients with tuberculosis and HIV infection. Anorexia is a common complaint of these patients.

Dehydration
- Assess skin turgor and look for sunken fontanels and orbits. Dehydration occurs rapidly in food poisoning (e.g., *E. coli*, *Salmonella*, and *Staphylococcus*).

Hygiene
- Impetigo, folliculitis, furuncles, and carbuncles are associated with poor hygiene. Poor dental hygiene is associated with Ludwig's angina.

FOCUSED NURSING ASSESSMENT

Nursing assessment should focus on ventilation, perfusion, mobility, mental status, and neurovascular status.

Ventilation
Airway
Maintain patency of the airway. Patients presenting with a
stiff jaw and dysphagia are at risk of aspiration as well as
laryngospasm. Suction equipment should be at the
bedside, and staff should be prepared to assist with
intubation and administer a neuromuscular blocking
agent.

Breath sounds
Consolidation may be present in pneumonia associated
with HIV infection and in TB. Wheezing may be present
in pertussis.

Perfusion
Apical heart rate
The auscultation of a murmur may indicate ARF. A systolic
mitral regurgitation murmur is best auscultated at the
apex using the diaphragm of the stethoscope while the
patient holds his/her breath after exhaling. A diastolic
aortic regurgitation murmur is best auscultated in the
third, left intercostal space. Diminished heart sounds
may indicate pericardial effusion (associated with ARF-
induced carditis). Palpitations and fainting may occur
because of conduction defects associated with
disseminated Lyme disease.

Neck veins
Congestive heart failure may be a complication of ARF.
Patients exhibit jugular venous distention and facial
edema. Neck veins may be flat and urine output
decreased in cases of hypovolemia as a result of fluid loss
from vomiting and diarrhea from food poisoning.

Mobility
Ataxia is present in some cases of food poisoning. Red,
swollen joints that are warm to touch may be present in
ARF.

Mental Status
Assess patient's level of responsiveness and record a
Glasgow coma scale score. Some infections may present
with central nervous system changes (e.g.,
cytomegalovirus, meningitis, encephalitis).

Neurovascular Integrity

Assess neurovascular status of all extremities. Several skin and soft tissue diseases have vascular implications (e.g., necrotizing fascitis, cellulitis, Kaposi's sarcoma). Vascular status of extremities can be assessed by noting the level at which the skin loses its hair and becomes shiny. The transition zone from warm to cold on palpation should be noted. Crepitus will be present on palpation in necrotizing fascitis. Because of the rapidity with which this disease progresses, patients with crepitus should be triaged immediately to the treatment area. Sensation should be assessed using pinprick or pinwheel. The points at which the patient begins to feel the prick and the point where the sensation turns to pain should be noted.

Risk Factors

1. Lyme disease mainly affects hikers or those involved in outdoor occupations such as farming and forestry. New England and mid-Atlantic states have a higher incidence of the disease.
2. Certain diseases are seasonal. Lyme disease has a higher incidence in summer and early fall.
3. Determine the proximity of pets and livestock to the patient. Tetanus occurs more frequently from wounds contaminated with soil where horses have resided. Lyme disease may occur in domestic animals with a higher incidence in cats.
4. Crowded living conditions, malnutrition, alcoholism, and drug addiction are associated with TB infection.
5. Certain eating situations pose higher risks for food poisoning. These include the following:
   * Picnics during warm weather with mayonnaise-based salads
   * Eating home-canned vegetables
   * Undercooked pork
   * Egg-based sauces
   * Fish
   * Fried rice
   * Eating ice, unpeeled fruits and vegetables when travelling in another country

6. Bisexual and homosexual men still have the highest rates of HIV infection and their rate of TB and DR-TB is rapidly increasing. Having received a blood transfusion before1985 increases one's risk for HIV.

Life Span Issues
Children

1. Children have fewer pulmonary symptoms with TB. They present with fever, malaise, and weight loss. They have a higher incidence of extrapulmonary TB involving the brain (meningitis), hematologic system (miliary TB), and bones (arthritis).
2. Infants between 1 and 2 months of age are at the highest risk for pertussis and its complications (seizures, encephalopathy, pneumonia). There is a higher rate in females than in males.
3. ARF rarely occurs initially in adults. School-age children are at greatest risk.
4. The older the child when developing ARF, the less likelihood of carditis developing as a complication.
5. Children with HIV infection may present with enlarged lymph glands, low platelet counts, and a history of recurrent otitis media, and/or pneumonia.
6. Hepatitis A and E in children are usually milder and have a shorter course of disease. Fever may be absent. However, hepatitis B, C, and D in infants progresses to chronic liver disease more frequently than in adults.
7. Children from 5 to 14 years of age have the highest incidence of Lyme disease.

Women and pregnancy

1. Most vaccines are contraindicated during pregnancy because they contain live virus/organism. Several communicable diseases during the first trimester result in a high incidence of fetal anomalies and death (e.g., rubella). Amniocentesis counseling may be appropriate.
2. Hepatitis E transmitted by fecal-oral route mainly in developing countries has a high mortality rate in pregnant women.
3. Women with cervical cancer, abnormal pap smears, genital warts, recurrent pelvic inflammatory disease, and vaginal candidiasis have a higher rate of HIV infection.

Adulthood

1. Mumps is more serious in an adult because complications of meningitis and epididymo-orchitis

(infection of the epididymis and testicles) are more common.

Geriatric

1. The geriatric population is at the highest risk of contracting tetanus. They may not be adequately immunized.
2. The geriatric population is at risk of developing TB because most had been exposed to TB early in the century when prevalence was high (reactivation of previously acquired disease). They may have outlived their initial infecting organism and are susceptible again to reinfection. TB may present as a pleural effusion in the geriatric population and initially be misdiagnosed as congestive heart failure.

INITIAL INTERVENTIONS

1. Measure and document the rash using a total body drawing or photograph the rash (with the patient's permission).
2. Initiate intravenous access in anticipation of fluid and medication administration for cases of suspected food poisoning or severe infection.
3. Initiate cardiac monitoring when extra heart sounds are auscultated, and hypotension, hypertension, or tachycardia are present.
4. Initiate pulse oximetry in cases of dysphagia, dyspnea, persistent coughing, and/or sputum production.

PRIORITY NURSING DIAGNOSES

Risk for fluid volume deficit
Risk for ineffective airway clearance
Risk for injury
Risk for decreased cardiac output

◆ **Fluid volume deficit** related to dehydration.
  INTERVENTIONS
  • Initiate IV access and administer crystalloids as ordered.
◆ **Ineffective airway clearance** related to excessive sputum production, inability to control secretions, laryngospasm, or nasopharyngeal edema.
  INTERVENTIONS
  • Insert nasopharyngeal or oral airway as condition indicates.
  • Suction airway.
◆ **Injury** related to infection and seizure activity.

INTERVENTIONS
- Administer antibiotics and anticonvulsant as ordered.
- Anticipate the administration of neuromuscular blocking agents.
- Initiate masking/isolation of patient if patient may be immunocompromised or infectious.

◆ **Decreased cardiac output** related to pericardial effusion or valve disease.
INTERVENTIONS
- Decrease oxygen demands by administering oxygen and minimizing activity.
- Administer diuretics as ordered.
- Anticipate surgical intervention.

PRIORITY DIAGNOSTIC TESTS

Laboratory

Aspartate transaminase (SGOT): This level may be elevated in hepatitis.

Alanine transaminase (SGPT): This level may be elevated in hepatitis.

Anergy Testing: Anergy testing may be initiated in the ED for geriatric and immunocompromised patients. These individuals may have a fading immune response to organisms to which they have been previously exposed. The person may react positively to inoculation with an organism, but the reaction may be so slight as to be misdiagnosed as negative. A battery of "control" antigens that all individuals are exposed to as part of life (e.g., candida) are administered along with the organism of concern (e.g., TB). Reactions to all inoculations are compared with one another to determine severity of reaction and subsequently infection. If the test is negative, a second dose is administered to elicit a booster or recall effect. A positive second test is as significant as an initially positive test. A negative TB test does not rule out TB. Immunocompromised individuals (e.g., HIV) may not be able to mount a reaction.

NURSING ALERT

Occasionally, a patient will want his/her TB test read in the ED. Reactions should be read within 72 hours after administration. Induration (the degree to which the tissue is hard on

palpation), not erythema, is significant. The following parameters should be used:
- 5 mm of induration is positive in (1) person with recent TB exposure, (2) HIV-positive individual, (3) person with chest film indicative of TB lesions
- 10 mm of induration is positive in: (1) high risk groups
- 15 mm of induration is positive in: (1) all groups

Rapid antigen tests: These tests detect cell wall antigen of dead or viable bacteria and viruses by means of latex agglutination or enzyme-linked immunosorbent assay. A positive test indicates current or previous infection.

Antibody tests: These tests can detect exposure to a particular organism if the patient is able to mobilize an immune response to the organism. The development of antibodies against a particular organism is a positive test. Antibody tests are used to detect exposure to hepatitis, *Streptococcus*, mumps, and several other diseases.

Bilirubin: Serum bilirubin levels are elevated in hepatitis.

CD4 count: This is a measurement of the number of helper T lymphocytes in the blood that bear the CD4 surface molecule, which is the cellular receptor for HIV.

CD8 count: This is a measurement of the number of suppressor lymphocytes. Non-HIV-infected persons tend to have more CD4 than CD8 lymphocytes.

Complete blood count (CBC): Leukocytosis may be present with increased lymphocyte count in children with pertussis or measles.

C-reactive protein: This value may be elevated in Lyme disease.

Culture and sensitivity testing: Wounds may be cultured for the presence of spirochetes (Lyme disease) and tetanus. Vesicles may be aspirated after cleansing with povidone-iodine solution and rinsing with alcohol, using a small gauge needle attached to a tuberculin syringe. Sputum cultures may be performed to test for acid-fast bacilli (tuberculosis). Nasopharyngeal cultures may be performed to detect *Streptococcus* and pertussis infection. Stool cultures may be obtained to identify causative organism in cases of suspected food poisoning.

Erythrocyte sedimentation rate: This value may be elevated in Lyme disease.

Monospot: This heterophil agglutination test detects antibodies to Epstein-Barr virus (the usual causal agent for mononucleosis).

Western Blot test: This test is used to confirm the presence of certain antibodies as a follow up to enzyme-linked immunosorbent assay testing. Viral proteins (e.g., HIV) are readily visualized.

Radiographic

Chest film: A chest film may be ordered to detect lesions in tuberculosis. Cardiac enlargement and pericardial effusion may be detected in cases of carditis with ARF.

Extremity films: These may be ordered in cases of skin and soft tissue infection to rule out osteomyelitis or the presence of a foreign body or pathologic fracture.

Radionuclide scans: These may be used to confirm osteomyelitis. Areas of increased radionuclide uptake are positive.

Other

Electrocardiogram: The P-R interval may be prolonged in carditis (associated with ARF) producing a first- or second-degree heart block.

Echocardiogram: An echocardiogram may be obtained to document pericardial effusion and valve disease associated with ARF.

Lumbar puncture with cerebrospinal fluid (CSF) analysis: Certain communicable diseases may result in encephalopathy and meningitis. CSF is examined for antibodies to specific organisms to confirm neurologic complications are related to progression of a specific disease.

COLLABORATIVE INTERVENTIONS

Overview

1. Obtain a wound/rash culture (sometimes a punch biopsy may need to be performed by the physician) before cleansing the wound/rash site.
2. Administer appropriate vaccine to provide active and/or passive immunity. Table 5-1 lists treatment for communicable and infectious diseases. Table 5-3 lists

TABLE 5-3 Vaccine Precautions

Vaccine	Side effects	Dose	Special considerations
Measles, mumps and rubella (MMR)	Rash, low-grade fever seizures, arthritis	0.5 ml SC	Contraindicated in pregnancy, persons allergic to eggs or have a hypersensitivity reaction to neomycin.
Diphtheria, tetanus, pertussis (DTP)	Fever, crying, irritability, seizures	0.5 ml IM	Persons with a known seizure history are at greater risk of experiencing a seizure after administration. 105°F temperature or greater, or persistent crying after previous administration should not receive another dose.
Tetanus toxoid (Td) diphtheria	Local redness and tenderness, headache, malaise	0.5 ml IM or SC	Contraindicated in persons with a known allergy to gamma globulin or thimerosal.
Tuberculin skin test	Local redness at injection site	0.1 ml of 5 tuberculin units of purified protein derivative IC	Induration (degree to which tissue is hard or firm), not erythema, is significant. Test should be read within 72 hours.

VACCINATION PEARLS OF WISDOM

1. Acellular pertussis vaccines have been developed that provide protective immunity with fewer side effects (fever, crying, irritability, seizures, encephalopathy).
2. The combination antigen vaccine DTP (diptheria, tetanus, pertussis) is used for children under 7 years of age, Td (tetatus and diphtheria) is recommended for individuals 7 years of age and older because side effects from pertussis vaccine are more severe in this age group.
3. If a series of immunizations are started but are interrupted, it is **not** necessary to restart the series or to give extra doses.
4. Patients who served in the armed forces since 1941 can be assumed to have received at least one dose of tetanus vaccine.
5. An episode of tetanus does not provide immunity so a complete series of immunizations is indicated.
6. Persons who received measles vaccine from 1957 to 1967 should receive additional vaccination or have a measles antibody titer drawn to confirm immunity.

---

precautions with selective vaccines. The box discusses misperceptions about vaccination to provide a resource for answering patient/parent questions.

Clinical Conditions
Acute rheumatic fever (ARF)
ARF only occurs after an upper respiratory infection of group A streptococci.

SYMPTOMS
- Arthritis and fever usually occur first.
- Cardiac involvement can range from minor dysrhythmias to severe congestive heart failure.
- Mitral and aortic valve disease may be present.
- A nonpruritic pink-red rash with a sharp outer edge (erythema marginatum) may appear on the trunk.
- Chorea (involuntary purposeless movements of the extremities and face) may occur in conjunction with heart problems.

DIAGNOSIS
- Diagnosis is based on the revised Jones' criteria (1).
- The patient must have evidence of a previous group A streptococcal infection, the presence of two major

REVISED JONES' CRITERIA FOR ARF

Major criteria

Carditis
Polyarthritis
Chorea
Erythema marginatum (skin rash)
Subcutaneous nodules

Minor criteria

Arthralgia
Fever
Prolonged P-R interval on ECG
Elevated erythrocyte sedimentation rate
Elevated C-reactive protein

criteria or the presence of one major criteria and two minor criteria (see the box).

TREATMENT

- ARF can be prevented by adequately treating the initial streptococcal infection. Once ARF occurs, it can reappear and secondary prophylaxis is indicated. Recurrences are less likely after puberty.
- Controversy exists over the length of time antibiotics should be administered. Suggestions range from until the individual reaches 18 years of age to lifetime administration.
- Patients with valve disease will require additional antibiotic preparation prior to dental and surgical procedures.
- Intramuscular antibiotic injections may be given monthly or daily oral medication may be used.
- In acute cases of ARF-induced carditis, diuretics and digoxin may be given in the ED.

Acute streptococcal infection

Acute streptococcal infection usually presents as a sore throat.

SYMPTOMS

- The patient may have a high fever, headache, nausea, and vomiting.
- Pharyngeal edema, exudative tonsillitis, and enlarged and tender cervical lymph glands may be present.

- The rash of scarlet fever (red, diffuse macules) may be present.

DIAGNOSIS

- Diagnosis is by a positive throat culture for group A beta-hemolytic *Streptococcus* or by increased serum level of antistreptolysin O or other antibodies to *Streptococcus.*

TREATMENT

- Antibiotic therapy is indicated for at least 10 days to prevent complications from strep infection such as acute rheumatic fever.
- Penicillin or erythromycin is recommended for penicillin-allergic individuals.

Cellulitis/skin and soft tissue infection

SYMPTOMS

- Erythema, tenderness, and hot, red, edematous skin with enlargement of regional lymph nodes are characteristic of cellulitis.
- Blisters may be present.
- In children, facial cellulitis may result from *Haemophilus influenzae* infection.
- The skin becomes dusky and purplish with facial edema.
- Ludwig's angina is a type of cellulitis that results from infection of the second and third lower molar. It is a rare but life-threatening illness characterized by tongue swelling, dysphagia, and drooling.

DIAGNOSIS

- Skin biopsy may be performed but in the ED setting, diagnosis is frequently based on clinical presentation.

TREATMENT

- Antibiotics are initiated.
- Surgical drainage may be used for abscesses.
- Analgesics will be administered before drainage.
- Cultures of drainage should be obtained before starting antibiotic therapy.
- Heat application may facilitate drainage and earlier healing.
- Elevation of the affected part decreases edema and pain.
- Bleeding wounds should be dressed in dry gauze until bleeding stops.
- Wet-to-dry saline dressing can be applied to draining wounds.
- In Ludwig's angina, treatment focuses on airway maintenance, IV antibiotic therapy, pain control, and nutritional support.

C

Diphtheria

Diphtheria is an acute infection of the skin or upper
respiratory tract. It is a rare disease in the United States.
For more information, please refer to a communicable
disease textbook or call the Centers for Disease Control
in Atlanta.

SYMPTOMS

- Diphtheria toxin destroys epithelium. A gray
  pseudomembrane forms over the tonsils and pharynx.
  The toxin may spread to other organs (e.g., lungs, heart,
  kidney) where it damages organ structure and function.

DIAGNOSIS

- Diagnosis is by clinical presentation.

TREATMENT

- Treatment is supportive by artificially maintaining organ
  function until the toxin clears.

Food poisoning

Food poisoning can occur from a variety of organisms (see
Table 5-2 for more information regarding incubation
periods and symptomatology). Food poisoning can be
classified as either gastrointestinal-based or neurologic-
based symptoms. Both kinds of poisoning can be life
threatening.

SYMPTOMS

- Food poisoning with neurologic effects will manifest
  itself by descending paralysis, ataxia, dizziness, pupillary
  changes and ultimately, respiratory compromise (e.g.,
  botulism, ciguatoxin).
- Gastrointestinal effects are nausea, vomiting, watery
  diarrhea, abdominal pain, and fever (e.g., *Staphylococcus*,
  Bacillus, *E. coli*, cholera, *Salmonella*, and trichinosis).

DIAGNOSIS

- Diagnosis is based on clinical and diet history.
- History of other individuals with similar symptoms who
  ate at the same function/restaurant is a significant
  factor.
- Stool cultures may be performed in cases where
  confirmation of organism is needed.

TREATMENT

- Oral glucose/electrolyte solutions may be used in
  patients who are not severely dehydrated.
- Intravenous fluids may be administered.
- Antiemetics and antimotility agents may be ordered.

- Antibiotics may be used if the patient is immunocompromised or toxic.
- Botulinum-trivalent antitoxin must be administered early before toxin confirmation in cases of suspected botulism.
- Endotracheal intubation and mechanical ventilation may be initiated.

Hepatitis

Hepatitis is an acute inflammation of the liver. It may be produced by a virus, chemical or drug reaction, and/or alcohol abuse. Viral hepatitis infection is either transmitted by a fecal-oral route (hepatitis A and E) or by a blood/sexual transmission route (hepatitis B, C, and D). Table 5-1 contrasts the various forms of hepatitis.

SYMPTOMS

- Regardless of the origin, symptoms are similar and include fever, malaise, anorexia, arthralgia, vomiting, diarrhea, right upper quadrant pain, and color changes in the stool (clay), urine (dark), and skin (jaundice).

DIAGNOSIS

- Diagnosis is based on elevation of liver enzymes, antibody testing (except in hepatitis E where no test is available), and liver biopsy.

TREATMENT

Treatment of hepatitis A is supportive, consisting of rest and fluids. Immune globulin is administered to all patient contacts and to the patient. Hepatitis B is experimentally treated with interferon but there is no cure. Hepatitis C is treated with 3 million units of interferon subcutaneously 3 times a week for 24 weeks. Acyclovir may be used. Hepatitis D infection can only occur if the patient has hepatitis B infection, therefore prevention of hepatitis B is the best prevention of hepatitis D. There is no treatment for hepatitis D or E. Fulminant hepatitis is treated with bed rest, low-protein diet, and neomycin or lactulose (orally or rectally as indicated) to decrease blood ammonia levels.

Human immunodeficiency virus

Patients may present to the ED with known HIV infection or with symptoms and unconfirmed disease. The goals of the ED visit should be to improve immune status and to prevent or treat opportunistic infections.

C

T HELPER CELL COUNTS AND OPPORTUNIST INFECTION SUSCEPTIBILITY

- T helper cell count 200-500/mm^3 = TB, Kaposi's sarcoma, thrush, and oral hairy leukoplakia
- T helper cell count 200-250/mm^3 = *Pneumocystis carinii* pneumonia (PCP), toxoplasmosis
- T helper cell count below 50/mm^3 = cytomegalovirus, lymphoma

---

SYMPTOMS
- Weight loss, fever, malaise, oral and skin lesions, visual changes, persistent coughing, and sore throat may be present depending on whether it is an initial HIV infection or opportunist infection with earlier diagnosed HIV infection. Specific discussion of all opportunist infections is beyond the scope of this book.

DIAGNOSIS
- HIV is confirmed by a positive ELISA and Western Blot test.
- Syphilis and TB testing may be performed because the three diseases often occur in tandem.
- WBC and T helper cell counts are predictive of opportunistic infections (see the box). Patients with suspected pneumocystis carinii pneumonia (PCP) who have an oxygen saturation <90% or a PO$_2$ 60 mm Hg usually require hospital admission.

TREATMENT
- Zidovudine is used to treat HIV infection (see Table 5-1) This drug may produce anemia and thrombocytopenia.
- Immunizations may be administered prophylactically.
- If the patient is diagnosed with PCP, steroids and pentamidine may be initiated in the ED.

Lyme disease
Lyme disease occurs from a spirochete that is transmitted by a tick bite. The spirochete may travel by the vascular or lymph system to any organ in the body.

SYMPTOMS
- There are three stages. Early localized infection is characterized by erythema migrans (expanding circular lesion usually occurring at the site of the tick bite).

- In early disseminated infection, patients may have joint and tendon pain.
- They complain of fatigue and malaise.
- Palpitations and fainting may occur because of atrioventricular conduction blocks.
- It may take a year or longer for chronic infection to occur.
- Chronic arthritis may develop.
- Encephalopathy may result in mood changes and memory and sleep disturbances.

DIAGNOSIS

- Testing for Lyme disease is most frequently conducted using antigen tests.
- The spirochete may be cultured from skin lesions.

TREATMENT

- Antibiotics, PO, or IV depending on severity of symptoms are given.
- Penicillin or tetracycline derivatives are prescribed.

Measles

SYMPTOMS

- Dry cough, headache, low-grade fever, sore throat, Koplik's spots, and a nonblanching, diffuse rash are characteristic of measles.
- A hacking cough, conjunctival irritation and photophobia may occur before the appearance of Koplik's spots.
- **Atypical measles** is a form of the disease that strikes individuals who received measles vaccine containing the killed measles virus instead of live attenuated virus. Persons immunized between 1957 and 1967 are at risk for atypical measles.
- Symptoms of atypical measles include high grade fever, edema of the feet and lips, and a rash that begins on the extremities and migrates to the head.

DIAGNOSIS

- Diagnosis is usually based on clinical presentation, exposure, and vaccination history.
- The WBC may be low with lymphocytosis present.

TREATMENT

- Treatment is symptomatic.
- Antipyretics and fluids are given.
- Rest in a darkened room may be suggested if photophobia is present.

- All exposed, susceptible persons such as other members of the household should receive measles vaccine within 72 hours of exposure.

Meningococcal infection

Meningococcal disease is transmitted by nasopharyngeal droplets. In most individuals, disease does not develop from infection. The disease can occur as acute meningitis or as fulminant meningococcemia characterized by disseminated intravascular coagulation (DIC) and septic shock.

SYMPTOMS

- If the organism produces meningitis, symptoms are fever, nuchal rigidity, and decreased LOC.
- Petechiae and purpura are common with both the meningitis and meningococcemia forms.
- The rash produces lesions on the extremities and trunk (Figure 5-1).
- They may be macules before becoming petechiae.
- In sepsis, malaise, hypotension, and pulmonary edema with congestive heart failure may occur.

DIAGNOSIS

- Diagnosis is by clinical presentation and history of viral upper respiratory infection.
- Cultures of blood, lesions, and cerebrospinal fluid will reveal meningococci.

TREATMENT

- Penicillin (300,000 U/kg/day IV) is the treatment of choice.
- Volume replacement and vasopressors may be required.
- Heparin may be used in cases of DIC.

Mononucleosis

Adolescents, college students, and military recruits are most susceptible to this disease. Transmission of the virus is by nasopharyngeal droplets.

SYMPTOMS

- Fever, swollen glands, sore throat, and lethargy are common.
- In some cases, the spleen is enlarged.

DIAGNOSIS

- A positive monospot test confirms the diagnosis.
- Liver enzymes may be elevated.
- Lymphocytosis may be present in the WBC.

TREATMENT
- Supportive treatment with fluids and rest is recommended.
- Contact sports and aspirin products should be avoided for up to 8 weeks to avoid splenic rupture and bleeding.

Mumps parotitis
SYMPTOMS
- The major symptom of mumps is nonsuppurative swelling and tenderness of the salivary glands.
- Fever is often present.

DIAGNOSIS
- Diagnosis is based on clinical presentation and antigen testing.
- A mumps infection confers lifelong immunity.

TREATMENT
- Treatment is supportive since there is no cure.
- Antipyretics and analgesics may be ordered.
- Topical warm or cold compresses may relieve discomfort.
- Males should be placed on bed rest until their temperatures return to normal.

Pertussis
SYMPTOMS
- Pertussis begins with low-grade fever, nasal congestion, and mild cough. After two weeks, the cough worsens.
- In adults, leukocytosis and lymphocytosis may be absent while it is frequently present in children with pertussis.
- Children have a greater incidence of protracted paroxysmal coughing that is worse at night.

DIAGNOSIS
- Diagnosis is confirmed by antipertussis–toxin antibody production.

TREATMENT
- Treatment is supportive using fluids and antipyretics.
- Antibiotics may be ordered to prevent a bacterial respiratory infection and pneumonia.

Rubella (German measles)
Rubella can be difficult to distinguish since it presents similarly to measles and scarlet fever.

SYMPTOMS
- Low-grade fever, sore throat, and a pink papular rash on the face and neck that spreads to the trunk and extremities are characteristic.

- Postauricular and suboccipital lymph nodes are enlarged and usually tender.
- The WBC is normal.

DIAGNOSIS

- Diagnosis is by rubella antibody assay tests.

TREATMENT

- Antipyretics and antipruritic medications may be ordered.

Tetanus

Tetanus is caused by a spore-forming rod found in contaminated soil. It most commonly follows an acute injury, but it can also infect chronic wounds (e.g., decubiti, skin abcesses). The spores can live in the body for months or years, producing disease at a time removed from initial injury.

SYMPTOMS

- Tetanus produces rigidity and spasms of skeletal muscle.
- The toxin spreads by way of the circulation.
- Nerves with the shortest axons are affected first.
- Symptoms begin in the facial muscles and jaw, progressing to the neck and trunk.
- Dyspnea and dysphagia are common.
- If the spasms are controlled by medication, overactivity of the sympathetic nervous system may result in dysrhythmias, tachycardia, peripheral vasoconstriction, and cardiac arrest.
- Urinary retention may occur.

DIAGNOSIS

- Diagnosis is usually based upon clinical presentation.

TREATMENT

- Rapid deterioration is expected; therefore, the patient is intubated and given neuromuscular blocking agents (e.g., pancuronium).
- To prevent further absorption of the toxin, tetanus immune globulin is administered.
- Wound/s should be debrided and antibiotics may be initiated.
- Patients will require immunization because the amount of toxin causing the disease is inadequate to confer immunity.

Tuberculosis

SYMPTOMS

- In persons <60 years of age, nightsweats, anorexia, and weight loss are the predominant symptoms.

- In those individuals 60 years and older, cough, sputum production, and weight loss are frequent symptoms.
- It is possible to have active disease without symptoms.

DIAGNOSIS

- Diagnosis is usually based upon a positive tuberculin skin test and lesions denoted on chest film.
- However, in immunocompromised individuals, diagnosis may be based on clinical presentation.

TREATMENT

- Isoniazid and rifampin are initially used to treat TB. For DR-TB, several drugs may need to be administered simultaneously.
- Generally, isoniazid, rifampin, pyrazinamide, and ethambutol or streptomycin are given (see Table 5-1).
- Steroids may be used in severe cases.
- Baseline liver function should be assessed before starting any TB medication because of their side effects.
- Visual acuity must be examined before and during ethambutol therapy.
- Because it is difficult to measure visual acuity in children, ethambutol is not recommended for pediatric use.

Varicella (chickenpox)

SYMPTOMS

- The rash associated with chickenpox is extremely pruritic and ranges from macules to papules to vesicles to crusted lesions simultaneously.
- A low-grade fever may be present.
- Reactivation of the varicella virus may occur in the form of herpes zoster (shingles).
- Vesicles are gray in appearance and are located along a dermatome (nerve fiber).

DIAGNOSIS

- Diagnosis is usually by clinical presentation although antibody testing may be done.

TREATMENT

- In immunocompromised individuals, varicella immunoglobulin can be administered within 96 hours of exposure to prevent or modify illness.
- The immunoglobulin will protect the person for 3 weeks.
- Analgesics, antihistamines and steroids may be given to provide relief from symptoms.

NURSING ALERT

Remember to warn patients/parents not to use aspirin or aspirin products if the patient is <21 years of age because of the association between Reye's syndrome and aspirin use.

NURSING SURVEILLANCE

1. Monitor cardiac pattern and treat potentially lethal dysrhythmias (e.g., second- and third-degree heart block may occur in ARF).
2. Trend temperature. Elevated temperature may further dehydrate a patient with fluid volume deficit.
3. Monitor urine output and color to assess core perfusion and liver dysfunction.
4. Trend oxygen saturation. Desaturation may occur in a patient who is not responding to drug therapy or requires artificial ventilation resulting from respiratory paralysis or spasm.
5. Monitor level of consciousness.

EXPECTED PATIENT OUTCOMES

1. Fever decreases or is absent.
2. Airway remains patent.
3. Breathing pattern is adequate (whether maintained by patient or artificially) as evidenced by oxygen > 94% and arterial blood gases normal for condition.

DISCHARGE IMPLICATIONS

Discharge instructions should be based on clinical diagnosis of patient. Refer to Table 5-1 for specific information regarding transmission routes, incubation periods, and complications associated with diseases. Some diseases require greater detail in discharge instruction and are discussed below.

1. *ARF:* Patients should be examined daily for the first weeks of the disease in order to detect carditis early prior to valve damage. The seriousness of this disease and the need for long term antibiotic therapy must be explained to the patient.
2. *Hepatitis:* Patients discharged with hepatitis should be instructed to rest and to anticipate low energy levels for up to 6 months. Alcoholic beverages should be avoided

for 6 to 12 months. Instruct the patient that immunity to one type of hepatitis does not confer immunity to another type of hepatitis.

3. *HIV:* If HIV testing has been performed (with written informed consent of the patient), certain counseling must be provided. Patients must be informed about the medical significance of the test (whether the test is negative or positive); test limitations; how HIV is spread; availability of medical and psychosocial care; and social consequences of testing (6). HIV-infected individuals should be referred to support groups and instructed on prevention of disease transmission to others.

4. *Lyme disease:* Patients should be instructed to wear light colored clothes, long sleeves and pants with wrist and ankle bands before entering tick-infested areas. Insect repellant may be used.

5. *Skin conditions:* Encourage all family members to wash with antibacterial soap and not to share razors or towels and washcloths.

6. *Tuberculosis:* Patients should be taught to report early signs of hepatitis because of the toxic liver effects of TB medications. Anorexia, nausea, weakness, jaundice, clay-colored stools, and dark urine should be reported quickly to their primary health care provider.

NURSING ALERT

Both ED and prehospital personnel should receive tuberculin skin testing every 3 to 6 months because of their high potential for exposure. Personnel should wear respiratory protection when suctioning high-risk individuals. Personnel should have a TB skin test immediately after known exposure.
Hepatitis B testing is recommended yearly to determine antibody level for personnel repeatedly exposed to blood. A booster vaccine should be administered if antibody levels fall below 10 (7).

References

1. American Heart Association: special writing group of the committee on rheumatic fever, endocarditis, and Kawasaki disease of the council on cardiovascular disease in the young: Guidelines for the diagnosis of rheumatic fever, *JAMA* 268:2069-2073, 1992.

2. Center for Disease Control: Resurgence of pertussis-United States, MMWR 42:952-960, 1993.
3. Dutt A and Stead W: Tuberculosis in the elderly, *Med Clin North Am,* 77:1353-1368, 1993.
4. Elpern E and Girzadas A: Tuberculosis update: new challenges of an old disease, *Medsurg Nurs,* 2:176-183, 1992.
5. Franckhauser M: Tuberculosis in the 1990s, *Nurse Pract Forum* 4:30-36, 1993.
6. Gold J: HIV-1 infection, *Med Clin North Am* 76:1-18, 1992.
7. Schiff E: Viral hepatitis today, *Emerg Med* 24:115-116, 119, 122-124, 126, 129-130, 132, 1992.

C

Chapter VI

Ear, Nose, Throat, and Facial/Dental Conditions

Mark Parshall

E

CLINICAL CONDITIONS

Epiglottitis
Croup (LTB—Laryngotracheobronchitis)
Le Fort II and III Fractures
Airway Foreign Bodies
Ludwig's Angina
Parapharyngeal Abscess and Peritonsillar Abscess
Epistaxis (Bleeding)
Facial Fractures (Altered Structural Integrity)
Mandibular Fractures
Dental Avulsions
Auricular and Nasal Septal Hematomas
Nasal Fractures
Facial Lacerations
Ménière's Disease and Acute Labyrinthitis (Vestibular Dysfunction)
Esophageal Foreign Body (Nonairway Foreign Bodies)
Nasal and Ear Foreign Bodies
Otitis Media (Infection)
Sinusitis
Otitis Externa
Odontalgia
Acute Necrotizing Ulcerative Gingivitis (ANUG)
Cerumen Impaction (Diminshed Auditory Acuity)

TRIAGE ASSESSMENT

Dental, facial, and ear, nose, and throat (ENT) emergencies range from life threatening to relatively minor. Emergent priority is given to upper airway injury or obstruction (as a result of bleeding, swelling, infection, burns, or foreign bodies), uncontrolled bleeding or hemodynamic instability, and to mixed presentations involving alterations in consciousness. In less emergent situations, attention is directed toward preservation or restoration of structural and functional integrity, pain reduction, and addressing adverse responses to actual or potential disfigurement.

> **NURSING ALERT**
>
> - Any patient presenting with airway symptoms, or a high energy injury to the face or neck with significant facial or neck swelling should be triaged directly to a resuscitation area.
> - Patients with high impact blunt or penetrating injuries above the level of the clavicles require emergent initiation of spinal precautions.

Airway and Breathing
Impaired ability to speak or swallow
Cardinal signs of acute airway compromise include impaired ability to speak or swallow, stridor, crowing, retractions, cyanosis, and, generally, obvious distress. Not all of these signs will be present in every instance.

Lethargy
A child who looks acutely ill but is lethargic, "too quiet," or apathetic should be triaged for emergent examination.

Position
If the patient assumes a "tripod" position, or is deliberately quiet in an effort to optimize air movement, suspect epiglottitis (17,18).

Dysphagia, drooling, dysphonia, and distress
Classic signs of epiglottitis have been termed the four D's—dysphagia, drooling, dysphonia (muffled voice), and distress (18). Drooling is not always present. Genuine difficulty swallowing (dysphagia) is accorded a higher triage priority than pain with swallowing (odynophagia) (12). The complaint of "difficulty swallowing" is often used by patients to describe painful swallowing.

Muffled speech, tongue protrusion, trismus, or torticollis
Cellulitis of the floor of the mouth, or soft tissues of the neck, or pharyngeal wall abscess should be triaged as a potential airway emergency if associated with muffled speech, tongue protrusion, trismus, or torticollis.

Mechanism of injury

High-energy blunt facial or soft-tissue neck injuries that are high risk for airway compromise or cervical spine injury include vehicular collisions (especially if unrestrained), motorcycle ejection, "clothesline" injuries, and being struck in the face or neck with a bat or truncheon.

Breathing patterns

Abnormalities in rate, depth, or symmetry of breathing related to facial, oral, or pharyngeal conditons, or high-energy mechanism of injury generally reflect incomplete airway obstruction. An altered breathing pattern when the airway is clear may be a sign of concomitant CNS problem (e.g., head injury or spinal cord injury).

Bleeding
Epistaxis

Bleeding from epistaxis, or facial or scalp wounds may be profuse. Although in most cases bleeding can be readily controlled with direct pressure, the patient's ability to understand and cooperate may be compromised by emotional distress, alcohol, or drugs.

Tachycardia, narrowed pulse pressure

Although epistaxis is relatively common in patients with hypertension, at triage the blood pressure is rarely so elevated as to have actually caused the bleeding episode (26). It is more common at triage to find the patient's vital signs consistent with mild or moderate blood loss (e.g., tachycardia and initially, a narrowed pulse pressure).

Syncope

The patient may respond to the sight of blood or presence of pain with a vasovagal syncopal episode. Accordingly, triage judgment with respect to bleeding involves more than vital signs and estimation of blood loss.

Other Triage Considerations
Symptom description

Information related to the rapidity of symptom onset, associated symptoms or complaints; medications, allergies, and tetanus status should be obtained in triage, or at the earliest possible juncture.

Ice

Ice should be applied to areas of traumatic facial swelling while the patient is waiting to be seen.

Domestic violence

Victims of domestic violence often present with facial injuries, and may need to be triaged as emergent for their safety, and to initiate crisis intervention, even when there is no threat to the airway or hemodynamic status.

Corrosive ingestions

Corrosive ingestions (e.g., battery acid or lye) require immediate triage to a resuscitation area (see Chapter 20).

Avulsed teeth

Avulsed teeth are accorded a higher triage priority than most other dental complaints (e.g., odontalgia) because of the limited window for replantation (see Collaborative Interventions) (13,14,23).

FOCUSED NURSING ASSESSMENT

Risk Factors
Injury

1. Soft tissue facial trauma is most commonly related to falls. Facial fractures are most commonly related to vehicular collisions and interpersonal violence (7).
2. Midfacial fractures (e.g., orbital blowout and Le Fort II and III fractures) increase the risk of permanent eye injury (9).
3. Facial trauma resulting from interpersonal violence is often associated with alcohol or drugs, and possible ongoing belligerence (7). It may be necessary to triage a patient to a secure area and have security personnel immediately at hand even in cases where the injuries themselves may not be emergent.

Life Span Issues
Infants and children

1. In children, airway structures are less rigid than in adults, and hence more likely to be compromised by swelling, infection, or trauma.
2. Infants below 3 months of age are obligate nose breathers, so even nasal congestion can lead to significant respiratory embarassment in this age group. Nasal flaring in infants is often a sign of significant respiratory compromise or distress.
3. Retractions in any age group are a potentially serious sign; in children, supraclavicular retractions are usually most indicative of severe effort.

4. Epiglottitis can occur in any age group, but is most prevalent in children between 3 to 6 years of age (12,17, 18,26).

5. Croup is most common from 3 months to 3 years of age (12,26).

6. The possibility of foreign body aspiration should be considered in a child with sudden onset of wheezing or stridor and retractions, or a child with chronic wheezing unrelieved by aerosolized bronchodilators.

7. Falls are the most common cause of facial injuries in children (7). The nurse should be alert to injuries that appear inconsistent with the mechanism reported or allegedly resulting from activities beyond the developmental abilities of the child.

8. Midfacial fractures are relatively uncommon in school-age and younger children. When present they suggest a high-energy mechanism of injury with an increased risk of intracranial injury.

9. Nasal foreign bodies occur most commonly in childhood, especially in toddlers. Foreign bodies of the ear are also common in childhood, but also are found in individuals of any age, often related to using various small objects to "clean" the ear canals.

Adults

1. In young adults, the most common cause of facial fractures is interpersonal violence. In males this tends to arise from altercations with strangers in settings where alcohol has been ingested. In females, assailants are more frequently known to the victim—often domestic partners (7).

2. Initial onset of Ménière's disease generally occurs between 30 and 50 years of age.

Geriatric

1. The most common cause of facial and head injuries in the geriatric population is falls (7). The nurse must be alert to an alleged mechanism of injury inconsistent with the injuries seen.

2. It is important in geriatric patients who have sustained falls to determine if there was a loss of consciousness either before or after the fall. Of particular concern is a history of several falls or increasing confusion over a span of several weeks, as this could indicate a subacute or chronic subdural hematoma.

3. Older adults are also more prone to posterior epistaxis (10,24) and profuse bleeding from facial and scalp wounds.
4. Ludwig's angina, a severe cellulitis of the oral cavity is most common in the geriatric patient with some degree of immune compromise (23).

INITIAL INTERVENTIONS

1. A patient with actual or potential airway compromise should be triaged directly to a treatment area where suction and intubation equipment are immediately at hand.
2. Cardiac and continuous pulse oximetry monitoring should be initiated if signs of airway compromise are present. (Epiglottitis in children may be an exception—see under Collaborative Interventions.)
3. Elevate the head of the bed when possible to facilitate air movement.
4. Bleeding should be controlled with direct pressure.
5. Large bore IV access should be established if the patient is hemodynamically unstable.
6. A patient with epistaxis should be triaged to an examination chair unless hypotensive or syncopal.

PRIORITY NURSING DIAGNOSES*

Risk for ineffective airway clearance
Risk for aspiration
Risk for cervical spine injury
Risk for impaired gas exchange
Risk for fluid volume deficit
Risk for brain injury
Risk for pain
Risk for sensory-perceptual alteration: auditory, visual, or proprioceptive
Risk for impaired skin or mucous membrane integrity
Risk for infection
Risk for body image disturbance
♦ **Ineffective airway clearance** related to trauma, swelling, infection, bleeding, or FB.

---

*Because of the heterogeneous nature of clinical conditions, nursing diagnoses in this chapter are stated in terms of related factors or risk factors. Interventions are discussed under Clinical Conditions.

E

◆ **Aspiration**
  RISK FACTORS
  - Positioning (e.g., spinal precautions)
  - Diminished level of responsiveness
  - Traumatic ileus
  - Nasal foreign body

◆ **Cervical spine injury**
  RISK FACTORS
  - High-energy blunt or penetrating mechanism of injury
  - Vehicular ejection
  - Injury above clavicles
  - "Clothesline" injury

◆ **Impaired gas exchange**
  RISK FACTORS
  - Upper airway swelling related to infection or trauma
  - Foreign body aspiration
  - Posterior nasal packing (8,10,24,26)

◆ **Fluid volume deficit** related to bleeding, vomiting, or impaired swallowing.

◆ **Brain injury**
  RISK FACTORS
  - High-energy blunt or penetrating mechanism of injury above clavicles
  - Known or suspected period of airway compromise/ hypoxia
  - Orbital cellulitis or severe sinusitis

◆ **Pain** related to trauma, infection, or inflammation.

◆ **Sensory-perceptual alteration: auditory, visual, or proprioceptive** related to trauma, infection, or vestibular dysfunction.

◆ **Impaired skin or mucous membrane integrity** related to trauma.

◆ **Infection**
  RISK FACTORS
  - Foreign body of ear or nose
  - Open facial fractures
  - Odontalgia or dental abscess
  - Open mandibular fractures
  - Nasal septal or auricular hematoma

◆ **Body image disturbance**
  RISK FACTORS
  - Facial trauma
  - Preoccupation with cosmetic consequences of injury

PRIORITY DIAGNOSTIC TESTS

Laboratory

Arterial blood gas: Useful in cases of partial airway obstruction or trauma. Avoid in suspected pediatric epiglottitis (see under Collaborative Interventions).

Blood studies as indicated or by trauma protocol: CBC, ethanol, chemistry panel, blood bank (type and screen or crossmatch and coagulation studies).[*]

Cultures: Blood cultures in orbital or pharyngeal cellulitis, or peritonsillar abscess; pharyngeal culture. Rapid strep cultures (i.e., 24 hours) have a lower false negative rate than latex agglutination (strep antibody) screens. (Never swab throat if epiglottitis is suspected.)

Radiographic

Plain radiographs: Cervical spine series (according to mechanism of injury and trauma protocols); lateral soft-tissue neck (foreign bodies and often in epiglottitis); facial films (choice of views depends on what needs to be visualized and whether or not the cervical spine has been cleared); chest x-ray; KUB; soft-tissue neck; or "babygram" (e.g., to localize a radiopaque foreign body).

CT scans: Useful in cases of facial injuries in multiple trauma or head injury; penetrating trauma/impalements; or orbital cellulitis or severe sinusitis.

Panorex:[†] For mandible injuries, multiple dental avulsions, and periodontal abscess.

Barium (Ba) swallow: For esophageal foreign body, particularly if due to food.[‡]

Other

Fiberoptic endoscopic procedures (laryngoscopy, bronchoscopy, esophagoscopy): Diagnostic as well as definitive treatment for foreign bodies.

---

[*]In posterior epistaxis, a baseline CBC, PT and PTT, and type and screen are often ordered in the ED. They are rarely necessary in anterior epistaxis.
[†]A patient must be able to sit up in a special chair for a Panorex. If the patient cannot tolerate sitting up, or the cervical spine has not been cleared, other studies, such as an AP face, reverse Waters' view and plain mandible films may be ordered.
[‡]Alternatively, a cotton pledget soaked in contrast may be swallowed (12).

Continuous pulse oximetry: Useful in cases of suspected airway compromise and to monitor response to oxygen therapy. A patient may have a "normal" SpO_2 and still require oxygen (e.g., if hemoglobin is low), therefore SpO_2 is more useful for trending; it should not be the sole criterion on which a decision to initiate oxygen therapy is made.

COLLABORATIVE INTERVENTIONS

Overview

Collaborative interventions are grouped by human response patterns to acute alterations in structure and function (e.g., risk of airway compromise or bleeding).

Clinical Conditions
Epiglottitis (supraglottitis)

Risk for airway compromise.

SYMPTOMS

- Epiglottitis is bacterial (usually Haemophilus influenzae) and is characterized by rapid onset of high fever (>39° C) and a toxic appearance.
- In addition to the classic signs previously discussed (see Triage), open-mouth breathing with tongue protrusion, a "sniffing" position, or a tripod position may be seen (12).
- Cyanosis or pallor may be present (17,18).
- Epiglottitis in adults may have a more indolent onset and may not be characterized by high fever.
- Often the chief complaint is of the worst sore throat of the patient's life (12).

DIAGNOSIS

- In children, epiglottitis is diagnosed primarily by clinical presentation and rapidity of onset.
- Lateral soft-tissue neck films may be helpful in ambiguous presentations, but are not always necessary.
- If a child is sent to x-ray, a parent should be allowed to remain with the child, a crash cart should be immediately available, and the child should be attended by an emergency nurse or physician.
- In adults, indirect laryngoscopy (e.g., with a mirror) can be performed (26) and lateral soft-tissue neck films may be more helpful.

TREATMENT
- *Children:* The child and parent should be triaged immediately to a resuscitation area, and the child should be allowed to remain in whatever position facilitates breathing (18).
- As soon as epiglottitis is suspected, the child should be continuously observed by an emergency nurse or physician (18).
- The child will not tolerate lying down and should not be made to do so (18,26).
- Because of the child's tenuous airway, the nurse should avoid, and protect the child from any intrusive procedures.
- Blow-by oxygen and a cardiac monitor may be used if the child will tolerate without increased distress, but no attempt should be made to secure a mask or nasal cannula to the child's face (17).
- Usually the airway will be secured under direct visualization by an otolaryngologist or anesthesiologist in the operating room, in case emergent tracheostomy is required (12,18,26).
- In crash situations in the field or ED, a cricothyrotomy may be necessary (18,26).
- Once the airway has been secured, attention can then be directed toward obtaining laboratory studies, initiating IV fluids, and administering antibiotics—usually a second- or third-generation cephalosporin or ampicillin/sulbactam (Unasyn) (21).
- *Adults:* Adults with epiglottitis are often treated with high-dose steroids in addition to antibiotics (12). Adults are less likely than children to need emergent intubation; development of stridor is a strong predictor of the need for intubation or tracheostomy in the adult (11).

Croup (laryngotracheobronchitis [LTB])
SYMPTOMS
- Croup can also be a cause of severe airway compromise.
- The child will have frequent paroxysms of the characteristic barking cough, inspiratory stridor, and retractions.
- Fever is often present, but usually not as high as what is seen in epiglottitis.
- Often, the symptoms are worse at night, and the parents frequently report that the child sounded worse at home

than on arrival in the ED (because of the soothing effect of cooler, moister air outside).

- Depending on the degree of distress, it is acceptable to attempt to measure vital signs and oxygen saturation in triage.
- In severe distress, triage is immediate. In older children, the coughing may be intermittent with relatively normal breathing in between.
- Depending on department volume and waiting times, it may be prudent to categorize even milder cases as emergent.

DIAGNOSIS

- Diagnosis of croup is based on clinical presentation and progression of symptoms.
- The cough is pathognomonic.
- In contrast to epiglottitis, the typical history is a respiratory infection of more insidious onset, often several days, which has degenerated.

TREATMENT

- Triage acuity and the rapidity with which treatment is instituted depend on the vital signs and degree of respiratory distress.
- If triage is immediate, oxygen should be started by whatever means the child will tolerate (e.g., blow-by) while vital signs are being taken.
- Continuous oxygen saturation monitoring should be initiated.
- Treatment is with cool mist and, in more severe cases, aerosolized racemic epinephrine.
- Patients who require racemic epinephrine generally will need to be admitted or, at least, placed on holding or observation status for several hours.
- Antibiotics are generally reserved for cases serious enough to warrant admission and are not a mainstay of emergent treatment.

Le Fort II and III fractures

SYMPTOMS

- Major midface fractures should be considered based on mechanism of injury.
- Le Fort II and III fractures are high-energy injuries from direct blows to the midface.
- They generally present with nasal and pharyngeal bleeding and massive swelling and ecchymosis around the eyes, nose maxilla, and upper oral cavity.

- Abnormal approximation of the teeth is common.
- The patient may be obtunded because of concomitant head injury.
- CSF rhinorrhea may be present, but may be obscured by bleeding.
- A "halo" test on a piece of filter paper is helpful.
- Le Fort I fractures are less serious, but loose or avulsed teeth may still represent an airway hazard.

Diagnosis
- The face may look elongated in a Le Fort II or III.
- Instability of the facial architecture is present.
- Definitive diagnosis is radiographic.
- A CT scan is usually necessary.
- The fractures are often complex, and may be mixed (e.g., a Le Fort II pattern on one side with a III pattern on the other).
- A Le Fort III fracture is a craniofacial separation. The fracture extends across the upper maxilla and nasal bones through the orbit and zygoma.
- A Le Fort II fracture is pyramidal and involves the maxilla, nasal bones, palate, and inferior or medial orbit.
- A Le Fort I is a linear maxillary alveolar fracture.

Treatment
- Le Fort fractures require surgical repair, but often on a delayed basis.
- From a nursing standpoint the anatomic distinctions are less important than the recognition of a high-impact injury that may communicate with intracranial structures.
- Based on mechanism of injury, the patient initially will require spinal precautions that increase the risk of aspiration.
- Yankauer or larger bore suction should be immediately at hand, and the patient may require intubation.
- Prophylactic intravenous antibiotics may be ordered.
- If a CSF leak is present, the patient will require neurosurgical consultation.

Airway foreign bodies
Symptoms
- Acute foreign body aspiration generally presents as moderate-to-severe distress with stridor, wheezing, or impaired phonation.

- Breath sounds may be diminished unilaterally or diffusely.
- An occult foreign body (e.g., one that was aspirated at some previous time and not recognized) may present with signs and symptoms of chronic cough, unequal breath sounds, and localized wheezing on forced expiration (27).

DIAGNOSIS

- Foreign bodies of the airway may be diagnosed by means of a history of sudden onset of distress, by radiograph (lateral neck or chest x-ray), fiberoptic laryngoscopy or bronchoscopy.
- Occult foreign body may be suspected in an individual who has suffered recurrent bouts of pneumonia (27).

TREATMENT

- Patients should be triaged to a resuscitation area and allowed to remain in whatever position breathing is most comfortable and least fatiguing—usually sitting up.
- A baseline O_2 saturation should be checked and high-flow cool mist oxygen per mask or blow-by should be initiated.
- The most common foreign body in adults is a food bolus.
- In children, small toys, buttons, coins, and nuts are common.
- Removal is generally performed with a fiberoptic laryngoscope and forceps, or via bronchoscopy.

Ludwig's angina

SYMPTOMS

- Ludwig's angina is a diffuse cellulitis of the sublingual, submental, and submandibular tissues characterized by high fever, tense, brawny edema of the submandibular area, and tongue protrusion (23).
- It can cause airway compromise and can extend to the mediastinum resulting in mediastinitis.

DIAGNOSIS

- This condition is usually seen in older adults, often with some degree of immune compromise (23).
- Diagnosis is based on the location and appearance of cellulitis.
- A CBC and blood cultures are generally ordered as a baseline septic workup.

- A lateral soft-tissue neck and chest x-ray may also be needed.

TREATMENT

- Involves admission and intravenous antibiotics, usually high-dose penicillin G and cefoxitin or metronidazole (21).
- Ampicillin/sulbactam or ticarcillin/clavulanate may also be used (21).

Parapharyngeal abscess and peritonsillar abscess

SYMPTOMS

- Both of these conditions cause severe retropharyngeal pain and dysphagia.
- Both are unilateral and cause uvular displacement and muffled ("hot potato") voice.
- Trismus may be present (12).
- A parapharyngeal abscess, however, also involves the lateral pharyngeal wall and often presents with torticollis (12).

DIAGNOSIS

- Diagnosis is by clinical symptoms.
- A peritonsillar abscess is more localized.
- The patient is usually symptomatic for 48 hours before the abscess becomes apparent (26).
- A parapharyngeal abscess usually extends down into the tissue planes of the neck and is the more serious, though less common, of the two.
- CT scans may be necessary to confirm the diagnosis (26).
- A baseline septic work-up may be ordered.

TREATMENT

- Patients with parapharyngeal abscess are admitted on high-dose antibiotic therapy.
- Peritonsillar abscesses are generally aspirated, or incised and drained in the ED; on occasion the patient may be discharged from the ED, but often will be admitted for a short stay and IV antibiotics.

Epistaxis (bleeding)

SYMPTOMS

- Active epistaxis is obvious. Even in cases where the patient appears to be bleeding from both nares, epistaxis is almost always unilateral.
- It is helpful in triage to have the patient identify on which side bleeding was first evident and whether the

direction in which bleeding was first noted was from the naris or in the pharynx (10,24).

- Unless syncopal, the patient should be triaged to an ENT examination room.

DIAGNOSIS

- The basic diagnostic question in epistaxis is the location of bleeding.
- The vast majority of epistaxis is anterior, most commonly from the mucosa of the anterior (cartilaginous) nasal septum (known as Kiesselbach's area or Little's area) (8,16).
- Identification of an anterior bleeding site is diagnostic. Anterior bleeds rarely require hematology and coagulation studies unless the patient is anticoagulated or uremic (26).
- Posterior epistaxis is more profuse and more difficult to control.
- Epistaxis unresponsive to pressure over Little's area is suspicious as is bleeding around or behind a preexisting anterior nasal pack.

TREATMENT

- Anterior epistaxis. The patient should sit upright, and apply firm, continuous bilateral pressure between thumb and forefinger to the septal cartilage just above the alae for about 10 minutes.
- Often it is helpful for the nurse to apply the pressure initially so the patient can aquire the "feel" for the location and amount of pressure.
- If the patient is unable to maintain the pressure, it should be maintained by the nurse.
- The patient should be supplied with a basin or suction for oral secretions, but should be instructed not to expectorate forcefully or blow the nose until immediately before the nasal examination.
- Typical supplies for a nasal examination include a head lamp, nasal speculum, bayonet forceps, a Frazier suction tip, silver nitrate applicators, and bacitracin ointment.
- Cocaine, diluted to a 4% or 5% solution is commonly used as a topical anesthetic and vasoconstrictor.
- Alternatively, a mixture of tetracaine (Pontocaine) or 4% lidocaine with phenylephrine or epinephrine can be used (10,24,26).

- At the beginning of the examination, the patient is instructed to blow out any clots from nares and suction with a Frazier tip should be immediately available.
- Anesthetic-moistened cotton pledgets are placed in the nasal vestibule by the physician using the bayonet forceps and should be left in place for 5 to 10 minutes after which any localized bleeding sources can be cauterized (10,24).
- Silver nitrate cautery is preferred over electrocautery as it is less likely to damage the septum (24).
- Once hemostasis has been achieved, an anterior pack with a long ribbon of vaseline gauze, or a cellulose (Merocel) tampon or Oxycel can be placed (8,10,24, 26).
- Vaseline or Merocel packing should be removed in 1 to 2 days in the ED or by the patient's private physician.
- Oxycel does not have to be removed; it dessicates and can be blown out in a few days.
- Patients should be counselled to avoid drinking beverages that are either very hot or very cold.
- They should also avoid aspirin and nonsteroidal antiinflammatory drugs for at least several days.
- Patients should be instructed not to lift heavy objects or engage in straining while a pack is in place.
- They may be more comfortable at home resting in an orthopneic position, e.g., with enough pillows to elevate the head and upper torso to the equivalent of a semi-fowler's position.

Posterior epistaxis

If an anterior site cannot be identified, or if bleeding continues in spite of packing, or returns after an anterior pack is in place, a posterior bleed is suspected (10,24). Posterior bleeds are usually from a branch of the ethmoid artery and can be profuse or intermittent (10). Generally a posterior bleed requires ENT consultation. If a posterior pack is placed, the patient should be admitted. Geriatric patients or those with COPD may require ICU admission because of a risk of hypoxemia or hypercapnia with a posterior pack in place (24,26). Ultimately, the patient may require surgical ligation. The most common means of tamponading a posterior bleed is a double balloon catheter (Naso-Stat or Epi-Stat) (8,10,24). The proximal balloon fills up the nasal cavity and the distal balloon is inflated in the nasopharynx to block retrograde bleeding and keep the larger, nasal balloon in place. The balloons may be inflated with sterile water or normal saline. A combination of vaseline gauze or Oxycel anterior packing may be utilized in conjunction with balloon tamponade (8).

Posterior gauze packs are rarely used any more as they are extremely uncomfortable, however, they are occasionally needed if balloon tamponade is ineffective. A posterior gauze pack consists of a wad of tightly folded gauze sponges that are firmly tied together by a minimum of three ties that are at least 6 inches long. A Robinson catheter is passed through to the nasopharynx and brought out through the mouth. Two of the ties are tied through the eyelet of the catheter and the third is taped to the cheek. The catheter is pulled back out the nose and traction is applied to the two ties until the pack lodges firmly in the nasopharynx. The two nasal ties are taped to the outside of the nose or the cheek. Systemic analgesics are usually needed for pain; some physicians may order a sedative as well. Patients on occasion will have a vasovagal episode resulting from the pain and stimulation of the pack.

Facial fractures (altered structural integrity)

The treatment of facial bone fractures varies with the location and the amount of bony displacement. Nasal and mandibular fractures are the most common. Ice should be applied acutely to any areas of facial swelling as soon as the patient has been triaged. Because most of the facial bones are nonmobile and it is difficult to assess the degree of deformity while acute swelling is present, many patients with facial fractures may be discharged with instructions to follow up with a plastic surgeon or ENT specialist after the swelling has gone down. Surgical intervention, if indicated, is often elective.

Mandibular fractures

SYMPTOMS

- Classic signs of mandibular fracture are malocclusion and inability to open the mouth completely.
- Forcible displacement of two or more adjacent lower teeth toward the tongue is another sign of probable mandibular fracture (23).

DIAGNOSIS
- Because of its shape, the mandible is frequently fractured in more than one location, hence the desirability of a Panorex film as this shows the entire mandible in the same plane (4,23).
- The most common fracture sites are the mandibular angle, body, and symphysis (4,23).
- If clinical signs of mandibular fracture are evident, it should be assumed that any intraoral laceration in the mandibular region is an open fracture (23).

TREATMENT
- Patients with mandibular fractures frequently need suction to help with removal of blood and oral secretions that can be especially problematic if spinal precautions are in place.
- Oftentimes, the patient or a family member can be given a Yankauer suction and shown how to use it; if the patient is too obtunded or uncooperative, the nurse should anticipate frequent suctioning.
- Recent literature suggests that open reduction and internal fixation is gaining favor over intermaxillary fixation (4).

Dental avulsions

SYMPTOMS
- A completely avulsed tooth is generally obvious.
- Often, intraoral bleeding or a bloody socket is present.
- A luxation is a displacement of a tooth.

DIAGNOSIS
- A luxation can be identified by manual examination.
- In complete avulsion, the tooth may be replantable, particularly if replantation occurs within 2 hours of injury.
- The best salvage rate for replantation occurs when extraoral time is <30 minutes (13,14). Therefore, it is important to establish the time of injury, and how the tooth has been handled.

TREATMENT
- While awaiting replantation, or en route to the hospital, it is best to keep the tooth in a container with milk or saline as a transport medium.
- Plain water should not be used because of its hypotonicity (13,14).

- Alternatively, the tooth may be carried by the patient in the sublingual or buccal sulcus, but only if the patient is alert and a suitable transport medium is unavailable (13). (Saliva is hypotonic and highly contaminated with bacteria.) There are commercially available tooth preservation sets that use Hank's solution, a buffered solution that contains glucose, Mg^{++}, and Ca^{++} in a small jar with a basket inside for holding the tooth (14).
- The root of the tooth should not be handled. Before replantation, the root of the tooth should be gently flushed with sterile saline.
- Early dental consultation is indicated.
- Dental fractures, on the other hand, are less urgent and have variable prognoses depending on what part of the tooth is involved.
- Higher priority should be accorded broken teeth that have exposed pulp that can be seen as a vascular core, or, at times, a pinkish-tinged pulsation visible through a dentinal surface (13).

Auricular and nasal septal hematomas

SYMPTOMS
- An auricular hematoma is caused by a blunt blow to the external ear.
- It is an obvious injury characterized by swelling and ecchymosis.
- Nasal septal hematoma is not obvious to gross inspection, but is a risk when the patient has a fractured nose.

DIAGNOSIS
- An auricular hematoma is diagnosed by direct observation.
- Nasal septal hematoma is diagnosed by direct inspection of the septum using a nasal speculum.

TREATMENT
- Cartilage is avascular and receives its blood supply from the perichondrium.
- A hematoma of the auricle or nasal septum threatens the viability of the underlying cartilage because the extravasated blood is between the cartilage and the perichondrium. This can result in avascular necrosis of the cartilage that causes either a "cauliflower ear" or saddle nose deformity (22,24).

- The treatment for either auricular or nasal septal hematoma is an incision and drainage (I and D) of the hematoma (22,24).
- Following the I and D, in the case of the auricle, the convolutions of the auricle are packed with vaseline gauze. Several gauze sponges are laced between the auricle and the scalp to hold it in a neutral position, then the entire area is padded with fluff gauze and secured with a roll gauze bandage that covers the dressed ear (24).
- In the case of the septal hematoma, following I and D, a small drain, such as a sterile rubber band is placed, and an anterior pack is inserted as with anterior epistaxis (24). In either case, the packing/dressing must be changed daily and the respective structures inspected for evidence of reaccumulation or infection.

Nasal fractures

SYMPTOMS
- Nasal fractures are the most common facial bone fracture and are characterized by pain, swelling, possible deformity, and epistaxis or clotted blood in the nares.

DIAGNOSIS
- Diagnosis of nasal fractures is generally on clinical grounds.
- The patient will need a nasal speculum examination to rule out septal hematoma.
- Radiographs are generally not necessary, and even when positive rarely influence treatment (19,22).

TREATMENT
- A fractured nose is generally nonurgent unless it is an open fracture or a septal hematoma is present.
- While the patient is awaiting treatment, ice should be applied.
- As with facial bone fractures, the necessity of repair for nasal fractures is generally evaluated after swelling has gone down 1 to 2 weeks after the injury.

Facial lacerations

Open facial wounds should be dressed with moist saline dressings or cleansed with saline or Shur-Clens. Betadine should not be applied directly to open facial wounds unless it is diluted because it is toxic to subcutaneous tissue and can increase scarring. Ice packs should be applied to areas of swelling. If the cervical spine is clear, elevation of the head is helpful to reduce swelling.

Ménière's disease and acute labyrinthitis (vestibular dysfunction)

SYMPTOMS

- Symptoms of Ménière's disease include tinnitus, rotational vertigo, and unilateral, progressive sensorineural hearing loss (6).
- During recurrent, acute episodes the vertigo and tinnitus become profound and may be associated with severe nausea and vomiting that can be sufficiently severe to cause dehydration and prostration.
- Acute labyrinthitis has a similar presentation, but is not characterized by chronic tinnitus or progressive hearing loss.

DIAGNOSIS

- Definitive diagnosis for Ménière's disease requires tests that are not performed on an emergent basis (e.g., audiometry, electronystagmography).
- Patients who give a history of multiple episodes of severe vertigo should be referred for work-up.

TREATMENT

- Treatment of an exacerbation of Ménière's disease is aimed at correcting fluid and electrolyte imbalances and relieving vertigo, nausea, and vomiting.
- Antiemetic drugs such as promethazine or droperidol may be necessary.
- Treatment for acute labyrinthitis is supportive and aimed at relieving symptoms.
- Oral meclizine is commonly prescribed to relieve vertigo, frequently in conjunction with a benzodiazepine such as diazepam that helps stabilize vestibular function (25).
- Patients need to be counseled to change positions gradually and to avoid sudden head movements.

Esophageal foreign body (nonairway foreign bodies)

SYMPTOMS

- Esophageal foreign bodies, while less serious, are extremely uncomfortable, and often it is difficult at triage to be certain a foreign body "in the throat" is, in fact, esophageal.
- If there is any doubt regarding the location of the foreign body (i.e., trachea vs. esophagus), it is safest to triage immediately to a treatment area.
- At times the patient can describe the sensation clearly enough that one can be reasonably certain.

- Phonation is generally not impaired and stridor should not be present.
- The patient may be retching without nausea.
- Esophageal foreign bodies commonly occur while eating, and may be associated with stricture, especially in older adults.

DIAGNOSIS
- Esophageal foreign bodies may be diagnosed by plain radiographs if the object is radiopaque.
- Food and radiolucent objects may be diagnosed by Ba swallow.

Treatment
- Often, an esophageal foreign body will gradually pass.
- Intravenous glucagon is occasionally helpful in relaxing the distal (smooth muscle) segment of the esophagus.
- Esophagoscopy is occasionally necessary.
- Depending on the size, nature, and location of the foreign body, it may be removed or pushed into the stomach by means of the endoscope.

Nasal and ear foreign bodies

SYMPTOMS
- Foreign bodies in children are frequently delayed presentations that mimic infections such as sinusitis or suppurative otitis.
- Foreign bodies of the ear often present as conductive hearing loss.
- Occasionally an insect crawls into the ear canal and can be extremely painful and distressing at any age.

DIAGNOSIS
- Foreign bodies of the nose may be visible on direct examination, but an index of suspicion must be maintained in cases of foul, purulent drainage.
- A foreign body of the ear can be seen via otoscopy, but if some time has elapsed since its introduction into the ear canal, it may be obscured by cerumen or purulent drainage.

TREATMENT
- With nasal foreign bodies, there is some degree of risk that the foreign body might get converted to an airway foreign body if pushed during a removal attempt.
- With ear foreign bodies, there is a risk of tympanic membrane rupture or laceration of the external auditory canal during removal (1).

- Because of these risks, it is best to set a time limit before undertaking a removal as more harm can be caused by determined removal attempts than has been caused by the foreign body itself.
- If the time limit has been reached without success, it is best to involve an ENT specialist (1,20,24).

E

- Foreign bodies of the nose or ear may be removed by means of alligator forceps, passing an ear curette or Fogarty catheter beyond the foreign body and gently pulling it out. Nursing responsibilities during removal consist primarily of assisting with the examination and removal. Small children will be frightened and often need to be secured with a sheet or on a papoose board. On occasion, conscious sedation may be ordered for a child before removal.
- Vegetable matter, such as beans or wood, is difficult to remove because it swells up and becomes too soft to be grasped with a forceps. Hard, spherical foreign bodies, such as beads, are also difficult to grasp.
- Insects in the ear canal can be killed by means of filling the ear canal with microscope immersion oil (highly refined mineral oil) (15), vegetable oil (15), or 4% topical lidocaine solution (24). Microscope immersion oil has recently been found the most rapid and effective in immobilizing and killing cockroaches in vitro (15). The killed insect can be removed by irrigation, suction, or with forceps (15,24).

Otitis media (infection)

SYMPTOMS

- Otitis media is most common in children below school age because of their short, relatively flat eustachian canals.
- Typically there is a history of several days of a URI followed by increasing fussiness, fever, pain, and emotional distress of child and parent alike. Symptoms may be unilateral or bilateral.

DIAGNOSIS

- Diagnosis is by otoscopic examination. The tympanic membrane is red and does not move normally with air insufflation.

TREATMENT

- Small children are often discomfited or frightened by ear examinations and may need to be held securely.

- Initially, the parent should hold the child seated in his/her lap with arms crossed over the child's arms.
- If the child is too restless or uncooperative, the child can be postioned supine, with the arms extended upward.
- The nurse should hold the child's upper arms at either side of the head, and a second person (staff or parent) should hold the child's thighs just above the knees. This permits the examiner to hold the head still gently with one hand while using the otoscope with the other.
- If the TM cannot be visualized because of cerumen, the ear canal is generally curetted by the physician.
- Treatment is with antibiotics. Amoxicillin is generally appropriate as a first-line agent for children or adults; trimethoprim-sulfamethoxazole or erythromycin are acceptable alternatives if the patient is allergic to penicillin (2,21,25).
- In general, a child with otitis media should be reexamined 1 to 2 weeks after completing a course of antibiotics to make sure the infection has been adequately treated. If the child is not improving within a few days of starting treatment, a reexamination and possibly a change in antibiotics is in order.

Sinusitis

SYMPTOMS

- Complaints of "sinus" congestion or headaches are extremely common, and it is essential to clarify more precisely what the patient's symptoms are.
- Sinusitis generally is accompanied by a sensation of pressure in the affected region and a purulent nasal discharge.
- The patient may be febrile.

DIAGNOSIS

- Definitive diagnosis can be made on x-ray or a CT scan, but often is presumptive, based on clinical presentation.
- Transillumination may be used as a diagnostic adjunct.

TREATMENT

- Untreated sinusitis can progress, and as with orbital cellulitis, lead to cavernous sinus thrombosis or other intracranial infections (5).
- Treatment usually consists of a broad spectrum antibiotic and a decongestant.
- To avoid inspissation of mucus, antihistamines should be avoided unless allergy is deemed a significant etiologic factor (24).

- Rarely, irrigation of the sinuses by an ENT specialist may be required.

Otitis externa

SYMPTOMS

- Infection of the external auditory canal can be quite painful. It is often related to swimming or diving, and is most common in adults and older children.

DIAGNOSIS

- Diagnosis is by otoscopy. The external auditory canal may be inflamed or contain exudative debris.

TREATMENT

- Consists of gentle debridement of the ear canal with a curette or calcium alginate swab and instillation of polymyxin B-neomycin-hydrocortisone drops (20,24).
- On occasion, a "wick" (an antibiotic-soaked strip of packing gauze) may be placed in the ear canal to help distribute the medication more evenly and prevent it from coming out of the canal.
- The patient should be instructed to avoid swimming or getting the ear canals wet for a period of about 2 weeks.
- At times, analgesic drops may be helpful.
- Older diabetics may develop malignant (Pseudomonas) otitis externa and may need to be hospitalized on parenteral antibiotics (20,21).

Odontalgia

SYMPTOMS

- Complaints of severe dental pain are particularly common at night and on weekends when patients may have difficulty accessing a dentist. If an abscess is the cause, the patient's jaw or cheek may be swollen on the affected side.
- The patient may be febrile.
- Frequently patients arrive believing they must be seen by a dentist immediately to have an emergent extraction, which is rarely necessary.
- It is helpful in triage to reorient the patient's expectations toward diagnosis of the problem, pain relief, determination of whether or not an antibiotic is indicated, and facilitating prompt follow-up.

DIAGNOSIS

- Odontalgia is a symptom. Diagnosis is directed toward establishing underlying cause and initiating appropriate treatment.
- Dental or Panorex radiographs may be needed.

- Common causes of odontalgia are abscesses and broken teeth with exposed dentin or pulp (13).

TREATMENT

- I and D of an abscess by the physician may be necessary.
- Nursing care is directed toward pain relief.
- The patient will generally be sent home on antibiotics and systemic analgesics.
- Patients with chipped or broken teeth may have them temporarily sealed with calcium hydroxide paste by the emergency physician if there is exposure of dentin or pulp (13).
- In facilities that do not have dentists on staff, it is helpful for the emergency department to have some arrangement with area dentists for follow-up of emergency department visits.

Acute necrotizing ulcerative gingivitis (ANUG)

SYMPTOMS

- This is a mixed anaerobic gingival infection often referred to as trench mouth or Vincent's angina.
- It is characterized by painful gingivostomatitis, headache, sore throat, anorexia, and halitosis.

DIAGNOSIS

- Diagnosis is by the characteristic appearance of the oral cavity.

TREATMENT

- Treatment is with oral penicillin, and bicarbonate or peroxide mouth rinses (12,13).
- Follow-up dental referral is recommended.
- Recurrences are common, and, on occasion, gingival debridement by a dentist may be necessary (13).

Cerumen impaction (diminished auditory acuity)

SYMPTOMS

- The typical presentation is a complaint of one ear, or occasionally both, feeling plugged or a sensation of fullness, and/or some degree of diminished auditory acuity (20,28).

DIAGNOSIS

- Impaction is easily noted on an otoscopic examination.

TREATMENT

- Removal may be by curette or more commonly by irrigation (see Procedure 13) (20,28).
- Irrigation should be avoided if there is suspicion of tympanic membrane (TM) rupture. Ordinarily, a

ruptured TM will not lead to hearing loss, but may be associated with vertigo (20).

- Patients often have mild discomfort during irrigation but should not experience vertigo, nausea, or severe pain.
- If a patient becomes increasingly symptomatic during irrigation, it should be discontinued and the physician should be notified.
- Removal may be attempted by curette, or the patient may be referred to a specialist.
- In all age groups, impacted cerumen is generally related to attempts to remove cerumen, usually with cotton swabs that tend to tamp it further into the ear canal. At times, patients hold a mistaken belief that cerumen is a pathological secretion, a belief that may contribute to inappropriately zealous removal attempts. Patients should be instructed not to attempt to remove wax with swabs, match sticks, paper clips, or other small objects.
- Cerumenolytic agents may be recommended to prevent recurrence. Anecdotally, over-the-counter (OTC) liquid docusate sodium (Colace liquid, 1% solution, 10 mg/ml)* instilled once a month is reported, to be more effective than either OTC or prescription cerumenolytics (Debrox or Cerumenex, respectively) (3). ENT follow-up is generally not indicated unless TM rupture has been found.

NURSING SURVEILLANCE

1. Airway maintenance.
2. Oxygen saturation monitoring and administration as indicated.
3. Control of bleeding and monitoring of fluid/blood replacement as indicated.
4. Vital signs as appropriate to condition and departmental policy.
5. Fever control/seizure prevention.
6. Adequacy of pain relief and evaluation of responses to other interventions.

EXPECTED PATIENT OUTCOMES

1. The airway shall be spontaneously maintainable or an artificial airway shall be in place.

---

*This product comes in a 30 ml bottle with a calibrated dropper. Docusate sodium syrup should never be used for this purpose.

2. Oxygen saturation should have remained above 91% throughout stabilization and vital signs should not have deteriorated.

3. In epistaxis, bleeding should be controlled and vital signs should be within normal range at time of admission or discharge. For the patient with a posterior pack, oxygen saturation monitoring and adequate intravenous access to permit administration of blood products, if needed, should be instituted.

4. For febrile children, a reduction in fever should be documented before discharge.

5. Nausea and vertigo should be improved at time of discharge. The patient should be tolerating clear liquids PO.

6. Certain types of pain, particularly resulting from otitis media and odontalgia, may not be completely controllable in the course of a brief visit, but should, at least, be reduced.

7. After disimpaction of cerumen, auditory acuity should be improved.

DISCHARGE IMPLICATIONS

1. The patient and family must understand the plan of care, expected self-care, medications, and expected time frames for symptom resolution and follow-up.

2. Means of providing humidified air (e.g., bedside humidifier or using the shower to steam up the bathroom) should be discussed with parents of children with croup if they are well enough to be discharged. Clear criteria that would warrant a return to the ED should be discussed as well.

3. Patients with anterior nasal packs should understand what to do if bleeding recurs and when to follow-up for packing removal.

4. Parents of children with otitis media or other febrile conditions must know how to measure a child's temperature, how to administer antipyretics and antibiotics, and how to recognize signs and symptoms of deterioration.

5. A patient with a nasal fracture should be instructed to follow-up with an ENT or plastic surgeon after the swelling has gone down (1 to 2 weeks) if it is difficult to

breathe out of one naris, or if not satisfied with the appearance of the nose.

6. Patients who have had an auricular or nasal septal hematoma incised and drained need to know when to return (or follow-up with a specialist) for dressing or packing changes and drain removal.

7. Patients with dental complaints should be helped to understand the importance of expeditious follow-up with a dentist or oral surgeon. The extent to which fear of dental procedures or financial constraints may have put the patient at risk for a given problem should be explored with the patient in a nonjudgmental fashion.

References

1. Bressler K, Shelton C: Ear foreign-body removal: a review of 98 consecutive cases, *Laryngoscope* 103(4):367, 1993.

2. Celin SE, Bluestone CD, Stevenson J, et al: Bacteriology of acute otitis media in adults, *JAMA* 266:2249, 1991.

3. Chen DA, Caparosa RJ: A nonprescription cerumenolytic, *Am J Otol* 12:475, 1991.

4. Chu L, Gussack GS, Muller T: A treatment protocol for mandible fractures, *J Trauma* 36:48, 1994.

5. Clayman GL, Adams GL, Paugh DR, Koopman CF Jr: Intracranial complications of paranasal sinusitis: a combined institutional review, *Laryngoscope* 101:234, 1991.

6. Emergency Nurses' Association: *Emergency nursing core curriculum*, ed 4, Philadelphia, 1994, WB Saunders.

7. Hussain K, Wijetunge DB, Grubnic S, Jackson IT: A comprehensive analysis of craniofacial trauma, *J Trauma* 36:34, 1994.

8. Jacobs EE, Ota HG, Turner PA: Control of epistaxis. In HL May, et al, editors: *Emergency medicine,* ed 2, Boston, 1992, Little, Brown, & Co.

9. Joseph E, et al: Predictors of blinding or serious eye injury in blunt trauma, *J Trauma* 33:19, 1992.

10. Josephson GD, Godley FA, Stierna P: Practical management of epistaxis, *Med Clin North Am* 75:1311, 1991.

11. Kass EG, McFadden EA, Jacobson S, Toohil RJ: Acute epiglottitis in the adult: experience with a seasonal presentation, *Laryngoscope* 103:841, 1993.

12. Kimmitz TP, Defries HO: Pharyngeal emergencies, *Top Emerg Med* 6(3): 66, 1984.

13. Klokkevold P: Common dental emergencies: evaluation and management for emergency physicians, *Emerg Med Clin North Am* 7:29, 1989.

14. Krasner PR: Treatment of tooth avulsion by nurses, *J Emerg Nurs* 16:29-35, 1990.

15. Leffler S, Cheney P, Tandberg D: Chemical immobilization and killing of intraaural roaches: an in vitro comparative study, *Ann Emerg Med* 22:1795, 1993.

16. McGarry GW, Moulton C: The first aid management of epistaxis by accident and emergency medicine staff, *Arch Emerg Med* 10(4):298, 1993.

17. Neff JA: Epiglottitis, *J Emerg Nurs* 13:184, 1987.

18. Nemes J, Schmidt E, Kelly L: Epiglottitis: ED nursing management, *J Emerg Nurs* 14:70, 1988.

19. Nigam A, Goni A, Benjamin A, Dasgupta AR: The value of radiographs in the management of the fractured nose, *Arch Emerg Med* 10(4):293, 1993.

20. Reich JJ, Turbiak TW: Otic emergencies. *Top Emerg Med* 6 (3):19, 1984.

21. Sanford JP: *Guide to antimicrobial therapy*, Dallas, 1993, Antimicrobial Therapy.

22. Sharp JF, Denholm S: Routine x-rays in nasal trauma: the influence of audit on clinical practice, *J R Soc Med* 87(3):153, March 1994.

23. Shesser R, Smith M: Oral emergencies, *Top Emerg Med* 6 (3):48, 1984.

24. Votey S, Dudley JP: Emergency ear nose and throat procedures. *Emerg Med Clin North Am* 7:117, 1989.

25. Weimert TA, Common ENT emergencies part 1: the acute ear, *Emerg Med* 24(5):134, April 15, 1992.

26. Weimert TA, Common ENT emergencies part 2: the acute nose and throat, *Emerg Med* 24(6):26, April 30, 1992.

27. Wolkove N, Kreisman H, Cohen C, Frank H: Occult foreign-body aspiration in adults, *JAMA* 248:1350, 1982.

28. Zivic RC, King S: Cerumen impaction management for clients of all ages, *Nurs Pract* 18(3):33, 1993.

Chapter VII

Endocrine Conditions

Pamela S. Kidd

E

CLINICAL CONDITIONS
Diabetic Ketoacidosis (DKA)
Hyperosmolar, NonKetotic Coma (HHNC)
Hypoglycemia
Thyrotoxicosis/Thyroid Storm
Myxedema
Acute Adrenal Insufficiency/Addison's Disease
Cushing's Disease
Syndrome of Inappropriate ADH Secretion (SIADH)

TRIAGE ASSESSMENT

Other than diabetes, endocrine conditions are extremely rare. Acute endocrine crises are life threatening and require rapid interventions. Patients may not realize they have an endocrine disorder, and the diagnosis may be made or suspected for the first time in the ED. Because hormones affect several target organs, symptoms are multiple and diverse. The goal of triage is to accurately detect a pattern of symptoms related to an endocrine disorder. Specific diagnosis and treatment of the problem will occur in the treatment area. The following questions should help to detect endocrine disorders.

Existing health problems

Asking about existing health problems will alert you if the patient is aware he/she has an endocrine problem. It also helps to rule out other etiologies of symptoms. For example, if the patient denies a heart problem but presents with tachycardia and palpitations, overproduction of thyroid hormone or hypoglycemia may be the cause.

Medication history

If the patient is taking medication, ask about the dosage. Insulin-dependent diabetic patients are at higher risk for ketoacidosis. Thiazide diuretics decrease serum potassium levels and induce hyperglycemia. Table 7-1

TABLE 7-1 Drugs That May Precipitate Endocrine Problems

Drug	Effect	Condition
Hydrochlorothiazide	Decreases insulin secretion and increases insulin resistance	DKA, HHNC
Beta-blocking agents (e.g., propanol)	Decreases insulin secretion	DKA
Dilantin	Decreases insulin secretion	DKA
Alcohol	Decreases insulin secretion	DKA
Calcium channel blockers (e.g., nifedipine)	Decreases insulin secretion	DKA
Cortisol	Increases insulin resistance	DKA, HHNC
Terbutaline	Increases insulin resistance	DKA
Sedatives	Decreases oxygen consumption	Hypothyroidism
Tranquilizers	Decreases oxygen consumption	Hypothyroidism
Diuretics	Decreases circulating blood volume	Hypothyroidism

DKA, Diabetic ketoacidosis; *HHNC*, hyperosmolar, nonketotic coma.

highlights commonly prescribed drugs that may precipitate endocrine problems.

Stress

Several endocrine disorders (e.g., ketoacidosis, Cushing's disease) are precipitated or exacerbated by stress resulting from cortisol secretion.

Dehydration

Assess if the patient has been vomiting, having diarrhea, urinating excessively, or not drinking fluids in a hot, humid environment. Vomiting is associated with diabetic ketoacidosis (DKA). All of these factors promote dehydration that can precipitate DKA and hyperosmolar, nonketotic coma (HHNC). Vomiting and diarrhea are associated with hyperthyroidism.

Thirst

Thirst is associated with diabetes.

Energy

Fatigue is associated with myxedema, Addison's disease, and diabetes.

Pain

Elicit a description of pain. Headaches are associated with hypoglycemia. Abdominal pain is associated with DKA and acute adrenal insufficiency.

Mood changes/insomnia

Mood changes and insomnia are characteristic of hyperthyroidism.

Weight

Weight loss is common in hyperthyroidism and Addison's disease.

Vital signs

- *Breathing pattern:* Kussmaul breathing (deep, accelerated, sighing respirations) indicates a pH below 7.2 and acidosis.
- *Blood pressure:* Hypotension is associated with dehydration and decreased circulating blood volume. Orthostatic changes in both blood pressure and pulse may be present. Diastolic hypertension is present in patients with chronic hypothyroidism (myxedema) resulting from peripheral vasoconstriction as an effort to maintain body core temperature. Systolic hypertension is associated with Cushing's disease related to fluid retention and oversecretion of catecholamines.
- *Heart rate:* Bradycardia is present in hypothyroidism. Tachycardia and palpitations occur in hyperthyroidism.
- *Fever:* Note any temperature elevation. Infection may be subtle and still increase insulin requirements beyond what the patient is capable of delivering precipitating hyperglycemia and hyperosmolarity. A temperature >104° F may be present in hyperthyroidism.

General Observations
Skin

- Assess the patient hydration status by examining skin turgor, mucous membranes, and orbits. Dry, hot skin is associated with addisonian crisis. Flushed, dry skin indicates dehydration. Dehydration is associated with Addison's disease, HHNC, and ketoacidosis. Flushed, wet skin is associated with hyperthyroidism.

- Cool, pale skin is associated with hypothyroidism.
- Darkly colored (hyperpigmented) skin in Caucasian patients suggests Addison's disease. Hyperpigmentation may be most visible on the back of the hands, elbows, and knees.

Goiter
- A goiter may be present in hyperthyroidism.

Exophthalmos
- Exophthalmos (bulging eyeballs) may be present in hyperthyroidism.

Diaphoresis
- Excessive diaphoresis may occur in hyperthyroidism.

Edema
- Generalized edema may be present in hypothyroidism and syndrome of inappropriate secretion of antidiuretic hormone (SIADH). People with Cushing's disease tend to have round, plump faces with fat pads on the shoulders.

Obesity
- Obesity is a symptom of Cushing's disease.

FOCUSED NURSING ASSESSMENT

The areas of ventilation, perfusion, cognition, and sexuality should be assessed in greater detail.

Ventilation

Auscultate breath sounds. Pulmonary edema, characterized by crackles, may occur in hypothyroidism. Diminished breath sounds may indicate infiltrates and possible infection as a precipitating cause of DKA, HHNC, and thyroid disorders.

Undress the patient and assess breathing pattern for symmetry and depth of excursion. As noted earlier, deep rapid respirations indicate acidosis.

Perfusion

Auscultate heart sounds. A murmur may be present in high-flow (e.g., Cushing's disease, hypothyroidism) or hyperdynamic (e.g., hyperthyroidism) states.

Assess peripheral pulses. Vasoconstriction is present in Cushing's disease. Diminished pulses may be present in dehydration.

Cognition

Perform a neurologic assessment and document a Glasgow coma scale score (GCS) for the patient (see Reference Guide 6). A person who is not oriented may be manifesting symptoms of cerebral edema from hyperosmolality or may be at risk for becoming dehydrated and precipitating hyperosmolarity. Cognition is almost always impaired in HHNC.

Assess the patient for tremors. Tremors and hyperreflexia occur frequently in hyperthyroidism.

Sexuality

Impotence and abnormal menses is associated with Cushing's disease.

Secondary sexual characteristics may be overpronounced (e.g., gynecomastia, breast development in males) in Cushing's disease.

There is a decrease in body and pubic hair in females in Addison's disease.

Risk Factors

1. A history of diabetes predisposes the patient to hypoglycemia and hyperosmolar coma whether related to ketoacidosis or HHNC.
2. Black males and Native Americans from the Pima tribe have the highest incidence of diabetes in the United States.
3. Obesity is a risk factor for non–insulin-dependent diabetes mellitus (NIDDM).
4. Oat cell lung cancer is frequently associated with SIADH.

Life Span Issues
Pregnancy

1. Pregnancy may potentiate DKA.
2. Pregnancy may stimulate hyperthyroidism. Failure to gain weight in pregnancy is an indicator of hyperthyroidism. Thyrotoxicosis may occur in the postpartum period.

Children

1. Peak onset of insulin-dependent diabetes mellitus (IDDM) is 11 to 13 years of age.

Adults

1. The risk of NIDDM increases over age 40.
2. Thyroid crisis or storm occurs more in females in the 30- to 50-year-old age range.

3. Addison's disease is more common in 30- to 50-year-old adults.

Geriatric

1. HHNC is more common in older individuals with NIDDM.
2. Hypothyroidism causes decreased oxygen consumption and heat generation. In the geriatric population, oxygen consumption and heat generation decline as part of aging. Myxedema is diagnosed more frequently in the geriatric population because symptoms are more pronounced because of less compensatory reserve.

INITIAL INTERVENTIONS

1. Administer low-flow oxygen as needed until laboratory tests return. Endocrine disorders affect metabolism, and oxygen administration promotes oxygen availability in both overproduction and underproduction of hormones.
2. Initiate pulse oximetry monitoring. Oxygen saturation readings can provide clues regarding acidosis, phosphate levels, and core body temperature. Increased affinity of oxygen to hemoglobin occurs in these states.
3. Initiate cardiac monitoring. Endocrine disorders may produce dysrhythmias, conduction defects, and congestive heart failure.
4. Initiate continuous blood pressure monitoring. Cardiovascular decompensation may occur as a result of the endocrine problem or in response to rapid treatment. Changes from baseline should be conveyed immediately.
5. Insert an intravenous catheter and obtain blood for potential tests (CBC, electrolyte levels, glucose level, and hormone function). An intermittent infusion device may be attached until further assessment is completed or laboratory data is returned, since overhydration may be a problem in some endocrine disorders. If dehydration is suspected, administer IV fluid.

PRIORITY NURSING DIAGNOSES

Risk for ineffective breathing patterns
Risk for decreased cardiac output
Risk for injury

The following nursing diagnoses apply to patients with endocrine disorders.

E

◆ **Ineffective breathing patterns** related to fatigue, acidosis, and/or electrolyte abnormality.

INTERVENTIONS

- Administer oxygen per physician order.
- Monitor oxygen saturation.
- Prepare for endotracheal intubation, neuromuscular blockade, and mechanical ventilation.

◆ **Decreased cardiac output** related to dehydration or decreased contractility resulting from chronic left ventricle overdistention.

INTERVENTIONS

- Administer volume or diuretics as case dictates per physician order.
- Decrease metabolic needs by treating fever, pain, and infection.
- Monitor intake and output.

◆ **Injury** related to electrolyte disturbances (usually hyponatremia, hypokalemia [except in Addison's disease], hypophosphatemia).

INTERVENTIONS

- Administer electrolyte replacement as laboratory values and patient condition indicates.
- Monitor intake and output.
- Perform frequent neurologic assessments.

PRIORITY DIAGNOSTIC TESTS

Laboratory

Quick bedside calculation of laboratory tests used in DKA and HHNC are located in Table 7-2.

Adrenocorticotrophic (ACTH) test: ACTH will be elevated in Cushing's disease.

Anion gap: An elevated anion gap indicates acidosis. An anion gap >20 mmol/L indicates DKA.

Arterial blood gases: pH values will be low in both ketoacidosis and HHNC. They will be below 7.2 in ketoacidosis. Bicarbonate levels will be below 15 mEq/L in DKA.

Cultures: Blood, urine, and sputum cultures may be needed to determine if infection is present in HHNC and DKA, since the WBC is normally elevated in these states.

Glucose: Glucose levels will be low in hypoglycemia, acute adrenal insufficiency, Addison's disease, and hypothyroidism. They will be elevated in ketoacidosis,

TABLE 7-2 Bedside Calculation of Lab Tests in DKA, HHNC

Type	Rationale	Formula
Sodium correction	Serum sodium levels appear lower than they actually are as hyperglycemia is corrected.	Add 2.8 mmol to the patient's reported sodium level for every 100 mg/dl increase in blood sugar above normal. Normal is considered 100 mg/dl. (Example: if blood glucose is 500 mg/dl, multiply $4 \times 2.8 = 11.2$. Add 11.2 mmol to the actual reported serum sodium value.)
Serum osmolality	Measured osmolality by laboratory includes all molecules. Calculated osmolality allows you to examine only the molecules that contribute to dehydration. If calculated osmolality is less than measured and the patient is comatose, there is another cause other than dehydration for the coma.	2(serum Na + serum K) + blood glucose ÷ 20 = calculated serum osmolality
Anion gap	Indicates an acidotic state but does not tell you what kinds of acids have produced the state (e.g., lactic acid vs. ketones).	Sodium − (chloride + bicarbonate) Normal range = 8-16 or Na + K − (chloride + bicarbonate) Normal range = 12-20.

HHNC, and Cushing's disease. A level >300 mg/dl
suggests dehydration or impaired renal function. The
highest levels (average = 1100 mg/dl) are in HHNC.

Potassium: Potassium will be high in Addison's disease
and untreated hyperosmolar states. As the patient is
rehydrated, potassium moves back into the cell and
levels may fall below normal.

Rapid synthetic corticotropin stimulation test: This test is
used to determine if adrenal dysfunction is causing
Addison's disease. Synthetic ACTH is administered IV
and cortisol levels are measured at 0, 30- and 60-
minute intervals after administration. Failure of
cortisol levels to increase indicate a primary adrenal
problem.

Serum osmolality: This value will be elevated in both
ketoacidosis and HHNC. A value >340 mOsm/L
produces a comatose state.

Sodium: Hyponatremia may be present in Addison's
disease and myxedema.

Triiodothyronine (T_3) level: T_3 is elevated in
hyperthyroidism.

Thyroxine (T_4) level: T_4 is elevated in hyperthyroidism.

Urine-free cortisol test: This 24-hour test detects cortisol
excretion in the urine commonly seen in Cushing's
disease. If the test is positive for cortisol,
adrenocorticotrophic hormone (ACTH) tests are
conducted to determine etiology of the disease.

Urine ketones: Ketones will be present in DKA but absent
in HHNC.

WBC: The WBC is normally elevated without infection in
diabetic patients. Levels of 40,000 cells/mm have been
noted in DKA without infection. Increased neutrophil
count indicates infection in diabetic patients.
Hypothyroid patients may be unable to elevate the
WBC in infection because of depressed bone marrow
activity. An elevated band count on the differential
indicates infection in these patients.

Radiographic

CT scan: Scans of the adrenal, pituitary, and thyroid
gland may be performed to identify gland enlargement
and/or tumors.

Other

ECG: T wave changes during fluid resuscitation for dehydration may indicate impending congestive heart failure. Sinus bradycardia, prolonged QT interval, and low voltage are seen on the ECG in hypothyroidism.

COLLABORATIVE INTERVENTIONS

Overview

1. Anticipate drug administration before return of laboratory data because of serious consequences from many endocrine disorders (Table 7-4).
2. Invasive hemodynamic monitoring may be initiated because of a need for monitoring vascular response to treatment. Assist with insertion and obtain measurements.
3. A urinary catheter is frequently inserted to monitor renal response to treatment.

Clinical Conditions
Diabetic ketoacidosis (DKA)

DKA can be present with or without hyperosmolar coma. The use of free fatty acids for energy vs. glucose produces ketoacids. The most frequent cause of DKA is undetected infection.

SYMPTOMS

- Hyperglycemia induces diuresis so the patient complains of polyuria, thirst, and fatigue.
- In order to differentiate DKA from HHNC, patients in DKA may complain of abdominal pain related to gastric dilatation, their respiratory rate may be rapid with deep breaths (Kussmaul's), and CNS changes may not be present.

DIAGNOSIS

- Ketones will be present in the urine.
- Arterial blood gases will reveal a pH below 7.35.
- Blood glucose levels will be elevated.
- Serum osmolarity will be high in some cases.

TREATMENT

- 0.9% normal saline (NS) is administered if the patient is hypotensive; otherwise 0.45% NS is given.
- Insulin is administered at a higher rate in DKA than HHNC (4 to 8 U/hr).

TABLE 7-3 Comparison of Treatment for DKA and HHNC

Rehydration	Correction of hyperglycemia
In both DKA and HHNC	**In DKA**
If serum sodium is > 165, administer 2.5% dextrose solution. If serum sodium is 145-165, administer 0.45% normal saline (NS). If serum sodium is < 145, administer 0.9% NS.	Administer regular insulin IV bolus of 0.1-0.2 U/kg. Follow with a 0.1-0.2 U/kg/hr IV drip until glucose level reaches 300 mg/dl.
Rate	**In HHNC**
2 L within first 2 hours followed by 1 L q 2 hr. Give ½ of fluid deficit within first 12 hr. Give last ½ of deficit over the next 24 hr. Start D₅NSS when glucose level reaches 300 mg/dl. If potassium level is 4.5 or less give 20-40 mEq of K⁺/L of fluid/hr for 3-4 hr of treatment. If pH is < 7.0, give 1 ampule (44 mEq) of bicarbonate unless the patient is comatose.	Administer 1-2 U/hr (not based on weight, takes much less insulin to correct problem).

- Potassium replacement may be necessary.
- Phosphate levels are typically lower with rehydration in DKA thus phosphate may be given. Table 7-3 compares treatment of DKA and HHNC.

Hyperosmolar, nonketotic coma (HHNC)

Patients who present with HHNC may not be diagnosed diabetics. Frequently HHNC is the first indicator of a chronic problem. Almost all cases are precipitated by infection.

SYMPTOMS
- Massive diuresis occurs. Patients complain of polyuria, thirst, and fatigue related to calcium, potassium, and magnesium losses.
- CNS symptoms are common as a result of high-serum osmolality.
- Patients complain of visual changes.
- They may be aphasic, stuporous, actively seizing and hallucinating.

DIAGNOSIS
- Serum glucose and osmolarity levels will be high.
- Urine ketones will be negative.
- Arterial pH will be >7.25.
- Urine may be positive for a urinary tract infection.
- Chest film may indicate pneumonia.

TREATMENT
- Rehydration is accomplished through administration of 0.45% NS.
- IV insulin is administered in dosages of 1 to 2 U/hr.
- Insulin is decreased once the glucose level drops to 300 mg/dl.
- Potassium and phosphate replacement may be necessary.

NURSING ALERT

In treating both DKA and HHNC, it is crucial for the nurse to reassess the patient's neurologic status and breath sounds frequently to detect impending fluid overload; too aggressive rehydration will cause cerebral and pulmonary edema.

Hypoglycemia

Hypoglycemia may occur in a diabetic patient because of inadequate food intake in relation to insulin dosage. Exercise, infection, and emotional stress may also alter blood glucose levels. Nondiabetic patients are also susceptible to hypoglycemia.

SYMPTOMS
- Symptoms are sudden in onset.
- The patient may complain of a headache, and dizziness, and appear confused.
- Diaphoresis, tachycardia, and palpitations may be present.

DIAGNOSIS
* Blood glucose level will usually be below 60 mg/dl.

TREATMENT
* Hypoglycemia is rapidly reversed with administration of intravenous glucose (50 cc of dextrose 50% solution) or oral glucose if patient is alert enough to prevent aspiration.

E

Thyrotoxicosis/Thyroid storm

Thyroid storm is a life-threatening illness resulting from the excessive release of thyroid hormones usually precipitated by infection or injury.

SYMPTOMS
* Symptoms represent elevated metabolism, tachycardia, diaphoresis, tremors, and hyperthermia.

DIAGNOSIS
* T_3 and T_4 levels are elevated.
* Hyperglycemia is present.
* Liver enzymes may also elevate.
* There is debate concerning when thyrotoxicosis becomes thyroid storm. The presence of mental status changes usually signals progression of the hyperthyroid state.
* Tachycardia (>140 beats/min) and fever (>106° F) indicate thyroid storm.

TREATMENT
* Antithyroid medication is administered (e.g., propylthiouracil, methimazole, see Table 7-4).
* Steroids may be given.
* Acetaminophen is administered and hypothermia measures are initiated.
* Beta-blocking agents (e.g., propranolol) may be given to decrease cardiac response to thyroid hormone.

Myxedema

Myxedema coma is an acute manifestation of hypothyroidism.

SYMPTOMS
* Altered mental status is present and may range from disorientation to psychosis.
* Hypothermia is another classic sign.
* A precipitating illness or event usually stimulates a hypothyroid crisis.
* Common associated conditions are stroke, infection, and traumatic injury.

DIAGNOSIS
- Diagnosis is based on the triad of symptoms discussed above.

TREATMENT
- IV levothyroxine is administered on suspicion of hypothyroidism, since it does not harm a euthyroid patient.
- Respiratory assistance may be needed because of the tendency to retain carbon dioxide. Intubation and mechanical ventilation may be initiated prophylactically because cardiovascular collapse occurs quickly with respiratory depression.
- A common complication is congestive heart failure. Diuretics and digoxin are used to treat this problem.
- Hypothermia is treated using core rewarming (e.g., warmed IVF, NG fluids, dialysis).

NURSING ALERT

External warming is avoided in the hypothyroid patient because peripheral vasodilation may produce cardiovascular collapse. Hypotension is a grave sign in hypothyroid patients.

Acute adrenal insufficiency/Addison's disease

Adrenal insufficiency is a devastating disease related to the effects of decreased glucocorticoids (energy availability), decreased mineralocorticoids (e.g., aldosterone) (dehydration), decreased androgens, and increased melanocyte-stimulating activity (hyperpigmentation). Rifampin, used to treat tuberculosis, may cause adrenal insufficiency.

SYMPTOMS
- General symptoms are fatigue, weight loss, dehydration related to nausea and vomiting, abdominal pain, and depression.

DIAGNOSIS
- Addison's disease may be caused by a primary adrenal problem or induced secondary to a hypothalamic or pituitary problem.
- ACTH levels will be low if a hypothalamic/pituitary problem exists.

- If cortisol production does not increase after administration of ACTH, an adrenal problem exists.

TREATMENT

- Hypovolemia and sodium depletion are treated with D_5NSS IV infusion. IV hydrocortisone is administered.
- Fludrocortisone is also administered to replace mineralocorticoids.

Cushing's disease

Cushing's disease is overproduction of cortisol as a result of overactivity of ACTH. Immune suppression resulting from cortisol overproduction increases the patient's risk for early death and masks signs of existing infection.

SYMPTOMS

- Obesity, hypertension, fatigue, abdominal pain, and osteoporosis are common symptoms.

DIAGNOSIS

- Urine-free cortisol test and measurement of the ACTH level are used to diagnose the disease.

TREATMENT

- Multiple medications are used in treating Cushing's disease (see Table 7-4). These medications have undesirable side effects and interfere with compliance.
- Surgery and pituitary irradiation may be used in some cases.

Syndrome of inappropriate secretion of (ADH) (SIADH)

SIADH is associated with lung cancer and central nervous system disorders.

SYMPTOMS

- Generalized edema with decreased urine output are frequent symptoms.
- Congestive heart failure and changes in level of consciousness are later signs.

DIAGNOSIS

- Thyroid and adrenal function are normal but serum osmolarity is decreased.
- Hyponatremia is present.

TREATMENT

- Fluid restriction is initiated.
- Demeclocycline is administered.
- Chemotherapy aimed at obliterating tumor/s may be indicated.

NURSING SURVEILLANCE

1. Monitor cardiac pattern and treat potentially lethal dysrhythmias (e.g., tall peak T waves indicating hyperkalemia, severe bradycardia, severe tachycardia).
2. Trend temperature. Administer antipyretics to decrease oxygen demands. Provide supportive warming in hypothyroidism. Beware of rapid rewarming and subsequent hypotension.
3. Monitor intake and output to determine renal response to volume replacement or diuresis.
4. Monitor level of consciousness as a result of increased susceptibility for cerebral edema from rapid reversal of hyperosmolar state.

EXPECTED PATIENT OUTCOMES

1. Temperature returns to normal.
2. Blood pressure and heart rate stabilizes.
3. Urine output is at least 30 cc/hr.
4. Glasgow coma scale score remains the same or improves.

DISCHARGE IMPLICATIONS

1. Patients on hormone replacement should be instructed to pay attention to signs of infection. Drug doses may need to be increased in cases of fever, diarrhea.
2. Dramatic changes in weight, the addition of other medications for other problems, and advancing age can alter dosage and should be reported to primary care provider.
3. In many cases of hormone replacement, dosage routines can be modified to fit patient response and comfort. For example, twice daily vs. three times daily dosage. Encourage patient to discuss dosage routines with primary care provider.
4. Patients taking steroids should be told to inform other physicians, dentists, etc., of their use before undergoing a procedure.
5. Patients with an endocrine disorder should wear a "Medic Alert" bracelet because changes in level of consciousness occur frequently; and some endocrine disorders are rare and may not be diagnosed by the care provider available during the acute crisis.

Addison's Disease

Patient should be furnished with a needle, syringe, and soluble corticosteroid preparation to use during an acute crisis when travelling to areas without easy health care access.

Diabetes

Diabetic patients generally will be discharged home after 4 hours of treatment if their pH is >7.35 and their bicarbonate levels are >20 mEq/L (1). Assure that the patient understands how to prevent dehydration. Have the patient demonstrate correct measurement of blood glucose and urine ketones using an appropriate device. Instruct the patient to either notify his/her primary provider or return to the ED if any of the following occur:

- Blood glucose level >250 mg/dl
- Urine ketones are positive
- Illness that lasts longer than 24 hours (2)

Instruct the patient on signs of hypoglycemia and hyperglycemia.

References

1. Fleckman A: Diabetic ketoacidosis, *Endocrinol Metab Clin North Am*, 22, (2):181-207, 1993.
2. Sauve D and Kessler C: Hyperglycemic emergencies, *AACN Clin Iss* 3:350-360, 1992.

TABLE 7-4 Drug Summary

Drug	Dose/Route	Use	Special considerations
Aminoglutethimide	1-2 g PO in divided doses	Cushing's disease	Causes rash, somnolence
Bromocriptine	2.5-15 mg PO	Cushing's disease	Causes nausea, headache, fatigue
Cyproheptadine	Up to 24 mg/day PO	Cushing's disease	Causes weight gain, somnolence
Demeclocycline	600-1200 mg/day PO	SIADH	Causes fever, headache, paresthesia
Fludrocortisone	50 mcg QOD —200 mcg/day PO	Addison's disease	Causes flushing, hypertension, headache
			Causes rash, itching
Hydrocortisone	In thyroid storm: 300 mg IVP followed by 100 mg q 8 hr IV	Thyroid storm, Addison's disease	
	In Addison's disease: -100 mg IV push followed by 100 mg q 6-8/hr IV		
Ketoconazole	600-1200 mg PO	Cushing's disease	Causes hepatotoxicity, nausea, and vomiting
Levothyroxine	500 mcg IV	Myxedema coma	Causes tachycardia, hypertension
Methimazole (MMI)	20 mg q 4 hr PO	Thyrotoxicosis	Causes nephrotoxicity and rash
Metyrapone	2-6 g PO	Cushing's disease	Causes nausea, headache, and rash
Mitotane	9-10 g PO	Cushing's disease	Causes vomiting
Potassium Iodide	1 g PO or NG or 5 drops q 6 hr	Thyroid storm	Do not give until new thyroid hormone synthesis has been blocked with MMI or PTU

| Propylthiouracil (PTU) | In thyrotoxicosis: 200-250 mg q 4 hr PO
In pregnancy: 300-450 mg PO
In thyroid storm: 1 g PO or NG tube | Thyrotoxicosis
Thyroid storm | Inhibits thyroid hormone synthesis and inhibits conversion of T_3 to T_4 |
| Sodium Iodide | 1-2 g IV over 24 hr | Thyroid storm | Do not give until new hormone synthesis has been blocked with MMI or PTU |

Environmental Conditions

Patty Sturt

E

TRIAGE ASSESSMENT

Common environmental conditions encountered in emergency department (ED) patients include heat-related, cold-related, and near-drowning emergencies. Depending on geographic location, other environmental emergencies can include high altitude illnesses; diving emergencies; venomous snake bites; arachnid envenomation; and bee, wasp, and red ant stings. The patient may present to triage with mild symptoms that progress quickly to life-threatening conditions. The following data can help to identify the type of environmental emergency and severity:

- Events and activities preceding and at time of onset of symptoms.
- Patient's age, weight, medical history, use of alcohol, and current medications. Infants and geriatric patients are highly susceptible to cold- and heat-related emergencies.

Alcohol and certain medications increase the risk of weather-related environmental emergencies.
- Weather conditions near or at time of onset of symptoms. This information may help in identifying cold- or heat-related emergencies.
- Recent animal bite or sting (suspect exposure to poisonous venom).

Vital Signs

- *Tachycardia and hypotension:* Tachycardia and hypotension may be related to a decreased circulating volume secondary to diaphoresis from a heat illness; cold diuresis from hypothermia; vasodilation from snake bite venom or anaphylaxis; or coagulation defects from pit viper envenomation.
- *Bradycardia:* Bradycardia may be related to myocardial depression secondary to hypothermia.
- *Fever:* Fever may be related to failure of the temperature regulatory mechanism in heat stroke.
- *Tachypnea:* Tachypnea is often related to acidosis and hypoxia, which may occur in heat stroke, animal envenomation, anaphylaxis, altitude illness, and diving emergencies.

General Observations
Respiratory distress
- Stridor, wheezing, and respiratory distress (suspect laryngeal edema and bronchospasm) may occur from anaphylaxis secondary to envenomation or from pulmonary edema secondary to near drowning.
Local skin changes
- Note the presence of localized erythema, ecchymosis, pain, and swelling (suspect bite or sting).
- Assess for the presence of red, painful skin areas (superficial reaction to an insect sting or bite).
- Note the presence of yellow waxy skin areas (suspect frostbite).
Diaphoresis
- Observe for presence of diaphoresis (suspect heat exhaustion or sympathetic nervous system [SNS] stimulation secondary to anaphylaxis).

Seizures

- Seizure activity may occur from brain hypoxia secondary to pulmonary changes from near drowning, diving, or high altitude emergencies.

FOCUSED NURSING ASSESSMENT

E

Nursing assessment should focus on oxygenation/ventilation, perfusion, and cognition.

Oxygenation/Ventilation
Airway

Stridor and/or wheezing may be present in anaphylaxis from animal envenomations, and in near drownings. The patient with a decreased level of consciousness is at risk for airway compromise.

Breath sounds

Wheezing and crackles frequently occur in near-drowning victims from alveolar-capillary membrane damage, decreased surfactant, and atelectasis. Crackles are present in high altitude pulmonary edema (HAPE), pulmonary edema from heat stroke, and air embolism in divers. Breath sounds will decrease in moderate-to-severe coral snake envenomation from respiratory muscle weakness and paralysis.

Heart rate and rhythm

Obtain apical pulse and place patient on cardiac monitor. Tachycardia is a common and early response to hypovolemia. Bradycardia, atrial fibrillation, ventricular fibrillation, and asystole are possible in hypothermic patients.

Blood pressure

Hypotension can become severe in anaphylaxis, heat stroke, and hypothermia. A doppler may be needed to obtain a blood pressure (BP) reading. Scorpion envenomation can produce hypertension (HTN) from stimulation of the adrenergic system with massive outpouring of catecholamines.

Peripheral circulation

Assess skin color, temperature, capillary refill, and peripheral pulses. Many environmental emergencies impair cardiac output from hypovolemia or vasodilation. Perfusion to the skin will be decreased as evidenced by pale and cool skin, delayed capillary refill, and weak peripheral pulses. In heat stroke the skin may be warm and dry. Assess perfusion of skin distal to areas with frostbite or edema from a venomous animal bite or sting.

Cognition
Level of consciousness
Increased intracranial pressure (ICP) from cerebral edema can occur in heat stroke, high altitude cerebral edema (HACE), arterial gas embolism from diving, near drowning cases, and hypoxic events. Increased ICP will be manifested by changes in level of consciousness and possible seizures.

Pupil size and reaction
Vasodilation and/or hypovolemia may impair perfusion to the brain. Assess pupil size and reactivity. Pupils are often fixed and dilated in severe hypothermia.

Risk Factors
Heat-related illnesses
1. Age: The geriatric population may have decreased functioning of the sweat glands and diminished cardiac reserves. Infants are unable to increase sweat gland activity for evaporation and heat loss.
2. Activity: Amateur athletes, military recruits, and laborers are prone to heat-related illnesses and often are not acclimated to the environmental conditions (5).
3. Environmental conditions: High heat, high humidity (decreases air evaporation so effective cooling is not maintained), closed work space, and occlusive clothing contribute to heat-related emergencies.
4. Medications: Phenothiazines (e.g., Sparine) impair hypothalamic function. Antihistamines and tricyclic antidepressants dull the sweating response. Beta-blockers decrease cardiac response to the increased body temperature. Cocaine and amphetamines stimulate the SNS and further elevate body temperature. Lithium, diuretics, and anticholinergic drugs have also been identified as risk factors associated with heat-related illnesses.
5. Past medical history/current illness: Status epilepticus generates a large quantity of heat from the intense muscle tension and activity. Alcoholism, obesity, and hyperthyroidism are other risk factors in heat-related illnesses.

Hypothermia

1. Age: Infants have a greater body surface area (BSA) for their weight, smaller amount of fat stores for insulation, and poor temperature-regulating mechanisms. The geriatric population may be less mobile and have chronic medical conditions. Geriatric individuals may not be able to sense cold well because of neuropathy and a decreased vasoconstriction response. Once stressed, geriatric individuals are unable to increase heat production.

2. Activity: Campers, hikers, and homeless individuals have greater exposure to environmental conditions associated with hypothermia and frostbite. Because of the high thermal conductivity of water, immersion can produce rapid hypothermia.

3. Environmental conditions: Wind speed above 5 MPH and exposure to an environment colder than one's body temperature is a basic requirement for hypothermia to occur (4).

4. Medications: Phenothiazines impair the ability to shiver. Barbiturates and other depressants decrease the victim's awareness of cold environments and may have vasodilatory effects. Ethanol is a major risk factor because of its central nervous system (CNS) depressant and vasodilatory effects. The vasodilation increases heat loss from radiation.

5. Past medical history/current illness: Hypothyroidism can depress core temperature and heat production. Hypoglycemia decreases ability to generate heat as a result of an inadequate supply of glucose to the CNS. Hypopituitarism and hypoadrenalism impair the body's ability to respond to a hypothermic state. Wernicke's encephalopathy and alcohol abuse cause decreased peripheral sensation and poor judgment that increase potential exposure times. Burn victims have greater evaporative loss.

6. Multiple injury: Victims of major trauma are at high risk for hypothermia from open wounds, cold intravenous fluids and blood products, unwarmed oxygen, and being exposed in an open treatment area.

Near drowning

Suicidal gestures, alcohol and/or drug use that impairs judgment, exhaustion, unsupervised children, reckless boating or water activities are risk factors for near drowning.

High altitude illness

High altitude begins at elevations above 8,000 feet. Ski enthusiasts and mountain climbers may be at risk for this illness. Plane passengers in pressurized cabins with preexisting hypoxia, cardiac, or pulmonary problems may have difficulty tolerating very high altitudes.

Diving illnesses

Inexperienced or exhausted divers, use of alcohol and/or drugs that impair judgment, and diving at depths of >33 feet are risk factors for diving illnesses.

Risk factors for various venomous animal bites and stings will be briefly discussed under collaborative interventions.

Life Span Issues
Children

1. Children younger than 4 years of age account for 40% of drownings (8).
2. Mortality from hypothermia is greatest in neonates.

Adults

1. Drowning is the fourth leading cause of accidental death and is second only to motor vehicle crash fatalities among males between the ages of 1 and 34 and females between the ages of 15 and 19 (7).
2. Hypothyroidism (a risk factor for hypothermia) is more common in women than in men.

INITIAL INTERVENTIONS

Regardless of the environmental condition, the following interventions should be considered.

1. Implement measures to maintain and protect the airway. These measures can include a chin lift–head tilt (if spinal trauma is not suspected), jaw thrust, nasopharyngeal airway, oropharyngeal airway if the patient is unresponsive or has no gag reflex, and/or preparing to assist with intubation. Have suction available to prevent aspiration.
2. Place the patient on a pulse oximeter to monitor oxygen saturation.
3. Initiate oxygen administration immediately if hypotension, tachycardia, or respiratory distress is present.
4. Initiate cardiac and blood pressure monitoring.
5. Seizures may occur with conditions that result in hypoxia. Utilize seizure precautions by padding side

rails, keeping side rails up at all times, and having suction equipment at the bedside.

6. Inform the patient of the plan of care. Patients with environmental conditions are often anxious and fearful.
7. Support edematous extremities for comfort.
8. Determine tetanus/diphtheria immunization status on any patient with altered skin integrity.

PRIORITY NURSING DIAGNOSES

Risk for ineffective airway clearance
Risk for impaired gas exchange
Risk for altered tissue perfusion
Risk for fluid volume deficit
Risk for knowledge deficit

◆ **Ineffective airway clearance** related to seizure activity.
   INTERVENTIONS
   • Techniques that can be used to maintain a patent airway include turning the head to the side to facilitate drainage, jaw thrust, suction, and insertion of a nasopharyngeal or oropharyngeal airway.

◆ **Impaired gas exchange** related to pulmonary edema or bronchospasms in near drowning, arterial gas embolism from diving emergencies, respiratory muscle paralysis from severe coral snake envenomation, or pulmonary edema from heat stroke.
   INTERVENTIONS
   • Assist with intubation as needed.
   • Administer 100% oxygen (see Chapter 17).
   • Anticipate need for arterial blood gases.
   • Monitor arterial blood gas results.

◆ **Altered tissue perfusion** related to severe edema with compression of neurovascular structures (from venomous bites), vasodilation, or coagulation abnormalities.
   INTERVENTIONS
   • Monitor amount of edema. Frequently assess pulses, capillary refill, color, sensation, movement, and pain distal to the edema.
   • Elevate the extremity.
   • Administer IV fluids and antivenin as ordered.

◆ **Fluid volume deficit** related to excessive diaphoresis, heat load, or inadequate fluid intake in hot/humid weather conditions.

INTERVENTIONS
- Oral balanced salt solutions can be administered if the patient is awake and alert.
- IV fluids should be given if the patient has a decreased level of consciousness or is hypotensive.

Knowledge deficit related to treatment of environmental condition and prevention of future occurrences.

INTERVENTIONS
- Keep the patient and family/friends informed of the treatment plan.
- Include information on prevention in discharge instructions.

PRIORITY DIAGNOSTIC TESTS

Arterial blood gases: Detects hypoxia and/or acidosis from hypothermia, heat stroke, near drowning, and arterial gas embolus.

Coagulation profile: Necessary in heat stroke and pit viper envenomation. Disseminated intravascular coagulation (DIC) may occur with these conditions.

Electrolytes and glucose level: Hyperkalemia and hypoglycemia occur in heat stroke. Baseline electrolyte levels are usually obtained on all patients with environmental emergencies.

Complete blood count: Obtained to assess white blood count, hemoglobin, and hematocrit levels. Hematocrit levels may elevate in heat-related emergencies. WBC may be elevated in reaction to a pulmonary inflammatory response.

Liver enzymes: These enzymes will be elevated in heat stroke.

Radiograph: A chest film may be ordered to assess lung fields for pulmonary edema. Pulmonary edema can occur in near drowning, heat stroke, and HAPE.

COLLABORATIVE INTERVENTIONS: CLINICAL CONDITIONS

Heat-Related Illnesses

There are a variety of clinical conditions that occur in heat illness. The symptoms appear as a result of the body's attempt to dissipate heat.

Heat cramps
SYMPTOMS
- Painful muscle spasms occur in heavily exerted muscle, most often the calves (12).

- Nausea occurs as a result of loss of sodium from sweating and salt-poor fluid intake.

DIAGNOSIS

- Diagnosis is based on history.
- Serum sodium level is often within normal range.

TREATMENT

- The patient should rest in a cool environment. An oral-balanced salt solution such as Gatorade is administered.
- Salt tablets are not recommended and may be dangerous for some patients.

Heat syncope

Fluid and electrolyte losses occur via sweating and there is shunting of blood to dilated peripheral vessels.

SYMPTOMS

- Headache, light-headedness, postural hypotension, and brief loss of consciousness may occur.

DIAGNOSIS

- Diagnosis is based on history and orthostatic vital signs.

TREATMENT

- The patient should rest in a cool environment.
- Oral salt solution is administered if the patient is not hypotensive.
- Modified Trendelenburg position (legs elevated) is the position of choice.
- Teach patient to avoid sudden or prolonged standing in a warm environment.

Heat exhaustion

Ineffective circulating blood volume caused by excess loss of body water and electrolytes from diaphoresis and inadequate fluid intake.

SYMPTOMS

- Headache, nausea, vomiting, malaise, thirst, tachycardia, anorexia, syncope, anxiety, slightly elevated temperature, cool/pale skin, hypotension, and diaphoresis may be present.

DIAGNOSIS

- Diagnosis is based on history.

TREATMENT

- The patient should rest in a cool environment. Oral hydration and/or IV fluids (NS, D_5NS of $D_5 \frac{1}{2}NS$ are frequently used).

Heat stroke

Heat stroke is a rare but life-threatening emergency.
Overexposure to high environmental temperatures,

especially when accompanied with high humidity and low-wind conditions, can impair the release of body heat and lead to an abnormal rise in body temperature. Temperature regulatory centers in the hypothalamus fail, which further increases body heat. Cellular breakdown begins and all organs can be affected.

SYMPTOMS

- Tachypnea, tachycardia, dysrhythmias, and hypotension may be present.
- The patient's skin may be warm and dry or clammy and diaphoretic.
- Confusion, decreasing level of consciousness, visual disturbances, seizures, decreased urine output, temperature ≥105° F, and pulmonary edema are additional signs and symptoms.

DIAGNOSIS

- Diagnosis is based on history and physical examination.

TREATMENT

- Airway, breathing, and circulation are supported. Intubation may be necessary.
- 100% oxygen is administered.
- The patient is placed on a cardiac monitor.
- Large bore IV.
- Fluid bolus of 200 to 300 cc if patient is hypotensive. Repeat as necessary.
- 50% dextrose IV push if decreased level of consciousness.
- Begin rapid cooling—ice packs to groin, neck, and axillae. Spray cool-to-lukewarm water over body. Place fans close to patient to facilitate evaporative heat loss. Place hypothermia (cooling) blankets over and under the patient. Cold saline peritoneal lavage may be used in refractory cases. Consider cold saline gastric lavage.

NURSING ALERT

Rapidly cool patient to 101° F. Once the temperature is 101° F, slow the cooling measures to prevent rebound hypothermia. Acetaminophen is not effective initially, since its use depends on a normal functioning hypothalamus. Shivering should be avoided, since it generates heat. Diazepam or lorazepam can be used to prevent or stop shivering. Thorazine is not recommended, since it is known to lower the seizure threshold and blood pressure. Continuously monitor temperature with a temperature-sensing urinary catheter or rectal probe.

E

Cold-Related Illnesses
Frostbite

Frostbite is tissue damage from cold. It can be superficial or deep.

SYMPTOMS

- Superficial frostbite produces redness followed by blister formation in 24 to 36 hours. Face, hands, and feet are commonly involved areas. Skin remains soft. Burning, tingling, and numbness may be present.
- In deep frostbite the skin may appear yellow and waxy. It may feel hard on palpation. The patient will complain of loss of sensation and a feeling of heaviness in the area. Edema may be present.

DIAGNOSIS

- Diagnosis is based on history and physical examination.

TREATMENT

- Warm soaks are applied or the affected area is immersed in warm water between 105°F and 115°F. Warming should continue for 20 to 40 minutes (9).
- Narcotic analgesics may be administered, since rewarming is usually painful.
- The area is gently dried after rewarming.
- A sterile dressing is applied to protect tissue.
- Blisters may be debrided.
- The area is elevated to prevent further swelling.
- Immunization status should be assessed.
- The tissue is handled gently because the frostbitten area will be fragile.

Hypothermia

SYMPTOMS

- See the box.

DIAGNOSIS

- Diagnosis is based on history, core temperature, and examination.

TREATMENT

- If intubation is necessary, it must be done gently to prevent unnecessary stimulation and the onset of

HYPOTHERMIA

Stage	Core temperature	Symptoms
Mild	90-95°F (32-35°C)	Tachypnea, tachycardia, ataxia, shivering, lethargy, confusion, occasional atrial fibrillation
Moderate	86-90°F (30-32.2°C)	Rigidity, hypoventilation, decreased level of consciousness, increased myocardial irritability, hypovolemia, blood sludging with metabolic acidosis, Osborne or J wave (positive deflection in the RT segment)
Severe	<86°F (30°C)	Loss of reflexes, coma, hypotension, acidosis, apnea, cyanosis, ventricular fibrillation, asystole

ventricular fibrillation. A good rule of thumb is to intubate the hypothermic patient as you would a patient with a possible cervical spine injury.
- Temperature is continuously monitored by rectal probe.
- IV access (two large bore) is initiated.
- Moderate-to-severe hypothermic patients should be protected from inadvertent rough handling. Aggressive handling may shunt acidotic, cold blood in the periphery to the core of the body.
- The patient is rewarmed by one or a combination of the following measures:
  Passive rewarming
- Results in spontaneous warming of the patient without use of additional heat beyond the patient's intrinsic heat production.
- Includes placing patient in a warm room, blankets, and preventing drafts.
- Used for mild hypothermia.

Active external rewarming

- Involves adding heat directly to the surface of the body.
- It includes heat packs, warming blankets, and overhead radiant warmers.
- External rewarming is used in mild and moderate hypothermia and in conjunction with active internal rewarming in severe hypothermia.

E

NURSING ALERT

Apply heat to the trunk of the body and not to the extremities. This will prevent vasodilation in the extremities that can result in hypotension and movement of acidotic, cold blood from the periphery to the core (6).

Active internal rewarming

- This is the most invasive method of treating hypothermia and provides the quickest rewarming times.
- It includes the following modalities: Application of warmed humidified oxygen, warmed gastric lavage, peritoneal lavage with dialysate warmed between 40.5°C and 42.5°C, closed pleural irrigation with warmed saline, and warmed IV fluids. Warmed IV fluids do not significantly raise core temperature but will prevent further heat loss.
- Active internal rewarming is used in moderate-to-severe hypothermia.

Near Drowning

Near drowning is defined as survival, at least temporarily, from submersion. Secondary drowning is death occurring minutes to days after the recovery. Near drowning can be categorized as wet or dry. Wet drowning indicates aspiration of fluid and occurs in 80% to 90% of submersions. Dry drowning accounts for 10% to 20% of cases. Dry drowning is defined as asphyxia secondary to laryngospasm (10). Near drowning from either fresh or salt water produces intrapulmonary shunting, decreased compliance, decreased functional capacity, pulmonary edema, and hypoxia.

SYMPTOMS

- Symptoms include shortness of breath, wheezing, crackles, altered level of consciousness, cardiac arrhythmias, chest pain, hypotension, and oliguria.

- Significant electrolyte imbalances do not occur in near drowning survivors.

NURSING ALERT

Cerebral edema can develop up to 24 hours after the insult. Frequent neurologic checks are necessary!

Initially the chest film may be normal. Pulmonary insufficiency related to pulmonary edema may not develop for up to 24 hours following the submersion. Frequent pulmonary assessments are a must (1)!!

DIAGNOSIS
- Diagnosis is based on history, symptoms, and chest films.

TREATMENT
- Maintain a patent airway.
- Administer 100% oxygen by nonrebreather mask.
- Assist with intubation if respirations are absent, minimal, the patient is comatose, and/or the patient is unable to maintain a PaO_2 of 60 to 90 mm Hg with high-flow oxygen by nonrebreather mask.
- PEEP may increase functional capacity of the alveoli.
- Bronchodilators are given to decrease wheezing.
- Prophylactic antibiotics (to prevent pulmonary infections) are not routinely used in near drowning victims.
- Insert urinary catheter to monitor urinary output.
- Anticipate need for osmotic diuretics if cerebral edema is suspected secondary to hypoxia.

NURSING ALERT

Always suspect the possibility of a cervical spine injury in a near drowning victim. Cervical spine injuries are a possibility with falls, diving, or skiing accidents.

High Altitude Illness

For most purposes, high altitude begins at elevations above 8,000 feet, the height at which most people's arterial oxygen saturation falls below 90% (13). In an unacclimated person, hyperventilation and increased erythropoietin secretion are insufficient to relieve the hypoxemia.

Acute mountain sickness (AMS)

Acute mountain sickness is a collection of symptoms brought on by acute exposure to high altitude.

SYMPTOMS

* Symptoms include headache, insomnia, anorexia, nausea, vomiting, dizziness, dyspnea, weakness, oliguria, cough, chest pain, difficulty sleeping, and/or peripheral edema.
* Symptoms peak 24 to 36 hours after onset and resolve over 1 to 4 days.
* Most cases are benign and transient.

High altitude pulmonary edema (HAPE)

High altitude pulmonary edema is a life-threatening form of altitude illness.

SYMPTOMS

* Symptoms include cough, dyspnea, wheezing, orthopnea, hemoptysis, tachycardia, tachypnea, and fever.
* Neck veins are usually flat and there is no hepatic engorgement.

High altitude cerebral edema (HACE)

High altitude cerebral edema is a life-threatening form of altitude illness that usually occurs at elevations above 12,000 feet.

SYMPTOMS

* Symptoms include severe headache, ataxia, altered mental status, vomiting, aphasia, seizures, and/or weakness of extremities.

DIAGNOSIS

* Diagnosis is based on history, examination, and symptoms.

TREATMENT

* Descent remains the definitive and most successful treatment for all forms of altitude illness. Even a 1,000 foot descent can result in reversal of mild-to-moderate symptoms.
* Mild AMS can be treated symptomatically with rest and supplemental oxygen.
* Other treatment measures include continuous positive airway pressure (CPAP), Acetazolamide (controversial), dexamethesone, diuretics, pulmonary vasodilators such as nifedipine, and analgesics to relieve the headache.

Diving Emergencies
Decompression sickness

As the depth and pressure increases during scuba diving, larger and larger amounts of nitrogen and oxygen dissolve in blood and tissue. Unlike oxygen, nitrogen is not metabolized by tissue and tends to accumulate. If ascent occurs too rapidly, nitrogen quickly escapes from the tissues as gas bubbles. It is the release of the gas bubbles and the site of release that determine the symptoms. Symptoms usually present on breaking the surface or within 4 hours of surfacing (3).

SYMPTOMS

- Symptoms include severe pain in or near joints, pruritus, rash, cough, dyspnea, chest discomfort, visual disturbances, weakness, vertigo, headache, aphasia, and coma.

DIAGNOSIS

- Diagnosis is based on history of diving and symptoms.

TREATMENT

- Place patient in left lateral decubitus position or supine with the head in neutral position.
- Administer 100% oxygen by nonrebreather mask.
- Follow ACLS protocols for dysrhythmias.
- Start one large bore IV with crystalloid infusion.
- Recompression is needed as soon as possible. Recompression is accomplished by the use of hyperbaric (high pressure) facilities or chambers (3).
- Patients with persistent symptoms may be treated with hyperbaric oxygen up to 7 days after the onset of symptoms.

Arterial Gas Embolism

If the breath is held on ascent or if air is trapped in the lung by bronchospasms during ascent, the volume of gas in the lung expands. When a pressure differential of 80 mm Hg is reached, air is forced from the alveoli through the pulmonary alveolar capillary membrane. This will result in air entering the interstitial space or arterial circulation. Embolized air bubbles transported by the arterial system may lodge in the heart, brain, or blood vessels (10).

SYMPTOMS

- Symptoms occur very rapidly and include decreased level of consciousness, seizure activity, blindness, confusion, headache, and paralysis.

- Symptoms of pneumothorax are shortness of breath, decreased breath sounds on affected side, and subcutaneous crepitus in chest and neck.

DIAGNOSIS
- Diagnosis is based on history and symptoms.

TREATMENT
- Administer 100% oxygen by nonrebreather mask.
- Assist with intubation if decreased level of consciousness or severe respiratory compromise.
- Start one large bore IV.
- Immediate recompression is a priority. Facilitate patient transfer to facility with a hyperbaric chamber.

Venomous Snake Bites

SYMPTOMS
- See box on p. 272.

DIAGNOSIS
- Diagnosis is based on the history, symptoms, and description of snake.

TREATMENT
- Measure circumference of bitten extremity.
- Immobilize extremity at or below the level of the heart.
- Remove any rings or constricting items from the involved extremity.
- Apply a compression dressing (over the bitten area) with an elastic wrap.
- Insert two large bore IVs.
- Anticipate the need for antivenin (Table 8-2) for those who experience moderate-to-severe envenomation.
- Administer oxygen by nasal cannula or mask.
- The performance of a fasciotomy is controversial in extremities with elevated compartment pressures. Many authorities are now becoming more conservative with the use of fasciotomy (2).
- Do not use ice.
- Incision and suction is not recommended in the ED.

Arachnid Envenomations

For symptoms and treatment, see Table 8-1.

DIAGNOSIS
- Based on history, description or physical characteristics of the animal, and patient's symptoms.

VENOMOUS SNAKE BITES

Pit vipers (rattlesnakes, cottonmouths, copperheads)

Characteristics: Pit midway between the eye and nostril on each side of the head; triangular shaped head; elliptic pupils; long, sharp, retractable fangs; single row of subcaudal plates

Venom: Primarily hematotoxic

Location: Found in every state but Maine, Alaska, and Hawaii; most common venomous snakes in the U.S.

Symptoms

- Fang punctures, edema, sharp, burning pain, and erythema of the site and adjacent tissues within 1-30 min of the bite. Edema may spread for 12-24 hr (2).
- Minimal envenomation may have regional lymphadenopathy and tenderness.
- Severe envenomation may be accompanied by hypotension and shock, paresthesias, anemia, DIC.

Coral snakes

Characteristics: Lack facial pits; black snouts; round pupils; broad bands of red and black, separated by yellow rings; short, fixed fangs

Venom: Primarily neurotoxic

Location: Arizona coral snake found primarily in Arizona and New Mexico. The eastern coral snake is found in North Carolina south to Florida and west through the gulf states to Texas (2).

Symptoms

- May be little or no swelling or pain immediately after the bite. Can be a delay of 1-5 hr before onset of systemic symptoms.
- Moderate envenomation: Fang punctures, minimal swelling; no complete respiratory paralysis.
- Severe envenomation: Complete paralysis within 36 hr after the bite.

From Gold BS, Barish RA: Venomous snake bites, *Emerg Med Clin North Am* 10(2):249-266, 1992.

TABLE 8-1 Arachnid Envenomations

Type	Location/Description	Symptoms	Treatment
Scorpion	Found mostly in the southwest U.S. (Arizona, New Mexico, and Texas).[*]	Intense pain with little or no erythema or swelling. One species (*Centruroides sculpturatus*) injects a lethal neurotoxic venom. Symptoms may include wheezing, stridor, profuse salivation, diaphoresis, confusion, seizures, hypertension, tachypnea, tachycardia.	Immobilize affected part. Do not apply a tourniquet. Antihypertensives. Ensure tetanus/diphtheria prophylaxis. Analgesic. Support ABCs.
Black widow spider	Common in California and other parts of the U.S. Usually found in outdoor buildings such as barns and under rocks. Black with red hourglass marking on abdomen.[*]	Venom is neurotoxic. Pain at the bite site may be sharp and stinging or resemble a light pinprick. Limb pain, local redness and swelling. Two tiny red marks may be present. Muscle spasms, headache, nausea, vomiting, hyperactive reflexes, ptosis, hypertension, diaphoresis, fever, seizures, shock.	100% oxygen/mask, IV access, diazepam and calcium gluconate (see Table 8-2) for muscle spasms. Antivenin (see Table 8-2) in seriously ill patient.[†] Immobilization of the limb and cool compresses. Avoid further trauma to area.
Brown recluse	Found in wood piles, attics, closets, and dark places. Found in southeastern, southcentral, and southwestern states. Light brown with dark brown violin shape on back.	Mild or no pain with bite, local edema, erythema, bleb formation, local ischemia. Severe ulcerative necrosis appears on third to fourth day. Fever, chills, malaise.	Determine tetanus/diphtheria immunization status. Antibiotics. Debridement of necrotic areas and sterile dressings.

[*]Allen C: Arachnid envenomations, *Emerg Med Clin North Am* 10(2): 269-297, 1992.
[†]Auerbach PS: Disorders due to physical and environmental agents. In Saunder CE and Ho MT editors: *Current emergency diagnosis and treatment,* 703-729, Norwalk, Conn, 1992, Appleton & Lange.

E

Bee, Wasp, and Fire Ant (Hymenoptera) Stings

These insects inject venom through a stinger connected to a venom reservoir (sac). Stings are common in summer months and usually involve the head, neck, and extremities.

SYMPTOMS

* Local reaction: Immediate pain at site of sting. Erythema, edema, and itching may be present.
* Systemic reaction: Hives, nausea, vomiting, conjunctivitis, rhinitis, facial swelling, abdominal pain, laryngeal edema (stridor), bronchospasms (wheezes), and anaphylactic shock (hypotension and tachycardia) may be seen in systemic reactions.

DIAGNOSIS

* Diagnosis is based on history of insect sting and symptoms.

TREATMENT

* Administer 100% oxygen by nonrebreather mask.
* Anticipate and prepare for a cricothyrotomy if severe stridor is present.
* Aerosolized albuterol or metaproterenol may be used for bronchospasms.
* Establish large bore IV access.
* Infuse normal saline or Ringer's lactate and administer fluid boluses as needed to maintain a systolic blood pressure of ≥90 mm Hg.
* Remove the stinger by scraping.
* Do not use forceps to grasp or pull the stinger out, since this may contract the venom sac and release more toxin (11).
* IV diphenhydramine (see Table 8-2) is often used in mild envenomations.
* For severe reactions, administer epinephrine (1:1000) subcutaneously, 0.3 ml in adults and 0.01 ml/kg in children (see Table 8-2).
* Hydrocortisone should be administered in severe cases (see Table 8-2).

NURSING SURVEILLANCE

1. Frequently assess airway patency, breath sounds, respiratory rate and pattern, skin perfusion, heart rate and rhythm, blood pressure, level of consciousness, and amount of edema in extremities.

EXPECTED PATIENT OUTCOMES

1. Patent airway.
2. Bilateral equal breath sounds with absence of stridor, wheezing, and shortness of breath.
3. Core body temperature between 97°F and 99°F.
4. Heart rate of 60 to 100 beats/min.
5. Absence of life-threatening dysrhythmias.
6. Systolic blood pressure of >90 mm Hg or at level needed to maintain adequate peripheral perfusion.
7. Normal mentation.
8. Urine output >30 ml/hr.
9. Decrease or no further progression of edema in extremities.

DISCHARGE IMPLICATIONS

Heat-Related Illnesses

1. Teach the need to increase intake of oral balanced salt solutions during hot, humid weather conditions.
2. Stress the need for frequent rest periods when participating in outdoor activities.

Cold-Related Illnesses

Frostbitten areas are very susceptible to further injury. Stress the importance of protecting the area from cold exposure and trauma. These patients may need to return to the ED or physician's office for dressing changes and reevaluation.

High Altitude Illness

Teach the need to gradually increase altitude. This is particularly important at elevations above 8,000 feet.

Diving Emergencies

Encourage divers to participate in certified diving programs and courses.

Near Drowning Emergencies

Teach parents the importance of constant and continuous monitoring of children near pools, ponds, lakes, and other areas with water or fluid.

Venomous Snake Bites

Stress the need to wear boots and pants during hiking or mountain climbing activities.

TABLE 8-2 Drug Summary

Drug	Dose/Route	Special considerations
Antivenin (Latrodectus mactans—black widow species antivenin)	Single dose of 6,000 U. Entire vial of antivenin (2.5 ml) is recommended for adults and children. IV—Each dose must be diluted with 2.5 ml sterile water for injection. Shake vial to dissolve contents completely. Further dilute in 50 ml of normal saline for injection. Administer over 15 min. Can be given IM.	Test for sensitivity to horse serum before using. Can do this with a skin or conjunctival test. • *Skin test:* Inject into the skin not more than 0.02 ml of the test material (1:10 dilution of normal horse serum in physiologic saline). *A similar injection of normal saline can be used as a control. Evaluate results in 10-20 minutes. An urticarial wheal surrounded by a zone of erythema is a positive reaction. • *Conjunctival test:* For adults instill into the conjunctival sac one drop of a 1:10 dilution of normal horse serum. For children, instill into the conjunctival sac one drop of a 1:100 dilution. Itching, redness, and tearing of the eye, usually within 10 to 30 minutes, is a positive reaction. Monitor vital signs closely, since acute anaphylaxis is possible.
Antivenin (Crotalidae) polyvalent (for treatment of envenomation caused by bites of pit vipers.)	Moderate-to-severe envenomation may require 30-150 ml (3-15 vials) depending on the severity and toxicity of the bite or bites. Infuse 5-10 ml IV over 5 min. If no reaction, the rest should be given over approximately 30 min to 2 hr.	Most effective within 4 hr of the bite and less effective after 8 hr. However, should be given even after 24 hr have lapsed. (see previous antivenin skin or conjunctival test (see previous antivenin drug) before giving the drug IV. Monitor closely, since acute anaphylaxis is possible.

Drug	Dose	Notes
Calcium gluconate (for muscle spasms associated with black widow envenomation)	Adult: 10% calcium gluconate, 1-2 ml/kg IV up to 10 ml per dose.† Do not exceed 2 ml/min.‡	For IV use only. Monitor for hypotension.
Dexamethasone (Decadron—used for AMS and HACE)	4-6 mg PO every 6 hr.§	—
Diphenhydramine (Benadryl—used for symptoms associated with stings)	25-50 mg IV or IM. IV—25 mg over 1 min or deep IM. Children 1 mg/kg	Drowsiness is a common side effect. Patient should not drive until effects wear off.
Epinephrine (1:1000) distress from anaphylaxis associated with stings)	Subcutaneously Adult: 0.3-0.5 ml. Pediatric: 0.01 mg/kg. IV Adult: 0.1 mg 0.1 ml diluted in 10 ml of normal saline§ IV—Administer over 10 min.	Administer with caution to the geriatric patient, those with cardiovascular disease, or hypertension. Cardiac arrhythmias are more likely to occur with these groups. Monitor patient for cardiac arrhythmias, chest pain, and hypertension.
Hydrocortisone (for severe reactions to hymenoptera stings)	100-250 mg or 2 mg/kg. IV—25 mg over 1 min.	Incompatible with aminophylline and Benadryl.

*Physician's Desk Reference, Medical economics, Montvale, NJ, 1995, pp 2643-2644.
†Allen C: Arachnid envenomations. *Emerg Med Clin North Am* 10(2): 269-297, 1992.
‡Gahart BL: Intravenous medications, St. Louis, 1994, Mosby.
§Auerbach PS: Disorders due to physical and environmental agents. In Saunders CE and Ho MT editors: *Current emergency diagnosis and treatment*, 703-729, Norwalk, Conn, 1992, Appleton & Lange.

References

1. Glankler DM: Caring for the victim of near drowning, *Crit Care Nurse* 13(4):25-32, 1993.

2. Gold BS and Barish RA: Venomous snake bites, *Emerg Med Clin North Am* 10(2):249-266, 1992.

3. Jerrard DA: Diving medicine, *Emerg Med Clin North Am* 10(2):329-340, 1992.

4. Jolly BT and Ghezzi KT: Accidental hypothermia, *Emerg Med Clin North Am* 10(2):329-337, 1992.

5. Merchandani H, Hameli AZ, Pressler R, Tobin JG, David JH and Melton V: Heat related deaths—United States, 1993, *JAMA* 270(7):810, 1993.

6. Michal DM: Nursing management of hypothermia in the multiple-trauma patient, *J Emerg Nurs* 15(5):416-421, 1989.

7. Neal JM: Near drowning, *J Emerg Med* 3:41-52, 1985.

8. Olshaker JS: Near drowning, *Emerg Med Clin North Am* 10(2):339-349, 1992.

9. Sheehy SB: Environmental emergencies, *Manual of emergency care*, St. Louis, 1990, Mosby.

10. Shinnick MA: Recognition of scuba diving accidents and the importance of oxygen first aid, *J Emerg Nurs* 20(2):105-110, 1994.

11. Sollars G: Thermoregulatory emergencies. In Kitt S and Kaiser J editors: *Emergency nursing*, 719-753, Philadelphia, 1990, WB Saunders.

12. Tek D and Olshaker JS: Heat illness, *Emerg Med Clin North Am* 10(2):299-309, 1992.

13. Tso E: High altitude illness, *Emerg Med Clin North Am* 10(2):231-245, 1992.

Extremity Trauma

Julia Fultz

TRIAGE ASSESSMENT

Musculoskeletal injuries are evaluated after airway, breathing, and circulation problems have been identified and treated. The only life-threatening injury associated with extremity trauma is hemorrhage that may be conspicuous or concealed internally. Hemorrhage is most frequently associated with pelvic, femur, and multiple fractures.

The goals of extremity injury management in the emergency department (ED) include the following.

- Hemorrhage control.
- Identification of vascular injuries before irreversible ischemia develops.
- Prevention of further tissue damage.
- Ensure peripheral perfusion.
- Reduction of pain.

Elicit a history from the patient. Family, friends, police, or emergency medical personnel may be able to provide valuable information.

1. *AMPLE* history (*A*llergies, *M*edications, *P*ast medical history, *L*ast meal, *E*vents preceding the injury).
2. Mechanism of injury to help predict injuries sustained.
3. Treatment before arrival at the hospital.
4. Any immediate or delayed dysfunction or pain experienced.
5. Prior history of musculoskeletal injury.
6. Before the event, did the patient use drugs or alcohol that may alter an assessment such as judgement of pain?
7. Tetanus toxoid history.
8. Advanced directives.

General Observations

- Expose the extremities and evaluate for hemorrhage that must be controlled by pressure dressings and/or pressure applied over the proximal artery (Figure 9-1). If an extremity cannot be exposed at triage for adequate assessment, the patient should be given priority for a treatment bed so the assessment can be completed.
- An initial assessment includes evaluation of the five P's that include pain, pallor, pulses, paresthesia, and paralysis. Compare the injured extremity with the noninjured extremity, if possible, and document findings.

Pain

Pain that is inconsistent with the extent of injury may indicate development of compartment syndrome. Pain distal to the level of the injury is uncommon unless there is neurovascular damage. Point tenderness may indicate an underlying fracture.

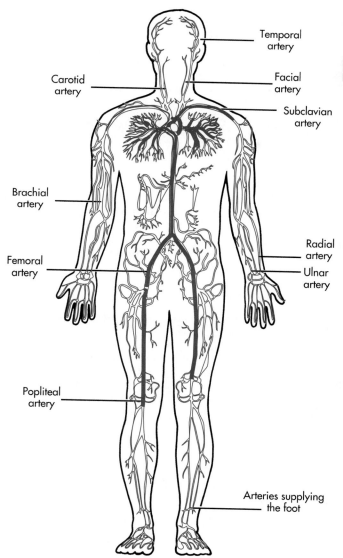

Figure 9-1   Pressure points for bleeding control.

NURSING ALERT

Compartment syndrome is a limb-threatening condition in which pressures in a muscle compartment rise high enough to interrupt the microvascular circulation causing ischemia and eventual irreversible tissue damage. Symptoms include severe progressive pain that does not parallel the injury sustained, pain on passive stretching of the muscle involved, tense swelling, and a diminished sensation to touch. It must be identified and treated swiftly. (See Compartment syndrome under Clinical Conditions.)

Pallor
Ischemia produces color and temperature changes.
Pulses
Pulses must be checked by palpation or by doppler if needed.
Paresthesia
Tingling or numbness is indicative of vascular and/or neurologic damage.
Paralysis
Indicative of neurologic injury.

NURSING ALERT

Vascular injuries associated with circulatory compromise pose an immediate or potential threat to extremity viability (2). The patient should be triaged directly to the treatment area. Pulses are the most important indicator of vascular injury (3); however, the presence of pulses does not rule out vascular injury (2) with some residual flow or compartment syndrome. Pulses must be reassessed at hourly intervals. An alert patient can be asked to inform the nurse if numbness or tingling develops in the extremity.

NURSING ALERT

Ten percent of the population lack one or both of the dorsalis pedis pulses (13).

- Note hematomas and document size.
- Note lacerations—evaluate depth, length, active bleeding, any blood around wound or soaked into clothing or temporary dressings.

- Note associated trauma such as angulations of the extremity, exposed bone, or damage to underlying structures.
- Place a clean, sterile dressing over open wounds. If the wound is actively bleeding, provide a pressure dressing. If the bleeding is pulsatile (indicative of arterial bleeding), hold a sterile dressing over the site, apply manual pressure, and triage the patient directly to the treatment area.
- Potential fractures should be immobilized if it has not already been done to prevent further tissue damage from the bone ends moving. (See Treatment under specific fractures for splinting techniques.) Angulated fractures and joints should be splinted as found during the triage assessment.
- Remove anything potentially constrictive from the injured extremity such as clothing, jewelry, or circumferential dressings.
- Ensure appropriate packaging of an amputated part (wrap in saline-soaked, sterile gauze, place in a plastic bag, and then place in a larger bag or container on top of a 50/50 mixture of ice and water) (2,15).

FOCUSED NURSING ASSESSMENT

It is imperative that assessments on multitraumatized patients begin with the ABCs and that life-threatening injuries are diagnosed and treated. Once identification and correction of these problems has been determined, a secondary assessment is performed and injuries involving the limbs and joints can be evaluated.

NURSING ALERT

In patients with injuries inclusive of lower extremity fractures, pelvic fractures, or multiple fractures, a sudden onset of shortness of breath may be caused by fat globules being released from the marrow into the circulation, then being trapped in the vascular bed of the lungs causing a fat embolism. Additional symptoms include a petechial rash, unexplained restlessness, pulmonary edema, or fever. Symptoms usually appear within 12 to 24 hours of the injury. Immediate immobilization of a fracture and limited movement of fractured bones help prevent fat embolism syndrome (14).

An examination of an extremity for injury, whether it is suspected or known to be injured, always involves exposure, inspection, and palpation of the extremity. Nursing assessment focuses on neurovascular integrity, mobility, and comfort.

Neurovascular Integrity

1. Inspect the exposed limbs for lacerations or avulsions. A laceration over a suspected fracture is treated as an open fracture until the assessment proves otherwise. Lacerations in close proximity to arterial pathways must be monitored for arterial bleeding (see Figure 9-1). Evaluate dressings for effectiveness in stopping any bleeding and reinforce the dressings as necessary.
2. Inspect hematomas, measure their size, and evaluate them for expansion.
3. Inspect each extremity for uniform color, mottling, cyanosis, and pallor, then compare extremities to each other.
4. Inspect for edema.
5. Evaluate extremity skin temperature. Note temperature by touch and compare extremities. Note temperature variances within the same limb.
6. Capillary refill in all extremities should be <2 seconds for pediatric patients and adult males. Adult female patients should have a capillary refill of <2.9 seconds and the geriatric patient <4.5 seconds (16).

NURSING ALERT

Capillary refill varies under certain circumstances. Environmental factors such as cold causes a delay in capillary refill as does certain medical conditions such as arterial insufficiency.

7. Palpate pulses in all extremities. Compare pulses distal to the injury to the pulses in the unaffected limb if possible.
8. Vascular injuries involving a suspected fracture must be immobilized and realigned followed by frequent assessment.

NURSING ALERT

Neurovascular compromise in the presence of an angulated fracture or joint dislocation often requires the knowledge and skill of an orthopedist. In the acute setting, there is a thin line between the decision to straighten an angulated fracture with neurovascular compromise and the decision to wait for more definitive care. Oftentimes fractures of joints involve associated dislocations and attempts to straighten an angulated fracture involving a joint without the benefits of radiologic evaluation and orthopedic consultation may worsen the injury beyond its original presentation.

9. Evaluate sensory function distal to the injury site.
   - *Touch:* Evaluate hypoesthesia (decreased sensitivity) and hyperesthesia (increased sensitivity) by touching the skin lightly with a fine wisp of cotton and differentiate between sharp and dull (use a sterile needle) or two-point discrimination.
   - *Proprioception:* Receptors respond to stretch, pressure, or position. Grasp the big toe or a finger and ask the patient to determine if you are moving it up or down. If patient is unable to determine, repeat with the ankle or wrist.
   - *Paresthesia (numbness and tingling):* Nerve involvement as a result of ischemia begins distally and travels proximally. Identify area of paresthesia and perform serial examinations.

Mobility

1. Loss of mobility can result from neurovascular damage as a consequence of trauma to tendons, ligaments, bone, muscles, or from pain.
2. Inspect the exposed limb for the following:
   - Abnormal angulations.
   - Shortening of the one extremity in comparison to the other.
   - External or internal rotation of an extremity.
   - Discolorations (erythema, ecchymosis, paleness, abrasions).
   - Edema.
   - Exposed bone, tendons, ligaments, or muscle.

3. Is there a limitation in the range of motion of the injured extremity?
4. Evaluate extremity muscle strength. Compare it with unaffected extremity if possible. Note any atrophy.
   • Can the patient raise the extremity without assistance?
   • Can the patient raise the extremity against gravity (dangle the leg over the bed or have the arm hang by the patient's side)?
   • Can the patient raise the extremity against resistance such as the examiner's hand?
   • Test flexion and extension by having the patient pull and push against the examiner's hand.
5. Palpate the extremity moving proximal to distal for tenderness, crepitus, and increased heat. If a fracture is known to be present, crepitus does not need to be purposefully elicited because of the additional injury that can result from the movement of the bone ends.

Comfort

1. The most reliable indicator of pain is the patient's own interpretation of what is being experienced (4).
2. Evaluate the following characteristics of pain:
   • *Location:* Generalized large area, localized small area, or a single point.
   • *Intensity:* The intensity of pain should be evaluated on a standardized scale that can be repeated to evaluate changes in level of pain such as a scale of "0" (no pain) to "10" (the worst pain possible) where the patient assigns the pain a number.
   • *Quality:* Prickling, burning, throbbing, aching, radiating.
   • *Onset:* Immediately after event or a delayed onset.
   • *Duration:* Continuous, steady, periodic, momentary.
   • *Variations:* What makes it worse? What makes it better?
3. Immobilization of the extremity frequently diminishes the amount of pain experienced by preventing bone ends from grating together when the muscle spasms.

Risk Factors

1. Repeated low intensity activity (joggers, dancers). Stress from repetitive activity is initially absorbed by muscles and soft tissue. As muscles begin to tire, more stress is

absorbed by the skeletal system that can lead to stress fractures, injured ligaments and joints (5).

2. Preexisting diseases that cause structural weakness of bones, joints, or muscles, such as osteoporosis, tumors, and Paget's disease.

3. High-risk sports activities such as skiing, rock climbing, motorcycle riding, or hockey.

4. Industrial/occupational work such as heavy machinery operator or a construction worker.

5. People of any age group in an abusive environment. Look for any injury to a limb that is incompatible with the explanation given for the injury, such as bruises at various stages of healing, inadequate care of a prior injury, bite marks, bilateral upper extremity bruising (from being held and shaken), or evidence of unset fractures.

6. In certain cases the existence of one type of fracture should lead the clinician to look for the presence of an associated fracture. The following are injury patterns common to specific fracture types (2):

   - *Fractures of the hip and pelvis:* Commonly associated with femoral shaft fractures.
   - *Patellar injuries:* May be associated with both a femur or tibial fracture.
   - *Calcaneal fractures:* Commonly the result of vertical deceleration injuries (fall). The transmission of force up through the body may lead to vertebral compression fractures.
   - *Suspected fractures of the radius and ulna:* May be associated with injuries to the elbow and wrist joints. The transmission of force may cause injury to the shoulder girdle.

Life Span Issues
Pediatric

1. Children who do not have completely developed motor skills are at an increased risk for injury.

2. A child's bones are more porous and more flexible than an adults, so children may sustain incomplete fractures (greenstick and buckle fractures).

3. The epiphyses are cartilaginous growth zones in children that can often be mistaken on radiographs for a fracture.

This area is relatively weak and separates before other structures are torn or broken (6). Fractures through the epiphysis with disruption of the growth plate can cause growth disturbances.

4. Fractures of the clavicles are the most prevalent of all pediatric fractures (17).

Geriatric

1. Geriatric patients who have decreased reaction times, decreased range of motion, decreased muscle strength, and problems with balance have an increased potential for injury.
2. Increased frequency of degenerative bone disease with advancing age increases the incidence of fractures.
3. Fractures may occur spontaneously in osteoporotic bone.
4. Geriatric patients are at an increased risk for pressure sores as a result of decreased mobility if bed rest is needed.

Pregnancy

The hormone relaxin causes the pelvic ligaments to loosen. This, along with a change in the center of gravity caused by the enlarged abdomen, predisposes the woman to loss of balance and falls, resulting in musculoskeletal injuries.

INITIAL INTERVENTIONS

1. Attend to any airway, breathing, or circulation problems.
2. Treat hemorrhage by direct pressure and pressure over the corresponding artery proximal to the injury.
3. Cover all open wounds with saline-soaked, sterile gauze.
4. Elevate injured extremities above the level of the heart to decrease edema unless compartment syndrome is suspected, then keep the extremity at the level of the heart to maximize tissue oxygenation.
5. Apply ice packs.
6. Immobilize suspected fractures. Include the joint above and the joint below the suspected fracture. Assess neurovascular function before, during, and after immobilization. (See Treatment under Specific Fractures for individual fracture immobilization techniques.)
7. Serial neurovascular checks.

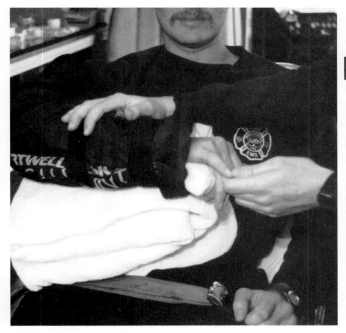

E

Figure 9-2 Vacuum splint.

NURSING ALERT

Never reposition or straighten an angulated joint fracture. Splint the extremity in the position in which it is found. A practical approach to splinting the angulated joint fracture is to use a conforming splint. An example of a conforming splint is the vacuum splint (Figure 9-2). The vacuum splint is unique because it is flexible until air is withdrawn from the device, which allows it to conform to the angulation. Then it becomes rigid, offering support to the extremity.

PRIORITY NURSING DIAGNOSES

Risk for fluid volume deficit
Risk for altered peripheral tissue perfusion
Risk for pain

Risk for impaired physical mobility
Risk for infection

◆ **Fluid volume deficit** related to fluid loss from fracture sites or amputations as evidenced by decreased capillary refill, elevated heart rate, hypotension, diaphoresis, tachypnea, altered mental status.

INTERVENTIONS
- Apply pressure dressings to active bleeding.
- Immobilize fractures to decrease blood loss from additional tissue damage.
- Insert two large bore IV catheters (14- to 16-gauge), attach to large bore trauma tubing with a maxi-drip chamber, and infuse crystalloid solution as ordered.

◆ **Altered peripheral tissue perfusion** related to neurovascular compromise as evidenced by decreased pulses, cool and/or pale skin, decreased motor and/or sensory function, and pain inconsistent with the extent of injury.

INTERVENTIONS
- Immobilization of injured extremity.
- Splint joint injuries and angulated fractures as found.
- Assess proximal and distal pulses every 30 to 60 minutes.
- Elevate extremity to promote venous return if not contraindicated as with compartment syndrome.

◆ **Pain** related to noxious stimuli from injury, tissue destruction, and invasive diagnostic procedures as evidenced by voiced complaints of pain, facial grimacing, skeletal muscle tension, irritability, restlessness, moaning, crying, anger, hostility, withdrawal.

INTERVENTIONS
- Immobilize fractures.
- Administer pain medication as ordered.
- Advise patient of what to expect with all procedures to be performed.
- Apply ice packs.
- Elevation of extremity if not contraindicated as with compartmental syndrome.

◆ **Impaired physical mobility** related to amputation, acute extremity pain, and extremity dysfunction as evidenced by difficulty walking, loss of manual dexterity, altered range of motion, paralysis, or paresthesia of extremities, verbalization of pain.

TABLE 9-1 Potential Local Blood Loss in Fractures

Injured area	Liters
Humerus	1.0-2.0
Elbow	0.5-1.5
Forearm	0.5-1.0
PELVIS	**1.5-4.5**
Hip	1.5-2.5
Femur	1.0-2.0
Knee	1.0-1.5
Tibia	0.5-1.5
Ankle	0.5-1.5
Spine/ribs	1.0-3.0

From Shires G: *Care of the trauma patient*, ed 2, New York, 1979, McGraw-Hill; Walt AJ, editor: *Early care of the injured patient*, ed 3, Philadelphia, 1982, WB Saunders.

INTERVENTIONS
- Immobilize fractures and splint joint injuries and angulated fractures as found.
- Administer pain medication as ordered.
- Serial evaluations for neurovascular compromise.
- Train for use of a mobility aid (crutches, walker, cane).

Infection related to altered skin integrity as evidenced by exposed underlying structures, gross debris, lacerations.
INTERVENTIONS
- Remove any gross debris gently; if resistance is met, discontinue.
- Cover any opening in the skin with a sterile dressing.
- Antibiotics as ordered.

PRIORITY DIAGNOSTIC TESTS

Hemoglobin and hematocrit: Used for those patients with fractures of the pelvis, femurs, or multiple fractures because of the potential blood loss (Table 9-1).

Type and crossmatch: Used for potential blood transfusion if significant blood loss from fractures is anticipated, or surgery to repair fractures.

Urine myoglobin: If severe muscle damage has occurred as in a crush injury or compartment syndrome.

Radiographs: Anteroposterior and lateral views to include the entire bone and both proximal and distal joints.

Arteriogram: Used to confirm or rule out a suspected vascular injury in the face of diminished or absent pulses.

CAT scan: Frequently used to identify acetabulum fractures and to evaluate the integrity of articulating surfaces such as the knee, hand, wrist, and ankle.

MRI: Identifies damage to bones, ligaments, cartilage, and menisci. This test is expensive and reserved for cases where the diagnosis is in doubt and treatment plan differs according to the test results.

COLLABORATIVE INTERVENTIONS
Overview

1. *Airway and breathing:* Be prepared to assist with the management of airway and breathing problems should they develop. Airway adjuncts and intubation equipment should be readily available.
2. *Oxygen:* Supply supplemental oxygen to avoid local tissue hypoxia in patients who are hypotensive, any multiple trauma patient who has fractures, any patient with multiple fractures, or those who have diminished or absent pulses to maximize tissue oxygenation. Monitor continuous pulse oximetry.
3. *Hypovolemia:* Crystalloid infusion via two large bore IV catheters (14 or 16 gauge, 1¼ inch long) attached to large bore tubing with a maxi-drip chamber. To increase speed of fluid administration, pressure bags may be applied. Be sure to eliminate air from the bag to prevent an air embolus. Do not use extension sets or stopcocks as both diminish fluid flow.
4. *Tetanus toxoid:* Administer PRN.
5. *Pain medication:* Administer as ordered.

Clinical Conditions
Fractures

The most significant skeletal injury that can occur is termed a fracture. In addition to the insult to the bone tissue, injury may occur to surrounding soft tissue, blood vessels, and nerves. Significant risk of complications such as infection are often associated with fractures involving major soft-tissue injury.

Fractures can be classified into two broad categories:

TABLE 9-2 Open Fracture Classification

Grade I	Small wound <1 cm long that has been punctured from below.
Grade II	Well-circumscribed wound up to 5 cm long with little or no contamination and no excessive soft-tissue damage or periosteal stripping.
Grade III	Wound >5 cm and is associated with contamination and/or significant soft-tissue injury (tissue loss, avulsion, crushing injury) and frequently includes a segmental fracture. Major vascular injury may be present or periosteal stripping.

Adapted from American College of Surgeons: *Advanced trauma life support,* student manual, ed 2, Chicago, 1993, The College.; Geiderman J M: Orthopedic injuries: management principles. In Rosen P, et al, editors: *Emergency medicine concepts and clinical practice,* ed 3, St Louis, 1992, Mosby.

Open fractures: Any fracture with an associated open soft-tissue injury. Open fractures can further be defined according to severity (Table 9-2).

Closed fractures: Any fracture without an associated open soft-tissue injury. The prognosis is generally better for closed fractures because of the limited risk of an infection occurring. Fractures are also classified according to their specific type, comminuted, compression impacted, greenstick, oblique, spiral, and transverse (Figure 9-3).

SYMPTOMS

- It is absolutely essential that a thorough mechanism of injury be obtained in order to identify potential orthopedic injuries that otherwise may be missed.
- The following symptoms are generally suggestive of a fracture. All need not be present to suspect a fracture (2).
- Pain at or around the site of injury.
- Swelling at or around the site of injury.
- Deformity of the extremity.
- Tenderness at or around the site of injury.
- Instability of the extremity.
- Crepitus (grating sound heard or felt when the ends of broken bones move together) on movement of the extremity.

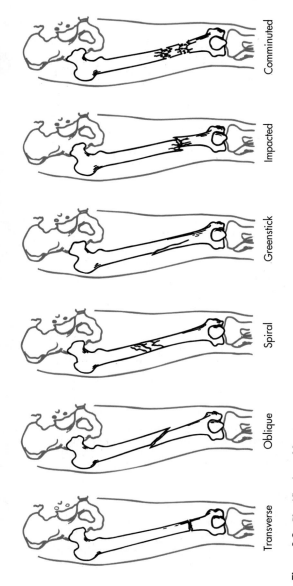

Figure 9-3 Classification of fractures.

Transverse Oblique Spiral Greenstick Impacted Comminuted

- Limited mobility and/or limited range of motion of the extremity.

> **NURSING ALERT**
>
> Signs and symptoms of extremity fractures are often grotesque in appearance. The site of a severely angulated fracture may lead to "tunnel vision." It is paramount to realize that fractures in general do not cause life-threatening situations, and that even though the injury may be "limb threatening," proper perspective and diagnosis/treatment of life-threatening injuries must take priority.

DIAGNOSIS
- The diagnosis of fractures is based on mechanism of injury, clinical presentation, radiographic studies.

Once diagnosed, certain orthopedic injuries can compromise organs, vasculature, and nerve networks. Generally, most orthopedic injuries involving the extremities are not life threatening, but the resulting trauma to body systems may be.

TREATMENT
The following list describes the priority of care for fractures:

Priority I
Suspected fractures of the vertebral column.

Priority II
Suspected fractures of the thoracic cage, pelvis, bilateral femurs, and head.

Priority III
Suspected fractures of the extremities (9).

Basic treatment of the fractured extremity involves:
- Control of hemorrhage with sterile pressure dressings.
- Manual immobilization.
- Cover open fracture wounds and exposed bone ends with saline-soaked, sterile gauze.
- Splint the injured extremity including the joint proximal and the joint distal to the injury.
- Apply ice packs.
- Elevation of the extremity above the level of the heart.
- Frequent evaluation of pulses.

In addition to general symptoms and treatments for fractures, specific extremity fractures may have distinct symptoms and treatment methods. These are described in this section.

Lower extremity fractures

Pelvic fracture: Usually the result of a great deal of force and represents a life-threatening injury resulting from hypovolemia (blood loss in excess of 4 liters may occur).

SYMPTOMS

- Pain when pressure is applied to the anterosuperior iliac crests.
- Impairment of distal circulation.
- Little external deformity may be present as a result of extensive overlying soft tissue.
- Blood at the meatus and blood on rectal examination. Rectal, urethral, and bladder injuries are complications of pelvic fractures.

TREATMENT

- Military antishock trousers (MAST) are used with low pressure (30 psi) to stabilize the pelvis. For use if a delay in definitive care is anticipated (such as a long transport), especially if hemodynamic instability is present. Some trousers have no air bladder in the posterior pelvis area. This may result in excessive pressure from the anterior compartment of the MAST and displace an otherwise stable fracture. MAST are often used in conjunction with a long spine board.
- Avoid unnecessary movement of patient.

Femur fracture: Bilateral femur fractures represent a life-threatening injury secondary to hypovolemia (blood loss in each femur may be as much as 2 liters).

SYMPTOMS

- Severe pain with midshaft femur fractures.
- Spasms of the quadriceps muscle as the result of bone ends overriding each other may cause extensive soft-tissue injury.
- Shortening of the affected extremity in comparison to the nonaffected extremity when parallel to each other.
- Distal femur fractures may involve the femoral or popliteal vessels causing diminished pulses.

TREATMENT

Principles of femur fracture management involve the use of a specialized splint called a traction splint. There are various types of traction splints currently available such as Thomas, Hare traction, Sager traction, each having their own unique application in the management of femoral fractures. Regardless of the brand of traction splint, the basic principles for its application are universal.

> **NURSING ALERT**
>
> Avoid the use of a traction splint if joint injuries are present on the ipsilateral side of the femur injury because further damage to the joint may result. The femur still needs to be immobilized using a nontraction splinting method such as a wire ladder splint or by securing the patient to a long board with necessary padding to stabilize the femur.

Knee fracture: Patellar fractures commonly occur with dislocations resulting from high-energy transmission (11) and may be associated with popliteal vessel injury. Direct transmission of force on the patella may result in a nondisplaced fracture (17).

SYMPTOMS

See Clinical Conditions, p. 293.

TREATMENT

- Do not attempt to straighten angulation of the knee. These fractures may coexist with dislocations.
- Immobilize knee fractures as found because of the proximity of joints both proximal and distal and the potential neurovascular compromise.

Air splint

For those devices that have zippers, apply by either slipping over the entire leg or by sliding it under the leg. As the name implies, the device is inflated by air until the splint is semirigid, but the clinician can easily place a finger in between the splint and the patient's skin. Use of the air splint requires detailed documentation of extremity assessment before its administration. Once the device is in place, assessment of the extremity is limited.

> **NURSING ALERT**
>
> Air splints can cause compartment syndrome (see section on Compartment syndrome).

Padded board splint, cardboard splint, ladder splints, velcro fastening splints

X-rays can be taken with air splints, board splints, and cardboard splints left in place. Ladder and velcro splints both have metal supports that interfere with visualization on radiographs.

Tibia and fibula fractures: Tibial and fibular fractures may occur together or independent of each other and are generally the result of a direct blow (e.g., pedestrian struck by an automobile). The tibia commonly fractures during falls because of its weight-bearing property.

SYMPTOMS

- Tibial fractures may remain "in line" if there is no insult to the fibula, however, weight bearing on the injured extremity is not possible.
- Proximal tibial fractures may be associated with the development of compartment syndrome. Evaluate for progressive pain that seems excessive in light of the injury sustained, such as tense swelling, diminished sensation, and weakness of the lower leg.
- Patients with a fibular fracture and a stable tibia may be able to place weight on the extremity. Posterior examination of the lower leg may reveal symptoms consistent with a fracture.

TREATMENT

- Splinting goals are aimed at providing stability while maintaining neurovascular function.
- At times, proximal tibial fractures may dictate the use of a traction device to reduce overriding bone ends, control internal hemorrhaging, decrease the possibility of compartment syndrome, and decrease pain (2,17).
- Any splint that immobilizes the lower leg can be employed. This is inclusive of the following splints:
1. Air splints
2. Ladder splints
3. Vacuum splints
4. Cardboard splints
5. Padded board splints
6. Velcro-fastened splints

Ankle fracture: Ankle fractures commonly exist with connective tissue injuries (ligaments).

SYMPTOMS

See Clinical Conditions, p. 293.

E

TREATMENT

- Fractures of the ankle may be accompanied by dislocations and attempts at reduction should be undertaken by a specialist.
- Immobilization of fractures of the "ankle" follow the same principles as immobilization of fractures involving joints. Immobilization of the ankle must be inclusive of the foot and the distal half of the lower leg.
- A common method of splinting the ankle is the use of a pillow splint. The pillow splint is a primitive but effective method to immobilize the ankle. It conforms to the ankle and elevates the foot, aiding in reduction of swelling to the joint. The pillow is placed under the ankle lengthwise and wrapped around the ankle. Triangular bandages are used as cravats to secure the device to the distal half of the lower leg and to the foot. Make sure the distal ends of the toes are exposed, so assessment of capillary refill and neurologic status of the extremity can be performed.

Foot fracture: Foot fractures are usually associated with dislocations and sprains, and it may be virtually impossible to differentiate the fractured foot from the sprained foot without the use of radiographs. Injuries secondary to axial loading may result in calcaneal (heel) fractures, and the energy may be transferred upwards resulting in spinal compression or burst fractures (2).

SYMPTOMS

See Clinical Conditions, p. 293.

TREATMENT

- Conforming splints such as the pillow splint or commercially designed splints specifically for application to the foot should be employed. Toes should be exposed as a means for continuous reassessment.

Upper extremity fractures

Scapula fracture: Suspect scapular fractures with significant soft-tissue injury to the shoulder and when the mechanism of injury suggests a high level of kinetic energy transmission. Scapular fractures mandate a careful evaluation for damage to surrounding structures because they are frequently associated with shoulder dislocations, pulmonary contusions, rib fractures with the potential for an underlying pneumothorax, vertebral compression fractures, and upper extremity fractures (1).

SYMPTOMS
- Patients frequently present with limited range of motion in the ipsilateral extremity.

NURSING ALERT

Life-threatening and limb-threatening injuries such as a hemothorax, pneumothorax, pulmonary contusion, or absent ipsilateral extremity pulses may be present with scapular fractures as a result of the blunt forces commonly associated with them. It is essential to exclude the possibility of these injuries early in patient management.

TREATMENT
- Rule out or treat potential life-threatening injuries.
- Application of a sling and swathe to immobilize the arm and shoulder, thereby decreasing movement of the scapula. The sling cradles the arm so the elbow is bent just under a 90 degree angle, thus preventing extension and to a certain extent, flexion. The swathe prevents abduction and adduction.
- If the sling is secured using a knot (such as with a cravat), tie the knot to one side of the neck to prevent discomfort.
- The swathe should be secured tightly enough around the ipsilateral arm and chest to prevent abduction. Both sling and swathe must be used together.
- Frequently assess neurovascular status.

Clavicle fracture
SYMPTOMS
- Often present with shoulder instability as a result of loss of support to the shoulder girdle.
- Frequently associated with neurovascular compromise. Examination distal to the injury is essential to ensure limb survivability (17).
- May be associated with pneumothorax, hemothorax, or brachial plexus compression.

NURSING ALERT

Clavicular fractures often cause damage to underlying structures such as the lung (pneumothorax, hemothorax), the subclavian vein, or the airway.

TREATMENT

- Rule out underlying structure damage.
- Treatment of clavicular fractures may include a figure-eight splint that takes the pressure from the rest of the shoulder girdle off the clavicle and maintains proper clavicular alignment.
- General procedure for application of the figure-eight clavicular splint.

1. With the patient erect, move both shoulders posteriorly as if standing "at attention." Pad areas of pressure.
2. Apply the splint while the patient maintains this position and tighten so the splint takes over the manual posterior action. See Procedure 27 for illustration of figure-eight splint.
3. Reassess the patient for airway and breathing compromise and neurovascular function.

Humerus fracture: Humeral fractures can be classified according to their anatomic location, proximal, shaft, and distal fractures. These fractures may be associated with damage to the brachial artery and damage to the radial, ulnar, and median nerves. Falls on the outstretched arm usually result in a spiral humeral shaft fracture, and direct blows usually cause a transverse humeral shaft fracture (17). Because of the anatomic location of the neurovascular bundles, suspected fractures of the distal humerus should have a thorough and documented neurovascular examination. Direct force to the olecranon process can result in indirect fractures to the distal humerus.

SYMPTOMS

See Clinical Conditions, p. 293.

TREATMENT

- Splint with a sling and swathe (see application description under Scapular Fractures).
- Proximal shaft fractures are splinted by applying the swathe using Velpeau's technique. Bring the lower arm up to an angle so that the hand of the injured extremity is in line with the opposite shoulder. This position allows relaxation of the pectoralis major.

Radius and ulna fractures

SYMPTOMS

- Concern for fractures near the elbow and wrist relate to neurovascular compromise and therefore require meticulous neurovascular evaluation and documentation.

- Colles' fracture is one of the more common fractures of the radius and ulna. It is commonly characterized as taking on a "silver-fork" type of appearance with the wrist turned up in relation to the radius and ulna.

TREATMENT

- Application of a rigid splint.
- When splinting for a Colles' or "silver-fork" fracture, utilize a conforming splint such as a ladder splint using roller gauze to pad void areas to provide stability.

Hand fracture: Fractures of the hand can have a devastating effect on the usage of the hand after injury. Position of the hand during injury is essential for the clinician to establish. This information may yield valuable insight to potential fracture sites, damage to tendons, and damage to the neurovascular system of the hand. An important aspect of potential hand fracture diagnosis is the conception of rotation. All parts of the hand must work together as one unit in order to provide optimal function.

SYMPTOMS

- Assess for rotational alignment. Normal rotational alignment occurs when the patient gently flexes the fingers in a loose fist and imaginary lines drawn down through the middle of the fingernail beds all meet in the area of the scaphoid. Digits may overlap if phalangeal or metacarpal fractures are present. Comparing the injured hand to the uninjured hand in this position also aids in this assessment (10).
- Frequently associated with soft-tissue injuries. Figure 9-4 lists anatomical landmarks useful in describing injury locations.

TREATMENT

- Remove rings promptly.
- Dress the soft-tissue injury appropriately.
- Place the hand in a position of function (fingers slightly flexed with the thumb abducted away from the palm), and place rolled gauze (kling, kerlex) in the patient's palm.
- Wrap the hand ensuring the fingertips are exposed for reassessment.

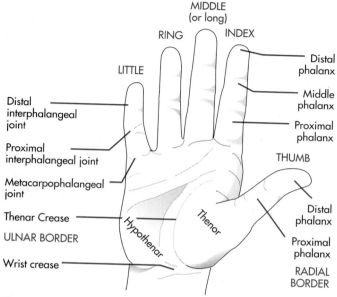

Figure 9-4 Volar view. Anatomical terminology useful in describing the hand.

- Apply a rigid splint or conforming splint taking care to place the splint distal to the wrist providing complete immobilization of the hand and preventing further injury.

Compartment syndrome

Compartment syndrome occurs when the pressure within a muscle compartment rises to a level that interferes with circulation and impairs the neurovascular integrity. Over a period of hours, the interstitial tissue pressures rise above that of the capillary bed, resulting in ischemia of nerve and muscle tissue. It most commonly results from edema or bleeding into the compartment space caused by a crushing injury, fractures, or prolonged compression of an extremity (from MAST, an automatic blood pressure cuff, or a cast or dressing that is too tight), burns (electrical or thermal), or bites (animal, human, snakes, spider) (2,8,12).

NURSING ALERT

Ischemia occurs within 5 hours (7) and irreversible damage occurs within 8 to 12 hours (13).

The most common sites include the following (Figure 9-5):
1. The four compartments of the lower leg.
2. The interosseous compartments of the hands.
3. Volar and dorsal compartments of the forearm.

NURSING ALERT

The most frequently affected compartment is the anterior compartment of the lower leg that is located lateral to the tibia.

SYMPTOMS
- Progressive and severe pain that is out of proportion with the underlying injury. Pain is aggravated by passive movement of the involved muscles.
- Diminished sensation to touch.
- Weakness of the involved extremity.
- Tense swelling.
- Pallor of the extremity (late sign).
- Loss of pulses (the cause of compartment syndrome occurs at the cellular level in the capillaries, so loss of pulses is a late sign if it is seen at all [18]).
- Delayed capillary refill (late sign).

DIAGNOSIS
- Clinical findings by examination.
- Direct compartment pressure measurement. Normal compartment pressure is <20 mm Hg. At 30 mm Hg, blood flow to the microcirculation is impaired (8). Tissue pressures >35 to 45 mm Hg are critical because of impairment of capillary blood flow (2).

TREATMENT
- Place the limb at the level of the heart.

NURSING ALERT

Do not raise the limb above the level of the heart because arterial and venous pressure, and therefore oxygenation of the tissue, could decrease further (7,18).

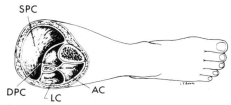

Four compartments of the leg: the anterior compartment (*AC*), the lateral compartment (*LC*), the superficial posterior compartment (*SPC*), and the deep posterior compartment (*DPC*).

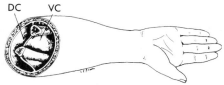

Two compartments of the forearm: the volar compartment (*VC*) and the dorsal compartment (*DC*).

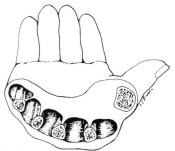

Five interosseous compartments of the hand.

Figure 9-5 Extremity compartments.

- Remove anything constricting the extremity (clothing, jewelry, cast material, circumferential dressings).
- Continue to monitor pulses, capillary refill, sensation, range of motion, skin temperature, pain.

- Subfascial injections of hyaluronidase. (Hyaluronidase affects the sheath of fibrous connective tissue that envelops each muscle by loosening collagen fibers. As the collagen fibers loosen, it allows fluid to pass through and decreases the intracompartmental pressure. These injections may need to be repeated [12,18]).
- Emergency fasciotomy of affected compartment.

Amputations

SYMPTOMS

- Amputations have the potential for major hemorrhage, however, in the complete amputation, bleeding is frequently controlled by arterial spasm and retraction or ordinary pressure applied to the stump (15).
- Obvious complete separation of the extremity or partial separation of extremity associated with no capillary refill, no sensation, no pulses, and no movement distal to the injury.
- Presence of vascular/neurologic function (capillary refill, pulses, sensation, movement) indicates an incomplete amputation.

> **NURSING ALERT**
>
> Differentiation must be made between the complete amputation and the incomplete amputation. If evidence of neurovascular activity is not present, the extremity distal to the injury should be treated as a complete amputation.

DIAGNOSIS

- Visualization of complete separation of the extremity at any level.
- Assessment to determine complete vs. incomplete amputation.

TREATMENT

- Two large bore IV catheters (14- or 16-gauge) 1¼ inches long should be placed in patients with a partial or complete amputation of an extremity.
- Pain management.
- Infection management includes antibiotics and tetanus toxoid. Wounds are usually tetanus prone, especially degloving and crushing injuries.

- Prepare to transport the patient with a complete amputation or partial amputation with neurovascular compromise to a reimplantation center.
  Complete amputation
Treatment involves two phases.
1. *The stump:*
- Apply direct pressure to control hemorrhage if needed.
- Remove gross dirt or debris by irrigation with Ringer's lactate or normal saline solution.
- Apply a sterile, moist dressing to the stump.
- Splint fractures.
- Elevation above the level of the heart.
- Monitor dressings for hemorrhage because active bleeding can be concealed.
- Volume replacement.
2. *The amputated part:*
- Rinse with Ringer's lactate or normal saline to remove gross contamination.
- Wrap the part in sterile, saline-soaked gauze and place in a dry plastic bag.
- Place the plastic bag with the amputated part in another plastic bag or larger container that contains equal parts of ice and water. The plastic bag with the part should rest on top of the ice water mixture. Ice and tissue should not come into direct contact. Cooling slows the chemical processes, and thereby increases viability and survival. Tissue tolerance of ischemia differs. Bone, tendon, and skin tolerates 8 to 12 hours of warm ischemia, 24 hours of cold ischemia. Muscle tolerates 6 hours of warm ischemia and 12 hours of cold ischemia (15).

NURSING ALERT

It is up to the surgeon who provides definitive care to decide if any, part, or all of the amputated part can be reimplanted. All amputated pieces and parts should accompany the patient to a reimplantation center.

Incomplete amputation
- Splint unstable fractures to prevent additional tissue damage.

- If no evidence of neurologic or vascular activity is found in the partially amputated extremity as determined by lack of pulses by palpation and doppler, and lack of motor movement and sensation, then cool the extremity(15). Cooling can be done with ice packs. Ice must not come into direct contact with tissue. The goal is to slow the chemical processes to increase viability of the tissue.
- If neurologic and/or vascular activity is present distal to the injury, then splint the extremity after applying dressings to the open wound.

Dislocations

Occurs when bone ends are displaced from the joints.

SYMPTOMS

- Pain to the joint area involved.
- Deformity of the joint.
- The extremity is "locked" in an abnormal position.
- Swelling of the joint.
- Complete loss of range of motion.
- Instability of limb if dislocation is accompanied by a fracture.
- Numbness, loss of sensation, and loss of pulses distal to the injury. (A dislocation can compromise the function of the arteries and nerves in close proximity.)

DIAGNOSIS

- Mechanism of injury.
- Clinical presentation.
- Radiographs.

TREATMENT

- Do not attempt to straighten any dislocated joint without radiographs and orthopedic consultation because straightening it may worsen the original injury.
- Immobilize the potential dislocation in the position found.
- Splint the affected extremity in the position found.
- Provide padding to fill void spots, and then take the weight off of the joint.
- Consider ice to reduce swelling in the joint area.
- Consider medication for pain control if not contraindicated by other injuries.

Sprains

A complete or partial tear of a ligament resulting from sudden stretching of the joint beyond normal range of motion.

SYMPTOMS

There are three grades of strains as follows:

Grade I

- Stretching or a small tear of the ligament.
- Minimal swelling, local tenderness.

Grade II

- Severe stretching and partial tearing of the ligament.
- Tenderness, edema, pain associated with weight bearing.

Grade III

- Complete disruption of ligaments.
- Joint may be obviously deformed.
- Marked tenderness and swelling.
- May be unable to bear weight.

DIAGNOSIS

- Radiographs

TREATMENT

Grade I

- Ice, elevation for 12 hours, a compression dressing, and light weight bearing.

Grade II

- Ice for 24 hours, immobilization if necessary, compression bandages, and light weight bearing with crutches.

Grade III

- Ice for 48 hours.
- Elevation and a compression dressing or cast for immobilization.
- Surgical repair may be necessary.
- No weight bearing.

Strains

Weakening or overstretching of a muscle where it attaches to a tendon.

SYMPTOMS

Mild strains

- Local pain, point tenderness, slight muscle spasm.

Moderate strains

- Local pain, point tenderness, swelling, discoloration, and inability to use limb for prolonged periods.

Severe strains

- Local pain, point tenderness, swelling, discoloration, and "heard a snapping noise."

DIAGNOSIS

- Radiographs

TREATMENT
Mild strain
- Intermittent cold pack, elevation above the heart and a compression bandage.
- Light weight bearing.

Moderate strain
- Cold packs for 24 hours, elevation above the heart, a compression bandage, light weight bearing only, and analgesics.

Severe strain
- Cold packs for 24 to 48 hours, elevation above the heart, a compression bandage, no weight bearing for 48 hours, and analgesics.

NURSING SURVEILLANCE

1. Monitor for airway and breathing problems in patients with fractures of long bones, the pelvis, or multiple fractures.
2. Monitor for continued hemorrhage and hypovolemia.
3. Evaluate hematomas for expansion.
4. Evaluate pulses.
5. Monitor skin color, temperature, and capillary refill.
6. Monitor sensory function distal to the injury.
7. Evaluate effectiveness of pain control.
8. Evaluate the effects of splint and traction splint application.
9. Monitor for fat embolism in patients with long-bone fractures, pelvic fractures, or multiple fractures.

EXPECTED PATIENT OUTCOMES

1. Neurovascular status does not deteriorate.
2. Patient reports a decrease in pain.
3. Hemorrhage is controlled.
4. Open wounds are protected from further contamination.
5. No further tissue damage occurs.
6. Alert patient verbalizes an understanding of procedures to be performed in the ED.
7. Patients with open fractures that require operative intervention (open pelvic, femur fractures) undergo surgery within 6 hours.
8. Patients with fractures that benefit from operative intervention undergo surgery within 24 hours.

References

1. Ada JR, Miller ME: Scapular fractures. Analysis of 113 cases, *Clin Orthop*, 269:174-180, 1991.

2. American College of Surgeons: *Advanced trauma life support*, student manual, ed 2, Chicago, 1993, The College.

3. Bowman, DA: Orthopedic and vascular emergencies. In Lee G, editor: *Flight nursing principle and practice*, St Louis, 1991, Mosby.

4. Christoph SB: Pain. In Kinney MR et al, editors: *AACN's clinical reference for critical care nursing*, ed 2, New York, 1988, McGraw-Hill.

5. Foss J: Orthopedic injuries. In Fincke MK, Lanros NE, editors: *Emergency nursing: a comprehensive review*, Rockville, Md, 1986, Aspen Publishers.

6. Geiderman JM: Orthopedic injuries: management principles. In Rosen P, et al, editors: *Emergency medicine concepts and clinical practice*, ed 3, St Louis, 1992, Mosby.

7. Gluchacki BK: Recognizing compartment syndrome, *Nursing 91* 21(10):33, 1991.

8. Good LP: Compartment syndrome: a closer look at etiology, treatment, *AORN J* 56(5):904-911, 1992.

9. Grant HD, Murray Jr, RH, Bergeron JD: *Emergency care* ed 6, Englewood Cliffs, NJ, 1991, Prentice Hall.

10. Overton DT, Uehara DT: Evaluation of the injured hand, *Emerg Med Clin North Am* 11(3):585-600, 1993.

11. Porter RS: Musculoskeletal injuries. In Porter RS, et al, editors: *Paramedic emergency care*, Englewood Cliffs, NJ, 1991, Prentice Hall.

12. Proehl JA: Compartment syndrome, *J Emerg Nurs* 14(5)283-290, 1988.

13. Proehl JA: Mobility. In Neff JA, Kidd PS, editors: *Trauma nursing*, St Louis, 1993, Mosby.

14. Reed LJ, Keegan MJ: Fat embolism syndrome: a complication of trauma, *Crit Care Nurs* 13(3):33-38, 1993.

15. Schlenker JD, Koulis CP: Amputations and replantations, *Emerg Med Clin North Am* 11(3):739-753, 1993.

16. Schriger D, Baroff L: Defining normal capillary refill: variations with age, sex, and temperature, *Ann Emerg Med* 17:932-935, 1988.

17. Simon RR, Koenigsknecht SJ: *Emergency orthopedics: the extremities*, ed 2, Norwalk, Conn, 1987, Appleton & Lange.

18. Syle DA: Orthopedic complications. Compartment syndrome, fat embolism syndrome, and venous thromboembolism, *Nurs Clin North Am* 26(1):113-132, 1991.

Eye Conditions

Mark Parshall

CLINICAL CONDITIONS
Chemical Burns
Noncorrosive Chemical Exposures
Open or Ruptured Globe and Impalement Injuries
Central Retinal Artery Occlusion
Amaurosis Fugax
Retinal Detachment
Hyphema
Orbital Blowout Fracture
Eyelid Lacerations
Iritis and Iridocyclitis (Anterior Uveitis)
Acute Glaucoma
Periorbital Cellulitis
Superficial Injuries
Ophthalmic Shingles (Herpes Zoster)
Conjunctivitis
Hordeolum (Stye)

For purposes of this chapter, eye conditions are organized according to the degree of risk for permanent visual impairment, rather than according to whether their etiology is traumatic or nontraumatic.

OCULAR ANATOMY

A detailed description of the anatomy and physiology of the eye is beyond the scope of this chapter, but a brief summary is necessary to clarify the risk of visual impairment associated with various conditions.

The interior of the globe is divided into aqueous and vitreous compartments. The vitreous compartment is bounded anteriorly by the back of the lens (3) and contains a clear, colloidal gel called vitreous humor. It is lined by the retina, a continuation of the optic nerve. The retina extends in all directions, lining the entire vitreous compartment including the posterior aspects of the ciliary body and iris (19). The choroid is a thin pigmented, vascular layer sandwiched between the retina and sclera. The sclera is the fibrous outer shell of the globe. It is continuous with the outer sheath of the optic nerve posteriorly and with the cornea anteriorly (3).

The aqueous compartment contains aqueous humor and is separated from the vitreous compartment by the lens and its suspensory ligaments (19). The aqueous compartment is divided into anterior and posterior chambers. The anterior chamber is bounded anteriorly by the cornea and posteriorly by the visible surface of the iris (3,19). Aqueous humor is secreted by cells in the ciliary body (7) and drains via the canals of Schlemm, which are located in the anterior chamber angle, near the corneoscleral junction (19). The posterior chamber is bounded anteriorly by the back of the iris and ciliary body and posteriorly by the front of the lens and its suspensory ligaments (Figure 10-1) (3*). The uveal layer of the eye consists of the iris, the ciliary body and muscle, and the choroid (3). The corneoscleral margin is called the limbus.

TRIAGE ASSESSMENT

NURSING ALERT

- True eye emergencies are those for which immediate triage to the treatment area and immediate intervention are necessary to preserve vision and are accorded a triage priority second only to immediate threats to life.
- True eye emergencies include: (1) corrosive chemical burns from acids, and alkali, (2) ruptured globe and penetrating ocular injuries, and (3) abrupt onset visual loss (e.g., central retinal artery occlusion).

---

*Reference 26 has a diagram (p 312) that incorrectly labels the vitreous compartment as the "posterior chamber filled with vitreous humor." A similar diagram, with the same error, can be found in the TNCC manuals through the 3rd edition, and in the slides for the TNCC Provider course (cf., Reference 13, pp 138-9). The vitreous, sclera, choroid, retina, and orbital portion of the optic nerve are collectively called the posterior *segment* of the eye (i.e., *not* the posterior chamber, which is entirely within the aqueous compartment).

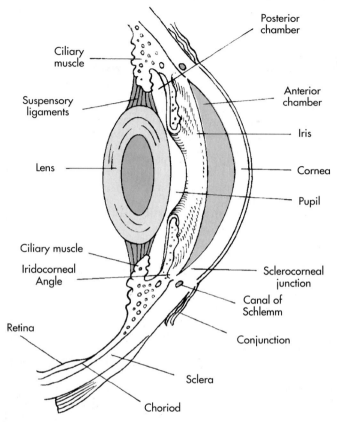

Figure 10-1 Occular anatomy.

Chemical burns

In the case of corrosive, acid, or alkaline chemical burns, high-volume irrigation, preferably with an eye shower, should begin immediately. Assessment of visual acuity should be deferred. It is acceptable at this stage to assess motion perception or light perception, but no time should be lost before commencing irrigation. If there is any doubt as to the corrosiveness or pH or a chemical injury, it is safest to presume in favor of immediate, high

volume irrigation during which time consultation with a
poison center may take place.

Open globe injuries/Ocular impalement

Treatment for an open globe should not be delayed for
visual acuity testing; determination of light perception or
hand motion perception, if any, is sufficient initially. (In
a majority of penetrating ocular injuries, initial visual
acuity is hand motion perception or worse [22]). The
patient should be brought to an acute treatment area
immediately. If possible, the head should be elevated.
No attempt should be made to assess ocular motility.
Topical anesthetics should never be administered if an
open globe is suspected. The injured eye should be
shielded at the earliest opportunity (see Initial
Interventions).

Sudden, atraumatic visual loss

A patient with sudden, atraumatic loss of vision should be
brought to an examination area for immediate
examination and treatment. The patient can be
screened in the treatment area for light perception and
consensual response.

NURSING ALERT

* Except in the case of true eye emergencies, triage assessment
  should note gross appearance of the eyes, any obvious differences or abnormalities of the globe, pupils, anterior chamber, iris, lens, lids, or periorbital tissues. Visual acuity, ocular
  motility, the severity and quality of pain, and pattern of redness should be noted.
* The patient with unequal pupil size or reactivity should be
  asked about any history of previous eye injury or surgery. If
  there is no history that accounts for the inequality, the
  patient should be assigned a higher priority.
* Depending on the amount of pain and usual and current
  waiting times for urgent problems, it is often necessary to
  raise eye conditions to a higher triage category.
* It is prudent to assign a greater urgency to any eye problem if
  it occurs in the better eye of a patient with useful vision in
  only one eye, or in an eye that previously has had surgery or
  significant injury.

Eye pain

* Pain from uveal structures (e.g., in iritis or acute glaucoma) is generally unilateral and deep. It may be described as a boring or aching sensation or as a headache behind or in the affected eye (9,21). This type of pain is not relieved by topical anesthetics, and, in general, the patient with this pain should be accorded a higher priority than one in whom pain is relieved by a topical anesthetic.
* Corneal pain is typically described as burning or searing (8,9). Pain resulting from corneal abrasion is generally described as a scratching, foreign body sensation. Pain resulting from corneal injury is promptly relieved by topical anesthetics.
* Pain resulting from conjunctivitis may be described as burning or itching.

Redness

* Redness associated with anterior uveitis—iritis or iridocyclitis—is often characterized by a "ciliary flush," a circular band of deeper redness at the corneoscleral limbus (8,11,17,21). In general, a ciliary flush indicates a more urgent condition than does diffuse injection.
* Redness (injection) from corneal injury or conjunctival inflammation or infection is diffuse with no ciliary flush.
* Conjunctival edema (chemosis), as well as injection, may be present in conjunctivitis. Table 10-1 summarizes common presentations of the painful and/or red eye in order to facilitate triage.

FOCUSED NURSING ASSESSMENT

Visual Acuity (Va) Testing

Depending on the layout of the emergency department (ED), it may not always be feasible to conduct a full Va examination in the triage area. Emergent problems that carry an immediate threat to vision can usually be identified in triage without a complete Va examination. However, all patients with eye complaints must have a Va examination of each eye separately and both together at the earliest feasible time (15,18). Assessment may be via a standard eye chart (at 20 feet), or a handheld card (at 14 inches). Patients with glasses or contact lenses should have their Va tested as corrected, if feasible. Except in cases of

TABLE 10-1 Triage of the Painful, Red Eye

Problem	Pain onset	Quality	Redness	Discharge	Other	Category
Noncorrosive chemical	Immediate	Intense burning	Diffuse	Watery, unilateral or bilateral	Unilateral or bilateral; blepharospasm	Urgent
Corneal foreign body (FB)	Immediate, progressive worsening	Scratching, FB sensation	Diffuse, but may have localized intensity	Tearing, watery usually unilateral	Usually unilateral; blepharospasm	Urgent
Hyphema	Immediate, progressive worsening	Dull, pressure (boring)	Blood in anterior chamber, +/- ciliary flush	+/-	Unilateral; often with periorbital hematoma; Lethargy	Urgent
Acute (angle closure) glaucoma	Gradual	Dull, like headache or pressure	Diffuse, often with ciliary flush; steamy cornea	+/-	Headache, nausea/vomiting scotoma, pupil dilated or midsized, possibly sluggish	Urgent
Anterior uveitis (iritis, iridocyclitis)	Gradual	Dull, intense, boring	Ciliary flush	Profuse tearing; usually unilateral	Pupil constricted, photophobia; usually unilateral	Urgent

Corneal abrasion	FB sensation that may have improved before worsening	Intense, burning	Diffuse, may have localized intensity	Tearing, watery; unilateral	Unilateral; blepharospasm; eye rubbing	Nonurgent as long as FB no longer present
Actinic keratitis (UV exposure)	Gradual onset, 8-12 hr after welding or sunlight exposure	Searing, burning, bilateral very intense	Diffuse, bilateral	Tearing, watery; usually bilateral	Photophobia, eye rubbing	Nonurgent
Conjuntivitis	Gradual	Burning, +/– photophobia. Itching (allergic)	Diffuse, unilateral or bilateral	Allergic— watery; viral—mucoid; bacterial— purulent	Chemosis, blepharospasm, possible fever; URI angioedema	Nonurgent
Subconjunctival hemorrhage	Usually painless	If pain present, consider other cause	Bloody, often localized	None	Usually asymptomatic, unless other problem present	Nonurgent

From Lawlor MC: Common ocular injuries and disorders, *J Emerg Nurs* 15:32, 1989; Miller SJH, editor: *Parson's diseases of the eye*, ed 18, Edinburgh, 1990, Churchill Livingstone; O'Brien JM, Albert DM, Foster CS: Anterior uveitis. In Albert DM, Jakobiec FA, editors: *Principles and practice of ophthalmology: clinical practice*, Philadelphia, 1994, WB Saunders; and Wagoner MD, Sadun AA, Beinfang DC: Acute disorders of the eye. In May HL, et al. editors, *Emergency medicine*, ed 2, Boston, 1992, Little Brown.

FB, Foreign body.

E

suspected penetrating trauma to the globe, it is acceptable, under physician order or written protocol, to administer a topical anesthetic before Va testing.

Each eye should be tested separately before testing consensual (OU) vision. It is helpful to adopt a standard sequence for conducting a Va examination usually OD, OS, OU (13,18). In conditions that affect one eye predominantly, it is acceptable to test either the "good" eye or the "bad" eye first. Some nurses feel it is best to start with the bad eye to prevent the patient from memorizing the chart (18). The author's preference is to start with the "good" eye first, since this is less stressful to the patient; memorization can be inhibited by having the patient start on a different line of the chart for each eye. It is important to reassure the patient that the purpose of the Va examination is to establish a baseline for subsequent examination or follow-up; a change from the patient's normal Va does not necessarily mean permanent impairment.

Documentation should include the best line the patient can discern with each eye and both together, whether or not corrective lenses were used, and the time at which the examination was performed. Missed letters/symbols on a line the patient is otherwise able to read can be indicated by a minus sign after the Va (e.g., OD: 20/40-2). If Va is <20/200 in either eye, the patient should be assessed for finger counting, hand motion perception, and light perception.

Risk Factors

1. *Occupation:* A high proportion of serious eye injuries are due to occupational activities, and could be prevented by use of protective eyewear (6,23,24). Twenty to twenty-five percent of all penetrating eye injuries are work-related (2). The highest-risk occupations are construction, auto repair, and agriculture (2,23,24). Approximately 15% of persons with serious work-related eye injuries have a history of prior on-the-job eye injury (2,24). Activities such as grinding or hammering may generate enough force to cause a shrapnel to penetrate the globe.

2. *Sports:* Recreational and sports activities are associated with hyphema, retinal detachment, and globe rupture (23,24,28). Risk of injury is not reduced by the skill or

experience of the individual, but can be sharply reduced with proper protective eyewear and headgear (24,25).

3. *Vehicular collisions and interpersonal violence:* Vehicular collisions are another common cause of eye injury, both minor and serious. Use of restraint devices reduces the risk of eye injury (23,24). Eye injuries resulting from intentional battery are among the most common seen in the ED. A much higher proportion of serious eye injuries resulting from vehicular collisions and fights are alcohol related (6,22). Risk of serious eye injury is increased if an orbital or midfacial fracture is present (12).

4. *Gender:* Males are two to six times at greater risk for eye injury across all ages (6,24). The highest incidence of eye injury is among young adult males, which reflects an aggregated risk from occupational and recreational causes, vehicular crashes, and battery (2).

NURSING ALERT

Anyone with a history of eye surgery or prior significant eye injury has a higher risk for serious ocular injury for any given energy level or mechanism of injury (12,14,24).

---

5. *Past medical history:* Anyone who has suffered a hyphema has an increased lifetime risk for developing glaucoma in that eye (27).

Iritis is commonly idiopathic but may be related to trauma or a wide variety of autoimmune, infectious, granulomatous, or neoplastic processes including juvenile rheumatoid arthritis, ankylosing spondylitis, Crohn's disease, Reiter's syndrome, Sjögren's syndrome, sarcoidosis, herpes, cytomegalovirus, syphillis, tuberculosis, chlamydia, leukemia, lymphoma, and malignant melanoma (21). Recreational nasal cocaine use has also been reported as a cause (31).

Life Span Issues
Children

Young children, especially toddlers, are relatively uncoordinated, lack judgment about hazards, and have developmental need to explore their world, thus, they have an increased risk of eye injury (10,23,24,25). Inadequate adult supervision is commonly related to pediatric eye injury. BB gun and fireworks injuries often cause devastating eye injury in children (9). Eye injuries are also commonly seen in cases of child abuse, and may be related to direct blows or shaking. Intraocular or retinal hemorrhage from head trauma in children are uncommon, except in child abuse (10,11).

Conjunctivitis may occur in any age group, but viral and bacterial conjunctivitis are far more prevalent in small children, probably related to droplet transmission and hand-to-face contact with inadequate handwashing (15,30).

Geriatric

Adults over the age of 65 have an increased risk of eye injury because of diminished visual and auditory acuity and changes in coordination and reflexes (20). Falls are the most common cause of serious eye injury in the geriatric patient. This increased risk may be related to the prevalence of prior eye surgery in the geriatric patient (14).

Glaucoma is most commonly a disease of the geriatric population but may occur in younger persons, particularly if hyphema or iritis is present, or there is a past history of eye injury or eye surgery. Central retinal artery or vein occlusion is also more common in the geriatric population but may occasionally occur as a complication of certain types of eye surgery. Giant cell arteritis (which can cause blindness) is primarily a disease of persons over 60 years of age (1).

INITIAL INTERVENTIONS

1. *Removal of contact lenses:* Patients who are alert and oriented generally prefer to remove their own lenses. If the patient does not have a lens holder, the lenses should be covered in plain sterile saline in separate, labeled (Left & Right) sterile containers. If the patient is unable, or too distressed, to remove the lenses, they can be removed by means of a small suction cup or manually. To remove hard lenses manually, the lids are opened beyond the margins of the contact lens and then closed with gentle, digital pressure that should pop the lens off the ocular surface. Soft lenses can be removed by gently pinching up the soft lens itself; the eye should be moist before removal.

NURSING ALERT

Topical anesthetics and fluorescein should not be instilled if contact lenses have not been removed.

E

2. *Eye irrigation:* Irrigation of one or both eyes is commonly performed. Except in corrosive chemical injuries, the eyes should be anesthetized topically before commencing and at intervals as needed (see Table 10-3). An eye fountain (eye shower) is preferred for rapid decontamination of chemical injuries. Irrigation (a minimum of 1 to 2 L) may also be performed with IV normal saline or Ringer's lactate via irrigating lenses (Morgan Lens) or manually via standard drip IV tubing (see Procedures). Small foreign bodies and fluorescein stain may be irrigated out with a small volume of ophthalmic irrigant such as Eye Stream.

3. *Eye shielding:* An open globe injury or hyphema should be protected by securing a metal or plastic eye shield or a disposable cup over the injured eye as soon as possible. The purpose of the shield is to prevent further injury as a result of rubbing or inadvertent contact, and to reduce stimulation from light or movement. The shield should be taped lightly to the adjacent skin in a manner that does not exert pressure on the injured eye. The unaffected eye should be patched lightly to reduce consensual movement in the injured eye.

4. *Comfort measures:* Patients with suspected iritis, glaucoma, hyphema, retinal detachment, or whose complaints involve photophobia should be placed, if possible, in an examination room that is quiet and can be darkened.

Patients with corneal injuries or conjunctival inflammation may have anesthetic drops administered while awaiting examination if standing protocols exist or if the nurse obtains an order. Inappropriate, excessive use of topical anesthetics can cause corneal injury and delay recognition of a worsening condition. Therefore patients are never discharged with topical anesthetics for self-administration. However, serial doses at appropriate intervals may be administered safely while the patient is in the ED.

PRIORITY NURSING DIAGNOSES*

Risk for acute visual impairment
Risk for visual impairment or loss
Risk for pain
Risk for fear
Risk for anxiety
Risk for impaired tissue integrity
Risk for infection
Risk for injury

♦ **Acute visual impairment† or loss** related to injury or impaired ocular perfusion.

♦ **Risk for visual impairment or loss**
  RISK FACTORS
  * Penetrating, chemical, or high-energy blunt mechanism of injury
  * Previous eye injury or eye surgery
  * Age (<10 years old or >65 years old) (10,12,14)
  * Nonuse of safety equipment (e.g., goggles, helmet, or vehicle restraints)
  * Increased intraocular pressure
  * Inflammatory or infectious precesses of the cornea or interior structures
  * Knowledge deficit‡

♦ **Pain** related to injury, inflammation or infection.

♦ **Fear** related to visual impairment or loss, pain, or circumstances surrounding injury.

♦ **Anxiety** related to potential decreased independence or interference with usual activities.

---

*Due to the variety of specific eye conditions, nursing diagnoses in this chapter are stated in terms of related factors or risk factors. Interventions are discussed under Clinical Conditions.

†The NANDA-approved nursing diagnosis "Sensory-Perceptual alteration: visual" is extremely broad, and subsumes problems as diverse as hemianopia, diabetic retinopathy, and visual hallucinations (16). To be meaningful, a nursing diagnosis should be stated at the level of specificity appropriate to the circumstances. The primary concerns in emergency care are limitation or prevention of visual impairment.

‡Due to the complexity of individual patient circumstances, it is more helpful to consider "knowledge deficit" a risk factor related to anxiety, compliance, functional outcome, and potential for recurrent injury, than as a nursing diagnosis for which the intervention is merely to dispense information.

◆ **Impaired tissue integrity** related to surface trauma, inflammation, or infection.
◆ **Risk for infection**
RISK FACTORS
- Corneal injuries
- Penetrating injuries
- Infectious lesions of the lids or periorbital tissues (e.g., shingles)
- Inadequate handwashing/infection control behaviors (e.g., conjunctivitis)
- Contact lenses (e.g., bacterial corneal ulcers)
◆ **Risk for injury**
RISK FACTORS
- Impaired visual acuity
- Impaired depth perception resulting from patching
- Risk-taking behavior/nonuse of protective eyewear
- Previous eye injury or eye surgery
- Knowledge deficit

PRIORITY DIAGNOSTIC TESTS

Slit lamp examination: A slit lamp (biomicroscope) is a binocular microscope that is used to diagnose anterior chamber inflammation/injury or depth of corneal injury. The patient must be cooperative and able to sit up for a slit lamp examination.* Children and toddlers usually need to be held in a parent's lap to accomplish the examination.

Direct ophthalmoscopy: Direct ophthalmoscopy examination is used to diagnose conditions of the vitreous compartment and retina, as well as intraocular manifestations of other conditions (e.g., papilledema).

Tonometry (Schiøtz or applanation): Normal intraocular pressure (IOP) is 12 to 21 mm Hg. IOP can be measured by any of several applanation tonometry devices or a Schiøtz tonometer. Before tonometry a topical anesthetic should be administered and the patient should be instructed not to rub the eye. Applanation tonometers, such as on a slit lamp, measure pressure directly and are most accurate. Fluorescein should be administered before

---

*For bedside examination, a Wood's lamp and magnifying loupe may be used.

the examination. Several handheld applanation tonometers are currently available that are more accurate, though more expensive, than a Schiøtz tonometer for beside use.[†] A Schiøtz tonometer measures pressure indirectly by displacement of a weighted plunger that moves an indicator needle along a calibrated scale. A conversion table, based on the plunger weight and scale reading, is necessary to determine the IOP in mm Hg. An applanation tonometry cone can be decontaminated by soaking for 10 minutes in a 1:10 bleach solution after which it should be rinsed off, blotted dry, and replaced. A Schiøtz tonometer can be swabbed off and decontaminated in its own sterilization unit. Department policies should indicate whether tonometer decontamination is a physician or nursing responsibility.

Fluorescein staining for Cobalt blue, Wood's lamp, or slit lamp examination. Fluorescein dye has increased uptake in an area of corneal defect (e.g., abrasion, keratitis). Fluorescein strips are preferred to drops for infection control reasons. A drop of topical anesthetic is placed on the end of the strip, the lower lid is retracted, and the strip is touched to the palpebral conjunctiva.

Plain radiographs: Plain films are helpful in the diagnosis of some orbital and midfacial injuries, but CT scan is more definitive.

CT scan: Computed tomography is preferred for complex facial injuries, orbital cellulitis, or suspected optic nerve trauma.

Cultures: Conjunctival cultures are helpful in cases of rapidly progressing conjunctivitis, or chronic conjunctivitis that has been refractory to treatment (30).

COLLABORATIVE INTERVENTIONS

Eye Patching

Patching keeps the lids shut over the cornea so that lid movements do not interfere with corneal reepithelialization. Before patching, any fluorescein in the eye should be irri-

---

[†]A Perkins tonometer (Midwest Ophthalmics, 1237 Naperville Dr., Romeoville, Il 60441; 1-800-831-1194) uses the same kind of cone as a slit-lamp tonometer. A Tono-Pen (Mentor O & O, 3000 Longwater Dr., Norwell, MA 02061; 1-800-927-0250) has single-use disposable tips and does not require fluorescein instillation.

gated out. Antibiotic ointment is commonly ordered prophylactically. A double-patch technique is used. The first patch
should be folded in half and placed on the closed eyelids. A
second patch (or more if the eye is deep set) is placed flat on
top of the folded patch. The patch is taped obliquely from
the forehead to the cheek with sufficient tension so that the
patient cannot open the eyelids beneath the patch. A prefab-
ricated plastic and foam patch that is secured by elastic
straps (Press-Patch) is an acceptable alternative. A patch
should be left in place for approximately 24 hours. A follow-
up examination in the ED or with an ophthalmologist
should be arranged to document evidence of healing or to
determine the need for further consultation. The patient
should be instructed not to drive while the eye is patched
because of diminished depth perception. Reading and
watching television should be discouraged while the eye is
patched because scanning movements of the unaffected eye
elicit consensual movements of the affected eye. Patients
with corneal injuries may also require oral narcotic pain
medication and the appropriate precautions for same. An
infected eye should not be patched because of the risk of
worsening infection or corneal ulceration.

Expediting Treatment, Consultation, and Transfer

Early nursing recognition (i.e., during triage or initial
assessment) of presentations likely to require ophthalmologic
or other specialty consultation expedites consultation and,
when indicated, transfer. Any of the true eye emergencies will
require immediate consultation or transfer. Less emergent
presentations that generally require urgent consultation or
transfer include hyphema, retinal detachment, corneal or
sceral lacerations, complex lid lacerations (e.g., disrupting a
lid margin or canthal region), orbital cellulitis, ophthalmic
shingles, and blowout fractures. Assuring that legal requirements for interfacility transfers are followed is a patient-
advocacy, as well as a medicolegal issue for emergency nurses.

Clinical Conditions
Chemical burns
SYMPTOMS

- The principal symptoms of a corrosive chemical burn to
  the eye(s) are severe, burning pain, rapid onset of visual

impairment, inflammation and swelling of the lids, and severe chemosis of the eye(s).
- Corneal haziness or opacification may be evident (29).

DIAGNOSIS

- Initial diagnosis of a chemical burn is presumptive, based upon symptoms, and known or suspected exposure.
- Common acids include sulfuric acid (car batteries), hydrochloric acid (drain openers), and muriatic acid (swimming pool chemical).
- Common alkali include lye (drain openers, oven cleaners), lime (plaster, concrete), and ammonia (29).
- Some detergents used for restaurant or institutional dishwashing contain bleach or alkaline corrosives; if constituents are not immediately known, they should be presumed corrosive.

TREATMENT

- If the chemical is in powder or crystalline form, it should be rapidly, but gently brushed from the ocular region and face before irrigating.
- Initial decontamination should employ whatever method of irrigation that achieves the highest volume in light of concomitant injuries (e.g., an eye shower would not be feasible for an unconscious patient, or if a cervical spine fracture has not been ruled out).
- Strong acids cause coagulation of proteins with which they come into contact, which limits the depth of injury (29). (An exception is hydrofluoric acid that burns more deeply than other acids) (8,11,29).
- Strong alkaline chemicals cause liquefaction of proteins with which they come into contact, and as such have a tendency to penetrate through to the anterior chamber where they can damage the iris, ciliary body, and lens (29). Therefore, alkaline ocular exposures often need a longer period of irrigation than acids.
- The patient with a chemical burn should be attended continuously during irrigation to provide emotional support and assure the adequacy of irrigation.
- Irrigation should be continued for as long as it takes to get the conjunctival pH to normal range (7.4-7.6) (11).
- The pH is tested by retracting the lower lid gently and touching a test strip to the conjunctiva (much in the manner of a fluorescein strip).

- After initial decontamination, anesthetic drops may be instilled as needed until the irrigation and initial examination are complete.
- The pH should be retested several times after irrigation to make sure the pH is not changing.
- Some particulates (e.g., plaster and concrete powders) may embed in the lids or conjunctival fornices and cause ongoing release. Fine forceps debridement of such particles by the physician may be necessary (29).
- Cycloplegic agents are generally ordered to reduce pain from ciliary spasm. Topical steroids are helpful in this setting, but should only be administered on the recommendation of the ophthalmologist (8,29).
- Acetazolamide (PO or IV) or topical beta-blockers may be ordered after irrigation to decrease intraocular pressure (29).
- Topical antibiotics and patching are commonly ordered.
- Systemic narcotic analgesics are often necessary (11).
- Tetanus prophylaxis should be administered if indicated.

Noncorrosive chemical exposures

Symptoms

- Other chemicals are painful, and irritating to the eyes, but less likely to cause permanent visual impairment.
- Symptoms generally include burning pain, blepharospasm and tearing.
- Visual acuity may be unaffected, or mildly diminished.
- Hyperemia (injection), but not chemosis, is usually present.

Diagnosis

- Common noncorrosive exposures involve petroleum distillates, alcohol-based products, and detergents. Even though, theoretically, the triage classification of noncorrosive chemical exposures is at a less emergent level, as a practical matter, the pain and emotional distress they cause often necessitates emergent treatment.

Treatment

- Again, if an eye shower is available, it is the best method of initial decontamination, followed by Morgan Lens irrigation.
- The physician may order a topical antibiotic and patch, as in a corneal abrasion or actinic injury.

On occasion, a patient may present who has gotten super glue in the eye that can cause the lids to adhere together. Usually this can be manually debrided by the physician.

Open or ruptured globe and impalement injuries

SYMPTOMS

- Signs of an open globe may include enophthalmos, proptosis (globe protrusion resulting from retrobulbar hemorrhage), obvious asymmetry of the globe, iridodialysis or pupil herniation (disruption of the iris at, respectively, the ciliary or pupillary margin), complete ("eight ball") hyphema, severe chemosis, and extrusion of aqueous or vitreous humor.
- Symptoms include severe pain and sudden, severe visual impairment or loss in the affected eye (22,28). Small, intraocular foreign bodies may be attended by more subtle visual impairment.

DIAGNOSIS

- The diagnosis of an open globe is primarily based on gross appearance, history, and mechanism of injury.
- Intraocular pressure may be decreased below 10 mm Hg.
- Intraocular metal or glass foreign bodies can be diagnosed radiographically.
- CT scanning is helpful to determine whether or not the optic nerve has been severed.

TREATMENT

- Open globe injuries should be covered with a metal or plastic eye shield or a paper cup (11).
- The unaffected eye should be patched or shielded to reduce consensual movement (5,11).
- Tetanus and preoperative antibiotic prophylaxis are indicated.
- If the patient presents with an impalement of the globe or orbit, manual stabilization of the impaling object should be immediate.
- As soon as concomitant threats to ABCs have been ruled out, or as they are being treated, dressings may be applied to stabilize the object in a manner that does not put pressure on the object or the globe.
- Removal should only be undertaken by the appropriate surgical specialist in the operating room.

Central retinal artery occlusion
SYMPTOMS
- Central retinal artery occlusion (CRAO) is a sudden, painless, unilateral visual loss caused by an embolus lodging in the central retinal artery.
- A sign of this condition is an absent direct, but normal consensual light reflex in the affected eye (8).

DIAGNOSIS
- The diagnosis is based on patient description of sudden onset unilateral visual loss that did not resolve within a few minutes of onset associated with characteristic funduscopic findings (e.g., an edematous, pale-milky retina with a "cherry red" fovea.)
- If the visual loss is associated with head pain, migraine, or temporal (giant cell), arteritis should be considered.
- If visual loss is bilateral, cerebrovascular disease or methanol ingestion should be considered (15).

TREATMENT
- With prompt recognition and treatment, a small percentage of patients can have useful vision restored, but salvage is rare after 2 hours from onset. Therefore this is a true ophthalmic emergency.
- If carbogen gas (95% O_2 + 5% CO_2) is available, it can be administered as a vasodilator for three 10-minute intervals with 5 minutes off between administrations.
- Otherwise, rebreathing into a paper bag may raise the patient's P_{CO_2}.
- Firm ocular massage through closed lids may be performed by the physician for 3 to 4 seconds with abrupt release of pressure in an attempt to dislodge a thrombus (8).
- Anterior chamber paracentesis, a pinhole puncture of the cornea at the limbal margin with a hypodermic needle or no. 11 scalpel blade may also be attempted (8). The purpose is to extrude a small amount of aqueous humor thereby suddenly lowering intraocular pressure.

Amaurosis fugax (fleeting blindness)
SYMPTOMS
- *Amaurosis fugax* is a transient, painless unilateral loss of vision ("transient monocular blindness"), most commonly related to ipsilateral carotid stenosis or microemboli.

- The patient describes a sensation of a curtain descending, then being raised (1).
- Unlike central retinal artery occlusion, there is spontaneous improvement, generally within minutes of onset.
- Unlike migraine, it is generally painless and not associated with fortification spectra (the scintillating, zig-zag scotoma of classic migraine) (1).

DIAGNOSIS
- The diagnosis is based on the rapid onset and resolution of the episode, and by funduscopic examination.

TREATMENT
- Amaurosis fugax is a symptom, not a disease. In essence, it is a visual TIA, and indicates the patient needs to be evaluated for the underlying cause, most commonly ipsilateral carotid disease.
- In patients with carotid stenosis, there is an increased risk of stroke, though not as great as with hemispheric TIAs.
- Noninvasive carotid flow studies may be ordered or scheduled, and the patient may be started on one 325 mg ASA q day (1).
- Vascular and ophthalmologic consultation or referral are indicated.
- Other, less common causes of transient, monocular blindness (e.g., giant cell arteritis) may call for different workups (e.g., an erythrocyte sedimentation rate for screening purposes) and referral (1,15).

Retinal detachment
SYMPTOMS
- Retinal detachment may be due to trauma or to degenerative changes associated with aging.
- It is painless and gradual in onset, unless associated with acute injury.
- The classic symptom description is clouded vision or the sensation of a veil or curtain interfering with vision (5).

DIAGNOSIS
- Diagnosis is based primarily on history, progression, and funduscopic examination.
- Specific funduscopic findings are beyond the scope of this chapter.

TREATMENT
- Ultimately the treatment for retinal detachment is surgical, but may be delayed.

TABLE 10-2 Grades of Hyphema

Grade	Blood level in anterior chamber
Microscopic	Blood-tinged aqueous humor—no layering
Grade I	≤⅛ anterior chamber height
Grade II	>⅛, but <½ of anterior chamber height
Grade III	≥½ of anterior chamber but not complete
Grade IV	Complete ("eight ball") hyphema

From Kitt S, Kaiser J: *Emergency nursing: a physiologic and clinical perspective*, Philadelphia, 1990, WB Saunders; Shingleton BJ, Hersh PS: Traumatic hyphema. In Shingleton BJ, Hersh PS, Kenyon KR, editors: *Eye trauma*, St. Louis, 1991, Mosby.

- Guidelines for treatment will depend, to some degree, on the preferences of the consultant, but may involve patching or shielding of both eyes to reduce eye movements (5).
- If the patient is to be discharged, a careful assessment must be made of what resources are available to the patient at home for assistance with self-care.

Hyphema

SYMPTOMS

- Hyphema is a collection of blood in the anterior chamber, usually caused by a direct blow to the globe, such as by a ball or a fist, which causes bleeding from the vessels of the ciliary body. Since the blood is denser than the aqueous humor, it tends to settle in the lower half of the anterior chamber and is visible as a distinct blood fluid level.
- A hyphema is graded according to how much of the anterior chamber is filled with blood (Table 10-2).
- Pain resulting from hyphema is a deep aching, but concomitant injury to the cornea or orbit may cause mixed pain presentations (9,27). The degree of visual impairment is proportional to the grade of hyphema.
- Hyphema is frequently accompanied by somnolence, particularly in children, the etiology of which is not certain (27).

DIAGNOSIS

- While it is usually quite easy to identify a hyphema, a few confounding circumstances may occur. Hyphemae are, at times, difficult to discern if a patient has dark brown eyes, because there is less contrast. Since it is a unilateral injury, comparison with the uninjured eye is always helpful.

- A second difficulty occurs if a patient is under spinal precautions or has been lying supine. In this instance, the blood may settle more diffusely in the anterior chamber, with a less distinct layering.

TREATMENT

- Clinical management of hyphema is directed toward preventing complications and reducing the risk of rebleeding.
- The injured eye should be shielded (not patched) to prevent further injury (e.g., from rubbing).
- If possible, the patient should be positioned sitting upright or with the head of the bed elevated.
- There is a risk of renewed bleeding, particularly 2 to 5 days after the injury.
- Although the blood is usually reabsorbed spontaneously, it can cause staining of the cornea.
- Cycloplegic or mydriatic drops may be ordered for ciliary spasm (27).
- A patient with a hyphema requires urgent ophthalmologic consultation.
- Higher grades of hyphema are hospitalized on bedrest.
- Some ophthalmologists will treat lesser grades of hyphema at home if the patient will comply with activity restriction and daily follow-up visits and is not on anticoagulants (11,27).
- A patient being discharged home should be advised not to take aspirin or nonsteroidal antiinflammatory medications (11).

Orbital blowout fracture

SYMPTOMS

- The classic symptoms of a blowout fracture are binocular diplopia and infraorbital anesthesia.
- Signs may include a gaze limitation as a result of entrapment of ocular muscles, or enophthalmos resulting from herniation of periorbital fat.
- Gaze limitation and enophthalmos may occur as late signs that may not be evident acutely, and may occur independently or in combination.
- The mechanism of injury is a blunt retrograde displacement of the globe that, since it is fluid filled, is relatively noncompressible. This can cause the orbital floor (ethmoid bone) or the lateral or medial orbital walls to fracture.

DIAGNOSIS

* Blowout fracture is suspected on the basis of mechanism of injury, signs and symptoms, and is confirmed radiographically by plain films or computed tomography.

TREATMENT

* An icepack to the orbital area is helpful.
* After the cervical spine has been cleared, the head should be elevated to reduce swelling.
* The patient should be instructed not to blow his nose.
* Specialty consultation by a plastic or maxillofacial surgeon is indicated, but surgical repair will not always be necessary, and is often performed on an elective basis after swelling has gone down.

Eyelid lacerations

The priority given to eyelid lacerations depends on their complexity, and whether or not a facility has ophthalmologists on staff. The lid lacerations that usually require specialty consultation are those that disrupt the tarsal plate or lid margin or involve the lateral or medial canthus of the eye (11).

Iritis and iridocyclitis (anterior uveitis)

SYMPTOMS

* Anterior uveitis is generally unilateral and associated with acute alteration of pupillary responsiveness.
* The pupil of the affected eye is constricted, and may be irregular.
* The affected iris may have a muddy grayish cast relative to the unaffected eye (17).
* The pain is of gradual onset, aching in nature, and associated with intense photophobia and watery discharge (17,21).
* Pain may also be increased in the affected eye when it responds consensually to elicitation of the light reflex in the unaffected eye.

DIAGNOSIS

* Patients with anterior uveitis will have inflammatory vasodilation and increased vascular permeability of the iris and ciliary body resulting in protein and fibrin exudation into the anterior chamber. This causes a characteristic flare on slit lamp examination that is diagnostic for the condition (8,17,21).
* A diagnosis of iridocyclitis implies that the ciliary body and iris are both involved. While this is more serious,

there is little difference in terms of initial evaluation
and treatment (17,21).

TREATMENT

- Fibrin deposits may cause formation of synechiae
  (adhesions) of the iris and ciliary body that can
  interfere with drainage of aqueous humor and lead to
  acute glaucoma (8,17,21).
- Treatment is administration of a long-acting cycloplegic
  agent such as homatropine hydrobromate 5% (Isopto-
  homatropine) or cyclopentolate HCI 1% (Cyclogyl)
  and referral for prompt ophthalmologic consultation.
- The eye should not be patched, but may be shielded or
  the patient may use dark glasses to decrease discomfort
  from light (8).
- Warm compresses may afford some symptomatic relief
  (8).
- The patient may need oral narcotics, and should be
  counseled not to drive while the eye is shielded or the
  pupil is dilated by cycloplegic medication.

Acute (angle closure) glaucoma

SYMPTOMS

- Acute glaucoma is also often characterized by a ciliary
  flush, but the pupil of the affected eye will be
  moderately dilated, or midposition and poorly reactive.
- The cornea may have a clouded or "steamy"
  appearance.
- The patient may report visual alterations such as
  diminished acuity, blurred vision, or halos around light
  sources.
- Often the pain is described as an intense, periorbital
  headache and may be associated with nausea and
  vomiting.
- As such, it will also need to be discriminated from
  migraine headache, which may also have symptoms of
  nausea, vomiting, and visual disturbance, but is not
  associated with altered appearance of the eye or
  increased intraocular pressure (15).

DIAGNOSIS

- An acute elevation of intraocular pressure above 20
  mm Hg is diagnostic for acute glaucoma.
- Determination of the acuity of the elevation is based
  upon the history and progression of symptoms.

TREATMENT

- If intraocular pressure has been found to be elevated, and the patient is not vomiting, oral glycerol (1 to 1.5 g/kg) may be ordered for its osmotic effects (4).
- If the patient is vomiting, IV mannitol (20%; 1.5 to 2 g/kg) may be administered (4).
- A topical beta-blocker such as timolol may be ordered (4).
- The carbonic anhydrase inhibitor acetazolamide (Diamox), up to 500 mg PO or IV, may be ordered to reduce the rate of production of aqueous humor (4).
- Pilocarpine drops (1% to 2%) may be ordered to constrict the pupil (4,8). Cycloplegic or mydriatic medications are contraindicated.
- Ophthalmologic consultation is necessary and may require transfer of the patient, but the patient may ultimately be discharged.
- Specific guidelines regarding medications, activity restrictions, and follow-up should be clarified with the consultant before discharge.

Periorbital cellulitis

SYMPTOMS

- Periorbital cellulitis is a potentially life-threatening infection because it can lead to cavernous sinus thrombosis and intracranial infection.
- The patient is usually febrile and has marked, unilateral periorbital erythema, swelling, and pain.

DIAGNOSIS

- A CT scan of the orbit is necessary to evaluate the depth of the infection.

TREATMENT

- Patients with periorbital cellulitis are usually admitted for administration of intravenous antibiotics (8,15).

Superficial injuries (corneal foreign bodies, abrasions, and actinic keratitis)

SYMPTOMS

See Table 10-1.

DIAGNOSIS

- Fluorescein staining and Wood's lamp, cobalt blue light, or slit lamp examination.

TREATMENT

- Superficial corneal foreign bodies may be removed by irrigation or with a cotton swab.

- Embedded foreign bodies can be removed by the physician with a spud or the bevel of a 25-gauge hypodermic needle. Often this is done under slit lamp visualization. This can be disquieting to the patient even though the cornea is anesthetized. It is often helpful for the nurse to remain with the patient during the removal to assist the patient to sit still.
- If the foreign body was metallic, it can leave a rust ring behind.
- Rust rings are often removed in the emergency department with a rotary burr.
- If the patient is deemed reliable and understands the necessity for follow-up, the eye can be patched with antibiotic ointment for 24 to 36 hours and the ring can be removed by an ophthalmologist the following day (11).
- Treatment for corneal abrasion or actinic injury involves antibiotic ointment, oral analgesics, and patching.
- Patients with contact lenses should be advised not to reinsert them until cleared by an ophthalmologist or optometrist.

Ophthalmic shingles (herpes zoster)
SYMPTOMS
- Ophthalmic shingles is characterized by unilateral intense pain with herpetic lesions disposed linearly along the distribution of one of the facial nerves.

DIAGNOSIS
- The distribution of the pain and lesions and the characteristic appearance of the lesions is diagnostic.
- A history of chickenpox supports, but doesn't make, the diagnosis.

TREATMENT
- Although it may be confined to extraocular tissues, there is a risk of corneal involvement that can lead to blindness.
- Ophthalmologic consultation is essential; hospitalization may be necessary.
- Treatment with oral acyclovir is common (4).
- While awaiting consultation, the patient will be more comfortable in a darkened room.

Conjunctivitis
SYMPTOMS
- Bacterial conjunctivitis is usually bilateral with a purulent, matting discharge that is usually worse upon awakening.

- Viral conjunctivitis is usually unilateral, has a more mucoid discharge, and often associated with fever and sore throat (8,15,30).
- Pain from infectious conjunctivitis is burning or itching, but less intense than corneal pain.
- The patient may complain of blurry vision resulting from blepharospasm or discharge, but visual acuity is generally unaffected (15).
- Allergic conjunctivitis may be unilateral or bilateral, and is generally associated with itching, puffy eyelids, and a watery-to-mucoid discharge (15,30).

DIAGNOSIS
- Diagnosis is by clinical presentation and progression.
- Cultures are indicated for infants, conjunctivitis of rapid onset and progression, and in chronic cases (28).

TREATMENT
- Viral conjunctivitis is self-limiting, but highly contagious. Treatment is focused on alleviation of discomfort with warm compresses and topical decongestants. Some practitioners prescribe topical antibiotic prophylaxis. Steroids and patching are contraindicated. Patients or parents should be advised of the importance of careful handwashing, and not sharing towels (30).
- Bacterial conjunctivitis is treated with antibiotic drops or ointments and warm compresses. Steroids and patching are contraindicated (30).
- Allergic conjunctivitis is treated with antihistamines and topical decongestants. Steroids are controversial and their use is discouraged in episodic care (30).

Hordeolum (stye)
SYMPTOMS
- A stye is a localized infection, usually staphylococcal, of any of several glands of the eyelid.
- It may involve the glands of Zeis or Moll's glands (external) or the meibomian glands (internal).
- The patient presents with a localized, tender erythematous swelling of the underside of the lid or lid margin.

DIAGNOSIS
- Based on clinical presentation.

TREATMENT
- Involves an antibiotic ointment and warm compresses.

NURSING SURVEILLANCE

1. Monitor pain relief and administer an analgesic or topical anesthesic as ordered.
2. Expedite examination and treatment.
3. Coaching, guiding, and teaching the patient and family throughout the emergency visit are essential. Concrete information about the eye examination and what sensations the patient is likely to experience facilitates coping by providing the patient with objective expectations against which the experience and any uncomfortable sensations can be gauged. Offering clear information about the nature of the eye problem and usual functional outcomes helps to reduce uncertainty as to what is in store in the short and long term.

EXPECTED PATIENT OUTCOMES

1. Reduction in pain and emotional distress (e.g., fear and anxiety).
2. Ocular pH is normal (7.4 to 7.6) in chemical injury.
3. No evidence of rebleeding in hyphema.
4. Intraocular pressure is stabilized.
5. The patient should feel secure in the ability to cope with the problem and treatment expectations.
6. The patient understands functional limitations imposed by treatment (e.g., cycloplegia or patching), as well as the plan of treatment and follow-up.

DISCHARGE IMPLICATIONS

1. The patient and family should understand expected time frames for improvement and the significance of any signs or symptoms that may represent a developing complication or other departure from the predicted course. It is important to establish with whom the patient should follow-up (e.g., ED, family physician, ophthalmologist) and whether follow-up is essential (e.g., hyphema) or merely "prn" (e.g., conjunctivitis).
2. The relation of the problem to risk-taking behaviors (such as failure to use protective eyewear) and measures the patient can take to prevent recurrent injury should be explored in a nonjudgmental fashion.
3. Patients with corneal injuries who wear contact lenses should be instructed not to reinsert their contacts until cleared in a follow-up examination.

TABLE 10-3 Topical Ophthalmic Agents Commonly Used In Eye Emergencies

Generic name	Proprietary name	Drug class/ Mechanism	% Solution	Dosage	Special considerations
Proparacaine HCl	Ophthaine Ophthetic	Topical anesthetic	0.5%	1 gtt, repeat prn	Onset in 20 sec, lasts 10-15 min.
Tetracaine HCL	Pontocaine	Topical anesthetic	0.5%	1 gtt, repeat prn	Onset in 1 min, lasts 15-20 min.
Phenylephrine HCL	Neo-Synephrine	Mydriatic/ Sympathomimetic	2.5% and 10%	1 gtt, repeat in 5-10 min	Onset <30 min, duration 2-3 hr. The 10% soln. is contraindicated in infants, and for patients with HTN, heart disease, or on TCAs.
Homatropine HBr	—	Cycloplegic/ parasympatholytic	2% and 5%	1 gtt, repeat q 10-15 min × 2-3 doses	Onset <30 min, peak effect lasts for about 3 hr. Some residual effect up to 48 hr.
Cyclopentolate HCl	Cyclogyl	Cycloplegic/ parasympatholytic	0.5%, 1% and 2%	1 gtt, repeat × 1 in 10 min	Onset 30-60 min, duration <24hr. Risk of neurotoxicity, especially in children.

Continued.

E

341

TABLE 10-3 Topical Ophthalmic Agents Commonly Used In Eye Emergencies (cont'd)

Generic name	Proprietary name	Drug class/ Mechanism	% Solution	Dosage	Special considerations
Tropicamide	Mydriacyl	Cycloplegic/ parasympatholytic	0.5%, 1%	1 gtt q 5 min × 2-3 doses	Maximum effect in 20-25 min and lasts for only 15-20 min. Usually used only to facilitate examination
Pilocarpine HCl	Pilocar, numerous others	Miotic/ cholinergic/ parasympathomimetic	0.25% to 10%	1 gtt up to 6×/day	Decreases IOP by promoting drainage of aqueous (2° to miosis).
Timolol maleate	Timoptic	β-adrenergic blocking agent	0.25% and 0.5%	1 gtt daily or bid	Decreases intraocular pressure for up to 24 hr. Does not affect pupil or Va. Caution in CHF, asthma, COPD or for patients already on systemic β-blockers.

From Ellis PP: Commonly used eye medications. In Vaughan DV, Asbury T, Riordan-Eva P, editors: *General ophthalmology*, ed 13, Norwalk, Conn, 1992, Appleton & Lange, Lawlor MC: Common ocular injuries and disorders, *J Emerg Nurs*, 15:32, 1989; and Wagoner MD, Sadun AA, Bienfang DC: Acute disorders of the eye. In May HL, et al, editors, *Emergency medicine*, ed 2, Boston, 1992, Little, Brown.

References

1. The Amaurosis Fugax Study Group: Current management of amaurosis fugax, *Stroke* 21:201, 1990.
2. Dannenberg AL, Parver LM, Brechner RJ, Khoo L: Penetrating eye injuries in the workplace: the national eye trauma system registry, *Arch Ophthal* 110:843, 1992.
3. *Dorland's illustrated medical dictionary*, ed 27, Philadelphia, 1988, WB Saunders.
4. Ellis PP: Commonly used eye medications. In Vaughan DV, Asbury T, Riordan-Eva P, editors: *General ophthalmology*, ed 13, Norwark, Conn, 1992, Appleton & Lange.
5. Emergency Nurses Association: *Emergency nursing core curriculum*, ed 4, Philadelphia, 1994, WB Saunders.
6. Feist RM, Farber MD: Ocular trauma epidemiology, *Arch Ophthal* 107: 503, 1989.
7. Ganong WF: *Review of medical physiology*, ed 16, Norwalk, Conn, 1993, Appleton & Lange.
8. Goodenberger D, Greer D: Ophthalmic emergencies, *Top Emerg Med* 6(3):1, 1984.
9. Hitchings R: Eye pain. In Wall PD, Melzack R, editors: *Textbook of pain*, ed 2, Edinburgh, 1989, Churchill Livingstone.
10. Hoover DL, Smith LEH: Evaluation and management strategies for the pediatric eye trauma patient. In Shingleton BJ, Hersh PS, Kenyon KR, editors: *Eye trauma*, St. Louis, 1991, Mosby.
11. Janda AM: Ocular trauma: triage and treatment, *Postgrad Med* 90(7), 51, July 1991.
12. Joseph E et al: Predictors of blinding or serious eye injury in blunt trauma, *J Trauma* 33:19, 1992.
13. Kitt S, Kaiser J: *Emergency nursing: a physiologic and clinical perspective*, Philadelphia, 1990, WB Saunders.
14. Klopfer J, Tielsch JM, Vitale S, See LC, Canner JK: Ocular trauma in the United States: eye injuries resulting in hospitalization, 1984 through 1987, *Arch Ophthal* 110:838, 1992.
15. Lawlor MC: Common ocular injuries and disorders, *J Emerg Nurs* 15:32, 1989.
16. McFarland GK, McFarlane EA, editors: *Nursing diagnosis and intervention*, ed 2, St. Louis, 1992, Mosby.
17. Miller SJH, editor: *Parson's diseases of the eye*, ed 18, Edinburgh, 1990, Churchill Livingstone.
18. Neff JA: Visual acuity testing, *J Emerg Nurs* 17:431, 1991.
19. Netter FH: *Atlas of human anatomy*, Summit, N.J., 1989, Ciba-Geigy.
20. Newman R: Trauma in the elderly. In Neff JA, Kidd PS, editors: *Trauma nursing: the art and science*, St. Louis, 1993, Mosby.

21. O'Brien JM, Albert DM, Foster CS: Anterior uveitis. In Albert DM, Jakobiec FA, editors: *Principles and practice of ophthalmology: clinical practice,* Philadelphia, 1994, WB Saunders.

22. Parver LM et al: Characteristics and causes of penetrating eye injuries reported to the national eye trauma system registry, 1985-91, *Pub Hlth Reports,* 108:625, 1993.

23. Schein OD: et al: The spectrum and burden of ocular injury, *Ophthalmology* 95:300, 1989.

24. Schein OD, Vinger PF: Epidemiology and prevention. In Shingleton BJ, Hersh PS, Kenyon KR, editors: *Eye trauma,* St. Louis, 1991, Mosby.

25. Semonin-Holleran R: Trauma in childhood. In Neff JA, Kidd PS, editors: *Trauma nursing: the art and science,* St. Louis, 1993, Mosby.

26. Sheehy SB: *Emergency nursing: principles and practice,* St. Louis, 1992, Mosby.

27. Shingleton BJ, Hersh PS: Traumatic hyphema. In Singleton BJ, Hersh PS, Kenyon KR, editors: *Eye trauma,* St. Louis, 1991, Mosby.

28. Sternberg P: Prognosis and outcomes for penetrating ocular trauma. In Shingleton BJ, Hersh PS, Kenyon KR, editors: *Eye trauma,* St. Louis, 1991, Mosby.

29. Wagoner MD, Kenyon, KR: Chemical injuries. In Shingleton BJ, Hersh PS, Kenyon KR, editors: *Eye trauma,* St. Louis, 1991, Mosby.

30. Wagoner MD, Sadun AA, Bienfang DC: Acute disorders of the eye. In May HL, et al. editors, *Emergency medicine,* ed 2, Boston, 1992, Little, Brown.

31. Wang ESJ: Cocaine induced iritis, *Ann Emerg Med* 20:192, 1991.

Chapter XI

Fluid Administration

George P. Glessner III
Pamela S. Kidd

F

CLINICAL CONDITIONS
Hypersensitivity/Transfusion Reaction
Hypovolemia

TRIAGE ASSESSMENT

The main goal at triage is to determine if a patient needs rapid intravenous (IV) fluid administration. An additional goal is deciding if the patient needs IV access for maintenance fluid or potential drug administration. The combination of patient history and clinical presentation will provide adequate clues regarding the need for IV fluids. In some situations, the need for fluid resuscitation is obvious (e.g., patient with decreased responsiveness with history of penetrating trauma). These patients are triaged immediately to the treatment area. In cases where fluid needs are not as apparent, the following questions should provide additional data.

Vomiting/Diarrhea

Has the patient had episodes of vomiting and/or diarrhea? If so, how often and over what time period? In infants, the number of wet diapers in a 24-hour period may be helpful information.

Bleeding

Has the patient noticed any bleeding? If so, from what site and for how long? Hematuria, hematemesis, and melena may be sufficient to decrease circulating blood volume.

Pain

Does the patient complain of pain? Assess the nature of the pain (PQRST, see Chapter 4). Shoulder pain without a known shoulder injury may indicate diaphragmatic irritation from peritoneal bleeding (Kehr's sign). Abdominal pain and tenderness with anorexia may also indicate peritoneal bleeding.

Poor oral intake

Is the patient susceptible for poor oral intake? Patients with a history of confusion and/or dementia may not be able to maintain daily fluid needs. In infants, assess the amount of formula and fluids the child has taken in a 24-hour period.

Past medical history

Does the patient have existing health problems that may influence fluid and electrolytes? For example, insulin-dependent diabetic patients are more susceptible for diabetic ketoacidosis and dehydration. Patients with congestive heart failure may be susceptible for dehydration from treatment of the condition, since diuretics are frequently administered.

Does the patient have signs or symptoms of an existing illness that may require IV medication administration on an emergent basis (e.g., acute chest pain, possible dehydration in a diabetic patient, respiratory difficulty)?

Environmental

Is there a history of prolonged exposure to either heat or cold, or excessive sweating?

Diet

Has the patient ingested fluids that may precipitate diuresis (e.g., alcohol, caffeine)?

Vital Signs

- *Respirations:* Hyperventilation may be an early sign of acidosis resulting from anaerobic metabolism related to decreased oxygen-carrying capacity of cells.
- *Heart rate:* Tachycardia may result from fever or be a compensatory effort to maintain cardiac output in cases of decreased blood volume.
- *Blood pressure:* Hypotension is a late sign of decreased vascular volume. If possible, blood pressure measurement should be taken in both arms in cases of suspected hypovolemia. These measurements will not be equal in a patient with a leaking or dissecting aortic aneurysm.
- *Fever:* Fever increases metabolic needs and may induce dehydration.
- *Orthostatic changes:* Although not typically obtained at triage, orthostatic vital signs may indicate hypovolemia

when a change occurs in heart rate (>20 beats/min) and/or systolic blood pressure (>20 mm Hg) between position changes. Treatment staff should be notified if orthostatic vital signs were not completed at triage.

General Observations
Injury
- Does the patient have wounds/burns that would allow leakage of fluid or hematomas that would allow fluid accumulation?

Skin
- What is the color, temperature, and turgor of the patient's skin? Cool, clammy skin indicates vasoconstriction and the need to shunt blood to core organs (e.g., kidney, brain). Pale skin progressing to cyanosis indicates decreased availability of hemoglobin. Lip margins may be faint and difficult to distinguish. Petechiae and purpura suggests thrombocytopenia and bleeding. Poor skin turgor suggests dehydration.
- Assess capillary refill. If it is >2 sec (unless the patient is a geriatric individual and noted to have peripheral vascular disease or is hypothermic), hypovolemia may be present.

FOCUSED NURSING ASSESSMENT

Nursing assessment should focus on ventilation, perfusion, cognition, and elimination. Reassessment must occur frequently because of subtle and rapid changes that may occur. "Normal" vital signs may indicate effective but temporary compensation to hypovolemia. Blood pressure changes occur late in hypovolemia, yet, tachycardia is often an early sign of hypovolemia in adults.

Ventilation
Breathing pattern
Rapid, deep breathing may indicate oxygen deprivation from inadequate hemoglobin. This same pattern may be associated with acidosis in diabetic patients suggesting dehydration (see Chapter 7).
Breath sounds
It is crucial that available hemoglobin receives oxygen for tissue transport. Unilateral, diminished, or absent breath

sounds indicates an underlying pulmonary problem that may need immediate treatment in order to enhance perfusion (e.g., placement of a chest tube, readjustment of an endotracheal tube). Basilar crackles may indicate underlying pulmonary or heart disease predisposing the patient to fluid overload with minimal volume replacement. Crackles may be present if the patient received too much volume replacement in the prehospital setting or at a transferring facility.

Oxygen saturation

Decreased oxygen saturation may indicate a decrease in circulating hemoglobin and not primary respiratory decompensation.

Perfusion

Neck veins

Flat neck veins are associated with hypovolemia. Distended neck veins indicate either hyperperfusion, increased pulmonary hypertension, or decreased cardiac contractility.

Peripheral pulses

Peripheral pulses may be difficult to palpate in hypovolemia or existing arterial insufficiency.

Heart sounds

In cases of hypovolemia, the apical pulse may be rapid and distant. A bounding, shifted apical pulse suggests heart failure and decreased ability to circulate blood volume effectively. The presence of a murmur suggests hyperperfusion whether due to a metabolic state (e.g., pregnancy, adolescence) or fluid administration.

Abdominal assessment

Although the abdomen is not traditionally viewed as an organ assessed for perfusion data, in cases of suspected hypovolemia, the abdomen should be examined as a potential bleeding source. A rigid abdomen, that is tender to palpation, with absent bowel sounds, and with or without ecchymotic areas suggests peritoneal bleeding.

Injury

After undressing the patient, reexamine the patient for obvious hemorrhage, burns, and potential infection sites (e.g., wounds) that may influence circulating blood volume.

NURSING ALERT

After immobilizing the cervical spine (if indicated, refer to Chapter 21), logroll the patient to examine the posterior surface. A retroperitoneal hematoma can produce hypovolemia very quickly. Assess the flank areas for bruising, edema, or pain on palpation.

F

Cognition

Restlessness and irritability are the first indications of decreasing blood volume. Lethargy and decreased responsiveness occurs later. Central nervous system changes are related to decreased cerebral oxygenation. A Glasgow coma scale score (see Reference Guide 6) should be documented and monitored throughout the ED stay.

Elimination
Urine output

The box lists expected urine output in a normovolemic state for both children and adults. Specific gravity should be checked to assess concentration of urine to preserve circulating fluid volume. Specific gravity >1.015 may be indicative of decreased fluid volume or an increase in solutes causing osmotic diuresis. Decreased urine output indicates either compensation induced by antidiuretic hormone in cases of hypovolemia or acute/chronic renal failure. Acute renal failure (ARF) can be induced by hypovolemia. ARF may also occur in cases of transfusion reaction. Hematuria may occur in transfusion reactions. It may also indicate the need for colloid replacement.

Stools

Monitor number, amount, consistency, and color of stools. Constipation may suggest dehydration. Diarrhea may indicate the need for fluid administration. Melena (tarry stools) may indicate the need for colloid administration.

Risk Factors

1. Positive medical history for gastrointestinal absorption problems predisposes the patient to dehydration (e.g., Crohn's disease, gastric bypass/stapling surgery, short-gut syndrome, ulcerative colitis).

FORMULAS USED IN FLUID ADMINISTRATION*

Basal fluid maintenance

1500 cc/m^2 BSA/24 hr = cc/24 hr (calculate as cc/hr)

General guidelines: Up to 10 kg = 100 cc/kg/24 hr
11-20 kg = 50 cc/kg/24 hr plus 100 cc/kg for first 10 kg
>20 kg = 20-25 cc/kg/24 hr plus 50 cc/kg for each kg 11 through 20 plus 100 cc/kg for first 10 kg

Volume replacement with crystalloids

Administer 3 cc for every cc lost. For fluid challenges administer:
IV bolus 20 cc/kg D5% RL in children
IV bolus of 200-300 cc RL in adult surgical patients
IV bolus of 200-300 cc NS in adult medical patients

Volume replacement with colloids

Administer 1 cc for every cc lost

Volume replacement for measured losses

Gastric Losses: Replace 1 cc for every cc lost q 4 hr. Use D$_5$ ½NS plus 30 mEq K/L

Intestinal Losses: Replace 1 cc for every cc lost q 4 hr. Use D5%LR.

Basal urine output

Up to 30 kg = 40 cc/kg/24 hr (2 cc/kg/hr)
>30 kg = 1200 cc/24 hr (17-18 cc/kg/hr)

*See Chapter 3 for burn resuscitation formulas.
NS = normal saline
RL = Ringer's lactate

2. Positive medical history for congestive heart failure, coronary artery disease, cardiovascular valve disease, pulmonary hypertension, hepatic insufficiency or failure, and chronic renal failure places the patient at risk for fluid overload.
3. Diabetic patients may experience dehydration with acidosis.
4. Fever, vomiting, and diarrhea increases fluid demands.

5. Warm, humid, environments may induce hyperthermia and result in dehydration.
6. Patients with a history of blunt or penetrating injury are at risk for hypovolemia as a result of hemorrhage (obvious or occult). Patients with spinal cord injury are at risk for neurogenic shock and relative hypovolemia resulting from vasodilation.
7. Patients with infection are at risk for relative hypovolemia.
8. Patients with electrical burns are at risk for greater occult fluid loss resulting from nonvisibility of tissue injury that causes vasodilation. They are also susceptible to fluid loss from draining wounds.
9. Patients with pulmonary burn injuries are at risk for under resuscitation as a result of the fear of inducing pulmonary edema.
10. Patients taking beta-blocking agents (e.g., propranolol) and calcium channel blockers (e.g., nifedipine) may not be able to circulate the amount of fluid administered in a fluid resuscitation situation precipitating congestive heart failure. These drugs also mask hypovolemia by blocking the normal compensatory response of tachycardia.

Life Span Issues
Children
Maintenance fluid requirements for children are greater than that for adults (Table 11-1). They become dehydrated more quickly from vomiting, diarrhea, fever, and heat exposure than adults. Children often exhibit clinical signs of fluid volume loss (e.g., increased heart rate, decreased blood pressure, agitation) very late. Astute ongoing assessment is essential to recognize early signs (e.g., decreased skin turgor, decreased urine output, lethargy) of fluid loss.

Pregnancy
Plasma volume increases by 50% during pregnancy. Hemoglobin and hematocrit decreases. Thus, the oxygen-carrying ability of the blood is less. Colloid replacement instead of crystalloid replacement may be used. Hyperemesis gravidarum (more common in the first trimester of pregnancy) can cause dehydration requiring fluid resuscitation.

TABLE 11-1 Administration of Maintenance IV Fluids

Solution type	Examples	Uses
Isotonic	0.9% Normal saline (NS)	Expands intravascular volume. Used for dehydration (e.g., diabetic ketoacidosis, hyperosmolar nonketotic coma) and for packed red blood cell administration.
	Ringer's lactate solution (RL)	Expands intravascular volume. Used for maintenance fluid when patient is NPO.
Hypotonic	NS 0.45% NS 0.2% Dextrose 5% and water (D_5W)	Shifts water into intracellular spaces. Useful in preventing dehydration and assessing renal status. D_5W may be used in adult patients for mixing IV medications. Used for maintenance fluid when patient is at risk for free water loss.
Hypertonic	Dextrose 5% in NS Dextrose 10% in NS Dextrose 10% in water Dextrose 5% in 0.45 NS Dextrose 20% in water	Shifts fluid from intracellular to extracellular space. Use in water intoxication states created by too much hypotonic fluid administration. Used for maintenance fluid to promote diuresis.

Geriatric

1. Ventricular compliance may decrease in the elderly. Rapid fluid resuscitation may result in heart failure and decreased cardiac output.
2. Malnutrition is more common in the geriatric population. Anemia may occur because of decreased red blood cell (RBC) formation related to nutritional deficiency. The use of blood products may be necessary in fluid resuscitation.
3. The normal changes in skin elasticity of the geriatric population makes assessment of skin turgor as a sign of hypovolemia unreliable. However, assessment of mucous membranes may be used when skin turgor is unreliable.

INITIAL INTERVENTIONS

Fluid Resuscitation

1. Initiate two large bore IV lines (14 to 16 gauge for adults, 22-gauge or greater for pediatric patients) with appropriate IV fluid (see Table 11-5). Obtain specimen for CBC (purple top tube), coagulation studies (blue top tube), electrolyte levels (red top tube), and possible type and crossmatch (large red top tube) simultaneously. (See Reference Guide 12 for minimal amount of blood needed to perform laboratory tests.) Secure IV lines.

> **NURSING ALERT**
>
> The need for fluid administration does not take precedence over airway and breathing. Efforts to gain IV access should not interfere with efforts to correct problems with airway or breathing.

Consider placement of intraosseous line in a child if unable to access a vein (see Procedure 21). The usual site for intraosseous infusion is the proximal tibia. The distal femur can be used in infants. Colloids, crystalloids, and medications can be administered through the intraosseous line. An intraosseous infusion site should be considered a temporary measure during emergencies/resuscitation. As soon as the patient is stabilized or resuscitated, venous access should be obtained, followed by discontinuing and removing the intraosseous infusion line. This will help decrease the possibility of osteomyelitis.

2. Anticipate need for administering blood products. Set up IV blood administration tubing and prime with normal saline. Obtain a blood warmer and/or rapid infusion device. If a blood warming device is being used for a pediatric patient receiving <750 cc/hr fluid replacement, the shortest IV tubing should be used without an extension in order for fluid to remain warm upon entry at a slower infusion rate (3).

In conditions where cell membrane integrity is altered (e.g., sepsis, burns), massive fluid shifts occur depleting circulating blood volume. Fluid administration is necessary, although administered fluid will also shift from the vascular space to the interstitial area to some degree. The use of natural and synthetic colloids (e.g., albumin, and hetastarch, respectively) may help fluid to be mobilized from the interstitial area into the vascular space. Pulmonary complications may occur from movement of fluid back into the vascular space if congestive heart failure is present.

Maintenance Fluid and/or IV Drug Administration

Insert a 20-gauge or larger intravenous catheter in the adult and a 24-gauge or larger IV catheter in infants and children (see Table 11-1) with appropriate IV fluid (see Table 11-5).

PRIORITY NURSING DIAGNOSES

Risk for fluid volume deficit
Risk for decreased cardiac output
Risk for alteration in tissue perfusion
Risk for injury

◆ **Fluid volume deficit** related to fluid shift or hemorrhage.
   INTERVENTIONS
   • Administer volume expanders.
   • Apply pressure to external bleeding sites.
   • Prepare for transport for diagnostic testing or to the operating suite if internal bleeding is suspected.

◆ **Decreased cardiac output** related to decreased circulating blood volume.
   INTERVENTIONS
   • Treat the underlying cause if decreased circulating blood volume.

- Administer crystalloids and colloids.
- Anticipate the use of vasopressors.

◆ **Alteration in tissue perfusion** related to shunting of blood to core organs

INTERVENTIONS
- Administer volume replacement to increase tissue perfusion and oxygen-carrying capacity.
- Decrease oxygen demands by keeping the patient warm, treating fever with acetaminophen and cooling blankets, relieving pain, and decreasing stressful stimuli.

◆ **Risk for injury** related to decreased cerebral oxygenation.

INTERVENTIONS
- Administer blood products as ordered.
- Administer oxygen as ordered.
- Monitor LOC.
- Keep side rails up and bed in lowest position.
- Anticipate seizure activity.

PRIORITY DIAGNOSTIC TESTS

Laboratory

Complete blood count: This test provides information on the number of RBCs and possible anemia. Elevation of WBCs may indicate an infection and subsequent fever and dehydration. Hemoglobin levels indicate the oxygen-carrying capacity of the blood. The hematocrit will indicate if dehydration is present (high level) or hemodilution (low level) or if hemorrhage has resulted in loss of RBCs.

Type and crossmatch: This test will be ordered if administration of blood products is anticipated. It will detect the blood grouping and Rh factor of the potential recipient.

Chest radiograph: A chest film will indicate if cardiomegaly and pulmonary edema is present as a result of fluid administration or fluid shifting.

COLLABORATIVE INTERVENTIONS

1. Assist with placement of central IV lines.
2. Assist with invasive hemodynamic monitoring (if indicated).
3. Insert a urinary catheter with urine meter.
4. Insert a nasogastric tube.
5. In traumatized patient, assist with placement of chest tubes. Prepare to assist with diagnostic peritoneal lavage and/or autotransfusion.

Clinical Conditions

Clinical conditions related to fluid administration are discussed in specific chapters (e.g., burns, DKA [endocrine]).

Hypersensitivity/Transfusion reaction

A transfusion reaction may be minor or severe. They are produced by the formation of antigen-antibody complexes between donor blood and recipient blood. A hypersensitivity reaction may occur with any blood product and synthetic colloids.

SYMPTOMS
- Symptoms are contrasted in Table 11-2.

DIAGNOSIS
- Diagnosis is confirmed by direct antiglobulin testing (positive Coombs' test) and separation of the offending antibody from red blood cells. For proper diagnosis, the steps in the box should be followed.

TREATMENT
- Treatment is outlined in Table 11-2.

Hypovolemia

It is impossible to discuss management of hypovolemia because treatment is dependent upon severity of fluid loss, preexisting health condition of the patient, and etiology of fluid loss. Controversies in fluid resuscitation at time of publication are listed in the box, since practice may change over the life of this book edition. Guidelines for blood component administration in adults are located in Table 11-3. Table 11-4 includes information on administering blood components in children.

NURSING SURVEILLANCE

1. Monitor for signs of fluid overload (see the box).
2. Monitor hemodynamic readings (if available).
3. Monitor urine output and specific gravity. High specific gravity indicates hypovolemia.

EXPECTED PATIENT OUTCOMES

1. IV lines remain patent for fluid administration.
2. Level of consciousness improves or remains at a GCS score of 15 or at baseline.
3. Urine output is adequate for weight.
4. Hemorrhage decreases or patient is transported quickly to operating suite.

TABLE 11-2 Comparison of Transfusion Reactions

Transfusion reaction	Symptoms	Treatment
Acute hemolytic reaction	• Hypotension • Burning in vein • Flushed face • Headache • Diffuse pain	• Stop transfusion • Start NS or RL • Consider diuretics • Monitor BUN, serum creatinine, LDH, and bilirubin levels
Minor incompatibility	Symptoms occur after transfusion is completed. • Mild jaundice • Failure to maintain expected hemoglobin level after transfusion	• No actions are indicated
Anaphylaxis	• Hypotension • Decreased responsiveness • Severe dyspnea • Generalized edema may be present	• Stop transfusion • Airway and breathing support (anticipate intubation) • Administer epinephrine • Start NS or RL
Hypersensitivity	• Urticaria • Pruitis • Hives • Facial edema • Fever • Nausea/vomiting • Dyspnea	• Stop transfusion • Administer antihistamine • Administer steroids • Administer acetaminophen

STEPS IN INVESTIGATING TRANSFUSION REACTIONS

1. Send (if available) prereaction recipient blood or get type and crossmatch results from prereaction recipient blood.
2. Send postreaction recipient blood specimen.
3. Send donor blood being administered at time of reaction.
4. Send posttransfusion urine sample.

TABLE 11-3 Blood Component Administration Guidelines in Adults

Blood component	Infusion rate	Filter	Volume	Comment
Whole blood	2-4 hr Max: 4 hr	Required	500 ml	Rapid infusion if need is urgent
Packed red blood cells	2-4 hr Max: 4 hr	Required	250 ml	Hgb rises 1 g/dl; Hct rises 3% after 1 U
Leukocyte-poor red blood cells	2 hr	Required	Variable	—
Fresh frozen plasma	1-2 hr, rapidly if bleeding	Use component filter	250 ml	Notify blood bank—takes 20 min to thaw
Platelets	Rapidly as patient tolerates	Use component filter	35-50 ml U	Usually 6-10 U are ordered. Request that blood bank pool all units
Albumin	1-2 ml/min in normovolemic patients	Special tubing	Varies	Comes in 5% and 25%; can increase intravascular volume quickly; infuse cautiously
Cryoprecipitate	30 min	Use component filter	10 ml/unit	Usually 6-10 U ordered. Request that blood bank pool units
Granulocytes	2-4 hr	Use component filter	300-400 ml	VS q 15 min during infusion Granulocytes have a short life span. Transfuse as soon after collection as possible.

TABLE 11-4 Blood Component Administration in Children

Blood component	Usual dose	Rate of infusion	Comments
Whole blood	20 ml/kg initially	As rapidly as necessary to restore volume and stabilize the child	Administration is usually reserved for massive hemorrhage.
Packed RBCs	10 ml/kg, not to exceed 15 ml/kg	5 ml/kg/hr or 2 ml/kg/hr if congestive heart failure develops	1 ml/kg will increase Hct approximately 1%. Infuse within 4 hr. If necessary, divide the unit into smaller volumes for infusion.
Platelets	1 unit for every 7-10 kg	Each unit over 5-10 min via syringe or pump	The usual dose will increase platelet count by 50,000/mm³.
Fresh frozen plasma	Hemorrhage: 15-30 ml/kg Clotting deficiency: 10-15 ml/kg	Hemorrhage: rapidly to stabilize the child Clotting deficiency: over 2-3 hr	Monitor for fluid overload.
Granulocytes	Dependent on WBC counts and clinical condition, 10 ml/kg/day initially	Slowly over 2-4 hr because of fever and chills, side effects commonly associated with infusion	Granulocytes have a short life span. Transfuse as soon after collection as possible.
Albumin 5%	1 g/kg or 20 ml/kg	1-2 ml/min or 60-120 ml/hr	Monitor for fluid overload. Type and crossmatch are not required.
Albumin 25%	1 g/kg or 4 ml/kg	0.2-0.4 ml/min or 12-24 ml/hr	Monitor for fluid overload. Type and crossmatch are not required.

F

CONTROVERSIES IN FLUID RESUSCITATION

1. Increasing the volume of crystalloid administered does not improve hepatocellular function in sepsis (8). Hepatocellular dysfunction is related to release of inflammatory cytokines and not hypoperfusion.
   Implication: Decrease replacement ratio for crystalloids in sepsis (currently 3:1 ratio).
2. Hypertonic saline produces a transient increase in blood volume (4).
   Implication: Optimal resuscitation may involve initial infusion of hypertonic saline followed by colloids, to maintain blood volume, or hypotonic solution to restore cellular hydration.
3. Hypertonic saline decreases cortical water content and intracranial pressure (6).
   Implication: Hypertonic saline may be most effective in the multiple-injury patient experiencing closed-head injury and hypovolemia (1).
4. Delayed fluid resuscitation in penetrating injury may be as effective as immediate fluid resuscitation because elevating the blood pressure before hemorrhage is controlled may be detrimental (5).
   Implication: Fluid resuscitation may begin in the operating suite and not in the prehospital setting or the ED in cases of penetrating trauma requiring surgical intervention.
5. No adverse effects have been noted in burn patients who receive blood transfusions at a hemoglobin level of 6-6.5 g/dl as compared to 10 g/dl (7).
   Implication: Hemoglobin levels will be lower before products are administered.

SIGNS OF FLUID OVERLOAD

- Dyspnea, crackles on auscultation
- Tachycardia, distended neck veins
- Diaphoresis, edema
- Increased central venous pressure and pulmonary wedge pressure (if measurement is available)

5. Acidosis improves as evidenced by arterial blood gases or venous carbon dioxide level.

6. Obtain supranormal values in cardiac index (>4.5 cc/min/m^2), oxygen delivery (Do$_2$ >800 cc/min/m^2, and oxygen use (VO$_2$ >170 cc/min/m^2) (2) if it is possible to measure mixed venous oxygen saturation and cardiac parameters.

DISCHARGE IMPLICATIONS

Most patients requiring fluid resuscitation will not be discharged from the ED. In cases where patients have received IV fluids for minor hypovolemia and have responded favorably to treatment, the following areas should be addressed:

1. Patients may have a delayed (7 to 10 days) reaction to blood transfusion. Delayed reactions are mild and do not require treatment. In delayed reactions, bilirubin levels rise producing jaundice, and possible frothy, dark urine.

2. Symptoms of fluid overload may not appear immediately after IV fluid administration. The development of edema, dyspnea, and tachycardia may indicate decreased ability of the heart to manage the circulating blood volume. Patients should be instructed to see their primary care provider or return to the ED if symptoms develop.

3. If vomiting, fever, and/or diarrhea returns, patients should increase their fluid intake, take prescribed antidiarrheal, antiemetic drugs, and return to the ED or their primary care provider if no improvement occurs.

4. Adult respiratory distress syndrome (ARDS), or disseminated intravascular coagulation (DIC), or multiple organ dysfunction may develop on a delayed basis after fluid administration particularly in high risk populations (e.g., geriatric patients with heart disease). Patients should be instructed to return to the ED if the following symptoms develop: respiratory distress, dyspnea, cough, decreased urination, hematuria, bleeding from mucous membranes, and/or fever.

TABLE 11-5 Fluid Resuscitation Summary*

Crystalloids	Description/ Indication	Action/s
0.9% Normal saline (NS)	Isotonic	• May produce fluid overload[†] • 25% of volume administered will remain in the vascular space
0.45% Normal saline	Hypotonic, moves fluid from vascular space to interstitial and intracellular spaces	• Decreases blood viscosity • May promote hypovolemia • May promote cerebral edema
5% Dextrose	Hypotonic	• 7.5 cc/100 cc infused will remain in vascular space • Inadequate for fluid resuscitation
Ringers' lactate solution	Isotonic, contains multiple electrolytes and lactate	• May produce fluid overload[†] • May promote lactic acidosis in prolonged hypoperfusion with decreased liver function • Lactate metabolizes to acetate, may produce metabolic alkalosis when large volumes are transfused
Hypertonic saline (7.5%)	Hypertonic, pulls fluid from interstitial and intracellular spaces into vascular space	• Requires smaller amount to restore blood volume • Increases cerebral oxygen dry while decreasing ICP • May promote hypernatremia • May promote intracellular dehydration • May promote osmotic diuresis • Controversial

*Dosages are not listed because of variability in patient response and need.

TABLE 11-5 (cont'd)

Synthetic colloids	Description	Action/s
Dextran	(Comes in 40, 70, and 75 molecular weight)	• Associated with anaphylaxis • Reduces Factor VIII, platelets, and fibrinogen function, so increases bleeding time • May interfere with blood crossmatching and typing, glucose, and erythrocyte sedimentation levels • Risk of fluid overload‡
Hetastarch		• May increase serum amylase levels • Associated with coagulopathy • Risk of fluid overload‡

Natural colloids	Description	Action/s
Fresh frozen plasma	Contains all clotting factors	• Potential to transmit blood-borne infection • Can cause hypersensitivity reaction • Blood volume expander
Plasma protein fraction (Plasmanate)	Does not contain clotting factors	• May cause hypersensitivity reaction • If given too rapidly, may cause hypotension • Blood volume expander

†Fluid overload using these agents may occur because of large amounts of fluid required for volume lost (3:1 ratio).
‡Fluid overload using these agents may occur in cases of preexisting pulmonary and/or heart disease.

TABLE 11-5 (cont'd)

Natural colloids	Description	Action/s
Albumin	5% iso-oncotic 25% hyperoncotic "salt poor"	• Preferred as volume expander when risk from producing interstitial edema is great (e.g., pulmonary and heart disease) • Hypocalcemia
Whole blood	Can be administered without normal saline; reduces donor exposure	• Hyperkalemia, hypothermia, and hypocalcemia • May require greater amount than packed RBCs to increase oxygen-carrying capacity of blood • Rarely used, not cost-effective
Packed RBCs	Administer with normal saline	• Deficient in 2, 3-diphosphoglycerate, so may increase oxygen affinity to hemoglobin and may decrease oxygen delivery to tissue • Hypothermia, hyperkalemia, and hypocalcemia

Experimental agents	Description	Action/s
Liposome encapsulated hemoglobin/ hypertonic saline (7.5%)	NOT APPROVED BY FDA	• Improves skeletal muscle oxygen tension • Expands vascular volume quickly • Improves tissue oxygenation
Hypertonic saline (7.5%) with Dextran 70	Combined crystalloid and colloid therapy	• Promotes rapid expansion of blood volume and promotes retention of volume in vascular space • Controversial

References

1. Battistella F and Wisner D: Combined hemorrhagic shock and head injury: effects of hypertonic saline resuscitation, 31:182-188, 1991.

2. Daleiden A: Physiology and treatment of hemorrhagic shock during the early postoperative period, *Crit Care Nurs Qtly* 16:45-59, 1993.

3. Faries G, Johnston C, Pruitt K, and Plouff R: *Ann Emerg Med* 20:1198-1200, 1991.

4. Gala G, Lilly M, Thomas S, and Gann D: Interaction of sodium and volume in fluid resuscitation after hemorrhage, *J Trauma* 31:545-556, 1991.

5. Martin R, Bickell W, Pepe P, Burch J, and Mattox K: Prospective evaluation of preoperative fluid resuscitation in hypotensive patients with penetrating truncal injury: a preliminary report, *J Trauma* 33:354-362, 1992.

6. Schmoker J, Zhuang J, and Shackford S: Hypertonic fluid resuscitation improves cerebral oxygen delivery and reduces intracranial pressure after hemorrhagic shock. *J Trauma* 31:1607-1613, 1991.

7. Sittig K, and Deitch E: Blood transfusions for the thermally injured or for the doctor? *J Trauma* 36:369-372, 1994.

8. Wang, P, Zheng F, Ayala A, and Chaudry I: Hepatocellular dysfunction persists during early sepsis despite increased volume of crystalloid resuscitation, *J Trauma* 32:389-397, 1992.

F

Chapter XII

Genitourinary Conditions

Pamela S. Kidd

CLINICAL CONDITIONS
Acute Cystitis
Acute Pyelonephritis
Sepsis
Urinary Calculi
Testicular Torsion
Epididymitis
GU Trauma
Renal Failure
Genitalia Injuries
Renal Transplant Rejection

G

TRIAGE ASSESSMENT

The most common genitourinary (GU) conditions encountered in the emergency department (ED) are genitourinary trauma, urinary tract infections (UTI), renal calculi, renal failure, and epididymitis. To differentiate among these conditions, you should elicit the following information from the patient at triage:
- History of fever (suspect infection).
- History of injury (suspect trauma).
- History of rapid weight gain, edema, increasing dyspnea (suspect renal failure).
- History of penile discharge (suspect genital problem).
- History of acute onset of pain, nausea/vomiting (suspect renal calculi or trauma).
- History of renal transplant.
- Pain changes with position (suspect genital problem).
- Bloody urine (suspect infection, trauma, calculi).

Vital Signs
- *Tachycardia:* Related to pain and/or increased fluid volume.

- *Hypertension:* Related to increased fluid volume.
- *Fever:* Related to infection.
- *Tachypnea:* Related to increased fluid volume.

General Observations

- Presence of jugular venous distention (JVD) (suspect renal failure).
- Audible crackles/rales with or without foamy sputum (suspect renal failure).
- Deep and rapid respirations (may indicate metabolic acidosis secondary to renal failure).
- Presence of diaphoresis, pale, clammy skin secondary to sympathetic nervous system action (suspect renal calculi, testicular torsion, epididymitis, GU trauma).

NURSING ALERT

Few GU conditions are medical emergencies. Patients with severe pain, tachypnea, or hypertension should be triaged immediately to the treatment area.

FOCUSED NURSING ASSESSMENT

Nursing assessment centers on perfusion, elimination, and sexuality.

Perfusion
Heart sounds
Presence of S_3 or S_4 may indicate acute heart failure related to fluid overload.

Breath sounds
Presence of rales/crackles that do not clear with coughing may indicate pulmonary edema related to heart failure secondary to fluid overload.

Mental status
Disorientation may occur related to decreased cerebral circulation secondary to heart failure and fluid overload or as a result of accumulated toxins.

Peripheral pulses
Weak peripheral pulses and moderate (3 to 4+) peripheral edema may be present as a result of fluid overload.

Vascular access devices

Presence of current or past vascular access devices may indicate previous renal deficiency. Assess patency if appropriate. Palpate the length of a graft for a strong thrill (constant vibration) indicating adequate blood flow. Auscultate for a bruit produced by blood flow through the graft. Maintain integrity of peripheral devices by not using the extremity for obtaining blood pressure measurement, blood specimen, or venous access.

Elimination
Pattern of elimination

Stopped urination stream may indicate obstruction. Increased frequency may indicate infection. Decreased urination (<400 cc in 24 hr) or diuresis (>4 to 5 L/24 hr) may indicate acute renal failure (ARF).

Pain on urination

If suprapubic in location, may indicate bladder or urethral trauma or lower UTI. If flank in location, may indicate renal or ureter trauma, upper UTI, or renal calculi.

Pain

Pain radiating to shoulder may indicate intraperitoneal extravasation of urine.

Hematuria

May be present in cases of infection, calculi, or trauma.

Retroperitoneal bleeding

Inspect flanks for ecchymotic areas and abrasions suggestive of renal trauma. If present, auscultate flank for presence of bruit suggestive of renal vascular trauma. Mark size of any hematoma.

Urinary meatus

Inspect urinary meatus for sign of bleeding associated with urethral injury.

Bruising

Inspect for bruising around the umbilicus and bruising over the flank resulting from a retroperitoneal hemorrhage (Grey Turner's sign). Positive bruising suggests renal trauma.

Bladder

Palpate bladder to assess if distention is present. Urgency, pain on voiding, and bladder distention suggest bladder and/or urethral injury.

Sexuality
Pain during or after intercourse
May be present in sexually transmitted diseases (STDs) (see Chapter 18) and in epididymitis.

Testicles
Unilateral testicular pain is associated with testicular torsion.

Scrotum
Scrotal pain occurs in epididymitis.

Penile discharge
May be present in STDs and epididymitis.

Testicular swelling
May be present in testicular torsion. Table 12-1 contrasts symptoms of torsion and epididymitis.

Genitalia
Inspect genitalia for presence of vaginal bleeding, penile discharge, or evidence of incontinence.

Risk Factors
1. *Exposure risk:* Multiple partners, bisexuality, homosexuality may expose the patient to HIV and STDs (see Chapters 5 and 18, respectively).
2. *Gender:* Genital trauma more common in males.
3. *Contact sports, heavy lifting:* Associated with renal trauma, bladder trauma, and testicular torsion.
4. *Acceleration/deceleration forces:* (e.g., falls, 1 car MVC where the car hits a stationary object such as a tree) are associated with renal trauma.
5. *Past medical history:* Diabetes, repeated UTIs, congenital renal abnormalities, and previous trauma are associated with chronic renal failure.
6. *Medication history:* Antibiotics (especially aminoglycosides), pesticide exposure (agricultural workers), and contrast media (recent diagnostic test) are associated with ARF.

Life Span Issues
1. *Youth:* Testicular torsion is more common in adolescence. Ureter rupture is more common in pediatric patients with blunt injuries (e.g., pedestrian rolled over by motor vehicle).
2. *Postmenopausal:* UTIs more common in young females and postmenopausal women.

TABLE 12-1 Differentiating Testicular Torsion and Epididymitis

	Torsion	**Epididymitis**
History	Previous episode common	Recent sexual activity
Pain	Sharp, sudden onset	Gradual onset
Fever	Absent	Present
Edema	Elevated testis (in order to assess this, stand at the foot of the patient's bed and have the patient fold his arms over his chest)	Swollen scrotum
Urethral discharge	Absent	Possible
CBC	Normal	Elevated WBCs
Urinalysis	Normal	Bacteriuria
Testicular scan	Hypoperfused	Hyperperfused
Prehn's sign (Amount of pain elicited on testis elevation)	Negative (pain increases)	Positive (pain decreases)

INITIAL INTERVENTIONS

Regardless of the source of the GU condition, the following interventions will not harm the patient and may be beneficial:

1. Head of bed, 30 degrees.
2. If patient can void, get a midstream clean-catch specimen. Split the specimen sterilely to provide for a urinalysis (UA) and a specimen for culture and sensitivity if the UA is positive for infection. Examine it for hematuria, protein, glucose, and pH using a clinical reagent strip. If available, examine it for the presence of leukocytes using a clinical reagent strip. Females on their menses should have a catheterized specimen obtained if

no sign of urethral injury is present. If the urine is negative for hematuria, a UA may not be obtained.

3. Initiate I/O recording.
4. In cases of testicular swelling, elevate scrotum on a pillow/towel and apply ice. Place a protective barrier between the ice and the skin.
5. If renal failure is suspected, get patient's weight. Measure circumference of edematous extremities. Initiate neurovascular checks of edematous extremities. Keep patient NPO until examined by physician.
6. Monitor vital signs every 30 minutes (or by policy) if renal failure is suspected.

PRIORITY NURSING DIAGNOSES

Risk for fluid volume excess
Risk for pain
Risk for altered patterns of urinary elimination: urge incontinence
Risk for urinary retention
Risk for infection

◆ **Fluid volume excess** related to primary renal damage or decreased cardiac output as evidenced by pulmonary, peripheral and/or generalized edema, hypertension, tachypnea, hyperphosphatemia, hyperkalemia, metabolic acidosis, JVD, ogiluria.

INTERVENTIONS
• Monitor breath sounds and oxygen saturation levels.
• Initiate intake and output measurement.
• Insert either an intermittent IV infusion device or limit IV fluids to keep vein open rate (30 cc/hr) per physician order.
• Anticipate administration of diuretics and urinary catheter insertion.

◆ **Pain** related to inflammation, tissue trauma, spasms as evidenced by tachycardia, facial expressions, frequent change in position, or refusal to change position.

INTERVENTIONS
• Place patient in position of comfort.
• Initiate imagery, relaxation exercises, and/or previous coping mechanisms identified by patient.
• Administer nonsteroidal antiinflammatory agents and narcotics per physician order.

◆ **Altered patterns of urinary elimination: urge incontinence** related to infection, trauma as evidenced by involuntary urine loss associated with urge to void.
INTERVENTIONS
- Monitor voiding patterns (precipitating factors, amount, time).
- Document any voiding mishaps (e.g., wet sheets).
- Assess associated symptoms with voiding.

◆ **Urinary retention** related to chronic obstruction as evidenced by bladder distention, decreased urine output.
INTERVENTIONS
- Assess breath sounds for crackles.
- Assess edema.
- Percuss/palpate bladder to determine degree of distention.
- Initiate intake and output measurement.
- Insert urinary catheter per physician order.

◆ **Risk for infection** related to anticipated invasive procedures, retention of urine, insertion of urinary catheter, and decreased immunocompetence.
INTERVENTIONS
- Maintain sterile technique for all invasive procedures.
- Document baseline temperature and route by which obtained.
- Assess for evidence of infection (urine integrity, quality of breath sounds, wound healing, as appropriate).

PRIORITY DIAGNOSTIC TESTS
Laboratory
If suspecting renal failure/fluid volume excess, obtain enough blood for CBC (purple top) and electrolytes (red top). If possible, fill an additional red top tube for potential type and crossmatch (transfusion may be necessary if anemia is severe). Clotting profiles may be needed, if so, fill a blue top tube. If suspecting infection or obstruction, CBC (purple top tube) should be adequate.

Complete blood count: Expect decreased hematocrit in chronic renal failure. Increased WBC in infection. If the infection is acute and bacterial in origin, increased neutrophils and decreased lymphocytes will be present.

UA and Urine C/S: Presence of casts indicates pyelonephritis (upper UTI). Presence of WBCs and

RBCs are nonspecific for infection and calculi. UTI may be the first manifestation of sepsis. Sepsis can be produced by gram-negative or gram-positive organisms. Urine-specific gravity and osmolality differ depending on origin of renal failure. Table 12-2 contrasts these differences.

BUN/creatinine: Differs according to origin of renal failure. See Table 12-2.

Electrolytes: Hyperkalemia may be present in renal failure. If so, assess for hyperactive reflexes and ECG changes (peaked T waves, prolonged PR interval and QRS duration).

ABGs: Metabolic acidosis (pH <7.35, HCO_3 <22, and $PaCO_2$ ≤35) may be present in renal failure.

NURSING ALERT

If hematocrit is low, anticipate obtaining specimen for type and crossmatch and initiating IV access (heparin lock is useful, since fluid restriction may be necessary). Use an 18-gauge or larger IV catheter.

If hyperkalemia and/or metabolic acidosis is present, anticipate dialysis. Initiate cardiac monitoring. Anticipate administration of sodium polystyrene sulfonate (Kayexalate), glucose with insulin, and/or sodium bicarbonate. IV access is necessary. Hyperphosphatemia requires administration of phosphate binders (aluminum hydroxide antacids [Amphojel]) or calcium antacids (Alternagel).

If increased WBCs are noted, no action may be necessary. However, if upper UTI/sepsis is suspected, IV antibiotics may be needed. Anticipate IV administration. Blood cultures may be ordered and can be initiated with IV insertion before antibiotic administration.

Radiographic

Intravenous pyelogram (IVP): Used to assess upper urinary tract function. Contrast medium is injected intravenously and serial x-ray films are obtained. Expect a 30 to 45 minute procedure. If blood pressure is unstable, nurse/physician should accompany patient if taken out of the department for test completion.

TABLE 12-2 Categories of Acute Renal Failure and Related Laboratory Values

	Prerenal	Intrarenal (ATN)	Postrenal
Urine			
Volume	Low	Low or high	Low or high
Sodium	<20 mEq/L	>20 mEq/L	>40 mEq/L
Osmolality	>350 mOsm	<300 mOsm (fixed)	<350 mOsm (varies)
Specific gravity	>1.020	<1.010	
Creatinine	~Normal	Low	Low
FEna	≤1%	>1%	
Plasma			
Urea (BUN)	High	High	High
Creatinine	~Normal	High	High
BUN: creatinine	20:1 or more	10:1 to 15:1	10:1

From Stillwell SB: *Mosby's critical care nursing reference*, St Louis, 1992, Mosby.

NURSING ALERT

Assess any allergies. Iodine and seafood allergies may require cancellation of IVP or premedication (steroids, antihistamines, acetaminophen) to minimize reaction.

Retrograde pyelogram: Used to assess ureter function. Dye is injected through catheters placed in ureters. Same concerns as with IVP.

Cystography: Used to assess bladder function. Radiopaque dye is injected through a urinary catheter. X-rays are obtained to assess if bladder is distended with dye or extravasated. Extravasation may be intraperitoneally or extraperitoneally. A cystogram is typically a 15 to 20 minute procedure.

> **NURSING ALERT**
>
> Patient may complain of severe burning and discomfort if bladder laceration/rupture is present. Prepare patient for this pain, and use distraction, imagery, and medication as appropriate to facilitate patient coping.

Retrograde urethrography: Usually performed in conjunction with cystography. Radiopaque dye is injected through a urinary catheter as the catheter is inserted to detect urethral lacerations. Same concerns as for IVP.

CT/renal scan: Rapidly replacing IVP and arteriography because it is noninvasive. Depending on type of scanner, procedure may take 15 to 30 minutes. Difficult to use in an agitated patient because clear films cannot be obtained with patient movement.

Renal angiography: Used when renal vascular injury is suspected. Patient has a mechanism of injury severe enough to cause renal damage (e.g., fracture of lower ribs) and unstable vital signs. If the IVP shows absent or poor visualization of contrast medium, an angiogram may be performed.

Renal ultrasonography: May be used to assess for obstruction and/or abscesses. Noninvasive procedure performed at bedside using reflection of high-frequency sound waves to produce organ image.

Radionuclide imaging: Radionuclide is IV administered, and a radioactivity detecting device records the radionuclide uptake to evaluate alterations in blood flow. Used for both renal and testicular problems.

> **NURSING ALERT**
>
> Use gloves when handling the patient's urine after this procedure, since the excretion of the radionuclide may take 24 hours.

COLLABORATIVE INTERVENTIONS

1. Semi-Fowler's position to facilitate urine drainage in urinary tract trauma.

2. A urinary catheter may be ordered to monitor urine output. If blood is present at the urinary meatus, the patient may have a pelvic fracture. If patient complains of suprapubic pain with or without perineal discoloration, do not pass the catheter until a retrograde urethrogram is performed.

3. In selecting a urinary catheter, examine the urethral opening and select an appropriate size for the opening (usually a size 12 to 16 Fr in adults). Age, weight, and gender are not useful criteria for choosing catheter size. If leakage occurs around the catheter, it is usually a result of the catheter being too large (4).

4. The patient may require rapid fluid removal using continuous arteriovenous hemofiltration, continuous venous-venous hemofiltration, hemodialysis, or peritoneal dialysis.

Clinical Conditions
Acute cystitis (lower UTI)
SYMPTOMS
- Irritability in children, dysuria, urinary frequency, suprapubic tenderness.

DIAGNOSIS
- UA has increased neutrophils.

TREATMENT
- Trimethoprim or trimethoprim-sulfamethoxazole PO (assess patient sensitivity to sulfa).
- Increased fluid intake and frequent resting periods may be ordered.

Acute pyelonephritis (upper UTI)
SYMPTOMS
- Same as cystitis plus fever, N/V, flank pain.

DIAGNOSIS
- Casts in urine.

TREATMENT
- Oral antibiotics if case is mild.
- If case is severe, or patient cannot tolerate PO meds secondary to N/V, IV antibiotics are administered.
- Cephalosporins, ampicillin, quinoline drugs (ciprofloxacin, ofloxacin, enoxacin, and norfloxacin), aminoglycosides, and IV trimethoprim may be ordered.
- Increased fluid intake and analgesics may be ordered.

Sepsis

SYMPTOMS
- Suprapubic pain, fever, change in vital signs without obvious cause, change in mental status.

DIAGNOSIS
- Blood cultures. However, blood cultures may be negative and systemic infection still be present.

TREATMENT
- Aminoglycosides may be ordered to treat urologic infections to reduce the frequency of gram-negative bacteremia.

Urinary calculi

SYMPTOMS
- Pain and extreme restlessness.
- N/V.
- Hematuria may be present.
- Fever is not present unless infection accompanies the calculi.

DIAGNOSIS
- Past history of calculi.
- IVP to identify site and renal function.
- Renal ultrasound may be used.
- Stone analysis if calculi passes.

TREATMENT
- Increase fluids to 2 qt/day.
- IV pain medication.
- Penicillamine to dissolve stones. Up to 5 mm may pass spontaneously.
- Extracorporeal shock wave lithotripsy may be used if calculi is in the renal collecting system or upper ureter and is <2 cm.
- Stones >2 cm in the upper renal poles or those >1 cm in lower renal poles may be removed by percutaneous nephrolithotomy.

Testicular torsion

SYMPTOMS (see Table 12-1, p. 371)
- Positive Prehn's sign.
- Increased pain when testis is elevated.
- Usually occurs after physical activity or during sleep.
- N/V.

DIAGNOSIS
- Result of a congenital defect.

- It is a surgical emergency and must be repaired within 6 hours to maintain testis viability.
- Decreased image on testicular ultrasonography. Doppler blood flow study shows diminished blood flow. Radionuclide testicular scan shows hypoperfused testis.

TREATMENT

- IV pain medication.
- Prepare patient for transfer to the operating suite.

Epididymitis

SYMPTOMS (see Table 12-1, p. 371)

- Swollen scrotum.
- Fever.
- Urethral discharge.
- Dysuria.
- Gradual onset.
- Recent history of sexual activity.

DIAGNOSIS

- Enhanced image on testicular ultrasound.
- Increased blood flow to testicular area using Doppler stethoscope.
- Radionuclide testicular scan shows hyperperfused testis.

TREATMENT

- Oral antibiotics.
- Ice packs to testes.
- Elevation of testes.
- Pain medication may be ordered.

GU trauma

SYMPTOMS

- Pain, swelling, ecchymoses in scrotum, perineum, and/or flank.
- Bladder distention.
- Pain on voiding.
- Hematuria, blood at the urinary meatus.
- Associated with pelvic fracture.
- Renal vascular injuries may present without hematuria (e.g., renal thrombosis).
- Gross hematuria does not indicate the severity of injury.
- Table 12-3 compares symptoms for upper and lower urinary tract trauma.

DIAGNOSIS

- IVP, retrograde pyelogram, cystography, retrograde urethrogram, CT scan.

TABLE 12-3 Comparison of Urologic Injuries

Nursing diagnosis	Renal injuries	Ureteral injuries	Bladder injuries	Urethral injuries
Pain	Mild, localized tenderness to severe discomfort in groin, flank, upper abdomen. May radiate to groin or thigh of affected side.	Flank, lower abdomen on affected side	Pelvic area, lower abdomen, suprapubic region. May radiate to shoulder.	Suprapubic region
Altered patterns of urinary elimination	Hematuria may be present (gross or microscopic).	Hematuria may be present. Possible anuria.	Small amount of bloody urine on catheterization. Strong urge to void but inability to do so.	May be slight hematuria initially. Difficulty voiding. High incidence of functional incontinence with urethral injuries in females and with posterior urethral injuries in males after trauma.
Fluid volume deficit	Possible	Possible	Possible	Unlikely
Altered genitourinary tissue perfusion related to infection	Possible	Possible	Unlikely	Unlikely

Infection as evidenced by N/V, abdominal distention and rigidity, absent bowel sounds, soft mass in flank	Possible	Possible	Possible with laceration of bladder fundus and penetrating trauma	Possible
High risk for altered renal tissue perfusion	AV fistula; hydronephrosis, hypertension	Ureteral compression leading to hydronephrosis	Unlikely	Unlikely
Sexual dysfunction	Unlikely	Unlikely	Unlikely	Higher incidence of impotence and infertility with posterior urethral injuries in males

From Kidd P: Elimination, metabolism and sexuality: genitourinary. In Neff J, Kidd P, editors: *Trauma nursing: the art and science*, St Louis, 1993, Mosby.

G

TREATMENT

- Usually conservative with drainage by urinary catheter or suprapubic catheter until hematuria clears.
- Renal vascular emergencies require surgical intervention. Prepare these patients for transfer to the operating suite.
- Expect patients with urinary tract trauma who are conservatively managed with urinary catheter placement and no surgical exploration to be admitted (2).
- Penetrating urinary tract trauma is usually surgically explored. Blunt bladder trauma with intraperitoneal extravasation is usually surgically explored.

Renal failure

SYMPTOMS

- ARF may have a prerenal, intrarenal, or postrenal cause.
- In the ED, the patient may present in a shock state and the ARF is secondary to hypoperfusion.
- Acute tubular necrosis is a form of intrarenal ARF. It may occur secondary to trauma or acute infection.
- Postrenal failure results from obstruction to urine flow, and in the emergency patient is usually related to a tumor or stone.
- Symptoms are diverse in nature with multisystem involvement. Table 12-4 lists system, symptom, and related pathophysiology.
- Patients present with oliguria initially. However, this is followed by a diuretic phase where urine output may increase to 3 to 5 L/24 hr.
- Patients presenting in the diuretic phase have fluid volume deficit and hypotension.
- Prerenal origin is related to decreased renal perfusion.

DIAGNOSIS

- Confirmed by BUN and creatinine levels.
- Table 12-2 compares the laboratory values in the three categories of ARF.

TREATMENT

- Depends on type of ARF.
- In prerenal origin, enhancing cardiac output and renal perfusion is a goal.
- Fluid challenge and low-dose dopamine may be used.
- Fluid restriction, diuretics, and dialysis may be used in intrarenal and postrenal etiologies.

TABLE 12-4 Clinical Manifestations of Acute Renal Failure

System	Symptom	Pathophysiology
Cardiovascular	Dysrhythmia	Hyperkalemia, hypocalcemia
	Heart failure	Hypertension, fluid retention
	Metabolic acidosis	Decreased H^+ secretion
		Decreased Na^+ reabsorption
		Decreased HCO_3 reabsorption/generation
	Hypertension	Increased Na^+ retention
		Activation of renin
Pulmonary	Pulmonary edema	Left ventricle dysfunction
		Increased capillary permeability
		Fluid retention
	Kussmaul's respirations	Metabolic acidosis
Hematopoietic	Anemia	Decreased erythropoietin
	Altered coagulation	Platelet dysfunction related to toxins
	Immuno-suppression	Decreased neutrophils
Gastrointestinal	Anorexia	Breakdown of urea, release of ammonia
	N/V	
	Gastritis/GI bleed	Ammonia produces ulcerations
Neuromuscular	Decreased LOC	Metabolic acidosis
		Uremic toxin accumulation
	Tremors, hyperreflexia	Hyperkalemia
Integumentary	Pallor	Anemia
	Yellow skin	Urochrome excretion
	Pruritus	Calcium and phosphate skin deposits
	Purpura	Platelet dysfunction
	Uremic frost	Terminal sign
		Urea skin crystals
Skeletal	Hypocalcemia	Hyperphosphatemia resulting from decreased excretion
		Decreased Ca^+ absorption resulting from decreased conservation of vitamin D

- Electrolyte abnormalities and metabolic acidosis must be treated.
- The most serious electrolyte abnormality encountered in the ED is usually hyperkalemia.
- Hyperphosphatemia and hypocalcemia may also be present.
- If the patient is in the diuretic phase of ARF, hypokalemia may occur. These patients require volume and potassium replacement.

Genitalia injuries

SYMPTOMS

- Severe pain, N/V.

DIAGNOSIS

- Most genitalia injuries are diagnosed by observation.
- Urethral injury may be present and is evaluated by retrograde urethrogram.
- Transillumination of the scrotum is performed to determine if the testis is ruptured.

TREATMENT

- Lacerations are treated by direct pressure.
- Crush injuries are treated with elevation and ice.
- Foreign bodies surrounding the penis may be removed with a ring cutter after relieving penile edema by irrigating the distal penis with heparinized saline or by making small incisions to allow fluid drainage.
- Most scrotum and vaginal lacerations are cleansed and repaired under anesthetic in the operating suite.

Renal transplant rejection

SYMPTOMS

- In addition to the symptoms seen in ARF, the patient will have fever.
- Urine output may drop suddenly.
- A 2 to 3 lb weight gain may be noted in a 24-hour period.

DIAGNOSIS

- Diagnosis is confirmed by renal biopsy, but a renal scan may be performed while the patient is in the ED to assess blood flow.

TREATMENT

- IV steroids may be administered.
- Immunosuppressant drug therapy is initiated.
- Drug therapy may include azathioprine (Imuran), cyclosporine (Sandimmune), and monoclonal

antibodies. These drugs require careful patient monitoring. See the company's drug insert for information.

NURSING SURVEILLANCE

1. Monitor hematuria.
2. Monitor vital signs.
3. Monitor I/O to assess fluid balance.
4. Observe and mark ecchymotic areas and/or expanding masses.

EXPECTED PATIENT OUTCOMES

1. Urinary output of 30 cc/hr or 1 cc/kg/hr in children is maintained.
2. Mean arterial pressure is maintained between 70 and 105 mm Hg.
3. Fever decreases.
4. Pain decreases in severity as documented by a pain scale.
5. Absence of N/V.
6. Diminished crackles/rales upon auscultation.
7. Electrolyte values trend toward normal limits.

DISCHARGE IMPLICATIONS

UTI

1. Teach good hygiene. Void after intercourse.
2. Stress follow-up after treatment in 7 to 14 days to examine for reinfection.
3. Vitamin C tablets (1 g/day) or three 8-oz glasses of cranberry juice daily decreases bacterial adherence to bladder wall and increases urine acidity (3).
4. Increase fluids to 2 qt/day.

Discharged with Indwelling Catheter

Patients with indwelling urinary catheters do not benefit from routine catheter changes (1). Irrigate a catheter only if decreased flow is noted. Catheters should be changed only if blockage is present. To decrease incidence of blockage, patients should consume 2 qt of fluids daily to dilute urine. Vitamin C tablets (1 g/day) or three 8-oz glasses of cranberry juice daily decreases encrustation on catheter surfaces thus, decreasing the incidence of blockage.

Renal Calculi

1. Stress increasing hydration to 2 qt/day.
2. Teach patient how to strain urine and provide strainer.
3. Inform patients that after analysis of the stone is performed, dietary changes need to be made (e.g., decreased calcium intake, decreased oxalate intake, low purine diet).

GU Trauma

1. Instruct patient to increase fluid intake.
2. Patient should return to ED if decreased urine output occurs. Patient can measure urine at home.
3. Bed rest is suggested until hematuria clears (if present).
4. Stress need for follow-up to assess renal function and potential complications such as hypertension.

References

1. Brechtelsbauer D: Care with an indwelling urinary catheter, *Postgrad Med* 92:127-132, 1992.
2. Hanno P, Cass A: The injured bladder, *Emerg Med* 347-351, March 15, 1992.
3. Moyle R, White R: Is choice of catheter size an important factor in patient discomfort? *Inforum* 12:9-10, 1991.
4. Roe B: Study of information given by nurses of catheter care to patients and their careers, *J Adv Nurs* 14:203-210, 1989.

Chapter XIII

Hematologic and Oncologic Conditions

Pamela S. Kidd

CLINICAL CONDITIONS
Hematologic
  Disseminated Intravascular Coagulation (DIC)
  Hemophilia
  Sickle-Cell Disease
    Acute Sickle-Cell Pain Crises
      Bone Crisis
      Chest Crisis
      Abdominal Crisis
      Joint Crisis
    Anemia
    Aplastic Crisis
    Acute Sequestration Syndrome
Oncologic
  Hypercalcemia
  Neoplastic Cardiac Tamponade
  Spinal Cord Compression
  Superior Vena Cava Syndrome (SVCS)
  Tumor Lysis Syndrome

TRIAGE ASSESSMENT

Most patients who present to the triage area with a hematologic or oncologic emergency will require urgent or emergent treatment. Patients with blood dyscrasias are usually very knowledgeable about their disease process and have sought emergency services only after trying multiple treatment strategies at home. Rarely are these patients initially diagnosed in the ED (see Life Span Issues). Oncology patients may not be as familiar with complications associated with their disease or the treatment of their disease but because of their chronic illness have a very small compensatory reserve.

Hematologic and Oncologic Conditions

Level of consciousness

If the patient is disoriented, suspect an intracranial bleed, metastatic tumor, or electrolyte abnormality and triage immediately to the treatment area. Sickle-cell anemia (SCA) patients are at risk for cerebrovascular attacks. Altered mental status or coma may occur as a result of cerebral hypoxia.

Pain

Back pain in a patient with cancer is a critical symptom. Pain is the first symptom in neoplastic spinal cord compression (SCC). The pain is usually localized and is increased when lying flat. Rest does not relieve the pain (Table 13-1). In hemophilia, pain will be present on rest and movement of an extremity or muscle group. Immobilization of affected area, and application of ice and a pressure dressing (elastic bandage) may relieve the pain. In SCA, pain may be precipitated by alcohol use, physical activity, changes in temperature and/or altitude, and emotional stress. Pain without joint swelling may be present in SCA.

Vascular access device

Does the patient have an indwelling central venous catheter or vascular access device? Infection and thrombosis may occur when these devices are present.

Hematologic Conditions

Injury history

Hemophiliacs and SCA patients develop symptoms inconsistent with a minor trauma history. In hemophiliac patients, no matter how trivial, all injury to the head and spinal column should be viewed as significant and triaged immediately to the treatment area (3).

Treatment prior to arrival

Ask what type of care was given at home. Hemophiliac patients may have administered several units of factor replacement at home, thus alerting ED personnel that additional medication/blood products may be necessary.

NURSING ALERT

Trust the patient. Many hemophiliacs will be able to detect bleeding before physical or radiographic signs. Because of the possibility of life-threatening or limb-threatening complications, triage the patient immediately to the treatment area.

TABLE 13-1 Oncologic Emergencies

Emergency	Symptoms	Triage clue
Acute tumor lysis syndrome		
Hyperuricemia	Dysuria, anuria, anorexia, vomiting, lethargy, pain and swelling of joints	Recent initiation of chemotherapy for treatment of leukemia or lymphoma
Hyperkalemia	Bradycardia, hypotension ECG changes: • Tall peaked T waves • Depressed ST segment • Widening of QRS diarrhea, muscle weakness	
Hyperphosphatemia/ hypocalcemia	Carpopedal spasms, hyperactive deep tendon reflexes, seizures, irritability, photophobia, diarrhea	
Hypercalcemia	N/V, constipation, abdominal pain, polyuria, bradycardia, mental changes ECG changes • Prolonged PR interval	History of breast cancer with bony metastatic disease
Spinal Cord Compression Cervical region: symptoms listed in order of appearance	Motor impairment of arm Motor impairment ipsilateral leg Motor impairment contralateral leg Motor impairment opposite arm	Pain is worse on lying down

Continued.

TABLE 13-1 Oncologic Emergencies (cont'd)

Emergency	Symptoms	Triage clue
Thoracic region	Stiff and weak legs Altered pain and temperature sensation on opposite side from maximum motor weakness Loss of bowel/bladder control	
Radicular or nerve root	Pain over affected spinal process that is aggravated with coughing, sneezing, or straight-leg raising, spasms, loss of deep tendon reflexes	
Superior vena cava syndrome	Edema, erythema of face and neck, visual changes, headache, conjunctival hemorrhage, engorged neck veins, dyspnea	Symptoms are worse on awakening; may have indwelling central venous catheter, since obstruction may be external from mass or internal from clot
Pericardial tamponade	Dyspnea, chest pain, cough, tachycardia, distant heart sounds (possible), jugular venous distention	Other typical symptoms of tamponade seen in traumatic injury (e.g., pulsus paradoxus, pericardial rub) may be absent
Anemia	Dyspnea, fatigue, dizziness, pallor, tachycardia	History of radiation to pelvis area and/or chemotherapy
Thrombocytopenia	Petechiae, GI/GU bleeding, epistaxis	History of radiation and/or chemotherapy
Disseminated intravascular coagulation	Fever, petechiae, conjunctival hemorrhage, melena, hematemesis, headache, change in mentation, hematuria	Bleeding from three unrelated sites

Factor type

If the patient is hemophiliac, ask what type of factor preparation he/she uses. If possible, get the batch number from the patient. This reduces the number of plasma donors to whom the patient is exposed.

Medications

Ask the patient what medications they take at home and if they have run out of medication. SCA patients may visit the ED for a renewal of analgesics.

Oncologic Conditions
Radiation/Chemotherapy

Assess if the patient has had radiation therapy and/or outpatient, as well as home, chemotherapy agents. Disseminated intravascular coagulation (DIC) and tumor lysis syndrome (TLS) may occur quickly after initiation of chemotherapy or radiation, especially first-time chemotherapy for leukemia. Symptoms may be related to chemotherapeutic agents the patient is receiving (Table 13-2).

Medical history

Certain cancerous cell types and tumor sites are associated with particular complications (Table 13-3).

Vital Sign Changes for Both Hematologic and Oncologic Conditions

- *Respirations:* Respiratory rate and pattern may be altered if airway compromise is occurring secondary to a retropharyngeal bleed. Hyperventilation may indicate acute chest crisis in SCA.
- *Blood pressure:* Hypotension will be present in acute sequestration syndrome in SCA. In this syndrome blood pools in an organ, depleting circulating blood volume. DIC may produce hypotension as a result of excessive bleeding. Hypotension may also occur in cases of hypercalcemia because of the polyuria it produces.
- *Fever:* A low-grade fever may be present in sickle-cell crisis and indicate infection as an etiology. Infection in the cancer patient is defined as one temperature ≥38.5° C (101° F) or three temperatures >38° C (100.4° F) in a 24-hour period (4).

TABLE 13-2 Complications of Chemotherapeutic Agents

Agent	Side effects	Use
Doxorubicin	Chemical pericarditis and dysrhythmia	Leukemia, breast cancer
Daunomycin	Chemical pericarditis and dysrhythmia	Leukemia, breast cancer
Cisplatin	Nephrotoxicity, neurotoxicity, and ototoxicity	Oat cell lung cancer, ovarian and testicular cancer
Cyclophosphamide	Hemorrhagic cystitis	Breast cancer, lymphoma
Methotrexate	Nephrotoxicity and hepatic toxicity, pulmonary fibrosis	Breast cancer, osteogenic sarcoma, lymphoma, leukemia
Bleomycin	Pulmonary fibrosis, Raynaud's phenomenon	
Interferon	Neurotoxicity, congestive heart failure	Hairy-cell leukemia
Interleukin-2	Hyperthermia, myocardial infarction, respiratory distress	

TABLE 13-3 Complications of Cancer

Primary cancer site/type	Associated oncologic emergency
Breast cancer	Hypercalcemia, neoplastic cardiac tamponade, SCC, SVCS, pleural effusion, brain tumor
Lung cancer	
Squamous cell	Pleural effusion, SCC, brain tumor, SVCS
Adenocarcinoma	Pleural effusion, SCC, brain tumor
Oat cell	SVCS, pleural effusion
Multiple myeloma	Hypercalcemia
Lymphoma	Hyperkalemia, hypercalcemia, neoplastic cardiac tamponade, TLS, SCC, SVCS, pleural effusion
Leukemia	Hypercalcemia, TLS, hyperkalemia, thrombocytopenia, hemorrhage
Prostate	SCC, brain tumor, DIC
Pancreatic	DIC, thrombocytosis
Bone	Hypercalcemia

SVCS, Superior vena cava syndrome; *SCC,* Spinal cord compression; *TLS,* Tumor lysis syndrome; *DIC,* Disseminated intravascular coagulation.

Vital Signs (Oncologic Conditions)

- *Pulsus Paradoxus:* An exaggerated decrease (>10 mm Hg) of the systolic blood pressure (BP) during inspiration (pulsus paradoxus) may be present in neoplastic cardiac tamponade.

Vital Signs (Hematologic Conditions)

- *Heart Rate:* Tachycardia will be present in acute sequestration syndrome to compensate for decreased circulating blood volume.

General Observations (Hematologic Conditions)
Hemorrhage

- Assess for signs of external hemorrhage (petechiae, ecchymoses, hematomas, swelling). If detected, pressure and cold should be applied to the site if possible. Elevation of the area is indicated and extremities should be immobilized at the triage area. The degree of swelling present is not a good indicator of the degree of bleeding.

Hyphema

- Assess for blood in the anterior chamber of the eyes (hyphema). Hyphema in SCA patients can have devastating complications because of the increased intraocular pressure resulting from blockage of outflow tracts by sickled cells. Triage these patients immediately to the treatment area.

General Observations (Oncologic Conditions)
Edema

- Assess for facial, neck, and periorbital edema. In superior vena cava syndrome (SVCS), edema in these areas may be present and worsen with bending over or lying down.

FOCUSED NURSING ASSESSMENT (HEMATOLOGIC AND ONCOLOGIC CONDITIONS)

Perfusion
Heart sounds

Muffled heart sounds may be present in neoplastic cardiac tamponade. Tamponade may result from primary or secondary tumors and mediastinal radiation treatment. A systolic murmur may be present in SCA as a result of chronic anemia. The apical pulse may be shifted in SCA because of congestive heart failure that develops from pulmonary hypertension secondary to repeated pulmonary infarcts. A pericardial rub may be heard in cardiac tamponade.

Neck veins

In SCA patients, neck veins may be distended because of cor pulmonale. In cancer patients, distended neck veins may suggest neoplastic cardiac tamponade or SVCS.

Cognition

Perform a neurologic assessment and assign the patient a Glasgow coma scale score (see Reference Guide 6). A patient with a score of <15 may need CT brain scanning. Assess neck rigidity, since meningitis is common in pediatric SCA patients. If present, anticipate performance of a lumbar puncture (see Procedure 22) and cerebrospinal fluid cultures.

Mobility

Stiffness of the joints, limited range of motion, and joint edema are common in hemarthroses (joint bleeding). Weakness on ambulation may be a sign of SCC and may be present for 4 to 6 weeks before the patient seeks treatment. Patients with SCC who are ambulatory at time of seeking treatment have a better chance of remaining mobile. Numbness and tingling of extremities may be another sign of SCC. Extension of the extremities may elicit an electrical sensation down the back.

FOCUSED NURSING ASSESSMENT (ONCOLOGIC CONDITIONS)

Ventilation
Breath sounds

Pleural effusions may develop in neoplastic cardiac tamponade and SVCS, diminishing breath sounds in the affected area.

Extremities

Examine the patient's extremities for deformity and angulation. Pathologic fractures may be present in malignancy. Pain is present on weight bearing.

FOCUSED NURSING ASSESSMENT (HEMATOLOGIC CONDITIONS)

Sexuality
Priapism

Priapism (painful sustained erection) may be present in SCA. Because erectile dysfunction and impotence may occur if left untreated, hydration and analgesia are initiated quickly.

Risk Factors for Both Hematologic and Oncologic Conditions
Infection

Many hemophiliacs have human immunodeficiency virus (HIV) because of having received blood products from multiple donors (HIV-contaminated blood products were used between 1978 and 1985 [2]). They may be immunosuppressed and have an active infection in addition to their presenting complaint.

Obstruction

SVCS is more likely to develop in a patient with right-sided vs. left-sided lung/bronchogenic cancer.

Life Span Issues (Hematologic Conditions)
Children

1. Hemophilia when not diagnosed at birth is usually detected when the child begins to walk and joint swelling occurs.
2. Cutting teeth and loss of deciduous teeth may precipitate bleeding in hemophilia.
3. Death in SCA patients between the ages of 1 and 3 years old is frequently related to pneumococcal sepsis and can be prevented with prophylactic penicillin. If the patient is receiving penicillin, this should be noted, since clinical presentation and bacterial studies may be altered in the presence of infection.
4. Acute chest crisis is more common in pediatric SCA patients.

Women

Postpartum bleeding may occur on a delayed basis after hospital discharge in women with von Willebrand's disease.

Adults

1. In adult hemophiliac patients, intracranial bleeding may occur spontaneously (without an injury history) in 50% of cases (3).
2. Adult SCA patients most frequently die from bone marrow and fat embolization and/or the effects of excessive narcotic use.

Life Span Issues (Oncologic Conditions)
Children

Bladder control regression may be the first symptom in children who have SCC from cancer.

INITIAL INTERVENTIONS (HEMATOLOGIC AND ONCOLOGIC CONDITIONS)

1. Initiate oxygen administration as needed to relieve dyspnea and impaired gas exchange. If dyspnea is present (as in suspected SVCS), elevate the head of bed and administer low-flow oxygen. Initiate pulse oximetry.

2. Initiate IV access. Oncologic and hematologic emergencies require either fluid resuscitation, factor replacement, pain control, electrolyte replacement or removal, or diuretics. Patients with SCA and hemophilia have had multiple IV catheters and their veins may be sclerosed. Ask the patient for the "best vein site," as well as the "best technique." Place the largest IV catheter that vein integrity will allow. Hydration in the SCA patient is initiated with D_5W because it allows free water to enter the cells and decreases the hemoglobin concentration, improving tissue oxygenation.

H

NURSING ALERT

For unsuccessful IV attempts, apply pressure to the puncture or injection site for at least 10 minutes in hemophiliac patients.

3. In hemophiliac patients, while starting the IV, obtain blood for complete blood count (CBC) (purple top tube) and coagulation studies (blue top tube). This allows for prediction of amount of factor replacement necessary based on severity and location of the bleed and degree of factor activity present.
4. Initiate pain control. Pain occurs in SCA from obstruction of blood flow and its resulting hypoxia and acidosis. SCA pain may be relieved by IV hydration. Ask the patient what usually relieves pain based on severity of episode. Distraction, imagery, and relaxation techniques can be initiated immediately. Seek an order for administration of acetaminophen, antiinflammatory agents, and narcotics.

NURSING ALERT

Aspirin products should not be administered to hemophiliac patients because of their interference with platelet function. Meperidine (Demerol) is not used in SCA patients because repeated doses are usually necessary resulting in accumulation of narcotic metabolites and subsequent respiratory depression. Ketorolac (Toradol) has had mixed success in treating SCA pain.

5. Institute infection control both for the patient and the health care worker. Hemophiliac patients have a high rate of HIV infection and hepatitis B. Cancer patients' white blood count (WBC) may be below 2,000 increasing their susceptibility for opportunistic and nosocomial infection. A mask may be placed on the patient and the patient placed in an isolation area (if available) until laboratory results are returned.

6. If the patient is complaining of chest pain, get an ECG. Several oncologic emergencies produce the symptom of chest pain (e.g., neoplastic cardiac tamponade and hypercalcemia).

PRIORITY NURSING DIAGNOSES

Risk for impaired gas exchange
Risk for pain
Risk for injury
Risk for impaired physical mobility

◆ **Impaired gas exchange** related to pulmonary infiltrates from microinfarctions in SCA, pleural effusion in malignancy, cor pulmonale in SVCS.
   INTERVENTIONS
   • Partial exchange transfusions and antibiotics may be administered.
   • Administer diuretics, oxygen, and vasoactive drugs as ordered.

◆ **Pain** related to nerve compression, inadequate cardiac output, or ischemia.
   INTERVENTIONS
   • Administer fluids and oxygen in cases of suspected ischemia as per physician order.
   • Use imagery, distraction, or relaxation techniques.
   • Administer narcotics, acetaminophen, or antiinflammatory drugs.

◆ **Injury** related to bleeding.
   INTERVENTIONS
   • Observe for hemorrhage.
   • Monitor mucous membranes, urine, sputum, and stool for blood.
   • Complete frequent neurologic and abdominal assessments.

◆ **Impaired physical mobility** related to joint bleeding and stiffness or SCC.

INTERVENTIONS
- Immobilize and elevate joints.
- Apply cold compresses to affected areas.
- Initiate and maintain spinal immobilization until radiographic tests are completed and results returned.

PRIORITY DIAGNOSTIC TESTS

Laboratory

Laboratory data diagnostic for hemophilia is located in Table 13-4.

Complete blood count (CBC): A CBC may be ordered to detect dehydration (high hematocrit) and infection in SCA. WBCs >20,000 have been associated with a higher infection and death rate in SCA. SCA patients typically have a WBC between 12,000 and 17,000 as a result of an active bone marrow. Hemoglobin levels will be extremely low in acute sequestration syndrome in SCA.

Electrolytes: Potassium and phosphorus may be elevated in tumor lysis syndrome. Calcium may be increased in malignancy and decreased in tumor lysis syndrome.

Fibrin split products: This level will be increased in DIC.

Hemoglobin S level: This level will be elevated in cases of acute crisis in SCA.

Platelets: Platelets will be decreased in DIC.

Prothrombin time: This level will be increased in DIC.

Partial thromboplastin time: This level will be increased in DIC.

Reticulocyte count: A reticulocyte count may be ordered in SCA to detect aplastic crisis. No reticulocytes will be present.

Uric acid: This level will be increased in tumor lysis syndrome.

Urinalysis: A urinalysis may be ordered to detect dehydration and/or infection in the SCA patient.

Radiographic

Lateral soft-tissue neck films: These films may be ordered to rule out retropharyngeal bleeding in hemophilia.

Chest film: A chest film may be ordered to rule out infection and infiltrates in SCA. A widened mediastinum may be present with SVCS.

CT scan: A scan may be used of the head to detect intracranial bleeding in hemophilia and SCA. A scan of the chest may show collateral circulation in SVCS.

TABLE 13-4 Laboratory Values in Bleeding Disorders

Condition	aPTT	Bleeding time	Factor VIII	Factor IX	vWF
Hemophilia A	Increased	Normal	Decreased	Normal	Normal
Hemophilia B	Increased	Normal	Normal	Decreased	Normal
von Willebrand's disease	Normal or increased	Increased	Decreased	Normal	Decreased

aPTT, Activated partial thromboplastin time; *vWF*, von Willebrand's factor.

Long bone films: These films may be obtained in hemophilia and SCA to detect acute joint effusions.

Spinal films: Most cases of vertebral body involvement by tumor (and SCC) can be identified using spinal films.

Other

Abdominal ultrasound: An ultrasound may be ordered to evaluate abdominal pain in SCA.

ECG: The direction of the QRS complex and T wave may alter with every other beat in cardiac tamponade. In hypercalcemia, first- or second-degree heart block may be present. In hyperkalemia associated with tumor lysis syndrome, tall peaked T waves may be present.

Echocardiogram: May be useful in diagnosing degree of pericardial effusions.

Venography: Venography may be used to identify the degree of obstruction in SVCS.

COLLABORATIVE INTERVENTIONS

1. Initiate blood product replacement. Hemophiliac patients may need factor replacement in cases where they present to the ED with a primary problem (e.g., laceration) and will require an invasive procedure (e.g., suturing). When in doubt, factor replacement should be initiated while awaiting laboratory results.
2. Simple or partial exchange transfusions may be administered in SCA to improve local blood flow to infarcted areas. A hemoglobin S level of <30% is desired.
3. In DIC, clotting factors may be replenished using platelets, fresh frozen plasma, or packed cells (see Chapter 11).

Clinical Conditions (Hematologic)
Disseminated intravascular coagulation

DIC may be associated with infection or as a complication of malignancy where tumors secrete substances that activate the clotting cascade or when antineoplastic therapy is lysing necrotic tumor cells. In DIC, the pace of the clotting cascade is accelerated and fibrinolysis is unable to keep pace with thrombus formation. Injury occurs from thrombi in the microcirculation and from bleeding as a result of the consumption of clotting factors in the microcirculation.

HOW TO CALCULATE
FACTOR REPLACEMENT

Amount of Factor VIII required = wt in kg × 0.5 × % change
desired in factor activity.*

Amount of Factor IX required = wt in kg × 1.0 × % change
desired in factor activity.*

*Table 13-5 includes factor activity treatment goals. Percent
(%) change is based on the difference between the degree
of factor activity present (by laboratory testing) and the
treatment goal.

SYMPTOMS
- Bleeding will generally occur from three or more sites.
- Petechiae, epistaxis, abdominal pain and distention,
  melena, hematuria, hemoptysis, and LOC changes may
  be present.
- The bleeding site(s) determine the symptoms.

DIAGNOSIS
- Laboratory data will show increased prothrombin and
  partial thromboplastin times.
- Fibrin split products will be elevated.
- Platelets and fibrinogen will be decreased.

TREATMENT
- Heparin therapy is used to block microthrombi
  formation.
- In malignancy, patients may be resistant to heparin
  therapy. Oncology patients with solid tumors usually
  suffer greater problems from hypercoagulability (1).
  Aspirin and dipyridamole may be used.
- Hemorrhage is more common in acute leukemias, bone
  marrow infiltration, and chemotherapy.
- Platelets (when the platelet count is <5000/mm³),
  packed red blood cells, fresh frozen plasma, or Factor
  VIII may be given.

Hemophilia

SYMPTOM
- Determine what type of clotting problem the patient has.
  If it is hemophilia A, Factor VIII is deficient. Ask if the
  patient has developed an inhibitor to human Factor VIII
  because agents with Factor VIII bypass activity will need
  to be administered.

TABLE 13-5 Comparison of Hemophilia Disorders

Condition	Treatment goal	von Willebrand's disease	Hemophilia A with inhibitors	Hemophilia A	Hemophilia B	Special considerations
Hematoma	Increase Factor VIII to 30%	FFP: 10 cc/kg Cryo: 2 bags/10 kg Factor VIII conc: 10 IU/kg DDAVP × 4 day	Factor IX conc: 50 IU/kg	Cryo: 2 bags/10 kg Factor VIII conc: 10 IU/kg*	FFP: 10 cc/kg Factor IX conc: 10 IU/kg	Cryo contains 60-125 U Factor VIII/bag Use microaggregate filter.
Hematuria	Increase Factor VIII to 30%	Steroids: 2 mg/kg FFP: 10 cc/kg DDAVP × 3 day Factor VIII conc: 10 IU/kg	Factor IX conc: 100 IU/kg Autoplex: 80-100 IU/kg Factor VIII: inhibitor bypass activity (FEIBA) 80-100 IU/kg Steroids: 2 mg/kg	Steroids: 2 mg/kg Cryo: 4 bags/10 kg Factor VIII conc: 40 IU/kg	Steroids: 2 mg/kg Factor VIII conc: 40 IU/kg	Factor VIII conc must be drawn up through a special filter needle.
Hemarthrosis	Increase Factor VIII to 30%	FFP: 5-10 cc/kg Cryo: 2 bags/10 kg DDAVP × 3 day Factor VIII conc: 10 IU/kg	Factor XI conc: 100-150 IU/kg Autoplex: 80-100 IU/kg Factor VIII: (FEIBA) 80-100 IU/kg Steroids: 2 mg/kg	Cryo: 3-4 bags/10 kg Factor VIII conc: 15-20 IU/kg	Factor IX conc: 15 IU/kg Prednisone: 2 mg/kg/day	—

Continued.

H

TABLE 13-5 Comparison of Hemophilia Disorders (cont'd)

Condition	Treatment goal	von Willebrand's disease	Hemophilia A with inhibitors	Hemophilia A	Hemophilia B	Special considerations
Mouth	Increase Factor VIII to 30%	DDAVP × 3 day Factor VIII conc: 20 IU/kg FFP: 20 cc/kg Amicar: 100 mg/kg q 6 hr Cyclokapron: 25 mg/kg q 6 hr	Amicar: 100 mg/kg q 6 hr Factor IX: 100 IU/kg Cyclokapron: 25 mg/kg q 6 hr	Cryo: 6 bags/10 kg Factor VIII conc: 40 IU/kg Amicar: 100 mg/kg q 6 hr Cyclokapron: 25 mg/kg q 6 hr	Factor IX conc: 20 IU/kg Amicar: 100 mg/kg q 6 hr Cyclokapron: 25 mg/kg q 6 hr	Amicar must be given slowly when given IV. Do not push!
Epistaxis	Increase Factor VIII to 30%	DDAVP × 5 day Factor VIII conc: 20 IU/kg FFP: 20 cc/kg Amicar: 100 mg/kg q 6 hr Cyclokapron: 25 mg/kg q 6 hr	Amicar: 100 mg/kg q 6 hr Factor IX: 100 IU/kg Cyclokapron: 25 mg/kg q 6 hr	Cryo: 6 bags/10 kg Factor VIII conc: 40 IU/kg Amicar: 100 mg/kg q 6 hr Cyclokapron: 25 mg/kg q 6 hr	Factor IX conc: 20 IU/kg Amicar: 100 mg/kg q 6 hr Cyclokapron: 25 mg/kg q 6 hr	—
Gastro-intestinal	Increase Factor VIII to 80%	FFP: 10 cc/kg Cryo: 2 bags/10 kg Factor VIII conc: 10 IU/kg	Factor IX conc: 100-150 IU/kg FEIBA or Autoplex: 50 IU/kg q 8 hr	Cryo: 6 bags/10 kg Factor VIII conc: 50 IU/kg	Factor IX conc: 40 IU/kg	—

Central nervous system	Increase Factor VIII to 100%	FFP: 15 cc/kg Cryo: 3 bags/10 kg Factor VIII conc: 15 IU/kg	Factor IX conc: 100-150 IU/kg FEIBA or Autoplex: 50 IU/kg q 8 hr	Cryo: 6 bags/10 kg Factor VIII conc: 50 IU/kg	Factor IX conc: 40 IU/kg	—
Retro-pharyngeal	Increase Factor VIII to 100%	FFP: 15 cc/kg Cryo: 3 bags/10 kg Factor VIII conc: 15 IU/kg	Factor IX conc: 100-150 IU/kg FEIBA or Autoplex: 50 IU/kg q 8 hr	Cryo: 6 bags/10 kg Factor VIII conc: 50 IU/kg	Factor IX conc: 40 IU/kg	—
Retro-peritoneal	Increase Factor VIII to 100%	FFP: 15 cc/kg Cryo: 3 bags/10 kg Factor VIII conc: 15 IU/kg	Factor IX conc: 100-150 IU/kg FEIBA or Autoplex: 50 IU/kg q 8 hr	Cryo: 6 bags/10 kg Factor VIII conc: 50 IU/kg	Factor IX conc: 40 IU/kg	—

Factor VIII conc, Factor VIII concentrate (Humate P, Hemofil, Koate); *Cryo,* cryoprecipitate; *Amicar,* ε-aminocaproic acid; *Cyclokapron,* tranexamic acid; *FFP,* fresh frozen plasma; *DDAVP,* desmopressin, can be administered IV, subcutaneously, intranasally. If given IV, dilute in 50 cc saline and give over 15-30 min.

- If the patient has hemophilia B, Factor IX is deficient.
- In cases of von Willebrand's disease, Factor VIII is synthesized but in inadequate amounts.
- Bleeding site and respective symptoms are listed in Table 13-6.

DIAGNOSIS

- Table 13-4 clarifies the laboratory values in most types of hemophilia.
- Factor levels need to be determined in order to calculate factor replacement that is adequate for the type and severity of factor deficiency and the type, severity, and location of the bleed.

TREATMENT

- Table 13-5 describes treatment alternatives based on location of bleeding.
- Bleeding of the mucous membranes of the mouth and nose is treated with both factor replacement and antifibrinolytic agents (e.g., Amicar) because saliva contains high levels of fibrinolytic enzymes making clots unstable.
- Ice, elastic bandages (pressure dressings), packing, and immobilization and elevation may be used in addition to medication/factor administration to control bleeding in joints, muscles, and nose.

Sickle-cell disease

SCA patients live in a balance between ongoing hemolysis of abnormal cells and accelerated erythropoiesis. The spleen is injured from multiple infarcts, increasing the patient's susceptibility to infection.

Acute Sickle-Cell Pain Crises: There are four types of crises: bone, chest, abdominal, and joint. There is no objective method of validating these crises. Treatment for each type of crisis is the same.

Bone crisis

SYMPTOMS

- Acute long bone pain.
- Back pain is common in pediatric patients.
- Nonpitting edema may be present.

DIAGNOSIS

- Diagnosis is by clinical presentation and patient history of SCA.

TREATMENT

- Hydration by mouth if tolerated or by IV route is indicated.

TABLE 13-6 Common Manifestations of Bleeding in Hemophilia Disorders

Bleeding site	Symptoms	Special considerations
Muscle	Pain at site on movement or rest. Numbness, tingling if nerve compression occurs. Decreased or absent DTRs.	Potential for compartment syndrome.
Hemarthrosis	Edema at site. Pain is usually in knee, elbow, shoulder, ankle, or wrist. Limited range of motion.	More factor replacement is required for weight bearing joints. Hypovolemia may occur if bleeding into shoulder or hips.
Central nervous system	Altered LOC, headache, vomiting, seizures.	May have 24 hr symptom-free interval after injury.
Gastrointestinal	Melena, hematemesis.	—
Retropharyngeal	Sore throat, dysphagia, dyspnea, change in voice quality.	Usually occurs after dental procedures.
Retroperitoneal	Tender RLQ. Absent bowel sounds. Rigid abdomen. Flank pain with hematoma. Hypovolemic signs.	—

DTRs, Deep tendon reflexes; *LOC*, level of consciousness.

H

- At least 3 to 4 L/24 hr is suggested for the adult SCA patient.
- Analgesics are administered.
- Supplemental oxygen has not been proven to be helpful regardless of the presence of hypoxia. However, oxygen may be administered to provide psychologic support.

Chest crisis
SYMPTOMS
- Pleuritic chest pain may be present in conjunction with dyspnea and hyperventilation.
- A nonproductive cough may be present.
- Hemoptysis suggests a pulmonary infarction.

DIAGNOSIS
- Diagnosis is by clinical presentation.
- Infiltrates may be present on a chest film.

TREATMENT
- Treatment is the same for all crisis states.
- For patients with a PaO_2 <60 mm Hg, partial exchange transfusion may be initiated.

Abdominal crisis
SYMPTOMS
- Patients complain of acute, constant abdominal pain with minimal tenderness on palpation.
- Nausea, vomiting, and diarrhea may be present.

DIAGNOSIS
- Diagnosis is by clinical presentation.

TREATMENT
- Treatment is the same for all crisis states.
- Antiemetic agents may be ordered if nausea and vomiting are present.

Joint crisis
SYMPTOMS
- Patients may complain of pain in one or multiple joints. Usually no joint swelling is present.

DIAGNOSIS
- Diagnosis is by clinical presentation.

TREATMENT
- Treatment is the same for all crisis states.

Anemia
Anemia in SCA occurs when the hemoglobin S levels fall below 18% because of illness, decreased erythropoiesis (aplastic crisis), or sequestration of RBCs in an organ.

Aplastic crisis

SYMPTOMS

- Fatigue and dyspnea are common.

DIAGNOSIS

- Decreased RBCs and hemoglobin on CBC.
- No reticulocytes are present.

TREATMENT

- Folate may be administered and in severe cases, a transfusion may be required.

Acute sequestration syndrome

SYMPTOMS

- Syncope and hypovolemic signs are common.
- Left-side abdominal pain may be present with abdominal distention.
- The involved organ, usually the liver or the spleen, will be enlarged and tender on palpation.

DIAGNOSIS

- Reticulocyte levels will be elevated.
- Hemoglobin levels will be extremely low (1 to 2 g/dl).

TREATMENT

- Vigorous fluid resuscitation and blood transfusion is necessary.

Clinical Conditions (Oncologic)

Hypercalcemia

Hypercalcemia in cancer may occur for the following reasons. The tumor produces a parathyroid hormone-like substance, hormonal treatment of primary cancer (e.g., tamoxifen), or the tumor produces direct bone destruction.

SYMPTOMS

- Nausea, vomiting, and polyuria are the initial signs and contribute to the hypovolemia associated with hypercalcemia.
- DTRs are diminished or absent.
- Decreased LOC may occur with hypoventilation.

DIAGNOSIS

- In malignancy, serum calcium levels have to be very high (e.g., 16 to 18 mg/dl) before symptoms occur.
- ECG changes of short ST segments, first- or second-degree heart block, and wide T waves may be present.

TREATMENT

- Treatment is discussed in Table 13-7.

TABLE 13-7 Drug Summary

Drug	Dose/Route	Special considerations	Use
Plicamycin	10-25 mcg/kg IV	—	Hypercalcemia
Mithramycin	15-25 mcg/kg IV q day × 2 days	Produces thrombocytopenia and rapid rebound of Ca^+ level after treatment	Hypercalcemia
Etidronate disodium (Didronel)	7.5 mg/kg IV q day × 3 days 400 mg PO bid	—	Hypercalcemia
Calcitonin	200-400 U IM or SC or 4 IU/kg q 12 hr IV	—	Hypercalcemia
Allupurinol	300-800 mg PO q day		Hyperuricemia
Sodium polystrene sulfonate (Kayexalate)	20-50 g PO	Potassium binding resin	Hyperkalemia
Calcium gluconate	5-10 cc of a 10% solution IV	—	Hyperkalemia
Sodium bicarbonate	44 mEq IVP over 5 min or 50-100 mEq in 1 L of 0.25% NS at 100-200 cc/hr IV	Encourages cellular expert of hydrogen and import of potassium	Hyperkalemia
Insulin and glucose	5-20 U regular insulin plus 25 g glucose IV (250 cc of 10-20% glucose solution)	Glucose will import potassium into the cell	Hyperkalemia

Aluminum hydroxide Furosemide	500 mg-2 g bid-qid PO 40-80 mg PO or IV q 4-6 hr	Must be titrated with normal saline IV administration	Hyperphosphatemia Hypercalcemia
Metoclopramide hydrochloride	2 mg/kg IV q 4-6 hr		Antiemetic for vomiting associated with chemotherapy
Gallium nitrate	100-200 mg/m^2 q day, infuse over 24 hr continuous IV infusion for 5 days	Do not use with other nephrotoxic drugs or in renal failure	Hypercalcemia

- Intravenous saline (0.9% alternating with 0.5%) is administered (2 to 5 L/day) or 250 to 500 cc/hr.
- Diuretics are given after volume is restored to assist in eliminating calcium.
- Medications aimed at preventing bone breakdown (e.g., calcitonin, plicamycin, gallium nitrate) are administered.
- Radiation and chemotherapy aimed at the primary tumor may be instituted.
- Dialysis may be used in patients with hypercalcemia and renal failure.

> **NURSING ALERT**
>
> Hypokalemia may occur with saline hydration and diuretic use in treating hypercalcemia. Monitor for muscle weakness, paralytic ileus, and flattening of the T wave (T wave inversion) on ECG.

Neoplastic cardiac tamponade
SYMPTOMS
- Signs of hypoperfusion exist.
- Decreased LOC, oliguria, hypotension, elevated central venous pressure, and muffled heart sounds may be present (Beck's triad).
DIAGNOSIS
- Diagnosis is made based on clinical presentation, ECG, and echocardiogram.
TREATMENT
- Pericardiocentesis is the treatment of choice (see Procedure 24).
- Continuous drainage by an indwelling catheter may be initiated until surgery can be performed.
- IV fluid administration and vasoactive medications (e.g., dopamine) may be used.
- Pericardial sclerosis may be instituted using chemotherapeutic agents.

Spinal cord compression (SCC)
SYMPTOMS
- Pain is localized, unrelieved by rest, and exacerbated by lying flat.
- Straining and coughing will also worsen pain.
- Motor ability is diminished first followed by sensation to pain and touch.

- Bowel and bladder dysfunction occurs last.
- Initially, deep tendon reflexes (DTRs) may be hyperreflexic but eventually DTRs are absent.

DIAGNOSIS

- Diagnosis is made based on clinical history, spine films, myelography, and MRI in some cases.

TREATMENT

- High-dose steroids may be given (100 mg/day dexamethasone IV).
- Radiation and surgery may be used.

Superior vena cava syndrome

The superior vena cava may be compressed externally by a mass or it may be obstructed internally by a thrombus (as in cases of indwelling central venous catheters) or direct invasion by the disease process.

SYMPTOMS

- Dyspnea, cough, dysphagia, hoarseness, and chest pain may occur.
- Edema of the face and neck may be present.
- In severe obstruction, syncope and decreased LOC occurs.
- Symptoms are worse upon rising in the morning or by bending over.

DIAGNOSIS

- Diagnosis is confirmed by chest film and venography.

TREATMENT

- If SVCS is caused by external compression, chemotherapy and radiation are used.
- If a thrombosis is present, urokinase (4,400 U/kg IV bolus followed by 4,400 U/kg/hr) or streptokinase (250,000 U IV bolus followed by 100,000 U/hr) or tissue plasminogen activator (check drug insert for proper dosage, since dosage varies) may be given.
- Surgery may be indicated.
- Diuretics may be given as a temporary measure.

Tumor lysis syndrome (TLS)

TLS is a positive indicator that therapy is effective. As tumor cells are killed, potassium, phosphate, and uric acid levels rise. Calcium levels will fall in response to the elevated phosphate levels.

SYMPTOMS

- Symptoms are listed in Table 13-1.
- Joint pain may occur secondary to accumulation of uric acid.

- Renal function may decrease because of uric acid crystal formation.
- Cardiac symptoms of tachycardia, hypotension, tall T waves, prolonged ST segment, and delayed conduction occur because of hypocalcemia and hyperkalemia.
- Hyperactive DTRs and muscle cramps may be present.

DIAGNOSIS

- Diagnosis is based on serum electrolyte levels and uric acid level.

TREATMENT

- IV hydration is started using 250 cc of 10% to 20% glucose with 10 to 20 U of regular insulin.
- Potassium is restricted in both IV fluids and diet.
- Calcium gluconate may be given.
- Cation exchange resins (Kayexalate and aluminum hydroxide) may be used to remove potassium and phosphate respectively, while allopurinol is used to remove the uric acid.
- Sodium bicarbonate may be given to decrease the likelihood of uric acid precipitation.

NURSING SURVEILLANCE

1. Monitor for complications of factor/blood replacement. Allergic reactions may range from wheezing, fever, chills, and hives to dyspnea. Flushing, tachycardia, nausea, and headaches may occur if the drugs are infused too rapidly (see Chapter 11).
2. Monitor for response to fluid administration. Fluid overload can result quickly in malignancy where radiation treatment has been administered to the mediastinum and chest. Hydration is a common treatment for oncologic emergencies (e.g., hypercalcemia, tumor lysis syndrome, cardiac tamponade). Fluid overload can also occur in SCA in cases of multiple pulmonary infarcts and pulmonary hypertension.
3. Monitor for changes in LOC.

EXPECTED PATIENT OUTCOMES

1. Factor activity levels are at least 50% (in cases of hemophilia).
2. Hemoglobin S level will be 30% or less.
3. LOC will remain unchanged or improve.
4. Seizure activity is diminished.

5. Serum electrolyte levels will normalize.
6. Pain will diminish.

DISCHARGE IMPLICATIONS (HEMATOLOGIC CONDITIONS)

1. Teach prevention of acute episodes.
2. In sickle-cell anemia, avoid changes in temperature, hydration, and stressful situations.
3. In hemophilia, avoid injury (e.g., wear protective devices such as helmets, knee pads as appropriate for activity) and aspirin-containing products. Home environments may need alteration to promote safety (e.g., playground areas). Electric razors only should be used. Good dental hygiene may prevent the need for tooth extractions and subsequent bleeding.
4. Teach recognition of acute episodes. Hemophiliacs should be taught how to examine their urine for microscopic hematuria (urine reagent strips). A tingling sensation may precede any objective signs of bleeding. Change in LOC, vomiting, severe headache, mood changes, and gait may signal intracranial bleeding. Pallor, weakness, and restlessness may indicate internal bleeding.
5. Encourage health care evaluation after what is perceived to be "minor" injury. Major bleeding may occur hours after minor trauma.
6. Help the patient obtain "Medic Alert" tag.

DISCHARGE IMPLICATIONS (ONCOLOGIC CONDITIONS)

1. Teach prevention of acute episodes.
2. Encourage patient mobility and fluid intake of 3 to 4 L of fluid/day to prevent hypercalcemia.

References

1. Bick R: Coagulation abnormalities in malignancy: a review, *Semin Thromb Hemost* 18:353-372, 1992.
2. Medical Advisory Council of the Florida State Chapter of the National Hemophilia Foundation (1993): Emergency room care for hemophiliac patients, *J Fla Med Assoc* 80:250-254, 1993.
3. Pfaff J and Geninatti M: Hemophilia, *Emerg Med Clin North A* 11:337-363, 1993.
4. Saleh T and Elfenbein G: Oncologic emergencies, *J Am Acad of Physic Assist* 4:7-20, 51A, 1991.

Chapter XIV

Mental Health Conditions

Celeste Shawler

CLINICAL CONDITIONS
Violent Behavior Toward Others
Violent Behavior Toward Self
Victims of Abuse
Anxiety
Individuals in Crisis

TRIAGE ASSESSMENT

Violent Behavior

Assessment of patients with the potential for violence toward self or others requires knowledge of the dynamics of crises and expert interventions that will provide for a safe and therapeutic environment in the emergency department (ED). Staff awareness and preventive practices must be incorporated into the ED nurse's daily routine (3,4). The manner in which the triage assessment is conducted is critical to elicit accurate data to identify the risk potential for violence toward self or others.

Manner of speech

Talk in a slow, calm voice, and avoid arguing or direct confrontation. REMEMBER: The patient is probably in emotional disequilibrium and very anxious.

Agitated patient

If the patient is agitated, quickly get them into a less stimulating section of the ED and do not make them wait for treatment. Waiting greatly increases frustration and potential for loss of control.

Topic of conversation

Pay attention to what the patient says and to how it is said.

Staff attitude

Be receptive to patients. Demonstrate care and concern. Let the patient know immediately you are concerned, you are here to help, and that the ED is a safe place. This will help to establish trust and credibility, stabilizing factors when interacting with those in crisis.

Staff protection

Utilize common sense and caution when interacting with someone who is violent toward others (13). Allow space between yourself and the patient and do not attempt to control violent behavior alone.

Victims of Abuse

Domestic violence

Should be considered when women seek treatment with either trauma or mental health problems (6). As many as 30% of women who are seen in the ED exhibit at least one or more symptoms of physical abuse (7).

Children

Children are frequently victims of abuse (see Focused Nursing Assessment).

Rape

Rape is a criminal offense. Understand that there is a stigma attached, so be extremely sensitive to the victim. Look for evidence indicating that force or coercion was used and that the sexual contact occurred against the victim's will (15).

Anxiety

Most patients admitted to the ED will have some degree of anxiety. An understanding of the continuum of anxiety from mild, moderate, severe, to panic and the interventions appropriate to each level will be outlined.

General Observations

Focus on the following assessment areas.

Violent behavior toward others

- *Acting out behaviors:* Assess acting out behaviors (present and past).
- *Signs of potential violence:* Does the patient have presence of drugs or alcohol? If yes, potential for violence increases. Signs include pacing, violent gestures, demanding, profane and threatening verbal language, and actively threatening language.
- *Reaction of patient to others:* Are there individuals present who calm or agitate the patient? If so, ask the ones that

calm the patient to remain with the patient and ask the others to remain at a distance from the patient.

- *Lethal weapons:* Are there lethal weapons in the possession of patient or visitors. If so, follow your institution's policy for obtaining the harmful item.

Violent behavior toward self

- Does the patient have a suicidal plan now?
- What is the history of suicide attempts?
- Is there presence of physical or psychiatric illnesses?
- Are there recent losses?
- What is the level and involvement of social support?
- Is there presence of alcohol or other drugs?

Victims of abuse

- Assess specific injuries.
- Ask how and when injuries occurred.
- Assess all physical complaints.
- Ask about stressors in life.
- Listen for consistency or lack of consistency in history. Lack of consistency may be due to high levels of anxiety.
- The patient should be interviewed alone.
- Begin to collect evidence as appropriate for policy and law.

Behavior indicating emotional crises

Any patient admitted to the ED has the potential to be in various stages of emotional crises.

- What recent stressful events have occurred in the life of this patient or family (8)?
- What has been the meaning of these events to the patient?
- Is there an actual or perceived threat to life?
- What is the medical emergency (overdose, drug reaction, high-risk medical condition, etc.) (21)?
- Is there a psychiatric emergency (21)? Does the patient need seclusion, restraints, crisis team, or security personnel?
- Assess patient's ability to care for self.

Disordered thought processes

- Individuals with delusions, hallucinations, and with a possible diagnosis of schizophrenia.
- Individuals who are severely depressed.
- Individuals who are psychotic (out of touch with current reality).

FOCUSED NURSING ASSESSMENT
Violent Behavior
Nursing assessment should center on behaviors, cognitive abilities, thought processes, and level of disequilibrium and disorganization.
Behaviors
- Describe present behavior (verbal and nonverbal).
- What is the level of motor activity (especially if pacing)?
- What is the physical appearance?
- How is patient attired (appropriate for weather, disheveled, etc.)?
- How much eye contact is there?
- What is the patient's verbal presentation? How does the patient communicate and what is the content of speech (quality, quantity, and organization)?
- Describe the mood and emotions of the patient.
- If the patient has a suicidal plan, are the means present (knife, pills, etc.)? Is it a well-defined or vague plan?

Thought processes/cognitive abilities
- Orientation.
- Perceptual abilities (hallucinations, illusions, etc.).
- Judgment and insight—understanding need for care.
- Memory.
- Thought processes—clarity, organization, symptomology.

Level of disequilibrium and disorganization
- How have life changes and stressful events affected their equilibrium?
- What is their perception of these events?
- Situational supports or lack of?
- Coping mechanisms in past and present?
- Triggering event, the "last straw."
- Need for immediate attention.

Victims of Abuse
Types of injuries in domestic violence
- Bleeding injuries, especially to the head, face, breasts, abdomen, and chest.
- Internal injuries, concussions, perforated eardrums, abdominal injuries, severe bruising, eye injuries, and strangulation marks on the neck.

- Back injuries.
- Broken or fractured jaws, arms, pelvis, ribs, clavicle, and legs.
- Burns from cigarettes, appliances, scalding liquids, or acids.
- Psychologic trauma, anxiety, attacks of hyperventilation, heart palpitations, severe crying spells, and suicidal tendencies.
- Miscarriages.
- Observe children for signs of stress caused by family violence. For example, emotional, behavioral, school, or sleep problems, or increased aggressive behavior (20).

Physical symptoms indicating possible spouse abuse (20)

Chief complaints (without physical cause):
- Headache.
- Abdominal pain.
- Choking sensation.
- Chest pain.
- Back pain.
- Dizziness.
- "Accidents."

Presenting problems

(Signs of high anxiety and chronic stress.)
- Agitation.
- Hyperventilation.
- Panic attacks.
- Gastrointestinal disturbances.
- Hypertension.
- Physical injuries.
- Eating disorders.
- Insomnia.

Anxiety
Mild or normal anxiety
- Provides the energy to get on with tasks.
- Is growth producing.
- Constructive.
- Necessary for survival.

Moderate anxiety
- Anxiety narrows the perceptual field.
- One can pay attention when directed to do so.

Severe anxiety
- High level of acute anxiety that occurs when stress is pervasive.
- Perceptual field is diminished to the point where person can attend to only one specific detail.
- Ability to solve problems is very limited.
- Efforts to relieve anxiety are likely to be random and not effective.

Panic level of anxiety
- Is the most intense and pervasive level of anxiety.
- Perceptual field is so limited by anxiety that person is no longer able to process any outside stimuli from the environment.
- Likely to disorganize and/or immobilize the patient.
- Panic does not extend over long periods of time (5).

Risk Factors
Violent behavior
1. Individuals with alcohol or drugs on board.
2. Individuals with history of agitated or disruptive behavior, especially under stress or stressful times.
3. Individuals with unstable or lack of supportive relationships.
4. Altered thought processes. Psychotic symptoms such as delusions, paranoia, hallucinations, etc.
5. Situational or maturational crises with an already fragile homeostasis.
6. Patients with a low tolerance for frustration and poor impulse control (2).
7. Patients with seizure disorders (especially during postictal states), organic brain syndromes such as dementia, confusional states resulting from metabolic disorders, head trauma, drug toxicities, and drug withdrawal (2).
8. Adolescents with previous suicide attempts, early sexual behavior, substance abuse, trouble at school and with the law, depression (18), social isolation, and impulsivity (19).

Victims of abuse
1. History of violence and abuse. Violence is a learned behavior.
2. Men who abuse believe in being in control, being dominant in the family, and abusing bolsters their low self-esteem.

3. Men who have extreme jealousy of their spouse may be more likely to abuse.
4. Violence is more likely to occur when alcohol or other drugs are used. However, alcohol and drugs are an excuse for the abuse, not a cause.

Life Span Issues

1. Centers for Disease Control and Prevention estimates that 300,000 high school students make a serious suicide attempt each year resulting in 4,000 ED visits. Follow-up studies suggest 6% to 50% of these adolescents make another attempt and as many as 11% eventually take their own lives (11,18).
2. Adolescents undergoing humiliating life experiences, having family conflict characterized by disruption and violence serve to increase risk of suicidal behavior (19).
3. Geriatric patients may need alternate assessment methods because of changes in hearing, speech, and mobility. Assess for organic mental disorders and contributing medical problems (21).
4. Pediatric patients need attention to family issues and developmental difficulties (21). Offer interventions to change and improve the family functioning. Commend the family on any strengths noted, offer information about parenting and community resources, encourage respite, support, and education for the parents, etc.

INITIAL INTERVENTIONS

Violent Behavior Toward Others

For preventive measures and initial interventions, see Table 14-1 and Priority Nursing Diagnoses and Interventions section.

1. Staff intervention should provide for the safety of the patient and others utilizing the least restrictive options as possible.
2. Realize physical aggression is an attempt to achieve security and control, thus, staff efforts to convey comfort, safety, and control reduce the risk of violence.
3. Talk with the patient calmly and respectfully using short concise explanations.

4. Allow patient a lot of space, beware of touching patient, and avoid physical entrapment of staff. Focus on wanting to "help" or work with the patient.

5. Do not wear loose or dangling jewelry or stethoscope around neck.

6. Do not have pockets full of scissors, clamps, etc. that are potential weapons against you.

7. Respect personal space of the patient.

8. Position self with patient so no obstacles exist between you and an exit.

9. Stand at about a 45 degree angle to patient and have good eye contact (3).

10. Attempt to control factors in environment that encourage development of previolent aggression (long waits, delays, stimulating environment, etc.) (14).

11. Use verbal strategies to de-escalate the patient with aggression (e.g., acknowledge anger). Say "we are not going to let you hurt yourself or others."

12. Implement teamwork with verbal strategies. "Show of concern" is a group of staff with one person talking to the patient.

13. Implement teamwork with physical control (16).

14. Initiate specific strategies when a patient is out of control and physical danger is imminent to staff (IV sedation, neuromuscular blocking agents after restraining patient).

15. Know your institution's policies and procedures for crises such as a panic button or notification of security/police/crises team.

Violent Behavior Toward Self

See Priority Nursing Diagnoses and Interventions section.

1. Get a verbal contract from the patient agreeing not to leave the ED.

2. Try to get a "no harm contract" from the patient. Patient is asked to verbalize intents regarding harm to self. Ability to do this or not affects acuity and interventions needed.

3. All safety measures are to be carried out in a respectful, informative manner to minimize patients' and visitors' potential discomfort.

4. Prepare room so that it is as free as possible of harmful objects. Arrange to have one or two rooms designated

as "safe" or that have the ability to be "safe" by rolling out carts, locking cabinets, etc.

5. Inform and explain the rationale for safety procedures.
6. Remove dangerous objects from patient (pills, weapons, etc.).
7. Put patient in hospital clothing in order to assess potential harmful objects or drugs hidden in clothing and to help assure that patient remains in ED. Pay attention to removal of clothes if patient is paranoid or if self-esteem and privacy is threatened and patient begins to decompensate even more than current state.

Victims of Abuse

See Chapter 2.

1. Provide a safe environment by allowing for privacy.
2. Acknowledge fears of patient and reassure about present safety.
3. Establish yourself and ED as reliable, caring, and concerned.
4. Assess your own responses to human abuse, so that own values and perceptions do not impede caring for the victims.
5. Be aware of institution's policies and procedures and state laws regarding documentation of injuries and collection of evidence.
6. For rape victims or other victims in psychologic crises, may need to call psychiatric personnel staff.
7. Call the rape crisis center for volunteers and information for follow-up care.
8. Report abuse to appropriate authorities in the institution and the state.

Anxiety

1. Maintain a calm, nonthreatening manner.
2. Reassure patient of their safety and security.
3. Use simple, brief messages.
4. Try to get in a low stimulating environment.
5. Pay attention to anything that causes fear in the patient.

Individuals in Crisis

1. Reduce sensory environment.
2. In acute crises, patient is often quite anxious, so direct questions to help patient define sequence and significance of events.

3. Offer reflective, acknowledging statements such as, "I can imagine with all the confusion and stress you have described, you feel quite overwhelmed."
4. Work toward finding something that will give immediate relief in at least one aspect of the patient's crises (12) (e.g., childcare, specific resources to attend to patient/family needs, voucher for some medications).

Disordered Thought Processes

Psychosis, schizophrenia, and major depression are characterized with major disturbances in thought processes. The patient may have a variety of symptoms from simple thinking to bizarre thinking. The individual is at high risk for harm to self because of inability to attend to self needs.

1. Generally a firm, consistent, gentle approach is most effective.
2. Give clear, brief directions.
3. Do not argue with patient about hallucinations or delusions—refer to "the voices." For example, "I believe you when you tell me you hear. . . . The voices must be troubling you . . . . We are here in the ED to help you. You are safe here."
4. Offer food, fluids, and other comfort measures.

PRIORITY NURSING DIAGNOSES

Risk for potential for violence directed at others
Risk for potential for self-directed violence
Risk for self-care deficit
Risk for alteration in thought processes
Risk for ineffective individual coping
Risk for anxiety

◆ **Potential for violence directed at others** related to self-concept, biochemical alterations, alterations in thought process, impairment of ability to control impulses, uncontrolled anger.

INTERVENTIONS

- Maintain low level of stimuli.
- Observe patient's behavior frequently (q 15 min), so interventions can be implemented as required.
- Place patient in a safe area.
- Remove all dangerous objects from environment.
- Respond matter of factly to verbal hostility and avoid arguing.

- Convey calm attitude.
- Have sufficient staff to indicate a "show of concern," if necessary.
- Administer tranquilizing medications prn.
- Observe for effectiveness and side effects of medications.
- If patient is in physical restraints, patient is highly vulnerable and needs constant observation.
- As agitation decreases, assess patient's readiness for restraint removal.

◆ **Potential for self-directed violence** related to depression, hopelessness, misinterpretation of reality, feelings of worthlessness, unresolved grief.
  INTERVENTIONS
  - Ask patient directly, "Have you thought about killing yourself? Do you have a plan? Do you have the means to do this?"
  - Ask specifics of plan.
  - Initiate a "no harm" contract. A short-term verbal contract with the patient that he or she will not harm self during a specific time frame.
  - If patient is unable to contract, increase level of observation and increase protection in environment.
  - Initiate frequent verbal contact with patient (q 15 min).
  - Maintain the patient in view of staff and in a safe environment.
  - Remove any potentially harmful objects from patient and environment.
  - Therapeutic interactions indicate learning of other ways to deal with problems other than harming self.

Self-care deficit related to perceptual or cognitive impairment.
  INTERVENTIONS
  - Offer nutritious snacks and fluids.
  - Assist patient to bathroom hourly and as needed.
  - If patient is paranoid about food, give in unopened container and let them open.
  - Ensure appropriate clothing for weather conditions.
  - Assist with personal hygiene if needed.

Alteration in thought processes related to impaired cognition, biochemical alterations.
  INTERVENTIONS
  - Accept content of patient's altered thinking.
  - Do not reinforce the altered thinking. Use "the voices" instead of words like "they."

M

- Reality orient (e.g., "Even though I realize the voices are real to you, I do not hear any voices speaking.").
- Reassure the patient they are safe.
- Try to identify persons in the patient's network that they know, can call, and may calm and reassure them. Sometimes a familiar voice, even on the phone, can calm the patient and help them reestablish some sense of control and balance.

◆ **Ineffective individual coping** related to poor support system, poor problem solving, lack of prior experience in dealing with similar crisis.

INTERVENTIONS

- Recognize that behavior is purposeful and attempt to reduce anxiety and insecurity.
- Help patient identify own strengths and resources and those in the community.

◆ **Anxiety (panic)** related to situational and maturational crises, threats to self-concept, threat of death.

INTERVENTIONS

- Maintain calm, nonthreatening manner.
- Reassure patient of their safety and security.
- Use simple words and brief messages.
- Keep immediate surroundings low in stimuli.
- Administer tranquilizing medications as ordered.

PRIORITY DIAGNOSTIC TESTS

Serum toxicology screening
Electrolyte levels
Blood ethanol levels
Urinalysis and urine drug screen
CAT scan (r/o tumors, space occupying lesions, aneurysms, etc.).
ED protocol for physical injury and evidence should be followed.

COLLABORATIVE INTERVENTIONS
Overview

In general, a crisis may occur when there have been stressors (situational, maturational, social, etc.) that exceed the individual, family, or community's coping abilities. The coping strategies that usually are effective fail to maintain the balance for those involved. The resulting disorganization, anxiety, and preoccupation with the difficulty often overwhelms those involved and many may seek the services of the ED.

Likewise, the ED is a place where a variety of crises are treated. Traumatic injuries, abuse, and suicidal attempts after losses are some examples of crises treated in the ED. Any individual with a perceived life-altering or life-threatening occurrence may be in a high-to-panic state of anxiety, and nursing interventions should reflect understanding of this. Because anxiety is contagious, the nurse should try to maintain a calm, nonthreatening manner when working with those in crises, so that the patient's feeling of security will be enhanced.

Clinical Conditions
Violent behavior toward others

Prevention measures are critical in the ED. The symptoms, diagnoses, and treatment of violent behavior are listed in order of acuity. Interventions for the protection of the patient are listed from least restrictive to most restrictive for the protection of the patient.

A designated safe, quiet area or room for psychiatric emergencies is needed (3,4). Staff must have education and practice in utilizing verbal strategies to de-escalate patients, nonviolent physical control techniques, and use of restraints. Available hospital staff and security should also be part of the ED resources. Teamwork is important.

It cannot be emphasized enough the importance of teaching and coaching the staff to be respectful of the patient's dignity as a human being NO matter the exhibited behavior. Hunt (9) emphasizes the importance of the ED nurse realizing that the patient is in the midst of a psychiatric emergency and needs to be reassured, checked frequently, and knowledgeable, sensitive nursing interventions utilized. She states, "I'd like to think if I or a friend or family member were in the ED, the nurse would . . . offer me a warm blanket, even though I am yelling and agitated, because you notice I am shivering."

In addition, the ED environment must be carefully monitored to prevent escalation of anxious, agitated persons. For example, long delays in treatment and an

M

overstimulating environment, for someone who has low impulse control or who is anxious and agitated, automatically increases their acuity and increases the chance of a psychiatric emergency occurring.

Table 14-1 outlines the symptoms, diagnosis, and treatments of the patient with behavior that is violent toward others. The table goes from low acuity and least restricted environment to high acuity and most protective environment.

Violent behavior toward self

For specific drug overdoses, see Chapter 20. Table 14-2 outlines the symptoms, diagnosis, and treatment of the patient with violent behavior toward self. The symptoms, diagnosis, and treatment of suicidal behavior are listed in order of acuity from least restrictive to most protective. Interventions for the safety of the patient are listed in the following table.

Victims of abuse

(See Chapter 2.)

RAPE

- Do not leave the person alone.
- Maintain nonjudgmental care.
- Maximize emotional support, stay with victim, show concern for victim's needs, encourage problem solving whenever possible.
- Ensure confidentiality.
- Encourage person to talk.
- Engage support system (family, friends) when appropriate (1).
- Obtaining proof of force includes the following:
  1. Writing physical injuries, taking pictures of injuries.
  2. Document direct quotes.
- Obtaining information for identifying assailant includes the following:
  1. Sperm and seminal fluid specimens from which DNA markers can be drawn.
  2. Head or pubic hair of assailant on victim.
- Proof of sexual contact includes the following:
  1. Presence of motile or nonmotile sperm on/in victim.
  2. Presence of acid phosphatase in vaginal fluid (highly suggestive of recent sexual contact because it is in high concentrations in seminal fluid and all but absent in vaginal fluids) (15).

TABLE 14-1 Care of the Violent Patient

Symptoms	Diagnosis	Treatment
• No history of violence. • Basically satisfactory support system. • Social drinker only and is not drinking now. • May be slightly agitated or impatient but is able to be redirected.	No predictable risk of violence	Utilize verbal interventions: 1. Talk with patient in calm, reassuring manner. 2. Ask patient to sit in a less stimulating environment. 3. Ask family or friends with stabilizing influence to stay with patient and those who provoke to stay away. 4. Encourage expression of anger verbally vs. acting out. Give positive feedback for appropriate verbal expressions of anger. 5. Offer patient choices when possible.
• Has occasional ideation of assault and violence (including paranoid ideas). • No history of assault or impulsive acting out. • Occasional drinking bouts and angry verbal outbursts. • Basically satisfactory support system.	Low risk of violence	Utilize verbal interventions 1-5 above.

M

Continued.

431

TABLE 14-1 Care of the Violent Patient (cont'd)

Symptoms	Diagnosis	Treatment
• No alcohol or drugs at present. • May be slightly agitated and verbalizing feeling out of control but able to be redirected.		
• Has frequent ideation of assault and violence but no specific plan. • Has history of impulsive acting out and verbal outburst while drinking or using other drugs. • Stormy relationships with periodic high-tension arguments. • Increased agitation (e.g., pacing, fist clenching, intensified facial expressions, raised voice, shouting). • Can be directed by an individual staff member or a group of staff.	Moderate risk of violence	Utilize 1-5 above, plus the following as needed: 6. Search for harmful objects and remove harmful objects from patient's room. 7. PRN medication may be indicated to decrease agitation and potential for violence. 8. Redirect patient with a group of staff: "verbal show of concern" if an individual cannot redirect the patient.
• Has plan for violence now. • Has history of frequent acting out against others.	High risk of violence	Utilize 1-8 above. 9. Anticipate and have ready a group of staff to provide verbal external control.

- Has used drugs or ETOH frequently and to excess.
- Has indicators of drugs and/or ETOH use on board.
- May have paranoia or hallucinations.
- Stormy relationships with much verbal fighting and occasional assaults.
- R/O organic etiology (e.g., basilar skull fracture).
- Body: Pacing, violent gestures.
- Verbal: Demanding, abusive, profane, threatening violence.
- May or may not be able to be redirected by a group of staff.

10. Physical control if patient unable to be redirected and patient progresses to an extremely high risk of violence. Proceed immediately with the next level of treatment (see below).

Extremely high risk of violence

- Has current high lethal plan.
- Has history of homicide attempts or impulsive acting out and strong urge to control and "get even" with someone.
- History of excessive and continual use of drugs and/or ETOH.
- Very likely intoxicated.

1. Psychiatric emergency: Requires immediate physical control to prevent harm to self and others.
2. Team effort to provide external physical control for patient.
3. "Assistance Please" code.
4. Team leader tells patient what team is going to do.

Continued.

M

433

TABLE 14-1 Care of the Violent Patient (cont'd)

Symptoms	Diagnosis	Treatment
• May have paranoia or hallucinations.		5. Five staff (one for each limb and one to protect patient's head).
• R/O organic (e.g., basilar skull fracture).		6. Four point restraint (see institution's policy). Patient is very vulnerable and requires constant observation.
• May arrive to ED in four point restraints or is actively threatening with violent gestures and/or a weapon.		• Apply restraints securely but not tight enough to interfere with circulation or respiration.
• Verbal: Demanding, abrasive, profane.		• Tie to bed frame, not rails.
		• Hourly respiration and circulation checks.
		• Elevate head of bed slightly if not contraindicated to prevent aspiration.
		• Constant observation.
		7. PRN medications as needed for safety and patient's comfort.
		8. If patient is threatening with a weapon, notify Security stat.

From Cahill CD, et al: *Iss Mental Health Nurs* 12(3):139-252, 1991; Carpenito LD: *Handbook of nursing diagnosis*, ed 4, Philadelphia, 1991, JB Lippincott; Green E: *J Emerg Nurs* 15(6):523-527, 1989; Hoff LA: *People in crisis: understanding and helping*, ed 3, Redwood City, 1989, Addison-Wesley; Kurlowicz L: *Am J Nurs* 90(9), 1990; Martin L, et al: *J Emerg Nurs* 17(6):395-401, 1991.

TABLE 14-2 Care of the Suicidal Patient

Symptoms	Diagnosis	Treatment
• No notion of suicide. • No history of attempts. • Has satisfactory social supports. • Close contact with significant others. • Engages in appropriate conversation. • Vague feelings of depression and helplessness. • No alcohol or drug problems. • EMV: 15 on the Glasgow coma scale. • Has considered low lethal methods of suicide.	No predictable risk of immediate suicide	• Verbally contract with the patient not to leave ED and document. • If leave, give information for follow-up. • Assign patient to a designated safe room where visible to staff. • Treat presenting complaint. • If possible, make follow-up appointment. • Discharge instructions to include resources for follow-up.
• No history of attempts. • No recent or serious losses. • Has satisfactory support network. • No withdrawal from social contacts. • May be mildly depressed. • No alcohol or drug problems. • Basically wants to live. • EMS: 15 on Glasgow coma scale.	Low risk of immediate suicide	• Contract not to leave ED and not to harm self and document. • Accompanied by family or friend who agrees not to let the patient leave. • If leave, give information for follow-up. • Assign patient to room where visible to staff. • Check patient hourly in waiting room or in treatment area and document. • If discharged, make follow-up appointment.
• Has considered suicide with moderate-to-high lethal method.	Moderate risk of immediate suicide	• Contract that will not leave or harm self and document.

M

Continued.

TABLE 14-2 Care of the Suicidal Patient (cont'd)

Symptoms	Diagnosis	Treatment
• No specific plan or has plan with low-lethal method. • History of low-lethal methods. • Some changes and/or losses. • Few or only one significant other. • Some feelings of helplessness, hopelessness, and withdrawal. • Moderate amount of depression. • Depends on ETOH or other drugs for stress relief. • Weighing the odds between life and death—may give no harm contract. • None to some disorientation/disorganization, confusion, or anxiety.		• Accompanied by friend or family member who agrees not to let leave. • 30 min checks by hospital staff while patient in lobby or family room. • If unable to do 30 min checks, take patient to treatment area. • Assign patient to safe room. • Continue 30 min checks. • Offer something to eat/drink. • Anticipate laboratory studies: ETOH and toxicity. • Anticipate psychiatric consult. • If discharged, make follow-up appointment.
• Has current high-lethal plan, obtainable means. • History of attempts with moderate-to-high lethality. • Some losses recently. • Only one or no significant others. • Unable to communicate with significant other. • Withdrawal.	High risk of immediate suicide	• Triage nurse takes patient to a safe room. • Register in back. • One-to-one with hospital staff. • Contract with patient for no self-harm if possible. • Offer something to eat/drink. • Anticipate laboratory studies: ETOH and toxicology. • Anticipate psychiatric consult.

- Moderate-to-high level of depression.
- Has used drugs or ETOH to excess.
- Depressed and wants to die—may not give no harm contract.
- Some-to-moderate disorientation, disorganization, confusion, disturbed thought process, or appears anxious.

- Has current high-lethal plan with available means.
- History of attempts with high lethality.
- Significant losses and/or changes.
- Cut off from resources/significant others.
- Psychosis with command hallucinations (e.g., "the voices tell me to hurt myself").
- Severe depression.
- Uses ETOH and other drugs continually and to excess.
- Wants to die.
- Probably will not give no self-harm contract.
- Marked disorientation, disorganization, confusion, or appears anxious.
- Severely disturbed thought processes.

Very high risk of immediate suicide

- Triage nurse takes patient to treatment area or requests assistance as needed.
- Register in back.
- One-to-one with hospital staff.
- STAT call to psychiatric consult team.
- Offer something to eat/drink.
- Anticipate laboratory studies: ETOH and toxicology.
- Psychiatric consult.

From Bradley V, Shawler C: One emergency department's guidelines for the care of suicidal patients, *J Emerg Nurs* 19(5):393-395, 1993.

M

DOMESTIC VIOLENCE

Women

1. Reassure victim of present safety.
2. Allow an open accepting interview so the patient feels more comfortable talking.
3. Reassure that intrafamily violence is not OK and treatment should be encouraged.
4. Offer treatment possibilities (couple counseling, information about shelters, counseling for the victim, community liaisons as supports to women, etc.).

Children

1. Collect and document data indicating abuse.
2. Report to appropriate institution and state authorities.
3. Discuss parenting challenges and suggest supports for parents.
4. Seek ways to meet needs of parents so that they may better parent.

Anxiety

1. Identify the severity of anxiety.
2. Panic requires immediate intervention as follows:
   - Remain with the patient.
   - Maintain a calm manner.
   - Utilize short, simple sentences.
   - Minimize environmental stimuli.
   - Suggest an antianxiety medication to relieve panic anxiety level.
3. Moderate-to-severe anxiety interventions as follows:
   - Walking or other use of large muscle groups.
   - Relaxation exercise with deep breathing and tensing and relaxing muscle groups (with direction from nurse).
   - Reduce external stimuli (sound, color, people, etc.) but do not isolate (5).

Individuals in crisis

The patients with mental health disturbances who enter the ED are in various states of disequilibrium and dysfunction. Indeed, if one uses a holistic view of patients, any insult to the patient's system has the potential to cause psychologic disequilibrium and dysfunction. Thus all patients admitted to the ED need assessment of and intervention for psychologic and psychosocial stressors.

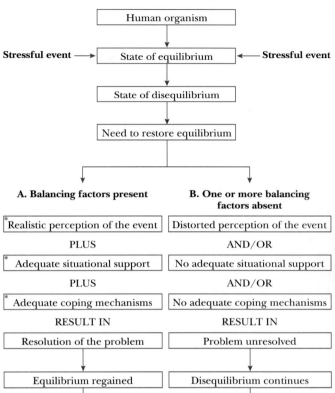

Human organism

Stressful event → State of equilibrium ← Stressful event

State of disequilibrium

Need to restore equilibrium

A. Balancing factors present

*Realistic perception of the event

PLUS

*Adequate situational support

PLUS

*Adequate coping mechanisms

RESULT IN

Resolution of the problem

Equilibrium regained

No crisis

B. One or more balancing factors absent

Distorted perception of the event

AND/OR

No adequate situational support

AND/OR

No adequate coping mechanisms

RESULT IN

Problem unresolved

Disequilibrium continues

CRISIS

*Balancing factors

Figure 14-1 Paradigm: the effect of balancing factors in a stressful event. (From Aguilera D, Messick J: *Crisis intervention theory and intervention,* ed 6, St. Louis, 1989, Mosby, p. 66.)

Recognition and prevention strategies for potential crises can greatly enhance functioning of patients and families. A model that focuses on crisis intervention and the problem-solving approach is illustrated in Figure 14-1. This model views human beings as being in a state of equilibrium until a stressful event occurs. The stressful event causes disequilibrium. For the problem to be resolved, the balancing factors must be present. If one or more of the balancing factors are absent, disequilibrium increases and the likelihood of crisis increases.

The first step in the nursing process is assessment of the problem using this model as a guide.

1. Assessing the meaning of the problem (sample questions):
   - How does this problem affect your life now?
   - How do you see this problem affecting your future?
   - Are others around you affected by this problem?
   - What does this problem mean to you and your life?
2. Assessing situational supports (sample questions):
   - With whom do you live?
   - Is there someone you are close to?
   - Do you have family and/or friends available to you?
   - Who do you trust?
   - Are you involved with a church?
   - Are you involved in any community activities?
3. Assessing coping skills (sample questions):
   - How do you usually cope with stress?
   - Can you do that now?
   - Is it working or not?
   - Has anything like this ever happened before?
   - What else do you think might help you now?

REMEMBER: All questions may not be appropriate for every patient, and other questions may be helpful in assessing the balancing factors.

This assessment helps with (1) prevention of potential crisis, and (2) interventions at various levels of disequilibrium.

Prevention of crisis: maintaining balancing factors
SYMPTOMS
- Situational stressor(s) such as chronic or acute physical illnesses, relocation, etc.
- Maturational and developmental events such as pregnancy, divorce, death of family or friend, new marriage or relationship, change in job/economic status, etc.

DIAGNOSIS
- Patient/family is in severe stress and is effectively coping but a crisis may be imminent.

- Watch and listen for cues that indicate ability to cope is waning such as:
  "I'm hanging in there, but I'm not sure how much longer I can do this."
  "My friends are helping me with all that's going on in my life, but they are getting tired too."
  "Even the little things take a lot of my energy."

TREATMENT
- Assist patient and family to identify strengths.
- Look for ways to expand support network.
- Find interventions that give immediate relief to one or more areas of patient's life.
- Recommend education classes (premarital counseling, prenatal classes, support groups, community support, etc.).
- Help to normalize thoughts and feelings related to distress.
- Help patients to pace themselves and delegate or delete unnecessary activities and expectations.

Disequilibrium continues: restoring balancing factors

SYMPTOMS
- Feeling anxious and helpless.
- Distress and crisis is perceived as overwhelming.
- Disorganized, unable to plan, reason or comprehend, frenzied activity.
- Acute somatic complaints (e.g., SOB, GI disturbances, fatigue).
- Attempts to use usual coping mechanisms fail.
- Coping mechanisms offer minimal and brief relief.

DIAGNOSIS
- Beginning of crisis.
- Balancing factors are not maintained.
- Disequilibrium is evident.

TREATMENT
- Listen actively and with concern.
- Help patient understand the crisis and that they are getting help and support now.
- Do strategies listed in "prevention" above and with consideration that anxiety is higher and cognitive functioning is decreased.
- Explore additional supports.
- Assist with expanding coping mechanisms.

M

Crisis apparent: emergent situation

SYMPTOMS

- Feeling increasingly tense, anxious, helpless, and panicky.
- Patient may engage in "wishful thinking" and denial, hoping to get relief.
- Using more unusual or primitive coping mechanisms in a "hit or miss" manner.
- Behavior and problem solving increasingly disorganized.
- Thoughts severely to completely disorganized.
- Coping efforts continue to fail.

DIAGNOSIS

- Emergency: crisis is evident.

TREATMENT

- Patient needs immediate help and interventions to restore equilibrium.
- The interventions are short-term and focus on solving the immediate problem.
- The patient may need a protective environment (hospitalization, designated stable and safe environment with family or significant others, frequent follow-up with home care, clinical appointments, etc.).

NURSING SURVEILLANCE

1. Monitor behaviors.
2. Trend behaviors, environmental factors affecting patient's behavior and various intervention strategies.
3. Assess biochemical imbalances and overdoses.
4. Recheck restraints:
   - Monitor the patient hourly.
   - Range of motion to all extremities at least every 4 hr by releasing one restraint at a time.
   - Skin care every shift.
   - Documentation (reason for restraint, restraint checks).
   - Trial release from restraints if patient's behavior indicates this is safe.
5. Reevaluate risks of harm to self or others.
6. Evaluate response to medications and other interventions.
7. Assess level of consciousness.
8. Vital signs as indicated.

EXPECTED PATIENT OUTCOMES

1. There is no evidence of violent behavior to self or others.
2. Patient makes no further suicide attempts during ED stay.
3. Patient is able to name resources outside hospital to utilize if feeling suicidal.
4. Patient is able to control impulses to prevent acts of violence against self or others with assistance from caregivers (family if discharged home, hospital staff if hospitalized) (22).
5. The patient verbalizes feelings of increased self-worth (17).
6. The patient can state some areas of their own strengths and weaknesses.
7. With assistance from caregivers, the patient can distinguish between reality- and non–reality-based thinking (22).
8. Patient is able to maintain anxiety at level where they can problem solve and function in daily living (22).
9. Patient is able to verbalize signs and symptoms of escalating anxiety and techniques for interrupting progression of anxiety.
10. Victims of abuse are able to make changes and take necessary actions to protect themselves and eliminate violence in their lives (6).

DISCHARGE IMPLICATIONS

1. Teach patient and family or significant others need for follow-up treatments.
2. Provide patient with information about community resources.
3. Instruct family or significant others to recognize signs of increased anxiety and agitation, strategies to decrease, and when to seek treatment at ED or other facilities.
4. Evaluate need for psychiatric nursing home care.
5. Make appointments for follow-up counseling.

TABLE 14-3 Drug Summary

Drug	Dose/Route	Special considerations
Haloperidol	3-5 mg bid/tid PO (adults) 2-5 mg q 4-8 hr IM (adults) 0.05-0.15 mg/kg/day PO (child)	Management of acute and chronic psychoses, agitated behavior. More severe symptoms of agitated behavior. May be administered as often as every 60 min depending on response. —
Chlordiazepoxide (Librium)	25-50 mg initial dose then q 1-2 hr IM (adult)	Minor tranquilizer or antianxiety agent.
Diazepam (Valium)	5-10 mg 1-2 hr up to 40 mg/day IM (adult)	Minor tranquilizer or antianxiety agent.
Oxazepam (Serax)	10-30 mg up to 120 mg/day PO (adult)	Effective with anxiety, tension, agitation, irritability, anxiety associated with depression.
Tricyclics: Amitriptyline (Elavil, Endep)	75-200 mg/day. Some patients may require as much as 300 mg/day. PO (adult)	Major depression associated with organic disease, schizophrenia, or alcoholism. Contraindicated with MAOIs and antiarrhythmics.
Imipramine (Tofranil, Janimine)	100-150 mg/day. After 2 weeks and symptomatic relief not achieved, may increase to 250-300 mg/day. PO (adult)	Major depression associated with organic disease, schizophrenia, or alcoholism.

Drug	Dosage	Indications/Contraindications
Monoamine oxidase inhibitors (MAOIs): Phenelzine (Nardil)	30-40 mg/day. Rarely exceed 100 mg/day. PO (adolescent, geriatrics) 45-90 mg/day PO (adult)	Contraindicated with MAOIs and antiarrhythmics. — Depression
Tranylcypromine (Parnate)	20-60 mg/day PO (adult)	Contraindicated in hypersensitivity to MAOIs, geriatric, hypertension, severe hepatic, cardiac, or renal disease. —
Serotonin reuptake inhibitors (SSRIs): Fluoxetine (Prozac)	10-40 mg PO (adult) Initial dose 20 mg/day in AM. Dosage may be increased after several weeks if no clinical improvement. Doses above 20 mg/day should be bid. Maximum dose 80 mg/day.	Major depression. Contraindicated with MAOIs.
Sertraline (Zoloft)	50-200 mg/day PO (adult)	Major depression. Not to be used within 14 days of MAOI. Use with caution with renal or hepatic impairment.

M

From USDHHS, PHS for Health Care Policy and Research: *Depression in primary care: detection, diagnosis, and treatment,* clinical practice guideline, AHCPR No. 93-0551, April 1993. See Sheehy, 1992; Skidmore-Roth, 1992; Townsend, 1990 in Bibliography.

References

1. Burgess A, Holstrom L: *Rape: victims of crisis,* Bowie, Md., 1975, Prentice Hall.
2. Cahill CD, Stuart GW, Laraia MT, Arana GW: Inpatient management of violent behavior: nursing prevention and intervention, *Iss Mental Health Nurs* 12(3):139-252, 1991
3. Glasson L: The care of psychiatric patients in the emergency department: preparation, staff awareness, preventive practices, and the psychiatric patient, *J Emerg Nurs* 19(5), Oct 1993.
4. Glasson L: RAP-DEE-responding to disruptive/violent behavior in the emergency department, *J Healthcare Protect Management* 1(2):112-114, 1992.
5. Haber J, Leach AN, Schedy SM, Sidler BF: *Comprehensive psychiatric nursing,* ed 2, New York, 1982, McGraw-Hill.
6. Hadley S: Clinical articles: working with battered women in the emergency department: a model program, *J Emerg Nurs* 18(1):18-23, Feb 1992.
7. Henry SL, Roth M, Gleis LH: Domestic violence—the medical community's legal duty, *KMA Journal* 90(4):163-169.
8. Hoff LA: *People in crisis: understanding and helping,* ed 3, Redwood City, 1989, Addison-Wesley.
9. Hunt E: Guest editorial: On avoiding "psych" patients, *J Emerg Nurs* 19(5):375-376, Oct 1993.
10. Hunt E: One emergency department's special observation record for documenting basic nursing interventions with psychosocial patients, *J Emerg Nurs* 19(5):422-425, Oct 1993.
11. Kalogerakis MG: Emergency evaluation of adolescents, *Hosp and Comm Psychiat* 43(6):617-621, June 1992.
12. Kercher EE: Crisis intervention in the emergency department, *Psychiat Aspects Emerg Med* 9(1):219-232, Feb 1991.
13. Kurlowicz L: Violence in the emergency department, *Am J Nurs* 90(9):35-40, Sept 1990.
14. Lavoie FW, et al: Emergency department violence in United States teaching hospitals, *Ann Emerg Med* 17(11):12-27, 33, Nov 1988.
15. Ledray LE: The sexual assault examination: overview and lessons learned in one program, *J Emerg Nurs* 18(3):223-230, June 1992.
16. Morton PG: Managing assault, *Am J Nurs* 86(10):1114-1116, Oct 1986.
17. Perrin KO, Williams-Burgess C: The suicidal patient in the CCU: nursing approaches, *Crit Care Nurse* 10(7):59-64, July/Aug 1990.
18. Piacentini J: Pediatric update: evaluating adolescent suicide attempters: what emergency nurses need to know, *J Emerg Nurs* 19(5):465-466, Oct 1993.

19. Srnec P: Children, violence, and intentional injuries, *Crit Care Nurs Clin North Am* 3(3):471-478, Sept 1991.
20. Swanson RW: Battered wife syndrome, *Can Med Assoc J* 130:709, 1984.
21. Talley S, King MD: *Psychiatric emergencies: nursing assessment and intervention,* New York, 1984, Macmillan.
22. Townsend MS: *Nursing diagnoses in psychiatric nursing,* Philadelphia, 1988, FA Davis.

Bibliography

Aguilera D, Messick J: *Crisis intervention theory and intervention,* ed 6, St. Louis, 1989, Mosby.

Alt-Grantham T, Duncalf A, Harms L, et al: A 38-year-old female trauma victim of a car bomb, *J Emerg Nurs* 18(1):14-17, Feb 1992.

Assey J: The suicide prevention contract, *Perspect Psychiatr Care* 23(3):99-103, 1985.

Back KJ: Critical incident stress management for care providers in the pediatric emergency department, *Crit Care Nurse* 12(1):78-79, 1992.

Bayley E, Turcke SA: *A comprehensive curriculum for trauma nursing,* Boston, 1992, Jones and Bartlett, 517-518.

Burns C, et al: Research: emergency nurses' perceptions of critical incidents and stress debriefing, *J Emerg Nurs* 19(5):431-436, Oct 1993.

Carpenito LD: *Handbook of nursing diagnosis,* ed 4, Philadelphia, 1991, JB Lippincott.

Cherpitel CJ: Alcohol and violence related injuries: an emergency room study, *Addictions* 88:79-88, 1993.

Curry JL: The care of psychiatric patients in the emergency department, *J Emerg Nurs* 19(5):396-407, Oct 1993.

Gibbs A: Aspects of communication with people who have attempted suicide, *J Adv Nurs* 15(11):1245-1249, 1990.

Green E: Patient care guidelines: management of violent behavior, *J Emerg Nurs* 15(6):523-527, Nov/Dec 1989.

Hogarty S, Rodaitis CM: A suicide precautions policy for the general hospital, *HONA* 17(10):36-42, 1987.

Lanza ML, Bantly A: Decision analysis: a method to improve quality care for nursing practice, *J Nurs Care Quality* 6(1):60-72, 1991.

Lavoie FW: Consent, involuntary treatment, and the use of force in an urban emergency department, *Ann Emerg Med* 21(1):25-32, Jan 1992.

Martin L, et al: A hospital-wide approach to crisis control: one inner-city hospital's experience, *J Emerg Nurs* 17(6):395-401, Dec 1991.

M

Nield-Anderson L, Doubrava J: Clinical article: defusing verbal abuse: a program for emergency department triage nurses, *J Emerg Nurs* 19(5), Oct 1993.

Salvatore NG: Restraints: a sampling of current practice, *J Emerg Nurs* 19(5):417-421, Oct 1993.

Sheehy SB: *Emergency nursing principles and practice,* St. Louis, 1992, Mosby.

Skidmore-Roth L: *Mosby's 1992 nursing drug reference,* St. Louis, 1992, Mosby.

Snyder JA: How we do it: documentation of nursing care of patients who have been restrained, *J Emerg Nurs* 19(5):461-464, Oct 1993.

Townsend MS: *Drug guide for psychiatric nursing,* Philadelphia, 1990, FA Davis.

U.S. Department of Health and Human Services, Public Health Service for Health Care Policy and Research: clinical practice guideline, *Depression in primary care: detection, diagnosis, and treatment,* AHCPR Publication No. 93-0551, April 1993.

Wright LM, Leahey M: *Nurses and families: a guide to family assessment and intervention,* Philadelphia, 1994, FA Davis.

Neurologic Conditions

Patty Sturt

N

TRIAGE ASSESSMENT

Neurologic emergencies can occur from trauma or disease processes that impair functioning of the brain and/or spinal cord. If the patient is not alert or oriented, it may be necessary to obtain the history from EMS personnel, family, friends, or witnesses. If the primary functions of airway, breathing, and circulation are intact, obtain the following data:

Recent trauma
A history of recent trauma involving the head, face, or
    spine should be elicited. Determine if there is a loss of

consciousness. Suspect increased intracranial pressure (ICP) from bleeding and/or edema with head trauma. Suspect spinal cord edema or partial-complete cord transection with spine trauma.

Neurologic history

Determine if there is a history of cerebrovascular accidents (CVAs), transient ischemic attacks (TIAs), seizures, syncope, tumors or masses involving the brain or spinal cord. These patients have a higher risk of cerebral edema, ischemia, or infarction.

Behavior

Behavior changes, sleepiness, memory loss, or confusion may indicate an increase in the ICP.

Headache

Headache is a symptom often associated with increased ICP from subarachnoid hemorrhage, head trauma, or an intracranial mass.

Sensation and movement

Numbness, decreased sensation, weakness, or paralysis in one or more extremities frequently occurs in patients experiencing a CVA or TIA.

Vomiting

Vomiting can occur from increased ICP resulting from a mass, intracranial hemorrhage, or head trauma.

Speech

Suspect a CVA, TIA, or intracranial mass if the patient has slurred speech or difficulty speaking.

Gait

A staggered gait and uncoordinated movements may be seen in patients with cerebellar dysfunction.

Ventricular peritoneal shunt

Increased ICP from excess cerebrospinal fluid (CSF) in the ventricles can occur if the shunt becomes dislodged, infected, or blocked.

Infections

Suspect meningitis or a brain abscess in patients with a recent history of infection involving the ears, sinuses, or respiratory tract.

Medications

Determine current medications. Ask about compliance of antihypertensives or anticonvulsants. Suspect ischemic CVA if noncompliant with antihypertensives. Suspect status epilepticus if noncompliant with anticonvulsant medications.

Vital Signs

- *Bradycardia:* Bradycardia is a late finding of increased ICP. Bradycardia related to unopposed parasympathetic nervous system stimulation occurs in spinal shock.
- *Hypertension:* Hypertension is a late finding of increased ICP. As ICP rises, the blood pressure rises reflexively to maintain cerebral blood flow.
- *Hypotension:* Hypotension is a symptom of spinal shock. Loss of vasomotor tone below the level of the injury causes vasodilation.
- *Respirations:* Respiratory irregularities are a late sign of increased ICP. An abnormal respiratory rate and pattern indicates impending herniation of the respiratory centers located in the brainstem.
- *Fever:* Fever is a symptom associated with lesions of the hypothalamus, increased ICP affecting the hypothalamus, central nervous system infections (meningitis, encephalitis), or status epilepticus.
- *Hypothermia:* Hypothermia may occur in spinal shock because of vasodilation and loss of ability to shiver below the level of the injury.

General Observations

- *Pupil size and reaction:* (see Focused Nursing Assessment).
- *Gait:* Staggered gait, uncoordinated movements, and ataxia are often indicative of cerebellar lesions.
- *Speech:* Slurred speech or difficulty expressing thoughts may indicate impairment of the Broca's area in the frontal lobe.
- *Eye movements:* Abnormal movements often occur with seizure activity.
- *Ecchymosis:* Ecchymosis around the eyes or behind the ear may be seen in some patients with a basilar skull fracture.
- *Drainage:* Basal skull fractures can transverse the paranasal air sinuses of the frontal bone or the middle ear within the temporal bone resulting in a dural tear. CSF can leak through the dural tear and drain from an ear or the nose.

FOCUSED NURSING ASSESSMENT

Nursing assessment should focus on perfusion, ventilation, mobility, and sensation.

Perfusion

Level of consciousness

Level of consciousness is the most important factor in the neurologic assessment. The Glasgow coma scale (GCS) is a tool that allows objective measurement of level of consciousness. There are three categories to be assessed—best eye opening, best motor response, and best verbal response. The range of possible scores is three to fifteen. Fifteen indicates a fully alert and oriented person. Three indicates a deep coma. Table 15-1 describes the three categories, possible findings in each category, and the scores.

> **NURSING ALERT**
>
> Inform the physician immediately if there is a decrease in the GCS. This may indicate an increase in ICP.

Pupils

Assess pupil size and reactivity to light. The millimeter scale is frequently used to record pupil size (Figure 15-1).

When light is shone into the eye, the pupil should immediately constrict. The terms used to describe the pupillary reaction include brisk, sluggish, nonreactive or fixed.

Pupils are normally equal. The box describes various pupil findings and their significance.

Respirations

Assess respiratory rate, depth, and rhythm. Abnormal respiratory patterns are frequently seen with lesions involving the pons and midbrain (respiratory centers of the brain).

Cheyne-Stokes: Rhythmic waxing and waning in the depth and rate of the respirations followed by apnea. Lesions are often bilateral and involve the basal ganglia, thalamus, or hypothalamus.

Central neurogenic hyperventilation: Respirations increased in depth and rate. Lesions are usually in the midbrain or upper pons.

Apneustic breathing: A pause of 2 to 3 seconds after a full or prolonged inspiration. Lesion located in lower pons.

Cluster breathing: Clusters of irregular breaths with periods of apnea at irregular intervals. Lesion located in lower pons or upper medulla.

TABLE 15-1 Glasgow Coma Scale

Category	Response	Description/Technique	Score
Best eye response	Opens eyes spontaneously	Opens eyes without verbal or tactile stimuli.	4
	Opens eyes to verbal stimuli	Opens eyes on command or when called by name. Start with a normal tone of voice and increase the loudness as necessary.	3
	Opens eyes to painful stimuli	Pinching the trapezius muscle, or pinching the inner aspect of the arm or thigh can be used. Do not rub the sternum with your knuckle, since the skin in this area is thin and fragile and bruises easily (especially in a geriatric patient). Avoid twisting or pinching the nipples. Do not apply pressure to the supraorbital area in head-injured patients. NOTE: These techniques to elicit pain also apply to the motor and verbal categories.	2
	No eye opening	Does not open eyes to painful stimuli.	1
Best motor response	Obeys simple commands	Raises arms or holds up specific number of fingers on request. Do not ask patients to grasp hand. Hand grasp may be a reflexive response.	6
	Localizes pain	Cannot follow commands but locates the painful stimulus and attempts to remove it with their hand.	5
	Withdraws from pain	Does not actually locate the source of pain with a hand but does withdraw from the pain. For example, may flex arm to withdraw from the painful stimulus of a pinch.	4

Continued.

453

TABLE 15-1 Glasgow Coma Scale (cont'd)

Category	Response	Description/Technique	Score
	Abnormal flexion (to noxious or painful stimuli)	Adducts shoulders, flexes and pronates arms, flexes wrist, makes a fist (decorticate posturing).	3
	Abnormal extension (to noxious or painful stimuli)	Adducts and internally rotates shoulders, extends forearm, flexes wrist (decerebrate posturing).	2
	No motor response	Flaccid. No response to maximally applied painful stimuli.	1
Best verbal response	Oriented	Able to converse, oriented to person, place, and time.	5
	Confused	Able to converse but is not fully oriented or demonstrates confusion.	4
	Inappropriate words	Words are recognizable but make little or no sense. Words verbalized in a disorganized manner.	3
	Incomprehensible sounds	Words are not recognizable—moans, groans.	2
	None	Does not make any sound in response to pain.	1

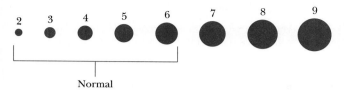

| 2 | 3 | 4 | 5 | 6 | 7 | 8 | 9 |

Normal

Figure 15-1 Pupil gauge in millimeters. (From Stillwell SB: *Mosby's critical care nursing reference*, St Louis, 1992, Mosby.)

COMMON ABNORMAL PUPILLARY RESPONSES

Oculomotor nerve compression

OBSERVATION

One pupil (R) is larger than the other (L), which is of normal size. The dilated pupil (R) does not react to light, although the other (L) pupil reacts normally.

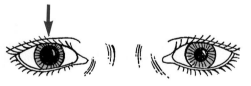

MEANING

A dilated, nonreactive (fixed) pupil indicates that the controls for pupillary constriction are not functioning. The parasympathetic fibers of the oculomotor nerve control pupillary constriction. The most common cause of interruption of this function is compression of the oculomotor nerve, usually against the tentorium or posterior cerebral artery.

The compression of the oculomotor nerve against these structures is caused by a lesion, such as a hematoma, tumor, or cerebral edema, on the same side of the brain as the dilated pupil. This causes downward pressure so that the uncus of the temporal lobe herniates, trapping the oculomotor nerve between it and the tentorium.

ACTION

The nurse will need to check previous assessments to determine what the pupil size and reaction to light have been in the past. If the dilated pupil is a new finding, it should immediately be reported to the physician because the process of rostral-caudal downward pressure must be treated without delay. It would be expected that changes would also be apparent in the level of consciousness, motor function, and other parameters of the neurologic assessment.

Bilateral diencephalic damage

OBSERVATION

Upon examination, the pupils appear small but equal in size, and both react briskly to direct light, contracting when light is introduced and dilating when light is withdrawn.

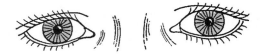

MEANING

The sympathetic pathway that begins in the hypothalamus is affected. Because both pupils are equal in size and respond equally to light, the damage is bilateral. Therefore, it can be assumed that there is bilateral injury in the diencephalon (thalamus and hypothalamus).

Because metabolic coma can also result in bilaterally small pupils that react to light, this diagnostic possibility must be ruled out.

ACTION

These findings should be compared to previous assessments to determine whether this is a new development. The possibility of metabolic coma should be considered by reviewing blood electrolyte and blood glucose levels. For example, diabetic acidosis may result in a metabolic coma because of an excessive amount of glucose in the blood. The abnormal glucose level would be evident by checking the blood glucose level.

A review of blood chemistry values is particularly important if the patient was a recent emergency admission, for which an adequate history may not have been collected. If the small, reactive pupils are a new finding, this information should be reported.

Horner's syndrome

OBSERVATION

One pupil (L) is smaller than the other (R), although both pupils react to light. The eyelid on the same side as the small pupil droops (ptosis). There may be a sweating deficiency (anhidrosis) on the same side of the face as the ptosis. The collective symptoms of a small reactive pupil, ptosis, and anhidrosis are called *Horner's syndrome*.

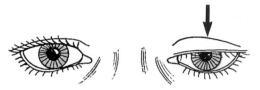

MEANING

There is an interruption of the ipsilateral sympathetic innervation to the pupil that can be caused by hypothalamic damage (posterior or ventrolateral portion), a lesion involving the lateral medulla or the ventrolateral cervical spinal cord, and sometimes, occlusion of the internal carotid artery. Downward displacement of the hypothalamus along with a unilateral Horner's syndrome may be an early sign of transtentorial herniation.

ACTION

If this is a new finding, it should be reported.

Midbrain damage

OBSERVATION

Both pupils are at midposition and are nonreactive to light.

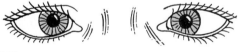

MEANING

When the pupils are midposition in size and nonreactive, neither the sympathetic nor parasympathetic innervation is operational. This finding is often associated with midbrain infarction or transtentorial herniation.

ACTION

The pupils should be evaluated in conjunction with other neurologic assessments. The change in pupil size and reaction should be reported if this represents a new finding.

Pontine damage

OBSERVATION

Very small (pinpoint), nonreactive pupils are seen.

Continued.

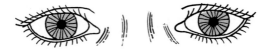

MEANING

Most often, this finding indicates hemorrhage into the pons, a very grave occurrence as the pons controls many motor pathways and vital functions. Bilateral pinpoint pupils may also occur with opiate drug overdose, so this possibility should be ruled out.

ACTION

Report this finding if it is new. The prognosis for patients with pontine damage is grave. Other changes in neurologic status, such as a decreased level of consciousness and respiratory abnormalities, would also be expected.

Dilated unreactive pupils

OBSERVATION

Both pupils are dilated and nonreactive (fixed).

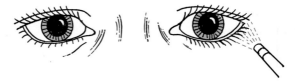

MEANING

This finding is characteristic of the terminal stages of severe anoxia, ischemia, and death. Since atropinelike drugs will cause dilated pupils, this possibility must be ruled out. In addition, an intact ciliospinal reflex can produce momentary bilateral dilation.

ACTION

Emergency action is necessary to reverse the anoxic state and prevent death. Oxygen therapy at high concentrations and a patent airway must be ensured to provide oxygen for the ischemic cerebral cells.

From Hickey JV: *The clinical practice of neurological and neurosurgical nursing,* Philadelphia, 1992, JB Lippincott, 128, 129.

Biot's (ataxic) breathing: Completely irregular, unpredictable pattern with deep and shallow random breaths and pauses. Lesion located in the medulla.

Circulation

Note the rate and quality of the pulses. Bradycardia can be seen in spinal shock. Atrial and ventricular arrhythmias can occur in patients with a subarachnoid hemorrhage (4). Obtain a blood pressure. Hypotension is seen in spinal shock.

Ventilation

Assess breath sounds for crackles and wheezes. Decreased breath sounds may indicate hypoventilation.

Assess chest and abdominal movement. Respiratory assessment is extremely important in patients with cervical spine injuries. Injury at C4 or above will impair phrenic nerve innervation and result in paralysis of the diaphragm. In these cases, air movement will be inadequate and mechanical ventilation will be necessary. Injuries involving T1 to T6 spare the diaphragm, but the intercostal muscles are impaired placing the patient at high risk for respiratory problems. Injuries involving T6 to T12 may impair the abdominal muscles and decrease the ability to generate a cough.

Mobility

Assess motor ability/strength. The motor assessment usually focuses on the arms and legs. The identification of changes is important for noting deterioration, improvement, or stabilization in condition. Always compare motor strength on one side with the other. To assess the upper extremities, extend the middle and index finger of your hands and ask the patient to squeeze with their hands. The grasps should be strong and equal. Next, have the patient attempt to move his/her shoulders, forearms, and wrist against resistance. To assess strength in their lower extremities, have the patient flex and extend the upper leg, knee, and ankle on each side to gravity and resistance. Instruct patient to press his/her feet against your hands. The following scale can be used to measure motor strength/movement:

0 = None	3 = Against gravity
1 = Trace	4 = Against some resistance
2 = Not against gravity	5 = Against strong resistance

TABLE 15-2 Motor Assessment of the Corticospinal Tract

Spinal level	Motor assessment
C5	Shoulder abduction
C5-6	Elbow flexion
C7	Finger and elbow extension
C6-7	Wrist dorsiflexion
C8	Thumb-finger pinch
L2-4	Hip flexion
L5-S1	Knee flexion
L2-4	Knee extension
L5	Foot dorsiflexion
S1	Foot plantar flexion

In spinal cord injury (SCI) patients, the motor assessment is helpful in identifying the level of injury and assessing function of the corticospinal tract within the cord. Table 15-2 indicates the level of the spinal cord and associated muscle function.

Sensation

Assessing the sensory function is helpful in identifying the level of involvement in SCI patients. Starting at the feet and systematically working upward and comparing both sides, determine the patient's ability to detect light touch and pain (pinprick). Ask the patient to tell you when the sensation is felt. Record the highest level of function on each side of the body. Figure 15-2 indicates the area of sensation with the level of the cord.

Risk Factors

1. TIAs, hypertension, hypercholesteremia, hypertriglyceridemia, diabetes mellitus, cigarette smoking, and alcoholism are all considered risk factors for CVAs.
2. History of atrial fibrillation increases the risk of cerebral emboli.
3. Medications such as anticoagulants and oral contraceptives place the patient at higher risk for neurologic problems.

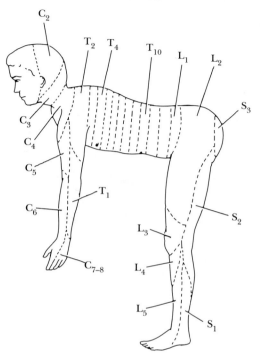

Figure 15-2 Arrangement of dermatomes is more easily understood when an individual is considered in quadruped (crouched) position. It is important to correlate the level of injury with the area of the body surface that is affected (dermatome). (Adapted from Zejdlik: *Management of spinal cord injury*, Boston, 1992, Jones & Bartlett.)

4. Driving while under the influence of alcohol or drugs increases the risk of motor vehicle crashes (MVCs). MVCs are the most frequent cause of head injuries and SCIs.

Life Span Issues
1. Head injury occurs most often in the 15- to 30-year-old age group. Males are affected more often than females (10).
2. Home falls contribute significantly to the incidence of head trauma, particularly in the geriatric population.
3. Sixty percent of SCIs occur in persons 16 to 30 years of age. The majority of those affected are males.

INITIAL INTERVENTIONS

1. Maintenance of a patent airway is the highest priority. Assume that the head-injured patient has a cervical spine injury. Open the airway with techniques that require no movement of the head. Such techniques include the jaw-thrust maneuver, nasotracheal intubation, placement of an oral or nasopharyngeal airway. A cricothyrotomy may be necessary if attempts at nasotracheal intubation fail.

NURSING ALERT

Any patient with an altered level of consciousness needs to be monitored carefully for airway compromise.

---

2. Support breathing with 100% oxygen/bag-valve mask device (BVMD) if the patient is hypoventilating or apneic. One hundred percent oxygen/nonrebreather mask should be used on those patients not requiring intubation.
3. Maintain patient in spinal immobilization until x-rays are taken and cleared by a physician. Patients should not be left on backboards for long periods of time. This promotes decubitus formation.
4. Have suction available at all times.
5. Insert two large bore IVs.
6. Anticipate the need for insertion of a ventricular drainage catheter in patients with signs and symptoms of increased ICP. The signs and symptoms of increased ICP include decreased level of consciousness, pupil changes, weakness, nausea, vomiting, headache, seizures, and an abnormal respiratory pattern.
7. Anticipate need for cervical traction in patients with a cervical fracture.
8. Anticipate need for CT scan. Notify CT scan technician.

NURSING ALERT

Complete spinal immobilization requires a rigid cervical collar of appropriate size, head immobilization devices, tape or straps across the forehead, straps across the shoulders, hips, and above the knees if the patient is on a backboard, and in-line spinal alignment.

PRIORITY NURSING DIAGNOSES

Risk for ineffective airway clearance
Risk for ineffective breathing pattern
Risk for altered cerebral tissue perfusion
Risk for potential for injury
Risk for altered tissue perfusion; peripheral, renal

◆ **Ineffective airway clearance** related to decreased level of consciousness, seizure activity.
  INTERVENTIONS
  • Maintain patient airway (jaw thrust, oral airway, nasopharyngeal airway, intubation).
  • Suction patient as needed.

◆ **Ineffective breathing pattern** related to increased ICP affecting the respiratory centers of the brain, SCI with impairment of the diaphragm and/or intercostal muscles.
  INTERVENTIONS
  • Administer 100% oxygen.
  • Assist breathing with BVMD as needed.
  • Prepare to assist with intubation if patient is hypoventilating or in respiratory distress.

◆ **Altered cerebral tissue perfusion** related to increased ICP.
  INTERVENTIONS
  • Maintain Pco_2 at 28 to 35 mm Hg.
  • Anticipate need to insert ventricular drainage catheter.
  • Closely monitor GCS score.

◆ **Potential for injury** related to cerebral edema, seizure activity, noncompliance with anticonvulsants.
  INTERVENTIONS
  • Pad side rails of bed.
  • Have suction and oxygen available at all times.
  • Administer anticonvulsants as ordered by physician.

Altered tissue perfusion; peripheral, renal related to hypotension associated with spinal shock.

N

INTERVENTIONS
- Insert two large bore IVs.
- Administer fluid boluses and vasopressors as ordered by physician.

PRIORITY DIAGNOSTIC TESTS

Laboratory

ABG: A P_{CO_2} of 28 to 35 should be maintained. Reducing the P_{CO_2} results in vasoconstriction of the cerebral arteries that reduces cerebral blood flow and ICP.

Complete blood count: Expect an increase in the white blood cell (WBC) count with central nervous system (CNS) infections such as meningitis.

Electrolyte levels: Mannitol (Table 15-3) can cause electrolyte imbalances (especially hypokalemia). Vomiting can cause hypokalemia and other electrolyte imbalances.

Type and crossmatch: This is necessary if the patient has other system involvement such as chest or pelvic injuries. Patients do not become hypovolemic from a closed-head injury.

ETOH level: A high serum alcohol level may alter the level of consciousness and decrease the patient's ability to cooperate with the examination and treatment.

Urine and serum drug screen: Many drugs can alter the level of consciousness and pupil size.

Cerebrospinal fluid (CSF): CSF may be obtained via a lumbar puncture or intraventricular catheter (IVC) to assess color, WBC count, protein content, glucose content, and culture and sensitivity.
- More than 5 to 10 WBC/mm³ indicates an inflammatory process such as meningitis. Cloudy fluid indicates infection.
- Normally, CSF glucose is approximately 80% of the blood glucose. A decreased CSF glucose level is suggestive of bacterial meningitis.
- The normal protein count is 15 to 45 mg/100 ml. The protein count may be elevated with tumors, viral meningitis, and hemorrhage.
- A culture can be obtained to identify the invading organism. Sensitivity can also be determined to identify the most effective drug therapy.

TABLE 15-3 Drug Summary

Drug	Dose/Route	Special considerations
Cefotaxime (Third-generation cephalosporin)	150-200 mg/kg in 4 divided doses or 1-2 g every 6 hr; not to exceed 12 g daily. *Pediatric:* 50-180 mg/kg/day in 4-6 divided doses. Dilute 50-100 mg/ml and administer IVPB over 15-30 min	Lower dose may be needed for renal impaired patients.
Ceftriaxone (Cephalosporin)	4 g in 2 divided doses. Total daily dose should not exceed 4 g. *Pediatric:* 50-100 mg/kg in 2 divided doses. Administer IVPB.	—
Diazepam (Benzodiazepine)	5-10 mg may be repeated every 5-10 min *Pediatric:* 0.1 to 0.3 mg/kg slow IV push 5 mg/min	Antagonist is Romazicon. Monitor for respiratory depression.
Furosemide (Diuretic)	20-40 mg IV Push over 1-2 min	Frequent administration may cause dehydration.
Hydralazine (Antihypertensive)	10-20 mg Slow IV Push at a rate of 10 mg/min.	Continuously monitor BP.
Lorazepam (Benzodiazepine)	2-4 mg IV Push. Rate should not exceed 2 mg/min.	Romazicon is antagonist.

Continued.

N

465

TABLE 15-3 Drug Summary (cont'd)

Drug	Dose/Route	Special considerations
Mannitol 20% (osmotic diuretic)	0.25 to 1 g/kg over 15-30 min. IVPB	Must be given in a line with a filter. Monitor for potential dehydration and increased serum osmolarity.
Methylprednisolone (Steroid)	For SCI patients: 30 mg/kg loading dose followed 5.4 mg/kg every hr for the next 23 hrs. Loading dose is IVP. Hourly infusion on pump.	Must be given within 8 hr of the injury.
Nitroprusside (Vasodilator)	50 mg in 250 cc of 5% dextrose in water for concentration of 200 mcg/ml. Start infusion of 0.5 mcg/kg/min. Titrate to desired BP. Maximum infusion rate is 10 mcg/kg/min. MUST be given with a continuous infusion pump.	IV bag must be wrapped with an opaque material or aluminum foil to protect it from light.
Penicillin G	20-24 million U in 6 divided doses. Administer IVPB over 30 min.	—
Phenobarbital (Anticonvulsant)	Pediatric: 20 mg/kg IV Do not exceed 50 mg/min	Monitor for respiratory depression and hypotension.
Phenytoin (Anticonvulsant)	15-18 mg/kg. 50 mg/min or slower by IV infusion*	Rapid infusion can precipitate cardiac arrhythmias and/or hypotension. Must be given in IV solution of normal saline.

*From Gahart BL: *Intravenous medications*, St Louis, 1994, Mosby. *IVP*, IV push; *IVPB*, IV piggyback.

Radiographic

Spine films: Cervical, thoracic, lumbar, and sacral views may be ordered to determine the presence of fractures and/or dislocations. C7 to T1 is often difficult to visualize in obese or heavily muscled patients. It may be necessary to pull the shoulders downward toward the feet while the x-ray is being conducted. The swimmer's view (one arm above the head) can also be helpful in visualizing the cervical spine. An open-mouth view can be used to visualize the odontoid process. The odontoid process is an upward extension of the body of C2.

Skull films: Used to rule out skull fractures. Include anteroposterior and lateral views.

CT scan: The CT scan is extremely useful in locating and diagnosing various cranial lesions such as abscesses, cysts, infarctions, hematomas, and tumors. Intravenous radiopaque material (contrast) may be given to improve the clarity of images.

MRI: The MRI is efficient in identifying cerebral and spinal cord edema, CNS ischemia or infarcted areas, hemorrhage, and tumors in the brain stem, basal skull, and spinal cord.

N

COLLABORATIVE INTERVENTIONS

Overview

Increased intracranial pressure

There are three main components that can exert pressure within the cranium. Of the total cranial volume the brain accounts for 80%, CSF accounts for 10%, and blood accounts for 10% (1). An increase in one must be accompanied by an equal decrease in one or more of the other components to maintain a constant intracranial volume and ICP. If there is not a decrease in one component when there is an increase in another, the ICP increases. Normal ICP is 0 to 15 mm Hg.

SYMPTOMS

- Symptoms may include a decrease in level of consciousness (see Table 15-1), pupil changes (see the box on pp. 455-458), abnormal respiratory patterns, nausea, vomiting, muscle weakness, hemiparesis, hemiplegia, seizures, headache, normal or elevated temperature, and an ICP of 15 to 20 mm Hg or greater.

- In severe increased ICP, a loss of brain stem reflexes occur, including the corneal, oculocephalic, and oculovestibular reflexes. The physician assesses the oculocephalic reflex (doll's eyes phenomenon) by rotating the head while holding the eyelids open. The reflex is intact if the eyes move in the opposite direction of the head. The oculovestibular reflex is assessed by injecting ice cold water into the external auditory canal. If the reflex is intact, the eyes will move toward the side being irrigated. This should be performed by the physician and not the nurse.

DIAGNOSIS

- The ICP is monitored by an intraventricular catheter (IVC) (see Procedure 20). Cerebral perfusion pressure (CPP) is also important to monitor if an IVC has been inserted. CPP = MAP − ICP. CPP is an indirect measurement of cerebral blood flow. Normal is 60 to 100 mm Hg. A CPP of at least 60 is necessary to maintain adequate brain perfusion (8).

  Many conditions can increase ICP. Brain volume can be increased by tumors, abscesses, intracranial bleeds, hematomas, and cerebral edema. Blood volume can be increased by hypercapnia and hyperthermia (heat-related illness) (12). For treatment of hyperthermia, see Chapter 8. CSF volume can be increased by hydrocephalus from tumors, subarachnoid hemorrhage, meningitis, and Guillain-Barré syndrome.

TREATMENT

- Maintain head in a neutral position to facilitate venous outflow.
- Avoid extreme hip and knee flexion. This can increase intraabdominal and intrathoracic pressures.
- Logroll when positioning patient.
- Hyperventilate with 100% O_2 via BVMD to achieve a P_{CO_2} of 28 to 35 mm Hg.
- Hyperventilate with 100% O_2 before and after suctioning.
- Suction for no longer than 10 to 15 seconds at a time. The number of suction passes should be limited to a maximum of two during any one suction episode (11).
- Position of the HOB is controversial. The HOB should be positioned based on the individual's ICP and CPP (7). If spinal injury has been ruled out, elevating the head of bed 30 to 45 degrees may facilitate venous outflow.
- Decrease loud stimuli and bright lights.

- Ask family members and visitors to speak softly.
- Drain CSF via the IVC per physician order or protocol.
- Administer mannitol and Lasix (see Table 15-3) as directed by the physician.
- Maintain seizure precautions.
- Insert a nasogastric tube.
- Insert a urinary catheter.

NURSING ALERT

It is imperative that symptoms of increased ICP be recognized and treated promptly to prevent herniation of brain tissue.

Clinical Conditions
Herniation syndrome
Herniation is the protrusion of brain tissue outside of its normal compartment (6).

SYMPTOMS
- See Table 15-4.

DIAGNOSIS
- Diagnosis is based on symptoms and CT scan.

TREATMENT
- Same as increased ICP. Specific treatment is based on location and cause of the increased ICP.

Seizures
Seizures are produced by intermittent, sudden, massive neuronal discharge (electrical activity) in various parts of the brain. The clinical manifestations depend on the type.

Generalized tonic-clonic (grand mal): Manifested by a sudden loss of consciousness with rigidity of the trunk and extremities. This is followed by a clonic phase with violent rhythmic muscular contractions. Apnea and cyanosis frequently occur. The seizure lasts approximately 2 to 5 minutes. Afterwards, the patient may experience a headache, confusion, weakness, and motor or sensory deficits. These persist for minutes to hours.

DIAGNOSIS
- Diagnosis is based on history (tonic-clonic seizures may occur with tumors, head injuries, overdoses, infections, electrolyte imbalances, ventriculo-peritoneal (VP) shunt malfunction, febrile illness in children, subtherapeutic anticonvulsant levels, or from hypoxic events), and symptoms.

N

TABLE 15-4 Herniation Syndrome

Type of herniation	Description	Symptoms
Supratentorial Cingulate herniation	An expanding lesion in one cerebral hemisphere causes pressure medially forcing the cingulate gyrus under the falx cerebri. Displacement of the falx compresses the internal cerebral vein. If untreated, can lead to central or uncal herniation.	Changes in mental status and level of consciousness. A midline shift may be present on the CT scan.
Central (transtentorial) herniation	Downward displacement of the cerebral hemispheres, basal ganglia, diencephalon, and midbrain through the tentorial notch.	Early signs: Decreased level of consciousness, small but reactive pupils, Cheyne-Stokes respirations, increased motor spasticity, hemiparesis. Late signs: Decorticate or decerebrate posturing, pupils progress from unequal and nonreactive to dilated and fixed.
Uncal (lateral transtentorial) herniation	A large lateral lesion at the middle fossa causes lateral displacement of the medial portion of the temporal lobe through the tentorial notch.	Early signs: Ipsilateral dilated pupil from pressure on the oculomotor nerve, contralateral hemiplegia, or hemiparesis, decreased level of consciousness, respiratory changes. Late signs: Unconsciousness, bilateral fixed dilated pupils, decorticate or decerebrate posturing, absence of oculocephalic and oculovestibular reflexes.
Subtentorial herniation	Can occur by either upward displacement of the cerebellum through the tentorial notch or downward movement of brain tissue (brain stem or cerebellar tonsils) through the foramen magnum.	Abnormal respiratory patterns and pupillary changes depending on area involved, coma, hemiparesis, hemiplegia, decorticate or decerebrate posturing.

- Carefully observe and record the activity associated with the seizure.

TREATMENT
- Maintain a patent airway by insertion of a nasopharyngeal airway and/or positioning patient on his or her side to facilitate drainage of secretions (see Chapter 17).
- If cause of the seizure is unknown, administer Narcan and dextrose 50% (dextrose 25% for children).
- Pad side rails to prevent injury. Keep the bed in low position.
- Establish IV access for medication administration.
- Administer anticonvulsants such as diazepam, lorazepam, and phenytoin as ordered. Phenobarbital is frequently used in children (see Table 15-3).
- Administer acetaminophen 10 to 15 mg/kg for febrile child.

Status epilepticus: Defined as continuous seizures or seizures that occur at a frequency that prevents the patient from fully recovering from one seizure before having another seizure.

DIAGNOSIS
- Diagnosis is based on history and examination.
- Common causes include sudden withdrawal of anticonvulsants, subtherapeutic levels of anticonvulsants, meningitis, encephalitis, hypoxia, or withdrawal from alcohol.

TREATMENT
- Same as under generalized tonic-clonic seizures.

Petit mal: Seizures generally occur in children 4 to 12 years of age. There is abrupt cessation of activity, a glassy stare, (the child may stare straight ahead for 5 to 30 seconds). The child resumes activity after the seizure.

DIAGNOSIS
- Diagnosis is based on history and symptoms.

TREATMENT
- Administer anticonvulsant medication as prescribed by physician.

Focal (Jacksonian): Seizures begin with slow, repetitive jerking of a body part that increases in strength and rate over a period of 5 to 15 seconds (3).

DIAGNOSIS
- Diagnosis is based on history and symptoms.

Treatment
- Protect patient from injury.
- Anticipate need for anticonvulsants.

Central nervous system infections

Meningitis: Meningitis is inflammation of the meninges (coverings of the brain and spinal cord) as a result of viral or bacterial invasion.

Symptoms
- Symptoms may include fever, severe headache, changes in level of consciousness, stiff neck, photophobia, seizure activity, increased ICP (because of cerebral exudate, cerebral edema, and hydrocephalus), and petechiae (seen in meningococcal meningitis).
- Infants may have bulging fontanels, irritability, temperature instability, and poor feeding.
- Geriatric patients may present with only low-grade fever and confusion (9).

Diagnosis
- Diagnosis is based on history (recent history of head trauma, ear infections, sinus infection, or respiratory illness), symptoms, and CSF analysis.

Treatment
- Maintenance of airway, breathing, and circulation.
- Initiate IV antibiotic therapy as soon as possible. Antibiotics used may include penicillin, cefotaxime, or ceftriaxone. Ampicillin may be used in infants and children.
- Decrease stimuli such as noise and lights.
- Initiate seizure precautions.
- Administer antipyretics and analgesics.

Encephalitis: Encephalitis is inflammation of the brain caused by viruses, bacteria, or parasites. Viruses are the most common cause.

Symptoms
- Symptoms may include fever, headache, stiff neck, changes in level of consciousness, hemiparesis, facial weakness, ataxia, nystagmus, and generalized seizures.

Diagnosis
- Diagnosis is based on symptoms and CSF analysis.

Treatment
- Decrease stimuli such as noise and lights.
- Administer analgesics and antipyretics.
- Initiate seizure precautions.
- Treat increased ICP.

- There is no definitive drug treatment for viral encephalitis. Steroids may decrease cerebral edema. Prophylactic anticonvulsants are frequently used to prevent seizures.

Head injuries

Concussion: Concussion is a transient, temporary loss of consciousness caused by mechanical force to the brain. Consciousness returns within minutes after the impact (2).

SYMPTOMS

- Symptoms may include amnesia, headache, loss of consciousness, dizziness, drowsiness, irritability, and visual disturbances.

DIAGNOSIS

- Diagnosis is based on history and symptoms.
- CT scan will be normal.

TREATMENT

- Monitor patient for changes in neurologic status.
- Administer nonnarcotic analgesics for headache.
- Give head injury instructions if patient is discharged from the ED (see Procedure 19).

Contusion: Contusion is a bruising of the brain. Swelling of brain tissue is a concern.

SYMPTOMS

- Symptoms are related to the amount of bruising and swelling and the area involved.
- Symptoms may include an altered level of consciousness, headache, nausea, vomiting, visual disturbances, seizures, and hemiparesis.

DIAGNOSIS

- Diagnosis is based on a history of head trauma, symptoms, and CT scan findings.

TREATMENT

- Treat increased ICP.
- Anticipate need for anticonvulsants.
- Initiate seizure precautions.

Epidural hematoma: Occurs from bleeding between the skull and dura mater (outer meningeal layer). Eighty-five percent of patients will have a skull fracture. Often there is a fracture in the temporal bone with a tear in the meningeal artery or vein under the bone.

SYMPTOMS

- Symptoms include an initial loss of consciousness followed by a lucid interval lasting a few hours.

- If a venous bleed is present, the lucid interval may last 1 to 2 days.
- The lucid interval is followed by a deterioration in the level of consciousness that can occur at a rapid rate. In at least 15% of patients, there is no lucid interval.
- Headache, dilated pupil, hemiparesis, and other symptoms of increased ICP may be present.

DIAGNOSIS
- Diagnosis is based on history, symptoms, and CT scan findings.

TREATMENT
- Treat increased ICP.
- Prepare patient for surgical evacuation of the clot.

NURSING ALERT

The ICP can increase quickly to a dangerous level in arterial epidural bleeds. Herniation is a concern. Death may result if surgery is delayed.

Subdural hematoma: Occurs when blood collects between the dura and arachnoid meningeal layers. The hematoma can develop from rupture of vessels or bleeding from contused or lacerated areas. Subdural hematomas are common in the geriatric population. There are three categories—acute, subacute, and chronic.
1. Acute: Associated with major cerebral trauma. Symptoms occur within 48 hours.
2. Subacute: Associated with less severe contusions. Symptoms appear within 2 days to 2 weeks.
3. Chronic: Symptoms occur from 2 weeks to several months.

SYMPTOMS
- Symptoms include headache (which gradually worsens), drowsiness, confusion, slow thought processess, hemiparesis (late sign), and seizures.

DIAGNOSIS
- Diagnosis is based on history, symptoms, and CT scan findings.

TREATMENT
- Treat increased ICP.
- Administer nonnarcotic and nonaspirin analgesics.

- Small hematomas rarely require surgery, since they are frequently absorbed.
- Larger hematomas require surgical evacuation.

Basal skull fractures: Involve the base of the skull. The frontal and temporal bones are frequently affected. The fracture can be linear, comminuted, or depressed. Fractures involving the sinus areas frequently result in CSF leaks.

SYMPTOMS

- Symptoms include drainage from ears or nose, periorbital ecchymosis (raccoon's eyes), ecchymosis over the mastoid bone (Battle's sign, does not usually develop for 24 hours), subconjunctival hemorrhage, hearing loss, agitation, headache, nausea, and vomiting.

DIAGNOSIS

- Diagnosis is based on history, symptoms, skull x-ray, and CT scan findings.
- The halo sign (blood encircled by a yellow stain on bed linens) is highly suggestive of CSF leak. Most leaks resolve in 2 to 10 days.

TREATMENT

- Anticipate need for prophylactic antibiotics if there is a CSF leak (prevent meningitis).
- Do not pack ears or nose.
- Instruct patient not to blow his/her nose.
- Ensure tetanus/diphtheria prophylaxis.
- Admit for observation.
- Monitor patient for symptoms of an epidural hematoma if fracture involves the temporal bone.
- Monitor for increased ICP from possible underlying tissue injury.

N

NURSING ALERT

Never insert a nasogastric tube in a patient with head or facial injuries with nasal drainage. The tube may transverse the sinuses and cribriform plate and enter the brain.

Vascular injuries

Subarachnoid hemorrhage (SAH): SAH, sudden bleeding into the subarachnoid space (SAS), most often results from the rupture of an aneurysm (5). An aneurysm is an outpouching of the wall of a blood vessel. Other causes include severe head injury and rupture of an arteriovenous malformation.

SYMPTOMS
- Symptoms include severe headache, sudden transient loss of consciousness (occurs in 45% of all SAH patients), nausea, vomiting, stiff neck, photophobia, signs of increased ICP, elevated temperature, and an elevated blood pressure (BP).

DIAGNOSIS
- Diagnosis is based on symptoms and CT scan findings.

TREATMENT
- Geared toward controlling the BP and ICP to prevent an aneurysmal rebleed until the patient goes to surgery (1 to 3 days after hemorrhage).
- Bed rest.
- Quiet environment.
- Maintain systolic BP at no more than 150 mm Hg. Systolic pressures above this level can be treated with hydralazine or nitroprusside (see Table 15-4).
- Anticonvulsants as prophylaxis against seizures.
- Analgesics to control headache.
- Monitor for complications such as diabetes insipidus.
- Treat increased ICP.

Stroke or CVA: Caused by thrombosis of a cerebral vessel or by cerebral embolism. The result is ischemia to the cerebral tissue. The box describes the symptoms based on the cerebral artery occluded.

DIAGNOSIS
- Diagnosis is based on history or risk factors for stroke, symptoms, and the results of diagnostic procedures including CT scan, angiography, and carotid studies.
- The CT scan may be normal initially.

TREATMENT
- Anticoagulant therapy may be needed to decrease further development of thrombi.
- Treat increased ICP as necessary.
- Supportive therapy such as supporting flaccid limbs and proper body alignment should be implemented.
- Elevate head of bed to facilitate drainage of oropharyngeal secretions.
- Thrombolytics are used experimentally for thrombotic strokes.

CORRELATION OF CEREBRAL ARTERY INVOLVEMENT AND COMMON MANIFESTATIONS

Internal carotid artery

Contralateral paresthesia (abnormal sensations) and hemiparesis (weakness) of arm, face, and leg.

Eventually complete contralateral hemiplegia (paralysis) and hemianesthesia (loss of sensation).

Visual blurring or changes, hemianopsia (loss of half of visual field), repeated attacks of blindness in the ipsilateral eye.

Dysphasia with dominant hemisphere involvement.

Anterior cerebral artery

Mental impairment such as perseveration, confusion, amnesia, and personality changes.

Contralateral hemiparesis or hemiplegia with leg loss > arm.

Sensory loss over toes, foot, and leg.

Ataxia (motor incoordination), impaired gait, incontinence, and akinetic mutism.

Middle cerebral artery

LOC varies from confusion to coma.

Contralateral hemiparesis or hemiplegia with face and arm loss > leg.

Sensory impairment over same areas of hemiplegia.

Aphasia (inability to express or interpret speech) or dysphasia (impaired speech) with dominant hemisphere involvement.

Homonymous hemianopsia (loss of vision on the same side of both visual fields), inability to turn eyes toward the paralyzed side.

Posterior cerebral artery

Contralateral hemiplegia with sensory loss.

Confusion, memory involvement, and receptive speech deficits with dominant hemisphere involvement.

Homonymous hemianopsia.

Vertebrobasilar artery

Dizziness, vertigo, nausea, ataxia, and syncope.

Visual disturbances, nystagmus, diplopia, field deficits, and blindness.

Numbness and paresis (face, tongue, mouth, one or more limbs), dysphagia (inability to swallow), and dysarthria (difficulty in articulation).

Spinal injuries

Cord transection: Complete transection of the spinal cord results in spinal shock with complete loss of motor, sensory, reflex, and autonomic function below the level of the injury. The severity of spinal shock is influenced by the level of the injury. Injuries above T6 will disrupt sympathetic nervous system (SNS) activity below the level of the injury. Thus there is unopposed parasympathetic nervous system (PNS) activity.

The extent of loss of function is less in partial cord transections. Varying degrees of spinal shock may be seen in cord injuries from contusions, compression, lacerations, and hemorrhage (13).

SYMPTOMS

- Loss of sensation below the level of the injury.
- Flaccid paralysis below the level of the injury.
- Hypotension.
- Vasodilation below level of injury.
- Bradycardia.
- Lack of sweating below the level of the injury.
- Loss of all spinal reflexes below the level of injury.
- Atonic bladder and bowel.

TREATMENT

- Maintain spinal immobilization.
- Maintain patent airway.
- Prepare to intubate patients with cervical cord injuries above C4.
- Administer 100% oxygen.
- Two large bore IVs with Ringer's lactate or normal saline.
- Maintain systolic BP at least 80-90 mm Hg or greater. Mental status and urine output are useful parameters in evaluating perfusion.
- Administer IV fluid bolus if BP is <80 mm Hg or inadequate to maintain perfusion.
- Titrate vasopressor agents such as dopamine or dobutamine if IV fluids not successful in maintaining BP.
- Place patient on cardiac monitor.
- Treat bradycardia with atropine. If necessary, isoproterenol can be used.
- Insert nasogastric tube to decrease risk of vomiting and aspiration.
- Insert urinary catheter to monitor urine output.

- Implement measures to keep patient warm (vasodilation and lack of ability to shiver can decrease body temperature).
- Assist with application of cervical skeletal traction. A general rule is to use 5 lbs of weight for each level of injury beginning with C1 (e.g., a fracture of C3 would require 15 lbs of weight). Weights should be free hanging.

Cord syndromes: See Figures 15-3 to 15-5.

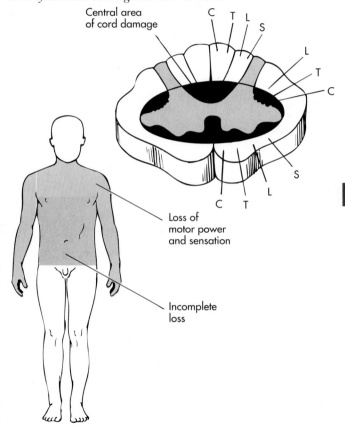

Central area of cord damage

Loss of motor power and sensation

Incomplete loss

Figure 15-3 Central cord syndrome. A cross section of the cord shows central damage and the associated motor and sensory loss (*C,* cervical; *T,* thoracic; *L,* lumbar, *S,* sacral). (Adapted from Hickey JV: *The clinical practice of neurological and neurosurgical nursing,* Philadelphia, 1992, JB Lippincott, 406, 407.)

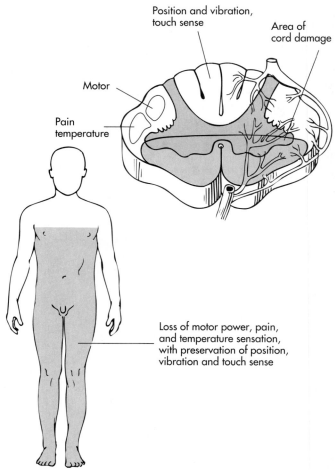

Figure 15-4 Anterior cord syndrome. Cord damage and associated motor and sensory loss are illustrated. (Adapted from Hickey JV: *The clinical practice of neurological and neurosurgical nursing,* Philadelphia, 1992, JB Lippincott, 406, 407.)

DIAGNOSIS
• Diagnosis is based on history of spinal trauma and symptoms.

TREATMENT
• Maintain spinal immobilization.

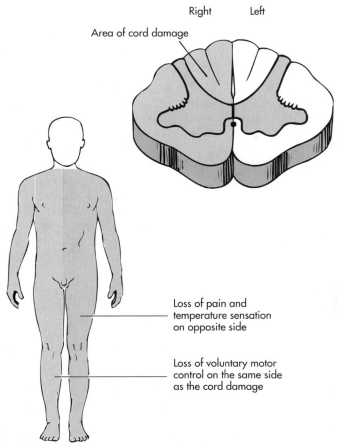

Right   Left

Area of cord damage

Loss of pain and
temperature sensation
on opposite side

Loss of voluntary motor
control on the same side
as the cord damage

Figure 15-5 Brown-Séquard syndrome. Cord damage and associated motor and sensory loss are illustrated. (Adapted from Hickey JV: *The clinical practice of neurological and neurosurgical nursing,* Philadelphia, 1992, JB Lippincott, 406, 407.)

- Administer 100% oxygen.
- Initiate two large bore IVs.
- Insert nasogastric tube and urinary catheter.
- Administer IV methylprednisolone (see Table 15-4).
- Assist with application of cervical skeletal traction or the halo immobilization device.

Autonomic hyperreflexia: (Also known as autonomic dysreflexia) is a serious hypertensive emergency that arises in the post-acute phase of SCI. This occurs in patients with injuries at or above T6 once reflex activity has returned. Autonomic hyperreflexia is caused by noxious stimuli that results in mass reflex stimulation of the sympathetic nerves below the level of the injury. Noxious stimuli are often caused by a distended bladder, constipation, fecal impaction, cystitis, urinary calculi pressure ulcers, and stimulation from skin lesions. If left untreated, this condition can lead to a CVA, seizure activity, or myocardial infarction.

SYMPTOMS

- Sudden hypertension is the primary symptom. The systolic BP may be as high as 240 to 300 mm Hg, or there may be significant rise in BP for that patient when compared with his or her usual baseline.
- Anxious appearance.
- Pounding headache.
- Blurred vision.
- Flushed face and neck.
- Profuse sweating above level of injury.
- Nasal congestion.
- Nausea.

DIAGNOSIS

- Diagnosis is based on history of previous SCI and symptoms.

TREATMENT

- Treatment is directed toward removal of the noxious stimuli and lowering the BP.
- If a urinary catheter is in place, attempt to irrigate if a plug or obstruction is suspected.
- Replace the catheter if irrigation does not remove the obstruction.
- Other treatment measures that should be considered include digital removal of fecal impaction and removal of pressure from areas of irritated or broken skin.
- Elevate the HOB and administer antihypertensive as ordered by physician.

NURSING SURVEILLANCE

1. Trend vital signs.
2. Trend GCS.

3. Trend pupil size and reactivity to light.
4. Trend ICP and CPP.
5. Trend motor and sensory function.
6. Trend urine output.

EXPECTED PATIENT OUTCOMES

1. Patent airway.
2. Bilateral equal breath sounds.
3. Systolic BP between 80 and 150 mm Hg or as needed to maintain perfusion.
4. Heart rate between 60 and 100 bpm.
5. Equal and reactive pupils.
6. No deterioration in level of consciousness.
7. ICP of 0 to 15 mm Hg.
8. CPP of 60 to 100 mm Hg.
9. Urine output of at least 30 cc/hr.
10. Normothermic.
11. No seizure activity.

DISCHARGE IMPLICATIONS

1. Instruct patient on importance of medication (anticonvulsant) compliance.
2. Teach geriatric patients to be aware of fall hazards—rugs, slick floors, similar colored floors and walls (contrasting colors better), and stairways.
3. Stress hazards of drinking alcohol before or during driving or swimming. Consider implementing injury prevention educational programs (for high risk groups).
4. Encourage the use of helmets when participating in recreational and sports activities.

Head Injuries
See Procedure 19.

References
1. Andrus C: Intracranial pressure: dynamics and nursing management, *J Neurosci Nurs* 23(2):85-91, 1991.
2. Bartkowski HM: Head trauma. In Saunders CE and HO MT, Editors: *Current emergency diagnosis and treatment,* Norwalk, Conn, 1992, Appleton & Lange, pp 239-249.
3. Hickey JV: *The clinical practice of neurological and neurosurgical nursing,* Philadelphia, 1992, JB Lippincott.

4. Keller C, Williams A: Cardiac dysrhythmias associated with central nervous system dysfunction, *J Neurosci Nurs* 25(6): 349-355, 1993.

5. MacDonald E: Aneurysmal subarachnoid hemorrhage, *J Neurosci Nurs* 21(5):315-321, 1989.

6. Marano Morrison CA: Brain herniation syndromes, *Crit Care Nurse* 7(5):35-51, 1987.

7. March K, Mitchell P, Grady S, and Winn R: Effect of bedrest position on cerebral perfusion pressure, *J Neurosci Nurs* 22(6):375-381, 1990.

8. McQuillan KA: Intracranial pressure monitoring: technical imperatives, *AACU Clin Iss* 2(4):623-636, 1991.

9. Nagani PH, Guze PA: Infectious disease emergencies. In Saunders CE and Ho MT Editors: *Current emergency diagnosis and treatment*, Norwalk Conn, 1992, Appleton & Lange, pp 614-615.

10. Olshaker JS, Whye DW: Head trauma, *Emerg Med Clin North Am* 11(1): 165-181, 1993.

11. Rudy EB, Turner BS, Baun M, Stone KS, and Brucia J: Endotracheal suctioning in adults with head injury, *Heart and Lung* 20(6):667-674, 1991.

12. Segatore, Milena: Fever after traumatic brain injury, *J Neurosci Nurs* 24(2):104-109, 1992.

13. Kidd PS: Emergency management of spinal cord injuries, *Crit Care Nurs Clin North Am* 2(3):349-355, 1990.

Chapter XVI

Obstetric and Gynecologic Conditions

Pamela S. Kidd

CLINICAL CONDITIONS
Ovarian Cysts
Dysfunctional Uterine Bleeding
Miscarriage
Ectopic Pregnancy
Preterm Labor
Abruptio Placentae
Placenta Previa
Ruptured Uterus
Pregnancy-Related Hypertensive Disorders (PRHD)
Emergency Delivery
Newborn Resuscitation
Postpartum Bleeding

TRIAGE ASSESSMENT
Gynecologic Conditions

Any source of bleeding can be potentially life threatening. Many patients present to the triage area with a chief complaint of vaginal bleeding. The clinician should assess to determine if the bleeding is associated with pregnancy, endocrine changes through the menstrual cycle, or a systemic problem such as hematologic disorder, use of anticoagulants, or traumatic injury.

The following are questions about the nature of vaginal bleeding that help the nurse to discriminate the type of gynecologic problem.

Vaginal bleeding

Ask the patient to compare present vaginal bleeding with normal menstrual flow. Asking for the number of pads or tampons used may be an indicator of the amount of bleeding. Assess if the patient has passed any tissue (hamburger-looking substance) or blood clots.

(Bleeding that is associated with clotting or lasts longer than 7 days is suggestive of substantial blood loss) (1).

Previous episode

Ask the patient if she has experienced the same symptoms at other times. (Bleeding that occurs at regular intervals associated with premenstrual symptoms such as breast tenderness and water weight gain is indicative of ovulatory bleeding.)

Last menstrual cycle

Ask the patient the date of her last menstrual cycle. (Irregular cycles are associated with uterine dysfunction.)

Pain

Ask if the patient is experiencing pain. (Uterine dysfunction is usually painless while endometriosis is painful.)

Contraceptive/Sexual activity history

Assess type of contraceptives used and sexual history. (Vaginal bleeding has been associated with intrauterine device use. It may also occur with some sexually transmitted diseases [STDs]). (See Chapter 18.)

Pregnancy history

Gravida is number of pregnancies, para is number of live births, and abortions include spontaneous, therapeutic, and elective abortions.

Medication history

Determine current medications used. (Anticoagulants, hormonal supplements, and oral contraceptives may induce vaginal bleeding.)

Vaginal discharge

Assess type and amount of vaginal discharge. Determine if this is different from normal vaginal discharge. (Vaginal discharge is associated with some STDs).

Obstetric Conditions

If a pregnant patient has suffered traumatic injury, establish a patent airway, administer oxygen and effective ventilation, support her circulation with IV fluids as necessary, and stop the source of bleeding. Complications of traumatic injury in pregnancy are uterine rupture, abruptio placentae, emergency delivery, and neonatal resuscitation (see Collaborative Interventions); liver and spleenic lacerations (see Chapter 21); and pelvic fractures (see

PHYSIOLOGIC CHANGES IN PREGNANCY

1. Increased heart rate
2. Increased cardiac output
3. Increased relative fluid volume
4. Decreased blood supply to the heart (vena cava compression)
5. Decreased blood pressure (BP) during first trimester
6. Increased BP during last 2 months of pregnancy (3-5mm Hg systolic change and 5-10 mm Hg diastolic change)
7. Increased oxygen consumption

From Harvey M, Troiano N: *NAACOGS Clin Iss in Perinatal and Women's Health Nurs* 3(3):52-59, 1992.

Chapter 9). To effectively assess abnormal clinical signs in pregnancy, the nurse must be aware of normal physiologic changes in pregnancy as related to airway, breathing, and circulation (see box above).

NURSING ALERT

Because of these physiologic changes, the pregnant patient will not demonstrate the classic signs of hypovolemic shock until the shock state is advanced. "Normal vital signs" may indicate a shunting of blood from the uterus in order to maintain core maternal body functions at the expense of fetal deterioration. Changes in fetal activity and heart rate may be the first signs of maternal hypovolemia.

Vaginal bleeding
Ask the patient to compare present vaginal bleeding with normal menstrual flow. Asking for the number of pads or tampons used may be an indicator of amount of bleeding. Assess if the patient has passed any tissue (hamburger-looking substance) or blood clots. (Bleeding that is associated with clotting or lasts longer than 7 days is suggestive of substantial blood loss (1). Tissue passing is associated with miscarriage.)

Last menstrual cycle
Ask the patient the date of her last menstrual cycle. (Bleeding may also be associated with self-induced abortion attempts.)

Pain

Ask if the patient is experiencing pain. (Placenta previa is
usually painless while ectopic pregnancy and abruptio
placentae are painful. Preterm labor is associated with
lower back pain. Term labor contractions are more
regular in timing.)

Pregnancy history

Gravida is number of pregnancies, para is number of live
births, abortions include spontaneous, therapeutic, and
elective abortions. Determine estimated date of
confinement (EDC). Calculate week of pregnancy
(abruptio placentae and placenta previa are more
prevalent in the last trimester).

NURSING ALERT

Fetal heart tones must be assessed, although they may not be
audible in the first trimester.

Fetal activity

Fetal activity escalates predictably 24 hours before labor.

Vital Signs (Gynecologic and Obstetric Conditions)

- *Heart rate:* Tachycardia related to hypovolemia and/or
  pain.
- *Blood pressure:* Hypotension related to hypovolemia.
  Hypertension related to pregnancy-induced vascular
  changes.
- *Respirations:* Tachypnea resulting from acidosis,
  secondary to anaerobic metabolism, related to a
  decrease in cellular oxygenation (in cases of
  hypovolemic shock related to abruptio placentae,
  placenta previa, ruptured ectopic pregnancy).
- *Fever:* Related to infection (STD, ruptured ectopic
  pregnancy, premature rupture of membranes in
  pregnancy).

General Observations
Skin

Assess the patient's skin for circulatory changes. Hypovolemia
is associated with cool, pale extremities. Pregnancy-related
hypertensive disorders (PRHD) may produce facial flushing.

FOCUSED NURSING ASSESSMENT (OBSTETRIC CONDITIONS)

Nursing assessment should focus on ventilation and perfusion.

Ventilation
Breath sounds

Pulmonary edema occurs rapidly in a pregnant patient with PRHD or in one who receives fluid resuscitation. Coarse or fine crackles may be auscultated.

Perfusion
Blood pressure and pulse

Assess fetal heart rate (FHR). Hemorrhage may occur and be concealed in ectopic pregnancy, abruptio placentae, or uterine rupture. FHR may decrease in situations where fetal hypoxia is occurring such as placenta previa, abruptio placentae, uterine rupture, and PRHD.

Vaginal discharge and bleeding

Mucoid, watery, or blood-tinged discharge is associated with preterm labor. The passage of tissue is suggestive of spontaneous abortion. Test the discharge for amniotic fluid (turns blue on contact with nitrazine paper). The presence of amniotic fluid indicates rupture of membranes and a higher risk for maternal infection and fetal deterioration. Meconium staining (green) of the amniotic fluid is associated with fetal problems.

Risk Factors (Obstetric Conditions)

1. Cigarette smoking increases the likelihood of premature labor, abruptio placentae, and placenta previa.
2. Age is a risk factor for hemorrhage in the last trimester of pregnancy. Women 35 years of age or older are at risk for placenta previa. Women under 20 years of age and over 30 years of age are at risk for abruptio placentae. Uterine rupture is common in older females.
3. Previous cesarean section (C section) is associated with uterine rupture and placenta previa (7).
4. Uterine trauma is associated with placenta previa, abruptio placentae, and uterine rupture.
5. Diabetes is associated with placenta previa and PRHD.
6. Alcohol consumption and cocaine use are associated with abruptio placentae.

7. Hypertension is associated with abruptio placentae.
8. History of infertility is associated with ectopic pregnancy.

Life Span Issues (Gynecologic Conditions)

1. Vaginal bleeding may occur in early adolescence because of irregular menstrual patterns and not pathology.
2. Vaginal bleeding may occur in middle age as a result of the beginning of menopause and not pathology.

INITIAL INTERVENTIONS

Gynecologic and Obstetric Conditions

1. Initiate IV access and send a blood specimen to the laboratory for a type and crossmatch and complete blood count (CBC) in all patients with vaginal bleeding and abnormal vital signs.
2. Initiate cardiac and BP monitoring in patients with significant vaginal bleeding.
3. Initiate pulse oximetry to monitor oxygen saturation.

Obstetric Conditions

1. Place all pregnant patients who are in their second trimester or greater on their left side to facilitate venous return. If the patient is on a backboard because of traumatic injury, elevate the right side of the backboard with a wedge.
2. If the patient is pregnant and hypertensive, anticipate seizure activity. Pad the siderails and keep the bed in low position. Have suction and airway materials available.
3. If available, initiate external fetal monitoring in pregnant patients with vaginal bleeding.
4. Treat pregnant patient's fear and anxiety by explaining all procedures and offering support by clergy, family, or significant others.

PRIORITY NURSING DIAGNOSES (GYNECOLOGIC AND OBSTETRIC CONDITIONS)

Risk for fluid volume deficit
Risk for pain
Risk for fear
Risk for anticipatory grieving
Risk for injury

◆ **Fluid volume deficit** related to hemorrhage.
   INTERVENTIONS
   • Initiate IV access.
   • Administer IV crystalloids and blood components as
     ordered.
   • Anticipate surgical intervention.
◆ **Pain** related to uterine contractions or peritoneal irritation.
   INTERVENTIONS
   • Administer analgesics as ordered.
   • Use imagery techniques and/or distraction if helpful to
     patient.
◆ **Fear** related to unknown pregnancy outcome.
   INTERVENTIONS
   • Allow mother to hear FHR.
   • Encourage participation in maternal tests and
     treatments by explaining benefits to fetus.
◆ **Anticipatory grieving** related to loss of pregnancy and/or
   reproductive abilities.
   INTERVENTIONS
   • Explain treatment options and probable consequences.
   • Maintain support base as identified by patient.
◆ **Injury** related to infection from peritoneal contamination
   or retained placental fragments.
   INTERVENTIONS
   • Administer antibiotics as ordered.
   • Anticipate dilatation and curettage (D and C) or surgery.
   • Monitor fever and leukocytosis.

PRIORITY DIAGNOSTIC TESTS
(GYNECOLOGIC AND OBSTETRIC CONDITIONS)

   (Many of the tests in this section are initiated in the ED
but results may take several days. The information is provided to support patient teaching.)

Laboratory
Complete blood count (CBC): May indicate infection if
   WBC is elevated or bleeding if hemoglobin and
   hematocrit are low.
Iron level: This level is low when vaginal bleeding has been
   excessive or chronic in nature.
Platelet level: This level may be low if the cause of vaginal
   bleeding is leukemia, idiopathic thrombocytopenic
   purpura, or disseminated intravascular coagulation (DIC).

Prothrombin time: This level may be high if vaginal bleeding is associated with von Willebrand's disease and other clotting disorders such as DIC associated with abruptio placentae and uterine rupture.

Human chorionic gonadotropin (HCG) test: Detection of HCG in the blood indicates pregnancy. The higher the level, the longer the gestation period. HCG levels in a woman with an ectopic pregnancy are lower than in a woman with an intrauterine pregnancy of the same gestation.

Type and crossmatch: May be ordered if blood transfusion is needed as a result of bleeding.

Serum gonadotropins

- Follicle stimulating hormone (FSH) and luteinizing hormone (LH): An FSH level >40 IU/L suggests impending ovarian failure (menopause). An LH: FSH ratio that is >2 IU/L suggests chronic anovulation.

Other

Endometrial biopsy: Used to determine presence of ovulation by measuring progesterone and estrogen levels in the endometrial lining.

Ultrasound: Used to identify ovarian cysts, early diagnosis of ovarian tumors, evaluation of abnormal uterine bleeding, ectopic pregnancy, and for guidance during aspiration procedures (e.g., pelvic and ovarian abscesses). A transabdominal scan may be performed using a full urinary bladder. The patient then voids and a transvaginal scan is conducted, if indicated.

NURSING ALERT

Determine type of ultrasound to be performed so patient can be instructed to void if needed. Transabdominal ultrasound requires a full bladder, transvaginal ultrasound requires an empty bladder.

Culdocentesis: Removal of >5 cc of nonclotting blood from the cul-de-sac indicates ectopic pregnancy. This test is very painful and is not used as frequently as ultrasound or CT scan to detect ectopic pregnancy.

COLLABORATIVE INTERVENTIONS
(GYNECOLOGIC AND OBSTETRIC CONDITIONS)

1. Administer high-flow oxygen using a nonrebreather mask at 10 to 15 L/min to compromised pregnant patients complaining of vaginal bleeding until diagnostic test results are back.
2. If not done earlier, initiate a large bore IV line for all patients complaining of vaginal bleeding.
3. Prepare the patient for a speculum examination. Obtain culture media, swabs, and specimen containers for conception products examination.

Clinical Conditions (Gynecologic)
Ovarian cysts

Ovarian cysts are difficult to identify on the physical examination. Their clinical presentation is very similar to ectopic pregnancy and appendicitis. Hormonal changes, endometriosis, or neoplasms may produce ovarian cysts.

SYMPTOMS

- Patients experience a wide range of pain severity with ovarian cysts.
- Generally the pain is worse during the latter half of the menstrual cycle.
- The pain may be localized to the right or left lower abdominal quadrant.
- The pain is increased with motion.
- If the cyst has ruptured, the patient experiences severe pain.

DIAGNOSIS

- Pelvic ultrasound is the diagnostic tool of choice.
- A CBC and HCG test may be performed.
- If rupture is suspected, a type and crossmatch and PT level may be ordered.
- Nausea and vomiting (N/V), fever, leukocytosis, and a firm-to-rigid abdomen without bowel sounds may be present.

TREATMENT

- Hormone supplements may be ordered.
- Pain medication is usually prescribed.
- Follow-up ultrasound is essential in order to detect enlargement.

- A ruptured ovarian cyst requires surgery for removal of products and irrigation of the peritoneal cavity.
- One or two large bore IV catheters should be inserted and Ringer's lactate or normal saline solution infused.
- IV antibiotics should be started in the ED.
- The patient must be monitored for shock (via BP, CVP [if available], base deficit [ABG], and urine output).
- Oxygen saturation levels are helpful.

Dysfunctional uterine bleeding

Dysfunctional uterine bleeding is usually associated with anovulation (most frequently during puberty and menopause).

SYMPTOMS

- The most common symptom is abnormal uterine bleeding associated with anovulation either acute (menarche and menopause) or chronic.

DIAGNOSIS

- Diagnosis is made by clinical findings and presentation.
- An endometrial biopsy may be performed.

TREATMENT

- If the bleeding is significant or the patient is hemodynamically unstable, a D and C should be performed in the operating suite. Estrogen and progesterone medications may be administered (see Table 16-2).

Clinical Conditions (Obstetric)
Miscarriage (spontaneous abortion)

A spontaneous abortion occurs before the 20th week of pregnancy. It may be threatened or complete.

SYMPTOMS

- Crampy abdominal pain may be present.
- Vaginal bleeding with or without the passage of tissue may occur.

DIAGNOSIS

- An HCG test is performed to confirm pregnancy.
- An ultrasound is performed to determine if a gestational sac is present and its location.
- A speculum examination is performed to determine if the cervix is dilatated and to assess source of bleeding.

TREATMENT

- Oxytocin or Methergine may be administered to promote expulsion of all material.

- Antibiotics and analgesics may be ordered.
- A D and C may need to be performed.
- The patient should be tested for Rh status, and Rh immunoglobulin administered if the mother is Rh negative.

Ectopic pregnancy

Ectopic pregnancy occurs when the fertilized ovum implants on tissue other than the uterine endometrium, usually because of impaired passage through the fallopian tubes.

SYMPTOMS

- Amenorrhea, pelvic or abdominal pain, and abnormal vaginal bleeding are the most common symptoms.
- A pelvic mass can be palpated in some cases.
- Symptoms most frequently occur at 4 to 6 weeks gestation.
- Ectopic rupture with intraperitoneal bleeding occurs at 6 to 10 weeks gestation. Thus, symptoms may include hypotension, tachycardia, N/V, rigid abdomen without bowel sounds, fever, and leukocytosis.

DIAGNOSIS

- An ultrasound may detect an ectopic pregnancy before clinical symptoms appear.
- Ultrasound findings are compared with HCG levels.
- Presence of nonclotting fluid in the cul-de-sac may be present upon culdocentesis.

TREATMENT

- Newer treatment strategies include transvaginal or laparoscopic injection of various agents or systemic chemotherapy using methotrexate (6).
- Surgery is usually performed to remove the products of conception and to repair the damaged fallopian tube.
- Rh testing of the mother should be performed and Rh immunoglobulin given if the patient is Rh negative.

Preterm labor

Many women ignore the signs of preterm labor and present to the ED after membranes have ruptured or cervical dilatation has occurred. Gestational age of the fetus may be reflected in baseline FHR, pattern of reactivity, and changes in the behavioral state of the fetus.

SYMPTOMS

- The symptoms associated with preterm labor may include elevated FHR (150 to 160 bpm) (3).

- If fetal monitoring is available in the ED, preterm fetuses have fewer number of accelerations and less amplitude with acceleration.
- Painless contractions and a change in vaginal discharge (mucoid, watery, or blood-tinged appearance) are the best predictors of preterm labor.

DIAGNOSIS

- Preterm labor is diagnosed by labor pattern and not by FHR alone.
- A speculum examination to rule out premature rupture of the membranes as causing the change in vaginal discharge is conducted, followed by a digital examination of the cervix to evaluate cervical dilatation and effacement.

TREATMENT

- Tocolytic agents (e.g., ritodrine, terbutaline, magnesium sulfate) are administered.
- The patient is placed on bed rest in the left lateral recumbent position.
- Fetal monitoring is used to detect activity and heart rate variability.

Abruptio placentae

Abruptio placentae usually occurs after 20 weeks gestation. It is a tearing and bleeding into the inner layer of the endometrium that compresses and impairs the functioning of the placenta. Abruptio may be concealed (rare) because of internal uterine bleeding or revealed/external (in 80% of cases) where bleeding dissects the membrane from the uterine wall (Figure 16-1) (4).

SYMPTOMS

- The patient complains of sharp, sudden generalized pain over the abdomen.
- Rapid, continuous, or intermittent uterine contractions may occur. Vaginal bleeding may be present. If present, it is usually dark in color.
- Fetal activity is less and FHR may decrease as fetal hypoxia occurs.
- Signs of hypovolemic shock may be present (decreased LOC, increased heart rate, decreased urine output, oxygen saturation, and BP).
- DIC is common with abruption.

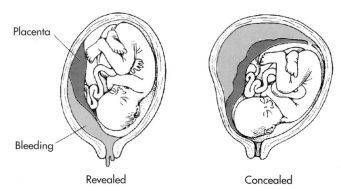

Placenta

Bleeding

Revealed   Concealed

Figure 16-1 Abruptio placentae. (From Murphy P: Problem pregnancies, *JEMS* 17(9): 48-49, 1992.)

DIAGNOSIS
- Diagnosis is usually made by clinical presentation.
- DIC may be confirmed by prolonged PT and the presence of fibrin degradation products.

TREATMENT
- The aim of treatment is to maintain maternal blood volume by fluid resuscitation with crystalloids and blood components (initially two large bore IV lines infusing Ringer's lactate solution).
- High-flow oxygen (10 to 15 L/min) is administered.
- The fetus is delivered and resuscitated as necessary.

Placenta previa
Placenta previa is a condition where the placenta is located either close to or over the internal os of the uterus. The placenta may cover the os partially or completely (Figure 16-2). The danger in placenta previa is a separation of the placenta from the uterine wall with subsequent hemorrhage. Perinatal mortality is greater because of decreased fetal perfusion both from the implanted placenta and from decreased circulating blood volume of the mother.

SYMPTOMS
- Almost half of all placenta previa patients have their first episode of bleeding before 30 weeks gestation.
- Initial bleeding is usually self-limiting.

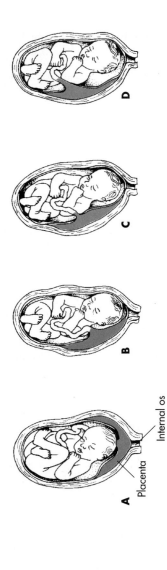

Figure 16-2 Placenta previa. **A,** *total placenta previa,* Internal cervical os is completely covered by the placenta; **B,** *partial previa,* internal os is partially covered by the placenta; **C,** *marginal previa,* edge of the placenta is at the margin of the internal os; **D,** *low lying previa,* placenta is implanted in the lower uterine section, and the edge is close to the internal os. (From Murphy P: Problem pregnancies, *JEMS* 17(9):48-49, 1992.)

- The earlier this episode occurs in the pregnancy, the less likely the pregnancy will reach term.
- Painless, bright red bleeding, not associated with contractions, are the most frequent clinical signs.

DIAGNOSIS
- A speculum examination may be performed, but digital examination is not advisable because of the potential for hemorrhage.
- Ultrasound is used to detect placental location.

TREATMENT
- The aim is to postpone labor to promote fetal maturation.
- Bed rest may be initiated.
- If the patient continues to bleed, the baby may be delivered by C section.
- Vaginal delivery is possible if previa is marginal.

Ruptured uterus

A ruptured uterus may be complete when a tear occurs through the uterus and peritoneal covering allowing intrauterine contents to be "spilled" into the peritoneal cavity. An incomplete tear may also occur (occult). Rupture of the healthy uterus most frequently occurs during labor with oxytocin administration. Rupture of a previously scarred uterus (e.g., C section) may occur as pregnancy advances.

SYMPTOMS
- Bleeding may be great if the tear is complete but not visible, thus the patient will have signs of hypovolemia (increased heart rate, decreased BP, decreased oxygen saturation).
- Parts of the fetus may be palpable in the abdomen.
- If the tear is partial, minor bleeding may occur and seal itself off by hematoma formation.
- Sharp, shooting abdominal pain or a tearing sensation may be present.
- Contractions may stop suddenly.
- Fetal mortality is high (50% to 75%).

DIAGNOSIS
- Diagnosis is made by clinical presentation.

TREATMENT
- Emergency surgical delivery C section is indicated for delivery of fetus and repair of peritoneum and uterus.

- Rapid fluid resuscitation is indicated.
- Two large bore IV lines are inserted and crystalloids and blood components administered.
- Administer high-flow oxygen (10 to 15 L/min).

Pregnancy-related hypertensive disorders (PRHD)

The four types of PRHD are: Chronic hypertension (hypertension diagnosed before pregnancy or that persists after forty-second week (postpartum), transient hypertension (increased blood pressure after 20 weeks or 24 hours after delivery), preeclampsia superimposed on chronic hypertension, and preeclampsia and eclampsia (2). Preeclampsia is defined as BP >140/90, a systolic increase of 30 mm Hg or greater, or a diastolic increase of 15 mm Hg or greater at two readings taken 6 or more hours apart. Edema and proteinuria are present. Eclampsia is the development of seizures in a preeclamptic patient (5). The arterial wall responds differently to angiotensin II and renin resulting in arterial spasms.

SYMPTOMS

- The patient may present with a variety of clinical signs.
- Patients may complain of visual changes, edema, persistent vomiting, or decreased urine output.
- A classic sign is in the second trimester; the mean arterial pressure (MAP) does not drop lower than the first trimester MAP.
- A 30 mm Hg or greater increase in systolic BP or a 15 mm Hg or greater increase in diastolic BP must be present to make the diagnosis.
- Papilledema and seizures may occur.
- In eclampsia, epigastric pain (occurring from liver edema) is associated with impending seizure and is a late sign.
- Fetal movement may decrease.
- Reflexes are hyperactive.

DIAGNOSIS

- BP changes occur as explained above.
- Urine protein levels increase (1^+ in mild cases, up to 3^+ or greater in severe cases).
- Platelet levels may be low, fibrin degradation products may be present, and liver enzymes may be elevated if the preeclampsia has progressed into HELLP (hemolysis, elevated enzymes, and low platelets) syndrome.

TREATMENT

- Seizures are treated as outlined in Chapter 15.

- Severe cases are treated with magnesium sulfate to prevent seizures, or valium, phenytoin, and phenobarbital are given when seizures occur.
- Hydralazine may be given for decreasing the BP.
- Terbutaline may be given for preventing contractions.
- Milder cases are treated with bed rest, no added salt diet, and home monitoring of BP and urine protein levels.
- Delivery is the last resort, since BP decreases after delivery.

Emergency delivery

The multiparous pregnant patient is at the greatest risk for imminent delivery.

SYMPTOMS

- Ask the patient if she is aware of when her bag of water ruptured. If so, was the fluid green or have a greenish tint?
- Green fluid (meconium) indicates infants that may need suctioning and intubation.
- The patient will have bloody show secondary to rapid dilatation of the cervix, a bulging anus and perineum indicating fetal descent, and crowning of the head.

STEPS IN EMERGENCY DELIVERY

1. Place the mother on left side to slow fetal descent.
2. Have the mother open her mouth and pant to slow progress.
3. Have a neonatal resuscitation bag and oxygen supply available. Suction equipment is also needed.
4. Wash your hands and glove.
5. Wash patient's perineum, reglove.
6. Ease perineum back until head emerges.
7. Suction the baby's mouth first, then the nose. Suctioning the nose first may elicit a reflex gasp of fluids in the lungs.
8. Place your hand under the cord as the baby emerges.
9. If the cord is extremely tight, clamp the cord with two clamps and cut between the clamps.
10. Keep the baby's head lower than its trunk during birthing to promote drainage.
11. Do not pull the baby out, allow baby to advance on its own.
12. Cut the cord after clamping 1½ inches from the infant's umbilicus after it stops pulsating. Use two clamps to prevent cord bleeding.
13. Document time of delivery and baby's APGAR score.

- If the baby's head remains visible between contractions, birth is imminent.

DIAGNOSIS
- Diagnosis is based on clinical presentation.

TREATMENT
- Follow the steps in the box for emergency delivery.

NURSING ALERT

If the cord prolapses before baby presents, place the mother in knee-chest position or Trendelenburg's position. Administer high-flow oxygen (10-15 L/min) to the mother.

Documentation
1. Record intrapartum and postpartum care. The box includes pertinent information to record.
2. Record neonatal assessment and treatments (Table 16-1 for scoring APGAR at 1 and 5 minutes). Neonatal ophthalmic medications vary according to state law. Beware that the infant is at risk for hypothermia and ineffective airway clearance.

Newborn resuscitation

An APGAR score of 5 or less is frequently a predictor of resuscitation need.

SYMPTOMS
- An APGAR score of <5 after 1 minute (because of poor ventilation and circulatory response) is usually present.

DIAGNOSIS
- There is no respiratory effort, the pulse is irregular, decreased, or absent.

TREATMENT
- 100 percent oxygen is administered after suctioning the infant using a bag-valve mask or blowby device.
- Intubation should follow immediately.
- Perform cardiac massage if heart rate is <100 bpm.
- Epinephrine 0.01 mg/kg of a 1:10,000 solution may be given endotracheally or through the umbilical cord in cardiac arrest.
- An IV line must be initiated (the umbilical cord may be used).
- Warming lights should be placed on the baby to prevent hypothermia.

PERTINENT DATA TO RECORD DURING THE INTRAPARTUM AND POSTPARTUM PERIODS

Intrapartum

1. Gravida, para, abortions, LMP, EDC
2. FHR
3. Membranes status
4. Vaginal bleeding: Amount
5. Percent effacement, centimeters of dilatation, station
6. Anesthetic agent/s, episiotomy, sutures
7. Amniotic fluid cultures

Postpartum

1. Time fetus delivered
2. Time placenta delivered
3. Cord blood samples obtained
4. Time placenta sent to laboratory for examination
5. Fundal massage and position q 15 min
6. Lochia color and amount q 15 min x 1 hr, then q 1 hr
7. Perineum assessment q 15 min x 1 hr, then q 1 hr

TABLE 16-1 APGAR Score

Sign	0	1	2
Heart rate	Absent	Slow/below 100 bpm	Above 100 bpm
Respirations	Absent	Slow/ irregular	Good crying
Muscle tone	Flaccid	Some flexion of extremities	Active motion
Reflex irritability	None	Grimace	Vigorous cry
Color	Pale blue	Body pink with blue extremities	Completely pink

Postpartum bleeding

Postpartum bleeding is defined as a blood loss >500 cc at delivery or during the first 24 hours after delivery. It is related to uterine atony or cervical/vaginal lacerations. However, in some cases postpartum bleeding may occur 2 to 4 weeks after delivery because of retained placental fragments.

SYMPTOMS

- Vaginal bleeding with clots and a soft uterus indicates atony.
- Tissue may be passed vaginally.
- Fever is present with leukocytosis if bleeding occurs several weeks after delivery.

DIAGNOSIS

- A speculum examination is made to determine the presence of cervical/vaginal lacerations.
- A CBC may be performed.
- Diagnosis is usually made by clinical presentation.

TREATMENT

- If the bleeding occurs early in the postpartum period, uterine massage may be performed by the physician with one hand externally massaging and the other gloved hand supporting the lower uterine segment through a vaginal approach (Figure 16-3).
- Oxytocic drugs are administered (e.g., Methergine, Ergotrate, Pitocin).
- Breastfeeding (if appropriate) helps the uterus to contract.
- Fluid resuscitation with two large bore IV lines infusing crystalloids or blood components may be indicated.
- High-flow oxygen (10 to 15 L/min) may be necessary.

NURSING SURVEILLANCE

1. Trend vital signs and oxygen saturation.
2. Monitor contractions for timing and duration.
3. Monitor FHR during contractions.
4. Monitor level of consciousness.
5. Trend pain.
6. Diligent pulmonary assessment is crucial in a pregnant patient who has been receiving IV fluids because of hemodilution and the chance of pulmonary edema occurring.

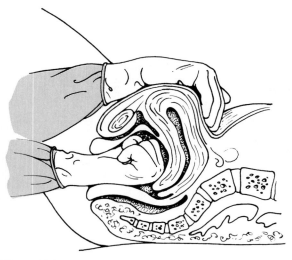

Figure 16-3   Bimanual compression of the uterus and massage with the abdominal hand usually will control hemorrhage from uterine atony. (From Cunningham FG, MacDonald PC, Gant NF: *Williams Obstetrics*, ed 19, Norwalk, Conn, 1993, Appleton & Lange.)

7. Monitor arterial blood gases, and beware of an increased CO_2 level, since respiratory alkalosis is normal for pregnancy.

EXPECTED PATIENT OUTCOMES

1. Patient's level of consciousness improves or remains stable.
2. Vaginal bleeding decreases in amount.
3. Pain decreases or is absent.
4. Urine output is >30 cc/hr.
5. Fever decreases or is absent.
6. Vital signs improve, systolic BP remains >90 mm Hg but <140 mm Hg.
7. No seizure activity.
8. FHR normal for gestational age.
9. Newborn infant's APGAR is >5 at 1 minute and improves at 5 minutes.

TABLE 16-2 Drug Summary

Drug	Dose/Route	Special considerations
Progesterone	100-200 mg IM	Used to treat dysfunctional uterine bleeding.
Medroxy-progesterone acetate	10-40 mg qd for 5-10 days PO	Used to treat active uterine bleeding.
Estrogen	25 mg q 4 hr x 3 doses IV	Used in persistent uterine bleeding. Progesterone is started after the estrogen is administered.
Oxytocin	Comes in 10 U/cc concentration. Add 10-40 U to 1,000 cc normal saline or Ringer's lactate for IV. 10 U IM	Titrate drug to achieve uterine contractions. Usually takes 200-500 cc/hr at the described concentration.
Ergonovine and Methylergonovine maleate	0.2 mg IM, repeat q 2-4 hr 0.2 mg IV	IV route is only used in life-threatening situations. Used to achieve uterine contractions.
Terbutaline sulfate	10 µg/min IV titrated up to a maximum of 80 µg/min for 4 hr, then switch to 2.5 mg PO q 4-6 hr	Used to stop premature labor. Cardiac monitoring of both mother and fetus should be instituted because of side effect of tachycardia. May cause hyperglycemia.

| Magnesium sulfate | 4 g in 250 cc D_5 W IV infused slowly, followed by 4-5 g IM in alternate buttocks q 4 hr. | Used to prevent seizures in HELLP syndrome, preeclampsia, and eclampsia. Also used to stop premature labor. Check reflexes and respiratory function before administration and during administration. May cause respiratory depression in mother and newborn. |
| Rh_0 Immune Globulin | Preferred dose is 1 vial within 3 hr but at least within 72 hr after ectopic pregnancy, abortion, miscarriage, amniocentesis. One vial within 72 hr of delivery in postpartum. | Used to prevent hemolytic disease of the newborn in a subsequent pregnancy. |

DISCHARGE IMPLICATIONS

1. All patients discharged with vaginal bleeding should be told to check their temperature qid and to return if fever occurs.
2. Tampons should be avoided until abnormal vaginal bleeding stops.
3. Patients with a threatened abortion should be told to abstain from sexual intercourse until bleeding stops. They should save all passed tissue for examination.
4. Pregnant patients with PIH should receive low salt or no added salt diet teaching. They should be taught how to take their BP and to perform urine reagent testing for protein content.
5. Patients who are found to be Rh negative should be told to wear a medical alert bracelet with this information.

References

1. Bayer S, DeCherney A: Clinical manifestations and treatment of dysfunctional uterine bleeding, *JAMA* 269:1823-1838, 1993.
2. Creasy R, Resnik R: *Maternal-fetal medicine, principles, and practice,* Philadelphia, 1992, WB Saunders.
3. Eganhouse D, Burnside JS: Nursing assessment and responsibility in monitoring the preterm pregnancy, *JOGN* 21:355-363, 1992.
4. Murphy P: Problem pregnancies, *JEMS* 17(9):44-60, 1992.
5. Silver J: Nursing care of the acutely ill obstetrical patient. In Kidd P, Wagner K, editors: *High acuity nursing: preparing to practice in today's health care settings,* Norwalk, Conn, 1992, Appleton & Lange.
6. Wade R: Gynecologic applications of real-time ultrasound, *Appl Radiol* 15-19, Feb 1993.
7. Zerbe M, Bashore R: Critical hemorrhage during pregnancy, *Crit Care Nurs Clin North Am* 4:729-736, 1992.

Chapter XVII

Respiratory Conditions

Darlene Welsh
Pamela S. Kidd

CLINICAL CONDITIONS
Asthma
Pulmonary Alveolar Edema (PAE)
   Noncardiogenic Pulmonary Alveolar Edema
   Cardiogenic Pulmonary Alveolar Edema
Pulmonary Embolism (PE)
Pneumonia
Chronic Obstructive Pulmonary Disease (COPD)
Spontaneous Pneumothorax

TRIAGE ASSESSMENT

Acutely ill emergency department (ED) patients may require airway management. Common respiratory conditions treated in the ED include asthma, pulmonary alveolar edema (PAE), pulmonary embolism (PE), pneumonia, spontaneous pneumothorax, and chronic obstructive pulmonary disease (COPD). COPD is usually a combination of two disease processes, chronic bronchitis and emphysema. Documenting patient complaints and medical history at triage assists with differentiating these conditions. Obtain the following patient information from transport personnel, patients, or family members:

Precipitating event
History of electrical injury, overdose, paralysis secondary to cerebrovascular attack or spinal cord injury, carbon monoxide poisoning, or smoke inhalation (suspect impending airway obstruction). Triage to treatment area immediately.

Previous need for intubation
History of intubation for respiratory failure is highly significant for fatal asthma. Triage to treatment area immediately.

Exercise ability, steroid use

History of exercise limitations, current use of steroids, prior hospitalization for acute asthma (suspect bronchoconstriction).

Dyspnea

History of paroxysmal nocturnal dyspnea, orthopnea, dyspnea upon exertion, lower extremity edema, unexplained fatigue, known cardiovascular disease (suspect cardiogenic PAE).

Burn/trauma history, altitude changes, near drowning

History of recent trauma, major burn, toxicant inhalation, hemorrhage (secondary to hypoperfusion and stimulation of the inflammatory response), drug overdose, altitude changes, massive infection, near drowning (suspect noncardiogenic PAE).

Potential for thrombus/emboli formation

History of venous insufficiency, deep vein thrombosis (DVT), orthopedic trauma or surgery, obesity, recent pregnancy or delivery, prolonged immobility, estrogen therapy (suspect PE).

Pneumothorax history

History of a spontaneous pneumothorax (suspect underlying pulmonary disease (e.g., COPD or spontaneous pneumothorax reoccurrence, particularly if original pneumothorax was treated with chest tube insertion or aspiration). The reoccurrence rate of spontaneous pneumothorax is at least 30% (2,7).

Infection

History of recent upper respiratory infection (URI), living in close proximity to others (as a result of increased exposure to the respiratory pathogens of others and to immobility), decreased level of consciousness, fever, leukocytosis, acquired immunodeficiency syndrome (AIDS) (suspect pneumonia).

Productive cough

History of productive cough (3 months duration for 2 to 3 consecutive years), wheezing, dyspnea, smoking, exposure to environmental pollution (suspect COPD).

Airway and breathing pattern signs

- Change in respiratory rate or pattern may be an early sign of respiratory insufficiency.
- Inward chest movement on inspiration.

- Outward abdominal movement on inspiration.
- Suprasternal, supraclavicular, and sternocleidomastoid muscle retractions.
- Retraction of intercostal spaces.
- Noisy inspiratory breathing (Table 17-1). Figure 17-1 shows the relationship between anatomy and type of stridor.

> **NURSING ALERT**
>
> When wheezing decreases while the patient is waiting for treatment, check to see if the patient is improving or if the patient's condition is worsening because of less airflow. Stridor indicates a life-threatening problem. It occurs when at least 75% of the airway is occluded. Triage immediately to the treatment area.

- Nasal flaring.
- Cyanosis (very late sign).
- Extreme anxiety.
- Decreased level of consciousness.

Vital Signs
- *Pulse:* Paradoxical pulse (a fall in systolic blood pressure [BP] of at least 12 mm Hg during inspiration) indicates severe asthma related to the negative intrapleural pressure created as an asthmatic patient inspires.
- *Tachycardia:* Related to fever, pain, change in cardiac output.
- *Bradycardia:* Related to ischemic heart disease.
- *Fever:* Related to infection.
- *Tachypnea:* Related to hypoxemia, impaired ventilation.
- *Blood pressure:* Hypotension related to heart failure, shock. Hypertension related to fluid volume overload.

Pain
- Chest pain that increases on inspiration and respiratory movement and is limited to one side (suspect spontaneous pneumothorax).
- Chest tightness is associated with airway inflammation and bronchoconstriction.

Dyspnea
- Continuous dyspnea unrelieved with rest (suspect spontaneous pneumothorax).

R

TABLE 17-1 Discriminating Source of Airway Obstruction

Origin	Etiology	Symptoms
Nasal		
• URI	Incidence may be increased during certain seasons if related to allergens/infection.	Absence of stridor
• Allergy	Related to inflammation of nares.	Rarely life threatening
• Foreign bodies/tumors		Patient presents with mouth breathing
Pharyngeal		
• Infection	Regurgitation of gastric contents	Snoring
• Foreign bodies	Dislodged/broken teeth	Inspiratory stridor
	Nasal, oral, pharyngeal bleeding	
	Occlusion of tongue in unconscious patient	
Laryngeal		
• Infection	Spasm may occur as a result of foreign material or suctioning.	Crowing
• Foreign bodies/tumors	Edema may occur as a result of intubation attempts, inhalation of caustic substances.	Inspiratory stridor is equal to expiratory stridor
• Trauma		
Tracheal		
• External pressure on trachea	Hematoma from repeated attempts at internal jugular cannulation	Inspiratory stridor is equal to expiratory stridor
	Compression of neck by hanging or strangling	
Bronchial		
• Inflammation	Exposure to allergens	Expiratory stridor/wheezing
	Exposure to caustic substances	
	Foreign body inhalation	

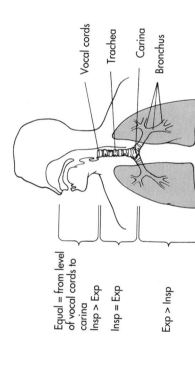

Figure 17-1 The airway. Types of stridor heard with obstruction of the airway. Insp = Inspiratory, Exp = Expiratory.

R

- Dyspnea that occurs during eating (suspect partial airway obstruction).
- Nocturnal dyspnea is associated with severe asthma and PAE.

NURSING ALERT

Most patients visit the ED as a last resort measure. Several home strategies have usually been unsuccessful. Take seriously any complaint of dyspnea.

General Observations

1. Patients in moderate-to-severe respiratory distress sit in high Fowler's position and cannot tolerate lying lower than 30 degrees (orthopnea).
2. Presence of jugular vein distention (JVD) suggests right heart failure, a common problem in those with PE, cardiogenic PAE, or severe COPD.
3. Patients with severe dyspnea are often extremely anxious, apprehensive, and afraid.
4. Pursed-lip breathing may be observed in those with pneumonia or COPD.
5. An increased anteroposterior diameter of the chest may be noted in patients with COPD.
6. Patients with emphysema are often thin and present with muscle wasting.

NURSING ALERT

Patients with respiratory conditions can quickly decompensate. Triage those with severe dyspnea, tachypnea, chest pain, or other signs of acute respiratory distress to the ED treatment area immediately. A spontaneous pneumothorax, if it is of significant size, can progress into a tension pneumothorax, which is a medical emergency (see Chapter 21).

FOCUSED NURSING ASSESSMENT

Nursing assessment of patients with respiratory conditions centers on ventilation, perfusion, cognition, and elimination.

Ventilation
Breath sounds

Crackles (rales) or wheezing can be heard in many respiratory conditions. Absent or diminished breath sounds are also significant findings and may indicate pneumothorax or some forms of alveolar consolidation. Crackles that do not clear with coughing may indicate heart failure. Breath sounds may be absent or diminished as a result of bronchoconstriction from foreign body aspiration. The right mainstem bronchus is a common site for foreign body lodgement or passage because of its lesser angle. Wheezing is not a reliable indicator of severity.

Respirations
Determine character of respirations. Patients with COPD frequently use accessory muscles to assist with breathing. Tripod positioning (upright with elbows placed on a supporting object) is common in those with respiratory distress. They may use the triage counter in this manner. Hyperventilation, tachypnea, and orthopnea are additional signs of respiratory distress.

Expiratory flow rate
If the patient has a history of COPD or asthma, obtain peak expiratory flow rate using a peak flow meter. If this value is <200 L/min, triage to the treatment area immediately.

Oxygen saturation
Determine S_{AO_2} levels with continuous pulse oximetry. S_{AO_2} of 91% or less is highly predictive of hospital admission (4).

Sputum
Describe sputum production. Pink, frothy sputum is a sign of cardiogenic PAE. Patients with pneumonia produce green, yellow, or rust-colored sputum. A change in sputum production or appearance in those with COPD indicates acute pulmonary infection.

Dyspnea
Assess dyspnea using a standardized scale (Figure 17-2).

Perfusion
Heart sounds
A third heart sound is often noted in heart failure.

Point of maximal impulse
Palpate the point of maximal impulse (PMI). Usually, the apex of the heart touches the anterior chest wall at or near the fifth left intercostal space, midclavicular line. Lateral displacement of the PMI is a clinical indicator of cardiac hypertrophy and possible heart failure (5).

R

Circle the Number That Best Matches Your Shortness of Breath	
0	None at all
0.5	Very, very slight (just noticeable)
1	Very slight
2	Slight
3	Moderate
4	Somewhat severe
5	Severe
6	
7	Very severe
8	
9	Very, very severe (almost maximal)
10	Maximal

Figure 17-2 Dyspnea scale.

Jugular vein distention

Determine the presence of JVD. Place the patient in semi-Fowler's position with the head turned to the right or the left. Observe the jugular vein at the posterior border of the sternocleidomastoid muscle. Right atrial congestion is suspected when jugular veins distend 2 inches or greater above the sternal notch (Figure 17-3). Jugular veins may be distended and the trachea shifted away from midline if a spontaneous pneumothorax has resulted in a tension pneumothorax.

Peripheral pulses/skin

Assess peripheral pulses, edema, skin temperature and color, and capillary refill. Observe for peripheral and central cyanosis. Indicators of venous insufficiency (a risk factor for PE) include pedal edema, brown, leathery extremity skin, and palpable pedal pulses. Pedal pulses are diminished or absent with arterial insufficiency.

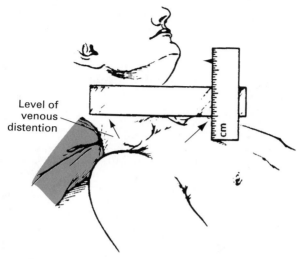

Figure 17-3 Jugular venous distention.

Cardiac rhythm

Identify cardiac rhythm. Patients with atrial fibrillation are at high risk for congestive heart failure (CHF) and subsequent PE. Suspect atrial fibrillation if there is a discrepancy between the radial and apical pulse. With atrial fibrillation, the rhythm is irregular without a pattern. When in doubt, place the patient on a cardiac monitor and run a rhythm strip. Individuals with cardiogenic PAE experience tachy or brady dysrhythmias.

Weight

Document weight in hemodynamically stable patients. If unstable, obtain baseline weight from patient or family. Many medications are dosed by weight.

Cognition

Perform a neurologic assessment using the Glasgow coma scale (GCS) (see Reference Guide 6). Medications (e.g., theophylline, Alupent) used to treat pulmonary disorders exert central nervous system effects such as nervousness, tachycardia, and agitation. Hypoxemia and hypercapnia can cause restlessness and decreased level of consciousness. Thrombolytics used to dissolve blood clots with some forms of PE can cause intracranial bleeding.

Elimination

Monitor urinary output. Patients with cardiogenic PAE can experience hypervolemia and decreased urine output. Hypovolemia or hypervolemia may occur in noncardiogenic PAE. Renal response to diuresis should be documented.

Risk Factors

1. *Exposure risk:* Homosexuality, multiple partners, IV drug abuse increase the risk of AIDS and *Pneumocystis carinii* pneumonia, (see Chapter 5). *Pneumocystis carinii* predisposes the patient to the development of spontaneous pneumothoraces. Smoking, air pollution, and occupational dust exposure lead to COPD development. An increased risk of spontaneous pneumothorax is associated with smoking.

2. *Gender:* Pregnancy or estrogen therapy can increase the possibility of PE.

3. *Past medical history:* People with cardiovascular disease such as CHF or atrial fibrillation are prone to cardiogenic PAE and PE. Those with deep vein thrombophlebitis are at high risk for PE.

4. *Environmental:* Institutionalized individuals are prone to pneumonia. Changes in altitude can precipitate noncardiogenic PAE.

5. *Situational:* Patients with prolonged immobility, obesity, or recent orthopedic surgery are at risk for PE. A depressed gag or cough reflex can result in aspiration pneumonia as encountered in some cerebral vascular accidents or patients with GCS scores <15. Neurologic injury, trauma, or burns are etiologies for noncardiogenic PAE.

6. *Anthropometric:* An increased height in proportion to decreased weight (tall and thin individuals) predisposes the individual to the development of spontaneous pneumothoraces resulting from a greater negative pleural pressure at the apex of the lung in this body type (7).

Life Span Issues
Pediatric
1. Newborns are at risk for spontaneous pneumothorax related to hyaline membrane disease and meconium aspiration.
2. Young children and adolescents experience noncardiogenic PAE secondary to trauma.
3. The incidence of staphylococcal pneumonia is greatest in children <2 years of age. Respiratory syncytial virus (RSV) is the most common cause of viral pneumonia in children (3).
4. Children with a history of cystic fibrosis have a higher incidence of spontaneous pneumothorax.
5. Infants and children exposed to passive smoking have a higher incidence of asthma.

Pregnancy
One third of pregnant women with asthma have increased symptom severity, particularly during the 19- to 36-weeks-gestation period.

Geriatric
1. COPD occurs mainly in middle-aged to older adults. It is frequently associated with asthma.
2. The geriatric patient is at risk for pneumonia.
3. Spontaneous pneumothorax in patients older than 40 years of age is associated with a history of COPD or pulmonary tuberculosis (1).
4. A blunted perception of breathlessness has been found in the geriatric patient. They may not be dyspneic with respiratory conditions. If they complain of dyspnea, their condition may be severe.

INITIAL INTERVENTIONS

R

Airway Obstruction
1. Perform the Heimlich maneuver if appropriate. Perform chin-lift or jaw-thrust maneuver to displace the mandible and move the tongue away from the back of the throat. Assume a cervical spine injury and do not tilt the head.
2. If patient is not ventilating, administer two breaths by pocket mask through the patient's mouth. If resistance is met, perform chin-lift or jaw-thrust maneuver a second time.

3. Insert an artificial airway. Artificial airways decrease gastric inflation. Oral airways are used to ventilate an unconscious patient. Have suction equipment available, since placement may stimulate the gag reflex producing vomitus. The proper size can be estimated by measuring from the external corner of the patient's mouth up to the tragus of the ear (protrusion above the earlobe). An oral airway inserts easier if it is wet before insertion. Do not tape the oral airway. The patient should be able to cough out the airway if the gag reflex returns. If they are alert enough to cough out the airway, they are alert enough to not need the airway. Ventilate the patient by applying a mask over the airway (pocket mask with one-way valve for mouth-to-mask ventilation). The most effective way of ventilating the patient is connecting the mask to a manual resuscitation bag with an oxygen reservoir attached. The bag should be connected to oxygen at a 10 to 15 L rate. Ventilate the patient 12 times a minute. Nasopharyngeal airways may be used if the patient is awake but not alert. The use of a nasopharyngeal airway is contraindicated when the patient is receiving anticoagulants. Apply local anesthetic ointment to the device before insertion. Figure 17-4 shows proper insertion technique. The nasopharyngeal airway can be connected to a manual resuscitation bag via an endotracheal tube adaptor inserted into the nares' end of the airway (Figure 17-5). The mouth and opposite nares must be occluded while squeezing the bag. Reference Guide 23 lists size of airway based on size of patient. If the patient's heart rate decreases during passage, suspect that the airway is too long, and it is compressing the epiglottis against the laryngeal entrance producing vagal stimulation (10).

NURSING ALERT

If resistance is encountered during ventilation, suspect obstruction and/or patient's preexisting illness has produced increased pulmonary resistance (e.g., CHF, bronchospasm, pneumothorax). The underlying cause must be treated. If no resistance is encountered, suspect a leak in the ventilation system. Check all tubing and connections, integrity of the manual resuscitation bag, and the fit of the mask (if appropriate).

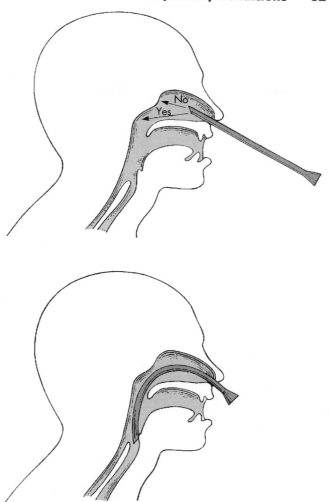

Figure 17-4 To insert a nasal airway. Insert the airway into the nostril and advance it along the floor of the nose (top)—not upward toward the frontal sinus, which will increase the risk of epistaxis. Slide it forward to place it in the posterior pharynx (bottom).

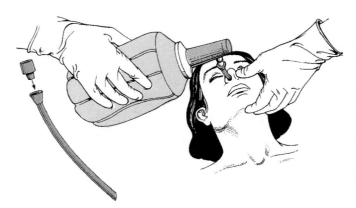

Figure 17-5 Nasal ventilation. When bag-and-mask ventilation is difficult, insert an endotracheal tube connector into a nasal airway (left), place the airway, close the opposite nostril and mouth, attach the bag, and ventilate (right).

4. In cases of massive emesis and/or bleeding associated with facial injuries, upper airway edema, or known cervical spine fracture, anticipate the performance of a cricothyroidotomy. This procedure is performed for airway obstruction at the level of the larynx or above. A 14 to 16 gauge IV catheter may be used to penetrate the cricothyroid membrane (Figure 17-6). This may be left in place and connected to a manual resuscitation bag. A larger incision may be made and a no. 4 Shiley tracheostomy tube or a no. 7 or smaller endotracheal tube (cut to fit) can be inserted (9). Extra vigor is needed for ventilation because of the small diameter of the catheter and passive gas escape from the mouth.
5. Obstruction below the larynx requires emergency bronchoscopy or surgery for foreign body removal.

General
1. Place the patient in high Fowler's position for maximal lung expansion. If heart failure is suspected, dangle lower extremities to decrease venous return.

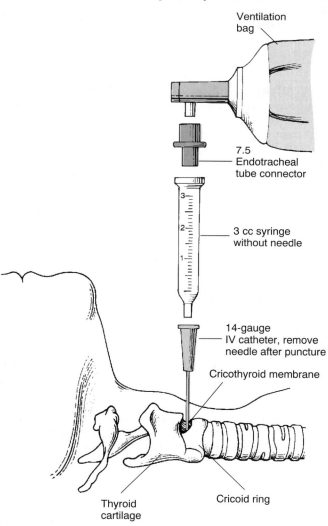

Figure 17-6 Emergency needle cricothyrotomy. Identify the cricothyroid membrane, and puncture it with a large intravenous catheter-over-needle. To attach the ventilation bag, place the connector from a no. 7.5 endotracheal tube into the barrel of a 3 cc syringe and attach that to the catheter hub.

> **NURSING ALERT**
>
> Do not place the patient supine with a pillow under the head, since this can precipitate airway obstruction.

2. Initiate cardiac monitoring.
3. Monitor oxygen saturation with continuous pulse oximetry.
4. Assess vital signs as acuity dictates.
5. Keep patient NPO until stabilized. In some instances, surgery or invasive tests may be required.
6. Monitor urine output.
7. Save a sputum sample in a sterile container. Sputum cultures may be ordered.
8. Suction the patient if appropriate. Hyperoxygenate and ventilate before suctioning.
9. Reassure the patient. Severe dyspnea frequently produces anxiety.

> **NURSING ALERT**
>
> Oxygen administration is controversial for some respiratory conditions. In situations where diminished breath sounds are auscultated (spontaneous pneumothorax), oxygen can be administered per device tolerated by the patient (e.g., nasal cannula, simple face mask). However, if the patient has a history of pulmonary disease (and the pneumothorax may be a secondary condition), administer a low concentration of oxygen, preferable 2 L or less. Reference Guide 14 lists oxygen devices and their possible oxygen delivery ranges. It is preferable to obtain a blood sample for arterial blood gas analysis before initiating oxygen administration, but patient distress should determine your sequence of actions.

PRIORITY NURSING DIAGNOSES

Risk for impaired gas exchange
Risk for ineffective airway clearance
Risk for altered tissue perfusion
Risk for ineffective breathing pattern
Risk for pain
Risk for infection (pulmonary)

Risk for activity intolerance
Risk for ineffective individual coping
Risk for knowledge deficit

◆ **Impaired gas exchange** related to decreased pulmonary ventilation/perfusion as evidenced by low PO_2 levels, elevated CO_2 levels, dyspnea, cyanosis, decreased oxygen saturation.

INTERVENTIONS
• Administer oxygen.
• Monitor arterial oxygen saturation via pulse oximetry.
• Report and treat significant changes in ABGs, (pH <7.35 or >7.45, PO_2 <80 mm Hg, PCO_2 <35 or >45 mm Hg, HCO_3 <22 or >26 mEq/L, and SaO_2 <95).
• Administer bronchodilators as ordered.

◆ **Ineffective airway clearance** related to obstruction, decreased mucociliary function, increased mucus production and viscosity, muscle weakness, and fatigue as evidenced by frequent nonproductive cough, adventitious or diminished breath sounds, airway noise, and tachypnea.

INTERVENTIONS
• Assist with coughing and deep breathing exercises.
• Endotracheal suctioning as ordered.
• Administer mucolytic and bronchodilating agents as ordered.
• For airway obstruction, see Initial Interventions in the triage assessment section.

◆ **Altered tissue perfusion** related to hypoxemia as evidenced by peripheral or central cyanosis, cool extremities, chest pain, and mental status changes.

INTERVENTIONS
• Administer vasodilators and oxygen as ordered.
• Limit activity to decrease myocardial oxygen demands.

◆ **Ineffective breathing pattern** related to muscle weakness, alveolar hyperinflation as evidenced by tachypnea, hyperventilation, dyspnea.

INTERVENTIONS
• Assist with breathing by placing patient in high Fowler's position.
• Supplemental oxygen as ordered.
• Coach breathing (see Discharge Implications for COPD).
• Promote nutritional status by encouraging high carbohydrate diet when appropriate.
• Encourage fluid intake.

R

- Decrease patient anxiety by acknowledging the patient's dyspnea.

Pain related to pleural irritation as evidenced by complaints of pleuritic (sharp) pain with respirations, chest wall tenderness, and restlessness.

INTERVENTIONS
- Administer analgesics as ordered.
- Teach splinting with cough.

◆ **Infection, pulmonary** related to bacterial or viral invasion of pulmonary system, immunosuppression, as evidenced by fever, positive sputum cultures, productive cough, dyspnea, and tachypnea.

INTERVENTIONS
- Administer antibiotics as ordered.
- Encourage dietary supplements as ordered.
- Administer antipyretics for fever >100° F, (38.3° C).

◆ **Activity intolerance** related to decreased pulmonary function as evidenced by shortness of breath, fatigue, chest pain, noncompensatory vital sign changes with activity.

INTERVENTIONS
- Gradually increase activity.
- Monitor for vital sign changes inappropriate for activity.
- Assist patient with movement using wheelchair as appropriate.
- Assess home environment for breathing demands (e.g., steps, transportation ability).
- Seek appropriate home health referral.

◆ **Ineffective individual coping** related to dyspnea, increased dependence, changes in body structure.

INTERVENTIONS
- Reassure patient.
- Include patient and family with treatment plan development when feasible.

◆ **Knowledge deficit** related to lack of information regarding disease process as evidenced by inability to describe home care, minimal participation in treatment plan, and verbalizing inaccurate information.

INTERVENTIONS
- Instruct patient and family on disease process and treatment plan.
- Determine patient/family understanding with nonthreatening questions.

PRIORITY DIAGNOSTIC TESTS

Laboratory

Serum electrolyte levels: Potassium, chloride, and sodium levels fluctuate with diuresis and impaired renal function. Diuretics are used to treat fluid volume excess in cardiogenic PAE.

Complete blood count: WBC counts are elevated or decreased in pulmonary inflammation or infection. Elevated hemoglobin may indicate polycythemia, a clinical indicator of prolonged hypoxemia.

Antibody titers and blood serology: Used to determine cause of pulmonary infection.

Arterial blood gases: Used to evaluate oxygenation, acid-base balance. Useful in most respiratory conditions. Not definitive for PE. Supplemental oxygen is adjusted according to ABG results and clinical symptoms. In asthma, respiratory alkalosis is common. If the Pco_2 starts to return to normal, it may indicate respiratory muscle fatigue.

Activated partial thromboplastin time (aPTT): Used to evaluate the effectiveness of heparin therapy in pulmonary embolism. Goal is to maintain aPTT 1.5 to 2 times the control.

Prothrombin time (PT): Used to evaluate the effectiveness of oral anticoagulation, (e.g., Coumadin). Goal is to maintain PT approximately 2.5 times the control. Coumadin is used to prevent clot formation in those at risk for PE.

Prealbumin, transferrin levels: Used to evaluate nutritional status.

Blood cultures: Used to diagnose bacteremia and causative agent in those with pneumonia.

Sputum culture and sensitivity: Used to determine causative agent of pneumonia and other respiratory infections. If pneumonia is suspected, broad-spectrum antibiotics are started before culture results return, in most instances. More organism-specific antibiotics are ordered when culture results become available.

Plasma DNA assay: Used to diagnose pulmonary embolism in the event of inconclusive lung scans (6).

R

Radiographic

Chest x-ray: Used to evaluate heart and lung structures. Nonspecific for pulmonary embolus. Infiltrates may be present with pneumonia. Hyperinflation, flattened diaphragm, cardiomegaly are present with COPD. Negative lung expansion is present in cases of spontaneous pneumothorax. Some foreign bodies may be radiopaque. Atelectasis of the involved lung may be present in foreign body aspiration.

Venography: Injection of dye into veins to detect DVT, a risk factor for pulmonary embolism. IV access is necessary for this procedure.

Pulmonary angiogram: Injection of dye into the pulmonary vasculature. Most definitive test for pulmonary embolism. Emergency medications may be administered if complications occur during the procedure, therefore IV access is required.

> **NURSING ALERT**
>
> Determine that the patient is not allergic to radiographic dye, iodine, or seafoods before dye tests. Premedication with Benadryl or Tylenol or the use of a less allergy-producing substance may be required.

Other

Ventilation/perfusion (V/Q) scan: A lung scan is performed after the inhalation of xenon 127. The perfusion scan is completed after the IV injection of technetium 97 macroaggregated albumin. Areas of poor ventilation and/or inadequate perfusion are identified.

Doppler ultrasonography: With doppler ultrasonography, a handheld transducer that produces high-frequency sound waves is moved across the skin of the extremity being examined. Audible tones proportional to blood velocity assist with detection of thrombi.

ECG: Used to detect heart failure, dysrhythmias, right heart strain.

Echocardiogram: Used to assess right ventricular function.

Bronchoscopy: Insertion of a fiberoptic or rigid scope to examine the internal structures of the airway and lungs. Premedication such as Demerol or atropine may be necessary to decrease secretions and discomfort during the procedure. Patient is NPO after the procedure until gag reflex returns. Rigid bronchoscopy is performed in the operating room. Bronchoscopy may be used to remove foreign bodies.

Peak expiratory flow rate (PEFR): This is the greatest flow that can be obtained during forced exhalation starting from full-lung inflation. A peak flow meter is used to measure this value. PEFR can be monitored by the patient at home. A normal peak flow ranges from 400 to 600 L/min. A peak flow <200 L/min indicates obstruction or respiratory fatigue. PEFR correlates well with forced expiratory volume (FEV_1) obtained by spirometry. Children may not be able to reliably obtain PEFR. Oxygen saturation values may be more useful in determining severity of the situation.

Spirometry (pulmonary function test): Use of a spirometer to determine lung capacities, lung volumes, and flow rates. Useful in determining the severity of airway obstruction in COPD and other respiratory problems. A reduced FEV in 1 second over forced vital capacity (FVC) ratio, FEV_1:FVC, confirms airway obstruction.

Bronchoprovocation testing: Airway response to histamine or methacholine is tested. If FEV_1 is <1,000 ml or PEFR is <200 L/min after medication administration, a diagnosis of asthma is made.

COLLABORATIVE INTERVENTIONS
Overview

1. Administer supplemental oxygen as ordered. The delivery system and amount of oxygen used for enhancing oxygenation outcomes depends on the severity of the disease process. Various types of oxygen delivery systems are described in Reference Guide 14. Be prepared for intubation, since respiratory conditions can rapidly deteriorate.
2. Initiate IV access with a large bore (20-gauge or larger) IV catheter. Two IV lines are preferable in severe respiratory distress. An intermittent infusion device may be substituted for continuous IV fluids if fluid volume overload is suspected.

ASTHMA CLASSIFICATION BY SEVERITY

Mild asthma

- <2 exacerbations weekly
- Good exercise tolerance
- Awakened from sleep with symptoms < twice monthly

Moderate asthma

- >2 exacerbations weekly
- <3 severe episodes requiring urgent care annually

Severe asthma

- Daily symptoms
- >3 episodes requiring urgent care annually
- >2 hospitalizations yearly

---

3. Place urinary catheter with physician's order. Patients with cardiogenic PAE require diuretics and accurate urinary output measurement.

Clinical Conditions
Asthma

Asthma is characterized by airway inflammation (mucous hypersecretion), increased airway responsiveness to stimuli (airway edema), and reversible airway obstruction. The aim of treatment is to decrease inflammation, thereby decreasing obstruction.

SYMPTOMS

- Wheezing, presence of paradoxical pulse, PEFR <400 L/m.
- The use of beta-blocking agents (e.g., propranolol, timolol, pindolol) may precipitate asthma in the geriatric patient.

DIAGNOSIS

- Diagnosis is based on clinical presentation. The box classifies asthma according to severity.

TREATMENT

- Although medications are addressed in Table 17-2, some medications used to treat asthma need further elaboration.
- Inhaled beta-agonist (e.g., albuterol) agents in either inhaler or nebulizer form are initially used. Continuous nebulization is more effective than intermittent in

patients with PEFR <200 L/min (8). Ipratropium bromide is used next in inhaler form. Steroids follow inhaled beta-agonists and ipratropium bromide in either IV, PO, or inhaler form. Use of xanthine derivatives (e.g., theophylline) is controversial, but they may be tried if symptoms persist.

- Beta-adrenergic agonist agents (e.g., subcutaneous epinephrine) are only used in younger asthmatic patients (<35 years old) whose airways are so narrowed because of bronchoconstriction that inhaled medication may not penetrate far enough into the lungs. They are not used to treat older patients or patients with a positive cardiac history because of their cardiovascular side effects (e.g., increased heart rate and contractility). Response to beta-agonists decreases with age.
- Children who are on chronic steroids need close monitoring for signs of adrenal suppression and decreased growth.
- Hospitalization is indicated for patients with the following:
  1. Respiratory rate >30/min.
  2. Heart rate >120/min (bradycardia may be present if severely hypoxic).
  3. PEFR <120 L/min.
  4. FEV_1 <1,000 ml.
  5. O_2Sat ≤91%.

The best indicator of good response to treatment is improvement in the PEFR or FEV_1 within 30 min of therapy.

NURSING ALERT

R

If an asthmatic patient requires intubation and mechanical ventilation, monitor the patient closely for barotrauma and pneumothorax. High airway pressure may be needed to ventilate the patient.

Pulmonary Alveolar Edema (PAE)
Noncardiogenic pulmonary alveolar edema
(Also known as adult respiratory distress syndrome.)
SYMPTOMS
- Respiratory distress with tachypnea, orthopnea, crackles, hypovolemia or hypervolemia, hypotension, low or high pulmonary artery pressures, faint heart sounds.

DIAGNOSIS

- Chest x-ray indicates infiltrates.
- Severe hypoxemia documented by ABGs.
- Low or high pulmonary artery pressures on pulmonary artery catheterization.
- History of risk factors for noncardiogenic PAE present (e.g., recent trauma, hemorrhage, drug overdose, infection).
- Clinical symptoms present.

TREATMENT

- Supplemental oxygen.
- Continuous positive airway pressure (CPAP) by mask or positive end-expiratory pressure (PEEP) and/or pressure support in the intubated patient may be necessary to improve alveolar inflation.
- Use of steroids is controversial.
- Careful diuresis or fluid replacement may be used depending upon preload measurements.

Cardiogenic pulmonary alveolar edema

SYMPTOMS

- Tachypnea, orthopnea, crackles, wheezes, pink, frothy sputum, high pulmonary artery pressures, hypervolemia, signs of heart failure (e.g., JVD, peripheral edema, organomegaly).

DIAGNOSIS

- Presence of clinical symptoms.
- Arterial blood analysis reveals hypoxemia.
- Infiltrates on chest x-ray.
- High pulmonary artery pressures on pulmonary artery catheterization.
- History of cardiovascular disease.

TREATMENT

- Supplemental oxygen, intubation, and mechanical ventilation in severe respiratory distress.
- Preload and afterload reduction by diuretics (e.g., furosemide), and vasodilators (e.g., nitroprusside, hydralazine [direct acting]), verapamil, diltiazem (calcium channel blockers), prazosin (alpha-adrenergic blocking agent), captopril (angiotensin-converting enzyme [ACE] inhibitor).
- Bronchodilators (e.g., theophylline) to enhance alveolar ventilation. Cardiac glycosides (e.g., digoxin) to improve cardiac contractility.

- IV morphine sulfate is administered to decrease venous return and alleviate anxiety.
- In some instances, rotating tourniquets are used in cases refractory to medical treatment (12).

Pulmonary embolism

SYMPTOMS

- Dyspnea, sudden pleuritic chest pain, cough, hemoptysis, diaphoresis, apprehension, tachypnea, tachycardia, crackles.
- Triad of petechiae (chest, axilla), dyspnea, and mental confusion is suspicious for fat emboli.

DIAGNOSIS

- V/Q scan, chest x-ray, pulmonary angiography, hypoxemia by ABG analysis, presence of clinical symptoms.
- Diagnostic tests such as doppler ultrasound of the lower extremities to assess for DVT.

TREATMENT

- Supplemental oxygen, intubation with mechanical ventilation in severe respiratory distress.
- Anticoagulation (e.g., heparin IV, then PO Coumadin).
- Thrombolytics (streptokinase, urokinase IV, or intrapulmonary) with severe PE.
- Immobilize lower extremity with DVT as applicable.
- Antiembolic devices on lower extremities in the absence of DVT (e.g., elastic, gradient, or intermittent compression stockings).

Pneumonia

SYMPTOMS

- Fever, shaking chills, pleuritic chest pain, tachypnea, diaphoresis, crackles, productive cough with purulent or rust-colored sputum.

DIAGNOSIS

- Infiltrates on chest x-ray, positive sputum cultures, CBC shows leukocytosis, presence of clinical symptoms.

TREATMENT

- Supplemental oxygen.
- Broad-spectrum antibiotics (e.g., penicillin, erythromycin).
- Bronchodilators and mucolytics such as theophylline and acetylcysteine to mobilize secretions.
- Analgesics for pleuritic chest pain.
- Chest physiotherapy.

R

- Nutritional support.
- Oral or IV hydration.
- Bed rest to decrease oxygen demands.

Chronic obstructive pulmonary disease (COPD)

SYMPTOMS

- Dyspnea, productive cough, wheezing, pursed-lip exhalation (see Discharge Implications), tripod positioning, use of accessory respiratory muscles, increased chest anteroposterior diameter, diminished breath sounds.

DIAGNOSIS

- Pulmonary function tests show reduced FEV_1:FVC ratio. ABGs indicate hypoxemia and hypercapnia.
- Chest x-ray reveals hyperinflation.
- Presence of clinical symptoms.

TREATMENT

- Supplemental oxygen based on ABG results.
- Inhaled anticholinergics, (e.g., ipratropium bromide (Atrovent) to bronchodilate.
- Antibiotics for infection.
- Use of steroids is controversial.
- Mucolytics to mobilize secretions.
- Beta-adrenergic agonists (e.g., albuterol) to bronchodilate.
- Subcutaneous epinephrine or terbutaline is administered for severe airway obstruction in those who are unable to receive aerosol bronchodilating agents.
- Oxygen may be administered using a Venturi mask with an oxygen concentration of 24% to 28%.
- If the patient is on home oxygen, the same dosage is used in the ED.

Spontaneous pneumothorax

Spontaneous pneumothorax may occur as a primary disorder, unassociated with pulmonary disease or as a secondary condition usually related to pulmonary fibrosis or the presence of pulmonary bullae and blebs. Symptoms for both types of spontaneous pneumothorax are similar, but severity is greater when the pneumothorax is due to a preexisting pulmonary condition.

SYMPTOMS

- Pain on inspiration on same side as pneumothorax.
- Dyspnea is present depending on the size of the pneumothorax and the remaining pulmonary reserve.

- In secondary spontaneous pneumothorax, the PaO_2 may be <55 mm Hg and the $PaCO_2$ may be >50 mm Hg.
- FEV_1 may be <1,000 ml.

DIAGNOSIS
- Size and location of pneumothorax is confirmed by chest radiography.

TREATMENT

Observation

If the patient is not dyspneic and the respiratory rate is within normal limits, observation may be preferred. Usually the pneumothorax is <15% of the hemithorax as confirmed by chest radiography (7). This type of treatment is used in first occurrences without presence of preexisting pulmonary disease.

Aspiration

Aspiration of air from the pleural space is more successful in patients with primary spontaneous pneumothorax. A guidewire is inserted over a 16-gauge needle. An 8 Fr aspiration catheter is then inserted over the guidewire and the guidewire removed. A 60 cc syringe is attached to the catheter by way of a three-way stopcock. Before removal, the stopcock is closed to the patient and a repeat chest radiograph is obtained. If no lung expansion occurs, a Heimlich valve is attached to the catheter. If there is still no lung reexpansion on another repeat chest radiograph, the Heimlich device is connected to a chest catheter draining system (e.g., Pleurovac) at a negative pressure of 20 cm water (7,11).

NURSING ALERT

R

Aspiration is rarely successful in cases of iatrogenic pneumothorax from central venous line placement. Anticipate the need for chest tube insertion.

Chest tube insertion

A 16 to 24 Fr thoracostomy tube may be placed in the 4th to 6th intercostal space, midaxillary line for air expulsion. The patient should be placed in supine position with head of bed elevated 30 degrees. The patient's arm, nearest the procedure, should be placed behind the patient's head. The tube is connected to a closed draining system (see Procedure 7).

> **NURSING ALERT**
>
> If reexpansion is not occurring after placement of the chest tube, check to see if the connecting tubing is kinked or clogged. Confirm that the tubing is connected to the suction apparatus correctly (if appropriate).

Chest tube insertion with instillation of sclerosing agent

A sclerosing agent (such as minocycline) may be injected through the chest tube. This is a very painful procedure! The patient should be sedated before instillation and lidocaine 4 mg/kg in 50 cc saline injected intrapleurally before instillation of sclerosing agent. The reoccurrence rate of spontaneous pneumothorax is less with this form of treatment.

Thoracoscopy

The patient may be admitted and thoracoscopy performed. After a thoracoscope is inserted, a sclerosing agent may be administered, bullae ligated, or blebs ablated by laser or resection.

Thoracotomy

The patient is admitted and surgical intervention is used. This treatment is rare and is associated with severe unilateral pneumothorax unresponsive to reexpansion by other modalities. It may also be used for simultaneous bilateral pneumothoraces.

> **NURSING ALERT**
>
> The size of the pneumothorax is not related to response to treatment. The longer the duration of symptoms, the easier the pneumothorax is to resolve.

NURSING SURVEILLANCE

1. Monitor respiratory function, including breath sounds.
2. Monitor dyspnea.
3. Trend vital signs and oxygenation status (SaO_2, PaO_2, PcO_2).
4. Monitor intake and output.

5. Monitor for cardiac dysrhythmias.
6. Analyze laboratory tests and report significant changes to physician.
7. Assess for therapeutic response and adverse reactions to medications.
8. Evaluate and support effective coping strategies.
9. Monitor PEFRs (if appropriate).

EXPECTED PATIENT OUTCOMES

1. Shortness of breath improves from initial assessment.
2. ABGs trend toward normal.
3. Heart rate ranges from 60 to 100 beats/min.
4. Mean arterial pressure remains 70 to 100 mm Hg.
5. Urinary output >30 ml/hr or >0.5 ml/kg/hr.
6. Absence of life-threatening dysrhythmias.
7. Effective coping strategies by patient and family.
8. Wheezing and stridor are absent and spontaneous ventilation present.

DISCHARGE IMPLICATIONS
General

1. Teach patients using oxygen at home about safety.
2. Guide the smoker to appropriate resources for smoking cessation. This may include medications, support groups, and relaxation training.
3. Encourage adequate nutrition to support respiratory function.
4. The geriatric population and those with COPD may benefit from annual influenza vaccines and in some instances from the one-time pneumococcal pneumonia vaccine (Pneumovax). The pneumococcal vaccine is contraindicated in those with active pulmonary infection. Assist the patient with appropriate referral.
5. Environmental pollutants should be avoided in those with or without respiratory disease.
6. Infection control can be supported by frequent handwashing, the use of tissues, and masks for those who are immunosuppressed.
7. Instruct patients regarding the home administration of medications.

R

PROPER METERED DOSE INHALER TECHNIQUE

- Shake canister.
- Hold the canister approximately 2 inches (4-5 cm) in front of the mouth.
- Completely exhale.
- Begin to inhale.
- Activate the canister.
- Continue to breathe deeply and hold your breath for 5 sec.
- Wait for response (1-10 min) depending on your symptoms.
- Repeat as needed.

Asthma

1. Involve children in the management of their asthma.
2. Teach use of metered dose inhalers (MDI). MDIs may be difficult to use for persons with impaired mental function, poor motor coordination, or weakened, arthritic hands. The use of spacers attached to the MDI allows the drug to be expelled into a large plastic chamber. The patient can inhale the medication from the chamber so there is not the need to coordinate activation of MDI with inhalation. Spacers also decrease the incidence of thrush and hoarseness associated with steroid MDI. The box explains proper technique.
3. Stress to pregnant asthma patients that hypoxia is of greater risk to the fetus than are inhaled medications.
4. Teach parents about the effect of passive smoking on children with asthma.
5. Teach home monitoring PEFR. Measurement or PEFR is best in the standing position while the patient breathes deep and blows out fast and hard through the peak flow meter. This maneuver is performed three times with the highest value being recorded. Portable peak expiratory flow meters should be calibrated regularly, since accurate readings depend upon a spring mechanism that can stretch over time. PEFR should be measured at the same time each day (twice daily up to four times daily during acute exacerbations). Morning values are usually lower than evening values.

6. Many patients believe that asthma medication is harmful and addictive. Stress that continuous use of medication is the key to prevention and is required for this chronic illness.
7. Teach when to seek urgent care. Classic symptoms are requiring frequent use (>4 times/day) of inhaler, frequent nocturnal awakening with symptoms, and drop in PEFR in the morning to 50% of evening value.
8. Avoid allergens by removing carpet, washing animals weekly, covering mattresses and pillows with impermeable covers.
9. Teach use of inhaler before exposure to known allergens.
10. Teach patients using steroid inhalers how to monitor their blood sugar and signs of gastrointestinal bleeding.
11. Warn patients that asthma is associated with aspirin and nonsteroidal inflammatory medication sensitivity. Acetaminophen should be used for pain and fever relief. Sulfite sensitivity may also be present. Sulfating agents are found in processed potatoes, shrimp, dried fruits, beer, and wine.

Pulmonary Alveolar Edema
1. Teach patient about home administration of respiratory and cardiac medications.
2. Patients with severe PAE are hospitalized.

Pulmonary Embolism
1. Advise patient to avoid long periods of immobility.
2. Instruct on home administration of Coumadin when applicable as follows:
   - Wear medical alert bracelet indicating anticoagulation.
   - Use electric razors, soft toothbrush.
   - Watch for bleeding, report black or maroon stools to physician.
   - Avoid foods high in vitamin K (e.g., green leafy vegetables, tomatoes, cauliflower, and fish) to maintain anticoagulation.
3. Encourage patient to wear loose fitting clothes.
4. Instruct on use of elastic or gradient stockings.

R

Pneumonia

1. Pneumonia is often slow to resolve especially in the geriatric patient. Instruct the patient to schedule frequent rest periods to minimize oxygenation needs.
2. Instruct patient to avoid those with URIs.
3. Determine that the patient understands home administration of antibiotics. Reinforce the importance of finishing antibiotic prescriptions.

Chronic Obstructive Pulmonary Disease

1. Ask patient to demonstrate use of inhaler to determine proper technique.
2. Teach breathing techniques to enhance oxygenation as follows:
   - Pursed-lip breathing—Breathe in slowly through nose, purse lips (as if to whistle), then breathe out slowly through pursed lips.
   - Diaphragmatic breathing—In upright position, place hand on abdomen just above waist, place the other hand on the upper chest, breathe in through nose and feel lower hand push out, hand on chest should not move, then breathe out through pursed lips and feel lower hand move in (3).

Spontaneous Pneumothorax

1. It may take up to 10 days for all symptoms to resolve.
2. Avoid air travel, scuba diving until total lung reexpansion is confirmed by chest radiography. Follow-up is recommended for 7 to 10 days after the event.
3. Alert patient that reoccurrences are likely and to seek treatment for return of symptoms.

TABLE 17-2   Drug Summary

Drug	Classifications	Dose/Route	Special considerations
Acetylcysteine (Mucomyst)	Mucolytic	*Inhalation:* Adult: 1-10 ml of 20% solution q 4-6 hr or 2-20 ml of 10% solution q 4-6 hr. *Direct instillation:* Adult: 1-2 ml or 10%-20% solution q 1-4 hr. Child: Same as adult.	Cautious use in patients with asthma, severe respiratory infections, and in geriatric patients. May be instilled directly into tracheostomy. Have suction apparatus ready for immediate use.
Albuterol (Proventil)	Beta-adrenergic agonist, bronchodilator	PO: 2-4 mg, 3-4 times/day. *Inhaled:* 1-2 inhal q 4-6 hr. Nebulizer: 2.5 mg in nebulized form.	SE include CNS stimulation. Proper use of inhaler necessary for therapeutic dosing.
Captopril* (Capoten)	Angiotensin-converting enzyme (ACE) inhibitor, vasodilator	PO: 6.25-12.5 mg tid up to 50 mg tid.	Exaggerated hypotension may occur with first dose.
Cromolyn sodium	Nonsteroidal antiinflammatory agent, inhibits release of mediators, prevents degranulation of mast cells.	Metered dose inhaler: 1 spray inhaled qid.	Not recommended in children under 6 years of age.

Continued.

R

541

TABLE 17-2 Drug Summary (cont'd)

Drug	Classifications	Dose/Route	Special considerations
Digoxin* (Lanoxin)	Cardiac glycoside	Initially, *PO* 10-15 mcg/kg in divided doses over 24-48 hr. *IV:* 10-15 mcg/kg in divided doses over 24 hr.	SE include AV block. Cautious use in geriatric patients, hypokalemia, cor pulmonale, lung disease.
Diltiazem* (Cardizem)	Calcium channel blocking agent, vasodilator	*PO:* 30 mg qid.	May cause headache, dizziness, light-headedness, advise patient to make slow position changes.
Epinephrine	Alpha- and beta-adrenergic agonist, bronchodilator	Asthma: Adult: SC 0.1-0.5 ml of 1:1000 q 20 min-4 hr. *Inhalation:* 1 inhal q 4 hr prn. Child: SC 0.01 ml/kg of 1:1000 q 20 min-4 hr. *Inhalation:* 1 inhal q 4 hr prn.	Use tuberculin syringe for greater accuracy. May cause CNS stimulation and cardiovascular side effects (increased heart rate). Errors in administration have caused fatalities.
Erythromycin (E-Mycin)	Antiinfective, antibiotic	Moderate-to-severe infections: Adult: *PO* 250-500 mg q 6 hr. Child: *PO* 30-50 mg/kg/day divided q 6 hr.	Administer on empty stomach. Can potentiate theophylline, Warfarin toxicity.

Furosemide* (Lasix)	Loop diuretic	Adult: *PO* 20-80 mg in one or more divided doses up to 600 mg/day. *IV/IM* 20-40 mg in one or more divided doses up to 600 mg/day.	Cautious use in geriatric patients, cardiogenic shock associated with acute MI. Adverse effects: postural hypotension, circulatory collapse, electrolyte imbalance.
Heparin	Anticoagulant	*IV*: 100 U/kg loading dose followed by maintenance or intermittent doses of 25,000-35,000 U/day.	Goal: aPTT of 1½-2 times control. Monitor for bleeding.
Hydralazine hydrochloride (Apresoline)	Nonnitrate vasodilator, antihypertensive	Adult: *PO* 10-50 mg qid. *IM* 10-50 mg q 4-6 hr. *IV* 10-20 mg q 4-6 hr. Child: *PO* 3-7.5 mg/kg/day in 4 divided doses.	Adverse effects include headache, orthostatic hypotension.
Ipratropium bromide (Atrovent)	Brochodilator, anticholinergic, inhibits bronchoconstricting vagal reflex.	*Inhalation*: 20 mcg ipratropium, 2-4 inhal 4 times/day.	Frequent PFTs to determine effectiveness. Used in chronic management of COPD, not in acute asthma. SE: Dry mouth.
Magnesium sulfate	Bronchial smooth muscle-relaxing agent	1.2 g *IV* over 20 min.	Still used experimentally in acute asthma. Mechanism of action not clear.

Continued.

R

TABLE 17-2 Drug Summary (cont'd)

Drug	Classifications	Dose/Route	Special considerations
Methylprednisolone	Corticosteroid	Adult: *PO* 40-60 mg/day. *IM* 240 mg, *IV* 60-80 mg up to 125 mg. Inhaler comes in a variety of forms: (e.g., beclomethasone): Adult: 0.84 mg/day (depending on concentration about 20 puffs/day). Child: 0.42 mg/day (depending on concentration about 10 puffs/day).	Used in treatment of acute severe asthma in IV form. Must be used cautiously in geriatric patients, since SE may exacerbate conditions of aging, (e.g., osteoporosis hypertension, diabetes). SE: thrush, hoarseness, inhaler use. SE can be prevented by rinsing mouth and throat after using inhaler or by using a spacer device.
Minocycline hydrochloride (Minocin)	Antiinfective, tetracycline antibiotic	*PO/IV:* Adult: 200 mg followed by 100 mg q 12 hr.	Use with pleural sclerosis: 5 mg/kg in total volume of 50 cc sterile water. Extremely painful for patient.
Morphine sulfate*	Narcotic (opiate) agonist	Adult: *IV* 2.5-15 mg q 4 hr or 0.8-10 mg/hr by continuous infusion.	Adverse effects include severe respiratory depression. *IV push:* May dilute in 4-5 ml of sterile water and give slowly over 4-5 min, undiluted: push slowly 1 mg/min.

Drug	Classification	Dosage	Nursing considerations
Nitroprusside,* sodium (Nipride)	Antihypertensive, nonnitrate vasodilator	*IV:* Adult: 0.5-10 mcg/kg min.	Must be diluted in 250-500 cc D$_5$W. Use infusion pump. Constant monitoring of BP indicated with use. Protect solution from light.
Penicillin G	Antiinfective, beta-lactam antibiotic	*PO:* Adult: 1.6-3.2 million U divided q 6 hr. Child: 25,000-100,000 U/kg divided q 6 hr. *IV/IM* Adult: 1.2-2.4 million U divided q 4 hr, Child: 25,000-300,000 U/kg divided q 4 hr.	Contraindicated in hypersensitivity to any penicillin. Monitor for signs of sensitivity to drug, allergy is unpredictable.
Pneumococcal vaccine (Pneumovax)	—	*SC/IM:* 0.5 ml in a single SC or IM dose, preferably in deltoid or lateral midthigh.	Should not be used with active infections. May cause local and systemic reactions including fever, local soreness, erythema, induration.
Prazosin* hydrochloride (Minipress)	Alpha-adrenergic antagonist, vasodilator	*PO:* 1 mg hs, then 1 mg bid or tid, may increase to 20 mg/day in divided doses.	Hypotensive effects increased with diuretics and other hypotensive agents. Monitor BP for hypotension.
Streptokinase	Thrombolytic enzyme	*IV:* 250,000 IU over 30 min loading dose, then 100,000 IU/hr for 48-72 hr.	Used in cases of severe hemodynamic compromise with pulmonary embolism. Avoid punctures, tissue trauma, observe for bleeding.

Continued.

R

545

TABLE 17-2 Drug Summary (cont'd)

Drug	Classifications	Dose/Route	Special considerations
Talc	Sclerosing agent	0.5 g talc in 250 cc isotonic saline for pleural sclerosis	Extremely painful for patient.
Terbutaline sulfate (Brethine)	Beta-adrenergic agonist, bronchodilator	Adult: *PO* 2.5-5 mg tid at 6 hr intervals. *SC:* 0.25 mg q 15-30 min up to 0.5 mg in 4 hr. *Inhaled* 2 inhalations separated by 60 sec q 4-6 hr.	May cause CNS stimulation. Monitor BP, HR.
Theophylline (Theo-Dur)	Bronchodilator	*PO/IV:* 400-2000 mg/day.	Observe for toxicity, GI upset, nervousness, insomnia, palpitations, dysrhythmias, seizures. Presence of CHF, cor pulmonale, hepatic disease, use of cimetidine, erythromycin, or ciprofloxacin decreases theophylline clearance and degradation, increasing the likelihood of toxicity.

Urokinase	Thrombolytic enzyme	IV: 4400 IU/kg diluted in 0.9% NaCl or D₅W infused over 10 min loading dose, followed by 4,400 IU/kg/hr for 12 hr.	Special filter required, see streptokinase for additional nursing implications.
Verapamil* hydrochloride (Calan)	Calcium channel blocker, vasodilator	PO: Adult: 40-80 mg tid or 90-240 mg sustained release 1-2 times/day up to 480 mg/day. IV 5-10 mg IV push, dilute in 5 ml sterile water, administer no faster than 10 mg/min.	Monitor BP, HR. Transient hypotension may occur with IV bolus.
Warfarin sodium* (Coumadin)	Oral anticoagulant	PO: 10-15 mg/day for 2-5 days, then 2-10 mg once/day to maintain a PT of 1.5-2.5 times control.	Observe for minor or major hemorrhage. Periodic PTs are measured.

---

*From Wilson BA, Shannon MT: In Govoni and Hayes Nurses' drug guide, 1993, Norwalk, Conn, 1993, Appleton & Lange.
CNS, Central nervous system; MI, Myocardial infarction; PFT, Pulmonary function test; SE, Side effect; HR, Heart rate; GI, gastrointestinal; AV, Atrioventricular.

R

References

1. Abolnik I, Lossos I, Gillis D, Breuer R: Primary spontaneous pneumothorax in men, *Am J Med Sci* 305:297-303, 1993.
2. Catena E, Pastore V: Spontaneous pneumothorax: medical or surgical treatment? *Monaldi Arch Chest Dis* 48:159-160, 1993.
3. Dettenmeier, PA: *Pulmonary nursing care*, St. Louis, 1992, Mosby.
4. Fleisher G, Surpure J, Rosenberg N, Kulick R: Management of asthma, *Pediat Emerg Care* 8:167-170, 1992.
5. Kozier B, Erb G, Olivieri R: *Fundamentals of nursing: concepts, process, and practice* ed 4, 1991, Addison-Wesley.
6. A lab test for pulmonary embolism, *Emerg Med* 45-46, June 15, 1990.
7. Light R: Management of spontaneous pneumothorax, *Am Rev Respir Dis* 148:245-248, 1993.
8. Rudnitsky G, Eberlein R, Schoffstall J, Mazur J, Spivey W: Comparison of intermittent and continuously nebulized albuterol for treatment of asthma in an urban emergency department, *Ann Emerg Med* 22:1842-1846, 1993.
9. Salvino C, Dries D, Murphy-Macabobby M, Marshall W: Emergency cricothroidotomy in trauma victims, *J Trauma* 34:503-505, 1993.
10. Somerson S, Sicilia M: Emergency oxygen administration and airway management, *Crit Care Nurse* 12(4):23-29, 1992.
11. Tomlanovich M: A stepwise approach to a collapsed lung, *Emerg Med* 45-48, 116, January 30, 1989.
12. White BS, Roberts SL: Pulmonary alveolar edema: preventing complications, *Dimensions Crit Care Nurs* 11(2):90-103, 1992.

Additional Readings

Pulmonary alveolar edema

A caveat in treating post-MI pulmonary edema, *Emerg Med* 114-116, April 30, 1990.

Gottesman, MH: Neurogenic pulmonary edema, *Emerg Med* 55-62, February 28, 1993.

Roberts SL, White B: Common nursing diagnoses for pulmonary alveolar edema patients, *Dimensions Crit Care Nurs* 11(1):13-27, 1992.

Pulmonary embolism

Balskus M, Niersbach C: Matters of life and breath, *Emerg* 21(4):12-14, 1989.

Bone RC: Pulmonary embolism new approaches to a complex problem, *Emerg Med* 144-152, October 15, 1992.

Councelman, FL: Best tests for pulmonary embolism, *Emerg Med* 67-86, December 15, 1990.

Currie DL: Pulmonary embolism: diagnosis and management, *Crit Care Nurs* 13(2):41-49, 1990.

Goldhaber SZ: Pulmonary embolism, *Hosp Med* 22-38, August, 1993.

Pneumonia

Blanchet KD: Current trends and future developments in the treatment of pneumocystis carinii pneumonia, *AIDS Patient Care* 258-263, 1992.

Granton JT, Grossman RF: Community-acquired pneumonia in the elderly patient, *Clin Chest Med* 14(3):537-553, 1993.

Niederman MS: Nosocomial pneumonia in the elderly patient, *Clin in chest med* 14(3):479-490, 1993.

Niederman MS: Pneumonia: the ongoing challenge, *Emerg Med* 77-86, April 15, 1989.

Woodhead MA: Management of pneumonia, *Respir Med* 86:459-469, 1992.

Chronic obstructive pulmonary disease

Edelman NH, Kaplan RM, Buist AS, Cohen AB, Hoffman LA, Kleinhenz ME, Snider GL, Speizer FE: Chronic obstructive pulmonary disease, *Chest* 102(3):243S-256S, 1992.

Emerman CL, Effron MD, Lukens TW: Spirometric criteria for hospital admission of patients with acute exacerbation of COPD, *Chest* 99(3):595-599, 1991.

Feinsilver SH: Respiratory failure in asthma and COPD, *Emerg Med* 90-96, April 15, 1989.

Listello D, Glauser F: COPD: primary care management with drug and oxygen therapies, *Geriatrics* 47(12):28-38, 1992.

Murphy TF, Sethi S: Preventing or treating COPD flare-ups, *Emerg Med* 65-68, March 1993.

Nesse RE: Pharmacologic treatment of COPD, *Postgrad Med* 91(1):71-84, 1992.

Rosen MJ: Treatment of exacerbations of COPD, *Am Fam Physic* 693-697, February, 1992.

Saroea HG: Chronic obstructive pulmonary disease: major objectives of management, *Postgrad Med* 94(2):113-122, 1993.

The risks of treating COPD, *Emerg Med* 114-118, October 15, 1989.

Update on treating asthma, *Nurses' Drug Alert* 6(17):45-46, 1993.

R

Chapter XVIII

Sexually Transmitted Diseases

Pamela S. Kidd

CLINICAL CONDITIONS
Candida
Chancroid
Chlamydia
Gonorrhea
Human Papillomavirus (HPV)
Pelvic Inflammatory Disease (PID)
Syphilis
Herpes Simplex Virus
Hepatitis B Virus
Trichomonas
Vaginitis

TRIAGE ASSESSMENT

Sexually transmitted diseases (STDs) can be divided into four etiologic categories: viral, bacterial, fungal, and protozoan. Bacterial diseases (e.g., syphilis, gonorrhea, *Chlamydia*, and chancroid) are easily treatable. The viral STDs (e.g., herpes, human papillomavirus [HPV], hepatitis B virus, human immunodeficiency virus [HIV]) are incurable, and the potential for transmission remains often for life. HIV and hepatitis B infection are discussed in detail in Chapter 5 because of their systemic effects beyond the genitalia. The usual chief complaints associated with STDs are abdominal pain, genital discharge or lesions, and/or vaginal itching. Patients may present with rashes and joint pain. The most frequently encountered STDs in the ED are *Chlamydia*, gonorrhea, syphilis, hepatitis B virus, herpes simplex, HIV, human papillomavirus, *Trichomonas,* and *Candida.* At triage it is not important to determine the causative agent of the problem. The focus should be on whether the disease is localized to the genitalia area or if it has ascended to the pelvic region. Patients with pelvic involvement have a higher incidence of ectopic pregnancy and ruptured ovarian cyst,

S

both of which are considered life threatening. At triage the following data are important to elicit:

Pain

Determine type and location of pain. The onset of low, bilateral abdominal pain is the first sign of ascending infection. The pain may be associated with menses and sexual intercourse (especially if gonorrhea is the causative agent).

Last menstrual period

Determine last menstrual period, present point in menstrual cycle, and degree of normality of menses. Protective properties of the cervical mucous against ascending infection are at their lowest during ovulation, menstruation, and immediately after abortion or postpartum. Abnormal menstrual flow and cycle is associated with many STDs.

Genital discharge

Purulent vaginal discharge that may be blood stained is associated with pelvic inflammatory disease (PID). Purulent urethral discharge may be present in males.

Initial or recurrent problem

Once infected, the genital tract may fail to recover its protective mechanisms and STDs recur frequently. PID is more common after an initial vaginal infection.

Medication history

Several medications may increase one's risk for STDs. Hormonal supplements such as progesterone and estrogen may alter the cervical area. Progesterone makes the cervical mucous more hostile to ascending microorganisms. Estrogen increases the cervical epithelium surface area, increasing the likelihood of gonorrhea and *Chlamydia,* since these organisms adhere to the epithelium. Thus, women who are on estrogen replacement after a hysterectomy are at greater risk for PID (5). Current antibiotic use may mask STD symptoms or alter diagnostic results of cultures. Conversely, contraceptive pill use is a protective mechanism against PID.

Birth control method

Birth control methods may increase susceptibility for some STDs while decreasing risk for others. Barrier methods (e.g., condoms, diaphragms) and oral contraceptives protect against ascending genital infection (4). The intrauterine device (IUD) increases risk for PID.

Dysuria
Males frequently complain of dysuria and frequency.

Systemic symptoms
Many STDs do not present with vaginal, penile, or abdominal symptoms. Patients may complain of sore throat, anal discomfort, or systemic symptoms (e.g., rash, fever).

General Observations
Gait
- Observe how the patient walks. Patients with PID may shuffle and walk bent over as a result of cervical and ovarian tenderness.

Skin
- Look for obvious lesions. Patients with syphilis may have a diffuse papular rash on their palms, soles of their feet, and face that resembles acne.

FOCUSED NURSING ASSESSMENT
Nursing assessment should center on pain, elimination, metabolic changes, and sexuality.

Pain
Where is the pain located? What are the characteristics of the pain? Auscultate bowel sounds, then palpate the abdomen for rigidity and tenderness. A rigid abdomen and absent bowel sounds may indicate PID, ruptured ectopic pregnancy (see Chapter 16), or a ruptured ovarian cyst. Alert the physician for the urgency to evaluate this patient.

Elimination
1. When was the last time the patient voided? A urinalysis (U/A) can detect nonspecific urethritis in men, if they have not voided for 1 hour.
2. If patient needs to void while waiting for evaluation and treatment, provide a sterile container and instructions on a clean-catch urine. Advise menstruating women that they may need to be catheterized to obtain a specimen.
3. Does the patient have constipation or rectal drainage? Advise the patient that a stool specimen may be needed and provide a proper container.

Metabolic/Vital Signs

A full set of vital signs including temperature should be obtained. Blood pressure (BP) may be decreased, and the patient's pulse elevated in cases of hemorrhage (rigid abdomen). Fever is common when the disease has progressed to salpingitis, particularly if the causative agent is gonorrhea. When genital infection has progressed to systemic sepsis, fever may be present depending upon the causative organism and the patient's immune status.

Sexuality

Depending on the privacy of the triage area, several of these questions may have been explored at triage. If the information has not been collected, ask about the following:

- Date of onset of sexual activity, last sexual activity.
- Number of partners/number of significant other's partners.
- Type of sexual activity (e.g., oral, anal).
- Type of protection used to prevent STDs and pregnancy.
- Last menstrual period.
- Any symptoms associated with the sexual activity.

Risk Factors

1. Vaginal douching has been associated with PID (4).
2. Smoking has been associated with PID (4).
3. Multiple sexual partners (defined as more than three in a lifetime [3]) increases risk for PID.
4. Diabetes is associated with a higher incidence of *Candida* infection.
5. The use of tight undergarments, feminine hygiene sprays, hyperglycemia and increased sugar intake are associated with vaginitis and *Candida*.
6. Early onset of sexual activity is associated with HPV.
7. Pregnancy may activate HPV and herpes.

Life Span Issues

Adolescent females (between the ages of 15 and 19) have the highest incidence of gonorrhea and *Chlamydia* (1). This is because gonorrhea preferentially infects columnar epithelial cells. In adolescence, these cells are everted over part of the ectocervix increasing the amount of susceptible tissue exposed during intercourse.

INITIAL INTERVENTIONS

1. If the patient has a fever and a rigid, painful abdomen, anticipate the need for a large bore IV catheter. Normal saline or Ringer's lactate solution may be administered at a keep-vein-open rate (e.g., 30 cc/hr). While starting the IV, obtain two large red top tubes and a purple top tube for possible type and crossmatch, RPR/VDRL testing, and CBC. Monitor vital signs closely.

2. Anticipate a pelvic examination. Communicate the possibility of a pelvic examination to the patient. Find out if the patient prefers to have certain individuals remain in the room during the examination. Prepare the patient by having the patient undress. Note any discharge on undergarments. Next, prepare the equipment (speculum, slide, slide cover, fixative, KOH, culture media for *Chlamydia,* gonorrhea, viral culturrete, bacterial culturrete, gauze sponges, swabs, wooden spatula/brush if a Pap smear is completed, lubrication for bimanual examination, hemoccult testing for stool). Make sure the bed allows for performing a pelvic examination (breaks down with stirrups). Have a high-powered light source available.

3. Obtain a urine specimen. If the patient is menstruating, a catheter specimen is obtained, otherwise, a clean-catch specimen is usually adequate. Test the specimen using a urinary reagent strip for blood, protein, pH, and glucose. Always split the specimen into two containers using sterile technique in anticipation for microscopic analysis and culture.

PRIORITY NURSING DIAGNOSES

Risk for pain
Risk for fluid volume deficit
Risk for impaired body image and self-concept
Risk for knowledge deficit

◆ **Pain** related to infection and inflammation.
   INTERVENTIONS
   • Analgesics by PO or IV route.
   • Warm compresses to genital lesions after diagnostic procedures are performed.

◆ **Fluid volume deficit** related to fluid shifts from infection and intraperitoneal hemorrhage.
  INTERVENTIONS
  • Administer IV fluid resuscitation (as indicated by vital signs and perfusion status) and antibiotics.
  • Prepare the patient for surgery, if indicated.
◆ **Impaired body image and self-concept** related to alteration in sexual function and/or reproductive abilities.
  INTERVENTIONS
  • Listen to the patient's concerns.
  • Explain measures to protect patient and partners.
  • Offer suggestions for alternative sexual activities during exacerbations.
  • In cases of decreased fertility from STD sequelae, initiate referral to infertility services.
◆ **Knowledge deficit** related to contraception and prevention of STDs.
  INTERVENTIONS
  • See Table 18-3.

COLLABORATIVE INTERVENTIONS

1. Perform/assist with pelvic examination and obtaining specimens. If a Pap smear is being performed, follow the procedure listed in the box.
2. Perform/assist with obtaining a wet smear using the technique listed in the box.

PAP SMEAR PROCEDURE

Nursing action

1. Warm the speculum and/or wet it with warm tap water. Do not use lubricants.

Physician actions

2. Use a cotton swab to remove excess discharge.
3. With a cytobrush or a wooden spatula, scrape the cervix.
4. Next use the cytobrush to brush the endocervical canal.
5. Smear the brush and/or spatula on a slide.

Nursing action

6. Spray the slide with a fixative (95% alcohol may be used).

WET SMEAR PROCEDURE

1. Place 1 drop of vaginal discharge on each end of a plain, unfrosted microscope slide or use two slides.
2. Add 1 drop of 10% KOH. Note the odor when KOH is applied. (A fishy smell is present in vaginitis.)
3. Cover the KOH drop with a coverslip.
4. Add enough saline to the remaining drop of vaginal secretion to dilute the specimen.
5. Place a coverslip over the saline specimen.

---

3. Obtain necessary cultures using appropriate technique. Refer to Priority Diagnostic Tests section for more information.

PRIORITY DIAGNOSTIC TESTS

Laboratory

Gram stain: Gram staining of cervical and urethral specimens (in men) is conducted to determine presence of gonorrhea. This test has a low sensitivity and is followed by culture. This test is also used to determine source of organism in vaginitis.

Blood cultures: May be conducted in suspected PID and disseminated gonorrhea.

DNA probe: DNA probe is the newest technique used to identify genital organisms. Both *Chlamydia* and gonorrhea may be identified by this technique.

Genital cultures: Vaginal, cervical, rectal, and urethral drainage may be cultured.

1. *Gonorrhea:* Thayer-Martin or Martin-Lewis culture media are commonly used and contain antibiotics against other organisms that commonly evade genital sites. Discharge is obtained on a swab and applied directly to the culture medium using a back-and-forth motion. The inoculated culture should be sent to the laboratory as soon as possible to be placed in a CO_2-rich environment/incubator.

2. *Chlamydia:* A special culture media is used for this organism. A cytologic brush-loop swab is used to obtain the specimen. The brush-loop swab is placed in the test tube of medium and cracked so the specimen fits within the tube. This specimen should be obtained

last during the pelvic examination because epithelial cells are needed and all discharge must be swabbed away. This specimen must be refrigerated quickly! Place the specimen in cup of ice until it is taken to the lab.

Throat culture: A throat culture is indicated with symptoms of pharyngitis in sexually active patients that engage in oral sex.

Rapid plasma reagin (RPR): Used to detect syphilis. Results yield a nonreactive or reactive state. A nonreactive reading does not rule out an incubating disease. If the disease is suspected, the RPR should be repeated at 1-week, 1-month, and 3-month intervals. A reactive test may indicate past infection inadequately treated or a new infection. Treated individuals should be retested at 3-month intervals for 1 year or until a nonreactive test occurs. If the RPR is positive, a VDRL test is performed because of its increased specificity for syphilis.

Venereal disease research laboratory (VDRL): Used to detect syphilis.

Erythrocyte sedimentation rate (ESR): Obtained in suspected PID. The value is elevated in any inflammatory condition.

Complete blood count (CBC): In cases of systemic symptoms (e.g., fever), a CBC is obtained to detect leukocytosis. The WBC count is elevated in PID.

Serum pregnancy test (HCG): A pregnancy test should be completed in all females with suspected STDs, since some treatments differ during pregnancy.

Direct fluorescent antibody test: Monoclonal antibodies are used to detect *Chlamydia.*

Urinalysis and/or urine culture: Several STDs may infect the urethra, as well as, other genital areas. Urethral leukocytosis with pyuria may be present in men with *Chlamydia* or gonorrhea.

Other

Joint aspiration: Indicated in cases of suspected disseminated gonorrhea with symptoms of joint pain and swelling, fever, and rash (gonorrheal arthritis).

Lumbar puncture (LP): An LP may be performed to obtain a cerebrospinal fluid specimen to test for syphilis if neurologic symptoms are present.

TABLE 18-1 Differential Diagnosis of STDs

Diagnosis	Nodes	Lesion
Syphilis	Firm, painless, usually not enlarged.	Single, painless lesion.
Herpes	Tender, bilateral inguinal node enlargement.	Multiple, tender vesicles that ulcerate.
Chancroid	Tender, unilateral, or bilateral nodes that may not be enlarged.	Multiple painful, leaking lesions.

Clinical Conditions

Several STDs produce enlarged inguinal lymph nodes and genital lesions. Table 18-1 compares several STDs on these symptoms. Treatment of STDs involve medication administration. Drugs used to treat common STDs are summarized in Table 18-2.

Candida

SYMPTOMS

- A thick, white, curdy vaginal discharge is present accompanied by vaginal itching and burning.

DIAGNOSIS

- Diagnosis is made by microscopic examination of a discharge with 10% KOH on a wet mount slide.

TREATMENT

- Miconazole nitrate or clotrimazole vaginal suppositories are prescribed.
- Reoccurrence is common.

Chancroid

Chancroid has been associated as a cofactor in HIV transmission. Serologic testing for HIV should be conducted.

SYMPTOMS

- Presence of lesions on external genitalia that begin as small papules and break down into painful exudative ulcers with ragged edges.
- Inguinal lymph nodes may be painful on palpation.

TABLE 18-2 Drug Summary

Condition	Drug	Dose/Route	Special considerations
Pelvic inflammatory disease	Inpatient: Cefoxitin or doxycycline Outpatient: Cefoxitin, doxycycline, ofloxacin, or clindamycin	Inpatient: Cefoxitin 2 g IV q 6 hr Doxycycline 100 mg IV or PO q 12 hr. Outpatient: Cefoxitin 2 g IM plus probenecid 1 g PO Doxycycline 100 mg PO bid × 14 days Ofloxacin 400 mg PO bid × 14 days Clindamycin 450 mg PO qid × 14 days	—
Syphilis	Penicillin G benzathine If penicillin-allergic, give doxycycline, tetracycline, or erythromycin	Penicillin G benzathine 2.4 million U IM Doxycycline 100 mg PO × 14 days Tetracycline 500 mg PO × 14 days Erythromycin 500 mg PO × 14 days	Dosage and route may vary according to stage of syphilis.
Gonorrhea	Ciprofloxacin Norfloxacin Ofloxacin Cefixime Ceftriaxone	Ciprofloxacin 500 mg PO × 1 Norfloxacin 800 mg PO × 1 Ofloxacin 400 mg PO × 1 Cefixime 400-800 mg PO × 1 Ceftriaxone 250 mg IM × 1	Ciprofloxacin is not recommended for persons under 17 years of age because it inhibits cartilage development. It is not approved for use in pregnancy.

Organism	Drug	Regimen	Comments
Chlamydia	Azithromycin Doxycycline Erythromycin	Azithromycin 1 g PO × 1 Doxycycline 100 mg PO bid × 7 days Erythromycin 500 mg qid × 7 days	Ceftriaxone is very painful and may be mixed with a 1% lidocaine solution for administration. —
Herpes	Acyclovir	First occurrence: Acyclovir 200 mg PO 5 × qd for 7-10 days or 800 mg bid × 5 days Repeat occurrence: Acyclovir 200 mg PO 2-5 × qd or 400 mg bid	—
HPV	Podophyllum	Podophyllum 0.5% solution applied bid × 3 days withheld for 4 days and then may be reapplied weekly × 3 weeks	
Candida	Micronazole Clotrimazole	Micronazole vaginal suppository 200 mg qd × 3 days Clotrimazole vaginal tablet qd × 3 days	Recommended for bedtime use.
Vaginitis	Doxycycline Tetracycline	Doxycycline 100 mg PO bid × 7 days Tetracycline 500 mg PO × 7 days	Erythromycin 500 mg PO qid × 7 days is recommended during pregnancy.

Continued.

S

TABLE 18-2 Drug Summary (cont'd)

Condition	Drug	Dose/Route	Special considerations
Chancroid	Erythromycin Ceftriaxone Azithromycin	Erythromycin 500 mg PO qid × 7 days or Ceftriaxone 250 mg IM × 1 Azithromycin 1 g PO × 1	—
Trichomonas	Metronidazole	Metronidazole 2 g PO × 1	Contraindicated in pregnancy.

DIAGNOSIS
- Diagnosis is made on clinical presentation.
- Usually four or less lesions are present.

TREATMENT
- Treatment is administration of ceftriaxone, azithromycin, or erythromycin.

Chlamydia

Chlamydia is the most common STD in the United States.

SYMPTOMS
- The majority of cases are asymptomatic and are detected on routine screening.

DIAGNOSIS
- Diagnosis is made by culture and DNA probe.

TREATMENT
- Sexual partners should be screened and treated.

Gonorrhea

Males have a higher transmission rate of gonorrhea than females because of the high-organism load in the ejaculate of an infected male.

SYMPTOMS
- Gonorrhea may be asymptomatic.
- Males may have urethral discharge, dysuria, and testicular tenderness. Men should be warned not to ignore a drop of urethral exudate seen on arising before urination.
- Females may have vaginal discharge, dysuria, abnormal menses, dyspareunia, and abdominal pain.
- Rectal pain and discharge may be present in both genders if anorectal gonorrhea is present.
- Gonococcal pharyngitis is possible after oral sexual exposure.
- Disseminated gonococcal infection may be present in untreated cases.
- Symptoms of fever and joint pain are common.
- A sparse pustular/blister-type rash may be present on extremities.

DIAGNOSIS
- Diagnosis is made by culture and DNA probe.

TREATMENT
- Sexual partners should be cultured and treated.
- Ceftriaxone or ciprofloxacin are administered.
- It is commonly resistant to penicillin.

S

Human papillomavirus (HPV)

This condition is commonly referred to as genital warts. The period from exposure to disease development varies from 1½ to 8 months. There is a positive relationship between HPV and the occurrence of cervical cancer. HPV also occurs in conjunction with HIV.

SYMPTOMS

- Warty growths (condylomata, cauliflower-like appearance) appear in moist genital areas where coital friction occurs. These growths are painless.

DIAGNOSIS

- Diagnosis is made on clinical presentation.
- No culture method is available.
- Cervical HPV infections are usually detected by Pap smear.
- Because of the possibility of neoplasia, all warts with atypical appearance, and that are pigmented, or located on the cervix should be biopsied.

TREATMENT

- This virus is very difficult to treat and reoccurrences are frequent.
- Liquid nitrogen may be applied.
- Podophyllum (podofilox, condylox) or trichloracetic acid may also be used.
- Lesions are removed by laser therapy in severe cases.
- Consider concurrent STDs as well.

Pelvic inflammatory disease (PID)

This condition refers to infection of the uterus, fallopian tubes, and adjacent pelvic structures. It may be called salpingitis. It ranges in severity from mild-to-life threatening. Infertility may occur because of tubal scarring and occlusion. Ectopic pregnancy may also occur for these same reasons.

SYMPTOMS

- Symptoms are not always apparent.
- The most common symptom is bilateral lower abdominal pain.
- Pain is also present with manipulation of the cervix and bimanual examination of ovaries.
- Abnormal vaginal discharge is present and varies depending on type of organism(s) involved.
- *N. gonorrhoeae* and *C. trachomatis* are most common.
- Fever and elevated WBC, ESR, and C-reactive protein level may be present if disease is severe.

DIAGNOSIS
- Diagnosis is based on clinical presentation.
- Fever, abnormal vaginal discharge, elevated ESR, and a mass on ultrasonography may be present.
- Because of the severity of possible sequelae, the diagnosis is made without confirmative endovaginal ultrasound or endometrial biopsy.
- Treatment is initiated on suspicion of the condition.
- A pregnancy test should be performed to minimize the possibility of missing an ectopic pregnancy (4).
- Hospitalization is indicated when possibility of a surgical emergency cannot be excluded, pelvic abscess is suspected, patient is pregnant, and/or an adolescent is unable to follow outpatient therapy or return for follow-up, or patient is HIV positive.

TREATMENT
- Antibiotics are the drug of choice (cefoxitin, doxycycline, clindamycin and ofloxacin are most commonly used).

Syphilis

Syphilis, caused by *Treponema pallidum,* has four stages. Symptoms vary according to stage. When associated with HIV, serologic testing is indicated. All patients with an STD are at risk for having asymptomatic syphilis. Syphilis can be contacted through blood and body fluids.

SYMPTOMS
- *Stage 1:* Painless, indurated chancre.
- *Stage 2:* This stage occurs 2 to 8 weeks after appearance of chancre. Skin rash and infectious lesions on mucous membranes are present in the early days of stage 2. Flu-like symptoms may be present.
- *Stage 3:* This is a latent, symptom-free stage where the disease is usually detected through routine laboratory screening procedures (e.g., prenatal, premarital).
- *Stage 4:* Neurologic and cardiovascular symptoms occur.

DIAGNOSIS
- In stages 1 and 2, genital scrapings are viewed under darkfield microscopy or fluorescent antibody techniques are used.
- RPR and VDRL titers detect the organism.

TREATMENT
- Penicillin remains the treatment of choice.
- In penicillin-allergic individuals, doxycyline, tetracycline, or erythromycin are recommended.

- Certain antibiotics prescribed for other STDs (antibiotics with beta-lactam resistance and tetracycline) are also effective against syphilis.
- Patients treated for an STD with antibiotics other than beta-lactams or tetracycline should be tested for syphilis 1 month later.

Herpes simplex virus

Herpes occurs from direct physical contact with infected secretions. Rectal herpes can occur from anorectal sex. During oral sex, fever blisters of the mouth can be transmitted to the genital area and vice versa. Although unlikely, transmission can occur through wet clothing and towels. These items should not be used by others during an outbreak. Contact lens wearers should cleanse their hands thoroughly before applying lenses, since the virus can multiply under the lens.

SYMPTOMS

- Single or multiple vesicles appear on the genitalia. These rupture and cause ulcers.
- Recurrent infections vary but are usually of shorter and milder duration.
- Prodromal signs of tenderness, burning, tingling, and itching may occur.
- Inguinal lymph nodes may be enlarged.
- Females have a higher incidence of systemic symptoms during their first occurrence.
- Fever, headache, and malaise may be present.

DIAGNOSIS

- Diagnosis is usually based on clinical presentation or viral culture.

TREATMENT

- Acyclovir accelerates healing, particularly in first occurrences, but its efficacy decreases with recurrent episodes.
- Warm compresses, sitz baths, and aspirin may help during outbreaks.

Hepatitis B virus

Sexual contact is the most frequently reported method of hepatitis B viral transmission and is especially prevalent among homosexuals (see Chapter 5).

SYMPTOMS

- Malaise, fatigue, jaundice, and abdominal pain are frequent complaints.

DIAGNOSIS
* Diagnosis is made by serologic testing.

TREATMENT
* Prevention is the key to treating this.
* A single dose of hepatitis B vaccine can be administered if treated within 24 hours of exposure, but a full series of three IM injections are still needed for protection.
* An HIV screen should be drawn before administration of vaccine.

Trichomonas

Trichomonas is caused by protozoa.

SYMPTOMS
* An odorous, frothy, and yellow-green discharge is present and associated with vulvar irritation.

DIAGNOSIS
* Motile organisms are identified on a normal saline smear of the discharge.

TREATMENT
* Metronidazole is the drug of choice.
* Sexual partners should be treated simultaneously.

Vaginitis

Vaginitis usually results from overgrowth of anaerobic organisms, rather than as a true infection.

SYMPTOMS
* Malodorous, gray-white, thin, adherent vaginal discharge associated with vulvar itching.

DIAGNOSIS
* Diagnosis is made on the presence of an amine odor to the vaginal discharge when mixed with 10% KOH.
* Vaginal pH is >4.5.

TREATMENT
* Treatment is initiated with metronidazole.
* Clindamycin may be used if the patient is pregnant.

S

NURSING SURVEILLANCE

1. Monitor pain level and changes.
2. Trend fever, vital signs, and urine output if abdomen is rigid.

EXPECTED PATIENT OUTCOMES

1. Pain decreases in intensity.
2. Patient understands differences in contraceptive methods and methods for preventing STDs.

DISCHARGE IMPLICATIONS

> **NURSING ALERT**
>
> Avoid using terms that assume marital status and sexual prefer-
> ence when conducting patient teaching. The term "partner" is
> preferred.

1. Sexual partners within the previous 30 days should be examined.
2. Follow-up cultures should be obtained from infected sites 3 to 7 days after completion of therapy.
3. Remind the patient to avoid intercourse until cured or adequately treated.
4. When discussing birth control options and STD prevention, warn patients that some diseases are not prevented by proper and consistent use of male condoms. Herpes, syphilis, HPV, and chancroid may be transmitted, despite condom use, depending on the site of lesions. Hepatitis B virus can be transmitted through natural skin condoms.
5. To encourage use of condoms, instruct patient on how to use the condom to increase excitement during the sexual act. For example, have the partner place the condom. The value of anticipating orgasm, relief from STD, and contraception protection may increase the involvement of both partners.
6. Teach the female patient about the need for Pap smears to detect dysplasia. All women beginning with the onset of sexual activity at age 21 should have regular Pap smears. Pap smears should be performed annually if the woman is sexually active. Two consecutive annual Pap smears should be obtained and thereafter a Pap smear every 3 years unless the patient has multiple partners (3). In cases where the woman has multiple partners, annual Pap smears are suggested. If the patient has known HPV disease, more frequent Pap smears are recommended because of the high risk for cervical cancer. Table 18-3 summarizes information related to contraception and partner/patient protection against STDs.

Candida

Treatment of male partners is not recommended.

TABLE 18-3 The Relationship Between Contraceptive Method, STD Protection, and Patient Education

Disease	Contraceptive method that provides protection	Information for follow-up
Chlamydia	Contraceptive sponge	Refer partner(s) for evaluation.
	Spermicide	
	Condom (male and female)	
	Diaphragm	
HPV	Condom (female better than male)	Have annual Pap smear. Examine partner(s) for warts. Weekly treatment until lesions resolve. Use condoms or abstain during treatment.
Gonorrhea	Condom (male and female)	Abstain until cured. Return for evaluation 2-3 days after treatment.
	Spermicide	
	Contraceptive sponge	Have partner/s treated.
Herpes	Condom (female better than male)	Abstain when lesions are present. Have an annual Pap smear. May transmit virus when asymptomatic, use condoms during sexual activity.
Syphilis	Condom (male and female)	Return for follow-up at 3-, 6-, 12-, and 24-month intervals. Refer partner(s) for evaluation.

Oral contraceptives and IUDs may increase risk of vaginitis and *Chlamydia*.

Herpes

Barrier methods should be used during sexual activity at all times. The condom must cover all infected places.
Female condoms cover more genital area than male

condoms. Sexual contact should be avoided during prodromal and symptomatic stages of the disease.

Pelvic Inflammatory Disease

Coitus should be avoided until inflammation and pain subsides. Intrauterine devices should be removed. Follow-up should be arranged 24 to 48 hours after ED discharge.

Vaginitis

Treatment of male partners is not recommended. The consumption of larger amounts of complex carbohydrates and less simple sugars has been helpful in some cases (2).

References

1. Alexander L: Sexually transmitted diseases: perspectives on this growing epidemic, *Nurse Pract,* 17 (10):31, 34, 37, 38, 41-42, 1992.
2. Crook W: Diet changes may aid vaginitis prophylaxis, *Nurse Pract* 18:13, 1993.
3. Matthews W: The ubiquitous humanpapillomavirus, *J Am Acad Physic Assist* 5, 500-505, 1992.
4. McCormick W: Pelvic inflammatory disease, *N Engl J Med* 330:115-119, 1994.
5. Williams D, Riddle J: Understanding salpingitis, *Prof Nurse* 6:217-20.

Chapter XIX

Surface Trauma

Chris Lindsey
Kimberly Short

CLINICAL CONDITIONS
Abrasions
Avulsions
Lacerations
Contusions
Puncture Wounds
Mammalian Bites

Surface trauma or trauma to the skin may be related to blunt or penetrating trauma and associated with falls, motor vehicle crashes, violence, mammalian bites, sporting, recreational or work-related incidents.

The skin protects the body by regulating body temperature, providing primary sensation, preserving and excreting body fluids, and producing vitamin D. The three basic layers of the skin are the epidermis, the dermis, and the subcutaneous layer. The epidermis, the surface layer, is avascular and the site for rapid cellular regeneration. The dermis is vascular and is the site of connective tissue, motor and sensory nerves, and the lymph nodes. The hair, nails, and the sebaceous and sweat glands begin in the dermis and protrude through the epidermis. The subcutaneous layer is composed of fatty tissue, which acts as an insulator and cushion for the body against trauma.

Many victims of surface trauma may have associated life-threatening injuries. It is essential that the airway, breathing, and circulation of all patients be assessed and proper interventions be implemented. For this reason many minor surface trauma injuries are low priority upon admission to the emergency department (ED) and given minimal attention initially.

s

TRIAGE ASSESSMENT
General Observations
Type of surface trauma
Is the wound open or closed?
- Open wounds may include abrasions and avulsions, lacerations, punctures, and mammalian bites.
- Closed wounds are contusions.

Severity of the injury
- Is there active bleeding?
- Using the five P's, assess the injured site for clues of concurrent neurovascular injuries:

  Pain. Location and the quality.

  Pallor. Color, warmth, and capillary refill.

  Pulses. Compare presence and quality bilaterally.

  Paresthesia. Absence or change in the sensation since the injury.

  Paralysis. Can the patient move the injured area? Did the patient move the injured area initially, and now there is a change? (After injury, edema begins and if unattended, may become severe enough to prevent movement, or worse, compromise neurovascular function, thus resulting in impaired range of motion.)

Past medical history
- Patients with a history of cardiac or respiratory diseases, diabetes, peripheral vascular disease, or blood dycrasias may have a greater risk for infection and delayed healing.
- Individuals who are on anticoagulation medications (e.g., Coumadin, Persantine, aspirin) may have prolonged bleeding times and greater blood loss.
- Alcohol dependence is associated with nutritional deficits and delayed healing.
- Smokers may have peripheral vasoconstriction and delayed healing.
- Individuals on immunosuppressive medications (e.g., prednisone, cyclosporin) and individuals receiving chemotherapy or radiation therapy may also have a greater risk for infection.

Prehospital treatment
- Bleeding control and wound cleansing measures may produce further damage if inappropriate (e.g., tourniquet).

Classification of the injury

1. *Emergency:* "Life or limb-threatening."
   - Uncontrolled arterial bleeding.
   - Injuries with associated hypovolemia.
   - Injuries with neurovascular impairment.
2. *Urgent:*
   - Injuries requiring suture closure.
   - Injuries that require debridement and/or foreign body removal.
3. *Nonurgent:*
   - Abrasions
   - Contusions (simple)
   - Small puncture wounds

FOCUSED NURSING ASSESSMENT

Mechanism of Injury

1. *How:* What object caused the injury and at what force (e.g., motor vehicle crash with facial lacerations from a windshield or large avulsion from an assault with a beer bottle)?
2. *When:* Time is of utmost importance in estimating wound contamination and influencing treatment. In general, wounds (lacerations) that are over 6 hours old may be considered contaminated (2). Lacerations over 8 hours old may not be sutured but allowed to heal by secondary intention and dressing changes. Facial lacerations may be sutured after 8 to 12 hours because of the greater disfigurement potential and the good vascularity of the face (1).
3. *Where:* A laceration to the arm is less contaminated and easier to clean than a complete lip laceration. Areas involving mucous membranes have a higher contamination risk (e.g., oral cavity and perineum).

Risk Factors
Drug and alcohol abuse

Any individual may have impaired cognition and perception under the influence of drugs. They may be a perpetrator of violence or the victims of violence. Drug-seeking places them at risk for trauma and also impairs their healing process. Many of these individuals are malnourished, have no families or support systems and spend their money on drugs and alcohol instead of purchasing supplies to help heal their injuries.

S

Smoking

Many burns are caused by the careless use of cigarettes such as falling asleep with a cigarette.

Abuse

Assess for signs of physical abuse or neglect (see Chapter 2). Note fear that may be exhibited by the patient in the presence of their caregivers and/or family. Stories that do not correlate with the injury should raise the index of suspicion.

Life Span Issues
Geriatric

1. The geriatric patient may have a decrease in mobility and sensation, thus increasing their susceptibility for injury. They may also have alteration in mental status or function that puts them at higher risk for injury and decreases their compliance with treatments.
2. Many geriatric patients are living in poverty and thus cannot pay for medications or dressing supplies. They may need a social worker referral and extra take-home supplies or medication dose packs before discharge.

Youth

1. Young adults may be involved in many recreational activities that increase their risk for surface trauma.
2. Children are always very curious and ready to explore. During some growth and development phases, they may be clumsy and are learning the definitions of hot, cold, yes and no.
3. Pediatric patients may need more anesthesia or may need to be physically or chemically restrained for the treatment of their injuries. Take time to communicate with the child at his level to make the experience as pleasant as possible.

INITIAL INTERVENTIONS

1. Control all bleeding.
2. Obtain vital signs.
3. Cleanse the wound and dress with a normal saline gauze.
4. Elevate the affected area.
5. Ice may be applied to the area, if area is edematous and/or bleeding. Be sure to use a thin cloth/gauze between ice pack and skin for protection from frostbite.

6. Remove all constrictive clothing and jewelry.
7. Document all palpated pulses.

PRIORITY NURSING DIAGNOSES

Risk for fluid volume deficit
Risk for pain
Risk for alteration in tissue perfusion
Risk for impaired skin integrity
Risk for infection
Risk for anxiety
Risk for impaired mobility

◆ **Fluid volume deficit** related to bleeding and/or serious fluid loss.
   INTERVENTION
   * Depending upon severity of the wound, place large bore IV (14 to 18 gauge) for fluid administration.
   * Apply pressure to site and/or pressure points (see Chapter 21).
   * Elevate site if possible.

◆ **Pain** related to surface trauma, wound irrigation, and treatment.
   INTERVENTION
   * Place a splint on injured area, provide ice pack, and elevate the injured extremity.
   * Mild analgesics may be ordered, as well as a local anesthetic such as topical adrenalin and cocaine (TAC) (see Table 19-2 and TAC Procedure 29).

◆ **Alteration in tissue perfusion** related to extremity vascular injury.
   INTERVENTION
   * Supplemental oxygen may be considered.

◆ **Impaired skin integrity** related to surface trauma.
   INTERVENTION
   * Prepare for wound closure by suture, stapling, or tape (Table 19-1).

◆ **Infection** related to contamination of wounds or preexisting conditions (e.g., diabetes, peripheral vascular disease, alcohol abuse, etc.).
   INTERVENTION
   * Cleanse wound (see Procedure 32) and apply dressing.
   * Administer diptheria tetanus as indicated (see Reference Guide 8).
   * Administer IV antibiotics as ordered.

S

TABLE 19-1 Wound Closure Methods

Method/Use	Advantages	Disadvantages
Steri-strips		
May be used for partial-thickness lacerations or small superficial lacerations without signs of adjacent tension.	Eliminates need for anesthetic. Decrease tissue trauma. Decrease risk for infection.	Potential for wound edge inversion. Less strength than sutures.
Approximate the wound edges, applying steri-strips uniformly. Use benzoin or mastisol on adjacent skin to secure adhesiveness of steri-strips.	—	—
Sutures		
May be used for simple and more involved lacerations. Closure of deep wounds is done in layers. Suture selection is a matter of individual choice.	Definite closure of wound edges. Patient able to shower and dressing is not always needed after 24 hrs.	Local anesthetic used. Follow-up appointment needed for suture removal.
Absorbable suture is used for deeper layers. Examples are plain or chromic catgut and the synthetics, Dexon and Vicryl.	—	—

Nonabsorbable suture is used for skin closure and must be removed.

Examples are silk or synthetics (nylon, polypropylene).

NOTE: The synthetics have a decreased wicking action that decreases the scarring potential.

—

Staples

May be used for linear lacerations to scalp, trunk, and extremities.*

Rapid method of closure. Produces less inflammation.

Provides less precise approximation. Should not be used when magnetic resonance imaging of the affected part may be conducted.

—

*From Markovchick V: Suture materials and mechanical after care, *Emerg Med Clin North Am* 10:673-689, 1992.

S

◆ **Anxiety** related to precipitating event of surface trauma, pain, and potential for disfigurement.
   INTERVENTION
   • Offer support and explain all procedures.

◆ **Potential for impaired mobility** related to severity and location of surface trauma.
   INTERVENTION
   • Splint and elevate injured area.
   • Continue to monitor neurovascular status.

PRIORITY DIAGNOSTIC TESTS

Radiographs: Used to rule out fractures and foreign bodies. (Organic objects such as seeds, beans, or wood are not radiopaque. Glass may be radiopaque.)

Complete blood count (CBC): May be obtained to monitor blood loss. An elevated WBC count may be present in infection, especially with old and/or contaminated wounds.

PT/PTT: May be obtained in patients with multiple injuries with blood loss or who have a history of anticoagulant use or blood dyscrasia.

Type and crossmatch: In multiple injury with hypovolemia, or a possible need for surgical intervention, a type and crossmatch for blood needs to be obtained.

Compartment pressure readings: Need to be recorded in severe cases of surface trauma with associated edema that is limb threatening (see Chapter 21).

COLLABORATIVE INTERVENTIONS

Clinical Conditions
Abrasions

An abrasion is impaired epidermis with some fluid loss and minimal to no bleeding (e.g., "road rash" from falls on pavement, rug or rope burns).

SYMPTOMS
• Pain is usually localized to the injured area.
• Localized edema may be present as a result of capillary vasodilation.
• Erythema is related to the inflammatory response.

DIAGNOSIS
• Diagnosis is by clinical presentation.

TREATMENT
• Wound cleansing procedure should be explained to include rationale (e.g., gravel and dirt must be removed

within 8 to 10 hours after injury or it will lead to "tattooing," darkening of the scar tissue) and to elicit cooperation.

- Premedicate the patient with a local topical anesthetic (see Procedure 29) such as TAC or an injectable form of anesthetic such as lidocaine (see Table 19-2). IV or oral analgesics may be indicated.
- Cleanse and/or debride wound (see Procedure 32).
- Consider applying a dressing to the wound, if it is draining, or is in an area of likely contamination (hands, feet, and elbows).
- Administer medications as appropriate (e.g., tetanus).

Avulsions

An avulsion is skin or full-thickness tissue that is torn away completely or left hanging as a flap and prevents wound edge approximation.

Symptoms

- Bleeding is usually present with pain.
- Underlying structures (e.g., bone, tendons, and muscles) may be exposed.

Diagnosis

- Diagnosis is by clinical presentation.

Treatment

- Bleeding is controlled by direct pressure, use of pressure points, or with a pressure dressing.
- The patient should be informed of procedures for wound care, debridement, and possible closure techniques in the ED or the operating room.
- Local anesthetic or IV-conscious sedation for wound care may be administered before cleansing and irrigating the wound. (See Procedures 8 and 32.)
- A dressing is applied to the wound after suturing.
- Medications are administered as needed (e.g., tetanus [see Chapter 5] and antibiotics).

Lacerations

Lacerations are open wounds in the skin and/or underlying structures produced by tearing or cutting.

Symptoms

- The amount of bleeding depends on depth, location, and involvement of structures.
- There is possible decreased extremity or digit function and sensation.
- Edema, erythema, crustation, and/or purulent drainage may be present depending on length of time since injury.

S

DIAGNOSIS
- Diagnosis is by clinical presentation.

TREATMENT
- Bleeding is controlled by above-stated measures and explained wound care.
- The patient is premedicated with anesthetics or analgesics for wound care, cleansing, and closure.
- The wound is cleansed before and dressed after wound closure (see Procedure 31).
- Medications are administered as ordered (e.g., analgesics, tetanus, and/or antibiotics).

Contusions

Contusions are characterized by bruising or blunt trauma to the skin and underlying structures.

SYMPTOMS
- Localized pain and edema are usually present.
- Discoloration of the surface of the skin produces general clues to the age of the contusion as follows:
  Blue/red: Within hours
  Purple: Within 1 week
  Greenish/yellow: Within 2 to 3 weeks
  Yellow/brown: Within 3 to 4 weeks

DIAGNOSIS
- Diagnosis is by clinical presentation.

TREATMENT
Treatment is aimed at providing comfort and preventing further edema and/or tissue damage.
- Ice is applied for the first 24 to 48 hours, then heat for 48 to 72 hours.
- The injured area may be elevated at or above the level of the heart.
- The affected extremity may be immobilized 24 to 48 hours after the injury depending on the location and severity of the injury (e.g., ace, splint, or sling).

Puncture wounds

Puncture wounds are small interruption(s) in the skin and/or the underlying structures with absent, hidden, or protruding foreign bodies (e.g., splinters, glass, or nails).

SYMPTOMS
- Bleeding and pain may be present.
- There may be signs and symptoms of infection (e.g., erythmea, warmth, edema, drainage).

- The deformity of the skin is related to the degree of foreign body penetration.

DIAGNOSIS

- Diagnosis is by clinical presentation and/or radiograph.

TREATMENT

- Bleeding should be controlled with previously stated measures.
- X-rays may be obtained to rule out foreign bodies.
- Wound care procedures including debridement and exploration should be explained.
- Analgesics or anesthetics may be administered for wound care, cleansing, and possible exploration.
- The wound is cleansed per protocol.
- A dressing is applied as indicated after wound exploration and closure.
- Medications are administered as directed (e.g., analgesics, tetanus, and/or antibiotics).

Mammalian bites

Mammalian bites are bites from humans or animals (most commonly dogs) that cause puncture wounds but may have associated abrasions, avulsions, contusions, and lacerations.

SYMPTOMS

- Bleeding may be present.
- Edema, erythema, and pain usually occur.
- Signs and symptoms of infection may be present.

DIAGNOSIS

- Diagnosis is by history and clinical presentation.

TREATMENT

- Bleeding is controlled.
- Analgesics or anesthetics may be administered for wound care, cleansing, and possible closure. Closure is controversial because of high incidence of infection. If sutured, a wound check should be scheduled within 24 hours.
- The wound is cleansed and dressed per protocol.
- Ice and elevation may be necessary for edema.
- The health department is notified for animal bites per local policy.
- Medications are administered as needed (e.g., analgesics and antibiotics).
- Rabies vaccination may be required, as well as tetanus (see Chapter 5).

NURSING SURVEILLANCE
Patient Observation
1. Response to wound care and participation in wound care.
2. Response to medications (e.g., analgesics, anesthetics, IV-conscious sedation). See Procedure 8. Monitor for allergic reactions (e.g., SOB, rash, elevated temperature).
3. Neurovascular integrity of affected area.

Wound Observation
1. Wound approximation.
2. Continued bleeding or drainage.
3. Appearance of dressings (e.g., intact, wet or dry, type of drainage).
4. Signs and symptoms of infection (e.g., erythema, edema, warmth at site, purulent drainage, unexplained temperature elevation).

Family Support or Significant Other
1. Keep them free from injury. Do not allow the member to watch wound care or suturing if potential for vasovagal response is present. If the family member insists on staying, recommend that they sit beside the stretcher.
2. Involve the family member in learning wound care instructions and discharge instructions.

EXPECTED PATIENT OUTCOMES
1. Bleeding is controlled and neurovascular status remains intact.
2. Patient states relief of pain within 30 minutes to 1 hour after pain medication is administered.
3. Patient verbalizes understanding of wound cleansing and closure.
4. Wound is approximated or protected by dressing before discharge.
5. Patient verbalizes signs and symptoms of infection.
6. Patient or significant other verbalizes understanding of wound care procedure.
7. Patient and/or significant other verbalizes knowledge of medications (e.g., analgesics, antibiotics, and immunizations) and potential side effects.
8. Patient verbalizes compliance with wound care and follow-up instructions.

TABLE 19-2 Drug Summary

Agent	Dose route (maximum recommended doses)	Special considerations
Lidocaine: With epinephrine*	7 mg/kg sc	Used as local anesthetic before wound procedure.
Lidocaine: Without epinephrine	4 mg/kg sc	Administer to wound edges only.
Procaine: With epinephrine*	14 mg/kg sc	Used as local anesthetic before wound procedure.
Procaine: Without epinephrine	8 mg/kg sc	Administer to wound edges only.
Bupivacaine: With epinephrine*	4 mg/kg sc	Used as local anesthetic before wound procedure.
Bupivacaine: Without epinephrine	1 mg/kg sc	Administer to wound edges only.

*Do not use agents with epinephrine in areas with decreased blood flow (e.g., digits).

9. Patient verbalizes understanding of follow-up examinations for wound checks and suture/staple removal, as well as, prn for signs of infection.

DISCHARGE INSTRUCTIONS

1. Keep the dressing clean and dry for 24 hours.
2. Wash hands thoroughly with soap and water before and after wound care.
3. After the first 24 hours, remove the dressing. Cleanse the wound gently of medication residue and wound exudate with soap and water. (Advise patient to have own bar of soap.) Advise patient to avoid prolonged immersion of wound in water (e.g., tub bath, swimming pool, or long showers).
4. Reapply a thin layer of antibiotic ointment. Antibiotic ointment protects the wounded area and decreases scarring.

S

5. Wound may be redressed or left open to air as appropriate. Factors to consider for redressing are location of wound (e.g., joints, hands, or feet), severity of wound, wound drainage, and potential for contamination.

6. Keep area elevated for 24 to 48 hours with ice pack application if needed to decrease edema or pain.

7. Verbalize signs and symptoms of infection such as redness, swelling, warmth, purulent drainage, and unexplained elevated temperature.

8. Take complete dose of antibiotics as prescribed. If rabies vaccination is indicated, the patient should be instructed to return for follow-up injections.

9. To return for wound check and suture removal as appropriate. Sutures are usually removed in 5 to 14 days. Animal and human bites should be rechecked in 24 hours because of potential for cellulitis.

10. Cover the affected area with a dressing or sunscreen for 1 year to minimize discoloration and scarring.

11. The nurse should assess socioeconomic factors before discharge.
    - Socioeconomic and environmental factors impact compliance with wound care at home. These factors include money for supplies and medications, personal hygiene habits, and the existence of running water or electricity in the home.

References

1. Edlich R, Rodeheaver G, Morgan R, Berman D, Thacker J: Principles of emergency wound management, *Ann Emerg Med* 17:1284-1302, 1988.
2. Robson M: Disturbances in wound healing, *Ann Emerg Med* 17:1274-1278, 1988.

Chapter XX

Toxicologic Conditions

Pamela S. Kidd

SPECIFIC OVERDOSES
Acetaminophen (Tylenol)
Salicylates (Aspirin)
Alcohol
Specific Alcohol Agents (Methanol/Ethylene Glycol)
Benzodiazepines
Tricyclic Antidepressants (TCAs)
Physostigmine (Antilirium)
Opioid (Codeine, Heroin)
Specific Opioid (Cocaine)
Hydrocarbons
Organophosphates
Iron
Lead
Anticholinergic and Antihistamine Drugs
Calcium Channel and Beta-Blockers
Cardiac Glycosides

TRIAGE ASSESSMENT

The most common agents involved in overdoses encountered in the emergency department (ED) are acetaminophen, alcohol, antihistamines, aspirin, tricyclic antidepressants (TCAs), and benzodiazepines. Calcium channel blockers and beta-blockers are increasingly being abused. At triage it is not important to determine what agent was abused, rather to determine if the patient's airway, breathing, and circulation are intact. Suspect an overdose in anyone who presents with an abrupt onset of multiple symptoms. Assuming that immediate life-saving interventions are not necessary, the following data are important to elicit:

Route of exposure (skin vs. IV vs. PO)
This determines where patient is placed in the ED (e.g., isolation room vs. resuscitation room). If exposure is through the skin (e.g., organophosphates), the patient's

skin requires flushing, and the health care providers are at risk for exposure.

Drug(s) ingested

Determine name of drug(s). Some drugs are slowly absorbed (digoxin, aspirin, phenytoin). Slow-release forms of drugs are treated differently.

Ingestion history

Determine how long ago and over what period of time the ingestion occurred. Lavage should be initiated within 1 hour of overdose to be effective.

Medical history

Determine patient's age, weight, height, medical history, and current medications. This information helps in drug calculations and to anticipate the patient's ability to metabolize drugs. Current medication history also helps determine treatment modality (e.g., if the patient takes furosemide, he/she may be potassium depleted before ingestion and use of a cathartic may further decrease the potassium level).

Patient's last meal

Determine amount and time of patient's last meal. Presence of food in the stomach may delay absorption.

Treatment before arrival

If ipecac has been given, emesis should occur within 30 minutes. Administration of ipecac may delay administration of oral antidotes and alter amount given. Vomiting may produce a vagal response and further decrease heart rate in a patient who has ingested cardiotoxic drugs.

Vital Signs

- *Tachycardia:* Related to sympathetic nervous system (SNS) stimulation (e.g., cocaine).
- *Bradycardia:* Related to myocardial depression or interference with calcium channels, SNS (e.g., beta-blocking and calcium channel blocking agents).
- *Hypotension:* Related to peripheral vasodilation or direct myocardial depression (e.g., opiates and tricyclic antidepressants).
- *Hypertension:* Related to SNS stimulation (e.g., cocaine, PCP).
- *Tachypnea:* Related to acidosis (e.g., salicylates).
- *Bradypnea:* Related to respiratory depression (e.g., narcotics, sedatives, tranquilizers).

- *Fever:* Related to anticholinergic effect or hypermetabolism (e.g., cocaine).
- *Hypothermia:* Related to hypometabolism (e.g., changes in glucose level).

General Observations
Pupil size and reaction
Constricted pupils may indicate organophosphate, opiates, or cocaine use. Dilated pupils (nonreactive) may indicate anticholinergic drugs, sympathomimetics, and mushrooms.
Skin
Inspect skin for needle track marks indicating IV drug use and/or multidrug overdose.

NURSING ALERT

All overdoses are potentially life threatening and should be treated as such. Patients should be triaged immediately to the ED treatment area. Symptoms occur later in patients who have ingested acetaminophen, sustained release drugs, and methanol/ethylene glycol. These are considered acute agents. Do not be fooled by a patient who is asymptomatic but may deteriorate in the ED waiting area.

The primary nurse should call the poison control center to determine definitive treatment.

FOCUSED NURSING ASSESSMENT

Nursing assessment should center on ventilation, perfusion, cognition, and elimination. The following should be assessed even if it was assessed at triage because changes occur rapidly.

Ventilation
Breath sounds
Pulmonary edema (PE) occurs frequently with hydrocarbon and opiate ingestion. Acute alcohol intoxication may also produce PE as a result of chronic alcohol abuse and its resulting congestive heart failure (CHF). Coarse or fine rales (crackles) may be auscultated.

Breathing pattern

Opiate overdoses produce respiratory depression and PE.
Respirations may be slow, shallow, and wet.
Hydrocarbons vaporize at low temperatures. They enter
the pulmonary tree easily producing bronchospasm, PE,
and aspiration pneumonitis. Salicylates produce
metabolic acidosis. Respirations are deep and slow,
related to direct stimulation of the respiratory center in
the brainstem.

Perfusion
Apical heart rate

Obtain an apical heart rate for 1 minute and compare this
rate and rhythm with a peripheral pulse. Many of the
commonly ingested drugs produce cardiovascular
effects. Calcium channel blocking and beta-blocking
agents decrease the heart rate and increase the
susceptibility for conduction blocks and ectopy.
Anticholinergic drugs and cocaine produce
tachydysrhythmias.

Blood pressure

Peripheral vasodilation and myocardial depression increase
as more of the ingested drug is absorbed.

Skin

Check skin color, temperature, capillary refill, and
peripheral pulses. Iron ingestion can produce gastric
hemorrhage and hypovolemic shock. Anticholinergic
agents produce hyperthermia, but the skin will be dry
because the patient is unable to sweat. Cocaine overdose
may produce diaphoresis.

Cognition
Mental status

Perform a neurologic assessment. Confusion and seizures
may occur at any time if the ingested amount of any
agent is great enough. The Glasgow coma scale (GCS)
(Reference Guide 6) should be used to document eye,
motor, and verbal response.

Hallucinations

You can hold up an imaginary piece of string and ask the
patient to tell you the color of the string. If they tell you
a color, they are having visual hallucinations.
Hallucinations are common with cocaine and lead
poisoning.

Unresponsive patient

If the patient is unresponsive, a coexisting traumatic injury (e.g., fall) may be present (see Chapter 22). Assess for evidence of trauma such as abrasions, bleeding, ecchymoses, edema, and deformity. Keep the patient flat with neck immobilized until cervical spine injury is ruled out.

Elimination
Bowel sounds

Absent bowel sounds are a good sign. This allows the drug to sit in the gut, slowing absorption.

Urinary output

Assess and measure urinary output. Has the patient voided since the ingestion? Some drugs may produce acute tubular necrosis (ATN) (e.g., methanol, ethylene glycol). Organophosphates overstimulate the parasympathetic nervous system resulting in urination and defecation.

Bowel movement

Assess stools. As noted above, organophosphates produce defecation. Bloody stools may result from iron ingestion.

Emesis

Assess and measure emesis. Are there pill fragments? Bloody emesis may occur with iron ingestion. If the patient has received ipecac, it is important to note the amount of emesis that occurs after administration.

Risk Factors

1. Young children who have access to medicine.
2. Geriatric patients with failing eyesight or memory.
3. People in pain or who are using drugs in chronic illness that may impair judgement.
4. Previous suicide attempts.

Life Span Issues
Adolescent

1. Fewer adolescents have mixed overdoses or use alcohol with the overdosed drug (1).
2. Adolescents tend to overdose on over-the-counter drugs instead of prescribed drugs.

Geriatric

1. The majority of overdoses in the nondepressed geriatric patient are the result of confusion, improper use of the

product, improper storage in container other than the original, or mistaken identity. This has discharge teaching implications.

2. Hemodialysis or hemoperfusion may be required at lower serum concentrations in the geriatric patient.

3. Geriatric patients are more likely to have chronic intoxication secondary to daily/multiple use of agents for other disorders (e.g., aspirin).

4. Geriatric suicide attempts are more likely to be successful (more serious attempt plus decreased ability to recover). Decreased hepatic and renal blood flow associated with aging decreases drug metabolism and excretion.

INITIAL INTERVENTIONS

Regardless of the drug ingested, the following interventions will not harm the patient and may be beneficial:

1. Implement measures to protect the patient's airway. If the patient is awake and cervical spine injury has been ruled out, place the patient in semi-Fowler's position. If the patient has decreased responsiveness, remove pillows. Insert a nasopharyngeal airway. If the patient is unresponsive, or has no gag reflex, insert an oral airway until the patient is intubated with an endotracheal tube (ET).

2. Anticipate aspiration. Have suction available. If the patient is unresponsive, place the patient in the left lateral recumbent position. This position allows the drug to remain in the curvature of the stomach and decreases drug absorption. It is easier to hear posterior breath sounds and to get a rectal temperature reading in this position.

3. Initiate pulse oximetry in order to monitor degree of oxygen saturation.

4. Initiate cardiac and blood pressure (BP) monitoring.

5. Protect the patient from injury. Seizures are common because of either the overdosed drug, hypoxia, and/or hypoglycemia. Pad the siderails. Keep the bed in low position. As noted above, have airway and suction materials available.

6. Do not punish the patient. Remember to ask why the patient took the overdose, not just what they took. The patient would not be in the ED if he/she knew a better way to manage problems.

PRIORITY NURSING DIAGNOSES

Risk for aspiration
Risk for impaired gas exchange
Risk for injury
Risk for altered tissue perfusion
Risk for decreased cardiac output
Risk for altered bowel elimination
Risk for fluid volume deficit
Risk for ineffective individual coping
Risk for knowledge deficit

◆ **Aspiration** related to depressed level of consciousness (LOC) and nausea/vomiting (N/V).

INTERVENTIONS
- Semi-Fowler's position if alert. Left lateral recumbent position if unresponsive.
- Insert airway adjunct as necessary.
- Suction prn.
- Administer the following agents as ordered: antiemetics, naloxone, thiamine, glucose, flumazenil.

◆ **Impaired gas exchange** related to altered serum pH, breathing pattern (salicylate), bronchospasm (beta-blocking agents).

INTERVENTIONS
- Apply pulse oximeter.
- Administer oxygen.
- Monitor respiratory effort, anticipate fatigue.

◆ **Injury** related to seizures (TCAs, flumazenil), change in body temperature (cocaine).

INTERVENTIONS
- Pad siderails, stretcher in low position.
- Suction prn.
- Administer anticonvulsant medications prophylactically as ordered.
- Administer the following agents as ordered: flumazenil slowly, dantrolene IV (as appropriate), antipyretics (as appropriate).
- Apply warming/cooling blanket (as appropriate).
- Use ice lavage (as appropriate).
- Warm, IV fluids (as appropriate).

◆ **Altered tissue perfusion** related to vasodilation and hypotension.

INTERVENTIONS
- Administer IV fluid cautiously.

- Administer vasopressors and diuretics as ordered.
- Assess capillary refill, pulse oximetry readings.

◆ **Decreased cardiac output** related to dysrhythmia, altered contractility, increased afterload (cocaine).

INTERVENTIONS
- Administer the following agents as ordered: calcium, sodium bicarbonate, glucagon, atropine, propanolol, esmolol (cocaine), vasodilators (cocaine).
- Anticipate external/internal pacing (calcium channel blockers).

◆ **Altered bowel elimination** related to cathartic use, decreased motility (anticholinergic drugs).

INTERVENTIONS
- Administer sorbitol and magnesium citrate as ordered.
- Monitor intake and output.
- Monitor electrolytes.
- Administer whole bowel irrigation for removal of drug packets, lithium, heavy metals, and sustained release medications.

◆ **Fluid volume deficit** related to forced diuresis, alkalinization of urine (salicylates), acute renal failure (ARF).

INTERVENTIONS
- Monitor vital signs.
- Monitor intake and output.

◆ **Ineffective individual coping** related to lack of perceived resources.

INTERVENTIONS
- Initiate psychologic/spiritual referral system.
- Ask why overdose was taken.
- Treat humanistically.

◆ **Knowledge deficit** related to improper use of medication.

INTERVENTIONS
- Clarify area of misunderstanding.
- Initiate patient teaching, once patient is stable.

PRIORITY DIAGNOSTIC TESTS

Laboratory
General considerations

Toxicology screening requires a large (10 cc) red top tube. An additional red top tube may be needed if cardiac enzymes or amylase level is ordered. If hemodialysis is necessary, a coagulation profile will be completed. This requires a blue top tube.

Serum toxicology screening: Toxicology screening may be performed, since acetaminophen, salicylate, lithium, theophylline, digoxin, and mercury levels may alter treatment plan (5).

Arterial blood gases: ABGs may be analyzed to check for anion gap acidosis associated with salicylate, ethylene glycol, and methanol ingestion.

Electrolyte levels: Baseline potassium, chloride, and sodium levels are usually obtained because treatments may produce electrolyte abnormalities.

Glucose level: May be ordered to rule out hypoglycemia as an associated factor in unresponsiveness.

Liver enzymes/amylase level: These may be elevated in acetaminophen overdoses as a result of hepatic necrosis.

Blood ethanol level: This is elevated in acute alcohol intoxication.

Cardiac enzyme and isoenzyme levels: These may be elevated in amphetamine, TCAs and cocaine overdoses.

BUN and creatinine: These may be obtained in cases where forced diuresis is a treatment modality to confirm normal renal function.

Urinalysis: A baseline urinalysis may be obtained in cases where forced diuresis is used as treatment modality to confirm normal renal function.

Urine toxicology screen: This may be ordered to help confirm the type(s) of drug ingested.

Gastric lavage screen: This may be ordered to help confirm the type(s) of drug ingested.

NURSING ALERT

If metabolic acidosis is present, anticipate the administration of IV sodium bicarbonate. Metabolic acidosis is common in TCAs, salicylate, and cocaine overdoses. An initial bolus is given followed by a continuous infusion titrated to achieve a serum pH of 7.50 to 7.55.

T

Radiographic

Abdominal films: Undissolved tablets (e.g., enteric-coated aspirin) may accumulate in the stomach, particularly if the patient has a gastric outlet disorder. This may be detected on film. Iron is radiopaque. Its presence can be detected by abdominal radiographs.

COLLABORATIVE INTERVENTIONS

1. Provide oxygen. Most drugs ingested induce acidosis. Use a mask until the patient is intubated.
2. Initiate IV access. Antidotes, antiemetics, fluids, and vasopressors may need to be administered.
3. Treat unresponsiveness. Dextrose is administered as 0.5 to 1.0 g/kg usually in $D_{25}W$ solution for the child and $D_{50}W$ solution for the adult. Glucagon 1 mg IM may be used if IV access is not possible (2). Naloxone 2 mg IV push (IVP) is administered in case the unresponsiveness is related to opiate overdose.
4. Maintain perfusion by promoting normal BP. Fluid is administered carefully (250 to 500 cc boluses) to avoid PE. In children, fluid is administered in 1 cc/kg doses. PE is a common complication after opiate, salicylate, pesticide, and hydrocarbon overdoses. Vasopressors are used as a last choice for hypotension, since they increase susceptibility for dysrhythmia in addition to the overdosed drug (6).
5. Impair drug absorption, modify drug metabolism, and enhance drug excretion.

Ipecac: Suggested doses are 30 ml for an adult and 15 ml for a child. It is contraindicated in children younger than 6 months (2). Ipecac may be used more successfully in children because they usually do not ingest substances that produce sedation. Ipecac directly stimulates the brain to induce emesis and irritates the gastric mucosa. Drinking water immediately after administration dilutes the ipecac and allows it to cover a larger surface area in the gut, producing greater emesis. Large items (e.g., iron pills) and heavy metals are best removed through emesis. It is contraindicated in hydrocarbon, TCAs, and multidrug ingestion. At best, ipecac can only remove 30% of gastric contents. It takes 20 to 30 minutes to work, and multiple doses may be required. Oral antidote administration may be delayed after using ipecac resulting from emesis. If a cardiotoxic drug (beta-blocker or calcium channel blocker) was ingested, the act of vomiting may cause a vagal response and further decrease heart rate. If overdose has occurred >1½ hours before being treated, ipecac or lavage is not helpful with most drugs. Ipecac is believed to be of little value in the ED (18).

Milk: Four to six oz may be given PO or via gastric tube if corrosive substance has been ingested (3).

Charcoal: Charcoal is administered in a 10:1 ratio (10 parts charcoal to 1 part drug). It may be used after emesis or lavage. A 50 to 100 g dose is used for adults. A 10 to 30 g or 1g/kg dose is suggested for a child. Charcoal may not be tolerated for 1 to 6 hours after ipecac administration. Combined therapy (charcoal after ipecac or charcoal after lavage) does not produce greater benefits and increases the risk of complications. ED stays are longer for patients receiving combined therapy (4). A large dose may be given before whole bowel irrigation. Soak the bottle in hot water for 10 to 15 minutes to make it easier to swallow/push. Water may be added to the charcoal and the solution shaken before administration.

Charcoal is not used in ingestion of corrosive substances, since it makes endoscopy impossible. Charcoal produces diarrhea and increases chance of aspiration. Charcoal aspiration produces prolonged severe bronchospasm. If the charcoal splatters in the eye, a corneal abrasion may occur. Charcoal does not absorb ethanol, hydrocarbons, or iron.

NURSING ALERT

Activated charcoal is often mixed in sorbitol (cathartic agent). When multiple doses of activated charcoal are given, make sure they are not administered in a sorbitol solution to avoid electrolyte abnormalities and death.

Gastric lavage: There is controversy over using gastric lavage without first inserting a cuffed ET tube because of potential aspiration. Lavage must be performed within 1 hour of ingestion of most drugs to be effective. After 1 hour, there is no difference in drug retrieval using lavage and charcoal rather than charcoal alone. If vomiting occurs before ED admission, lavage may not remove any additional drug, and it may force gastric contents into the small intestine. The procedure is to administer tap water or normal saline until returns through the orogastric tube are clear (1.5 to 20 liters for adults, 10 cc/kg for children). A large orogastric tube (36 to 42 Fr for adults) (26 to 28 Fr for children) should be inserted. A double lumen tube allows for simultaneous delivery and aspiration.

Cathartics: Cathartics are frequently used to help remove drug packets and iron. They should only be used with the first dose of charcoal, especially in children and geriatric patients because of potential electrolyte abnormalities.

- Sorbitol: Sorbitol is an oral cathartic available as a 70% solution that is diluted to 35% with water. A 0.5 to 1 g/kg dose (usually 2 to 3 cc/kg) is given to a maximum dose of 50 g (2). Sorbitol produces less electrolyte abnormalities and has the shortest gastrointestinal (GI) transit time of all cathartics. It works faster than magnesium citrate. Sorbitol gives charcoal a sweet taste and decreases the grittiness, so charcoal is more palatable.

- Magnesium sulfate/citrate: Magnesium sulfate and citrate are cathartic agents. They should not be used in patients with CHF secondary to increased saline load. Magnesium cathartics are contraindicated in patients with impaired renal function (17).

Cation exchange resins: Sodium polystyrene sulfonate is a cation exchange resin used to bind lithium. A side effect of this treatment is hypokalemia. Cation exchange resins may be used until dialysis is available.

Forced diuresis: Forced diuresis is used if an agent is distributed mainly within the extracellular fluid with minimal protein binding, and it is excreted in the urine. This treatment is controversial because of potential dehydration and electrolyte imbalances.

Altering urine and serum pH: The aim of this intervention is to change the agent into a less absorbable ionized form. Acidic agents (e.g., salicylate and phenobarbital) clear more rapidly in alkaline urine. A pH level of 7.45 is desired. It is true that basic agents (PCP and amphetamines) clear more rapidly in acidic urine, but acidic urine may result in acute tubular necrosis (ATN). Thus treatment is usually not initiated to make urine more acidic. If initiated, ascorbic acid is administered.

Hemodialysis: Hemodialysis is used if the ingested drug is distributed primarily within the extracellular fluid, and it is able to penetrate the dialysis membrane. This intervention is preferred for drugs distributed in extracellular water (5). Lithium, ethylene glycol, methanol, theophylline, and salicylate may be removed using dialysis. Dialysis can reverse metabolic acidosis if it is used early before the drug diffuses into the tissue. It can correct electrolyte problems. Hemodialysis requires anticoagulation.

Hemoperfusion: This intervention is used in overdoses of digoxin, paraquat, TCAs, glutethimide, barbiturates, and acetaminophen. Hemoperfusion is used to remove lipid soluble drugs. Charcoal and ionic exchange resins serve as filters that blood passes through. This filter adsorbs the drug. Acetaminophen may be removed by hemoperfusion, decreasing the degree of hepatic toxicity associated with the drug. Hemoperfusion causes greater hemolysis than hemodialysis. It is preferred for drugs that are highly protein bound. It uses direct exposure of blood to adsorbent particles.

Continuous arteriovenous hemofiltration (CAVH): CAVH may be used with lithium toxicity. An advantage of this procedure is that hemodialysis facilities are not needed. It is a very slow process. It is used to remove agents that remain in the blood for a long period of time.

Exchange transfusion: Exchange transfusions may be used in children with lead poisoning and drugs that produce hemolytic anemia. A series of three complete transfusions may be needed to exchange and remove drugs.

Whole bowel irrigation: The aim of whole bowel irrigation is to flush pill fragments through the GI tract. Opponents argue that this procedure may distribute pills throughout the GI tract enhancing absorption. Polyethylene glycol-electrolyte solution (PEG-ELS) (Go-Lytely) is infused via a nasogastric or orogastric tube at rates varying from 200 to 2000 cc/hr for 5 hours. Up to 40 liters have been administered. This intervention can cause electrolyte abnormalities. It is good for treating sustained release drug overdoses (e.g., theophylline), metals (iron, zinc, and lead), foreign bodies, "body packers"/cocaine smuggling, and lithium. If administered with charcoal, the solution may bind with charcoal, decreasing the charcoal's ability to bind with the overdosed drug (14).

Antidotes are summarized in Table 20-1.

TABLE 20-1 Common Overdoses in the ED

Drug	Symptoms	Treatment
Acetaminophen	None initially, RUQ pain, N/V, pallor, diaphoresis 48-72 hr later	Acetylcysteine, antiemetic, cimetidine, activated charcoal
Salicylate	N/V, rapid, deep respirations, tinnitus	Sodium bicarbonate, hemodialysis, whole bowel irrigation
Alcohol	Tachycardia, hypoventilation, confusion, diplopia	Benzodiazepine, hemodialysis, lavage
Benzodiazepines	Hypotension, tachycardia, respiratory depression	Flumazenil
Tricyclic antidepressants	Bradycardia, blocks, hypotension, seizures	Lavage, activated charcoal, sodium bicarbonate, physostigmine
Opiates	Constricted pupils, hypotension, PE, bradycardia	Naloxone
Hydrocarbons	Bronchospasm, PE	Lavage
Methanol/ethylene glycol	Delayed symptoms (coma, ARF), tachycardia confusion	Ethanol IV, hemodialysis
Organophosphates	Salivation, lacrimation, urination, defecation, N/V, constricted pupils, muscle weakness	Pralidoxime chloride IV, atropine, skin/eye irrigation
Iron	Bloody vomit/stools	Deferoxamine chelating agent

Anticholinergic drugs (antihistamines, decongestants, sleeping pills)	Blurred and double vision, nonreactive dilated pupils, unable to sweat, hyperthermia, tachycardia	Physostigmine in cases of cardiac instability, lavage, activated charcoal
Calcium channel blockers	Bradycardia, blocks	Calcium, dopamine, pacemaker
Lead	Confusion, anemia	2,3-dimercaptosuccinic acid (DMSA)
Cocaine	Tachycardia, hypertension, dilated pupils, dyspnea, chest pain, thrombosis, hyperthermia, hallucinations	Whole bowel irrigation for body packets, sodium bicarbonate, alpha- / beta-blocking agents, vasodialators, ACE inhibitors, calcium channel blockers, activated charcoal, lavage
Beta-blocking agents	Bradycardia, blocks	Atropine, glucagon, whole bowel irrigation

ACE, Angiotensin-converting enzyme; *PE*, pulmonary edema.

Specific Overdoses
Acetaminophen (Tylenol)

Acetaminophen is one of the most common pharmaceutical agents involved in overdoses in the United States (13).

SYMPTOMS

- These patients look good in the ED and symptoms do not occur until later (up to 12 hours after ingestion [6]).
- Initial symptoms of acetaminophen overdose are N/V, pallor, and diaphoresis.
- They may arrive at the ED 48 to 72 hours after ingestion with right upper quadrant (RUQ) pain related to liver failure.

DIAGNOSIS

- A serum level of 140 mg/kg or greater is toxic.
- It takes at least 4 hours after ingestion for the level to be dependable.

TREATMENT

- Acetylcysteine (Mucomyst) should be given for 1 to 2 days (17 doses at 70 mg/kg or until acetaminophen level is 0) after ingestion to prevent hepatic failure (defined as AST/AAT; SGPT/SGOT >1000 IU/L). Acetylcysteine protects the liver by enhancing glutathione synthesis. Hepatic enzymes need to be monitored. When given PO, it can make the patient vomit because of smell. It may be mixed with cola or orange juice to enhance palatability.
- Antiemetics may be administered.
- Patients may also be treated with activated charcoal, since it is highly effective in binding the drug. Activated charcoal may bind acetylcysteine, but there is no evidence that it makes acetylcysteine ineffective (2,8).
- Administration of acetylcysteine has priority over the administration of charcoal. The dosing of both agents (if multiple doses of charcoal are used) can be alternated every 2 hours.
- If the patient presents >2 hours after ingestion, activated charcoal is not helpful.
- Beware if patient has preexisting liver disease because toxicity occurs at a lower level.
- Cimetidine (300 to 800 mg q 6 hr) may be used to decrease hepatotoxicity.
- The patient should not be discharged until an acetaminophen level is back.

- A liver transplant is indicated if there is early metabolic acidosis, renal failure, and prolonged prothrombin time (PT) (>100 seconds).

Salicylates (aspirin)

Salicylates are used chronically by many people; therefore, chronic as well as acute overdosage is possible, especially if they have gastric outlet problem or use an antacid.

SYMPTOMS

- N/V, tinnitus, rapid, deep respirations (secondary to metabolic acidosis and direct stimulation of respiratory center in the brainstem) occurs in salicylate overdose.

DIAGNOSIS

- Determined by serum level using a Done nomogram (Figure 20-1).

TREATMENT

- Treatment depends upon salicylate level. If the level is >30 but <60, multiple doses of charcoal are administered.
- For levels between 60 mg/dl and 125 mg/dl, alkaline diuresis is initiated.
- Hemodialysis is used in cases where the salicylate level exceeds 125 mg/dl.
- Salicylates can form large clumps (bezoars) that clog orogastric tubes. These clumps may be dialyzed. Alkalinization of the urine and serum with the use of IV sodium bicarbonate enhances excretion. The clumps may be removed by surgery.
- In cases of enteric-coated aspirin overdose, absorption may be delayed.
- Whole bowel irrigation and lavage with sodium bicarbonate may also be initiated.
- Hypertonic IV solutions are given to correct dehydration.
- Glucose is administered to correct ketosis and hypoglycemia.
- Vitamin K may be administered to treat hypoprothrombinemia and bleeding tendencies.

Alcohol

SYMPTOMS

- Alcohol intoxication produces tachycardia, hypoventilation, confusion, and seizures related to hypoglycemia.
- Diplopia is first sign of thiamine deficiency.

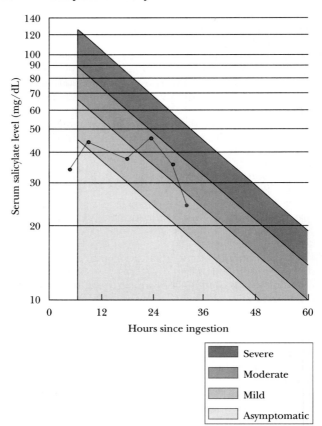

Figure 20-1 The Done nomogram showing sequential serum salicylate levels in patient who ingested toxic dose of enteric-coated aspirin. (From Pierce R, Gazewood J, Blake R: Salicylate poisoning from enteric coated aspirin: delayed absorption may complicate management, *Postgrad Med* 89(5):62.)

DIAGNOSIS
• Diagnosis is based on serum ethanol level.
TREATMENT
• Alcohol overdose is usually treated with lavage. Lavage is most effective if the patient presents <1 hour after ingestion.

- High-dose flumazenil (2 to 5 mg IVP) is being investigated.
- Hemodialysis can be used in large overdoses.
- Benzodiazepine may be given to prevent withdrawal side effects.
- In alcohol intoxication, thiamine is administered before glucose. Thiamine is used as a cofactor to make adenosine triphosphate (ATP). If you give glucose, the only available thiamine (which is already deficient) is depleted to break down the glucose. Wernicke-Korsakoff encephalopathy can occur with permanent psychosis. Chronic alcohol abusers may also have gastritis, pancreatitis, and liver disease.

Specific alcohol agent (methanol/ethylene glycol)

Methanol (e.g., antifreeze, windshield wiper fluid, paint thinner, and "boot leg" whiskey)/ethylene glycol (e.g., antifreeze, cosmetics, solvents, and paint). These agents produce delayed toxicity.

SYMPTOMS

- Symptoms are similar to alcohol intoxication.
- Slurred speech, ataxia, confusion, and tremors may be present.
- These substances may produce renal damage and metabolic coma.

DIAGNOSIS

- Diagnosis is confirmed by a specific serum methanol/ ethylene glycol level.

TREATMENT

- Ethanol may be given IV to block the conversion of methanol into more toxic substances (e.g., formaldehyde) until hemodialysis can be performed.

Benzodiazepines

(e.g., diazepam, lorazepam, and midazolam).

SYMPTOMS

- Hypotension, tachycardia, ataxia, slurred speech, respiratory depression, and hypothermia are frequently associated with benzodiazepine overdose.

DIAGNOSIS

- Positive benzodiazepine serum levels confirm the overdose.

TREATMENT

- Flumazenil (Romazicon) reverses benzodiazpenes. This medicine is administered slowly or it may cause seizures. An initial dose of 0.1 mg over 60 seconds is given.

Usually the patient regains consciousness in 5 to 15 minutes. In cases of mixed drug overdose, larger doses are needed. The dose can be repeated in 10 minutes. Most patients respond to a 3 mg dose or less.

- Before administering flumazenil, life support equipment should be at the bedside. After 30 to 45 minutes, 65% of patients become resedated.
- This antidote can be given PO, IM, IVP, or used as a continuous infusion. Side effects of seizures and dysrhythmia have been noted.
- Seizure activity may be related to quick withdrawal from chronically used benzodiazepines and not because of flumazenil administration (16). Controversy exists regarding flumazenil administration in a patient with a positive seizure history or in a mixed overdose involving TCAs because of dysrhythmia associated with TCA overdose.
- Because benzodiazepines may have a therapeutic effect in mixed overdoses involving convulsive agents (e.g., cocaine), flumazenil may not be administered to reverse sedation. Flumazenil may be used as a diagnostic aid in unexplained coma.

Tricyclic antidepressants (TCAs)

(e.g., amitriptyline, doxepin, and imipramine). These drugs vary in dose creating toxic effects and varying in absorption. It is difficult to predict an individual's response to an overdose.

SYMPTOMS

- Anticholinergic effect, produces respiratory depression, ventricular tachycardia, blocks, hypotension, seizures, agitation, hyperreflexia, arrest, and rapid deterioration without notice.
- Seizures usually occur right before cardiac arrest.

DIAGNOSIS

- Blood plasma, urine, and gastric contents are analyzed for TCA presence.

TREATMENT

- TCAs are highly bound to plasma proteins so dialysis and forced diuresis is not helpful (11).
- Lavage followed with charcoal, cathartics, and alkalinizing the blood are treatments.
- Gastric lavage is used 12 to 24 hours after ingestion because anticholinergic effect delays gastric emptying,

and TCA may be secreted back into the gut from the circulation.

- Ipecac is contraindicated as a result of the patient's rapidly deteriorating LOC.
- Sodium bicarbonate may be administered, since the effects of TCAs are diminished in an alkaline environment.
- Although controversial, physostigmine (Antilirium) may be administered. This medicine can produce seizures, bronchospasm, bradycardia, and profound atropine-like effects. A dose of 0.5 to 1 mg/min is administered IV.
- Seizures are treated with benzodiazepines followed by Dilantin (phenytoin) because it improves cardiac conduction.
- Norepinephrine is more effective in reversing hypotension than other vasopressors (dopamine is less effective because of catecholamine depletion).

Opioid (codeine and heroin)

Symptoms

- Constricted pupils, vomiting, seizures, hypotension, bradycardia, PE, respiratory depression, and coma.
- Complications arising from a heroin overdose is usually evident on arrival in the ED.
- Heroin is rapidly metabolized to morphine with an action of 4 to 5 hours.
- If patient is awake, alert, and without pulmonary complications in ED, he/she probably does not require hospitalization (7).

Diagnosis

- A urine toxicology screen is the most sensitive detecting device.
- A positive response to naloxone administration is confirmatory.

Treatment

- Naloxone 2 mg IVP is used initially. It can be administered SC, IM, or through an ET if necessary. The amount of naloxone given varies.
- Some agents (e.g., codeine, fentanyl) require large doses (approximately 35 mg) of naloxone to reverse. This should be given in 2 to 5 mg boluses.
- Naloxone drips can be used (as in methadone overdoses), but be sure you watch the patient for potential agitation.

T

- In some opiate overdoses, 12 to 18 hours after discontinuing the naloxone drip, poisoning occurs again.

Specific opioid (cocaine)

Cocaine may be administered nasally, IV, or by SC injection. Cocaine interferes with sodium permeability during depolarization, and it produces neurologic blockade of impulses.

SYMPTOMS

- Cocaine increases serum catecholamines, thus it has sympathetic nervous system effects. In the brain, cocaine blocks the uptake of dopamine and norepinephrine. In acute use, this excessive dopamine produces hyperstimulation. In chronic use, dopamine and norepinephrine are depleted in the cell because of lack of cellular uptake (10).
- Physiologically, cocaine produces increased systemic vascular resistance (hypertension), and subsequently myocardial ischemia resulting from increased afterload.
- Chest pain is a common complaint of cocaine users.
- Pupils dilate.
- Hyperthermia may result.
- Coronary vasospasm and thrombosis may result from increased platelet aggregability secondary to epinephrine release and increased thromboxane production.
- The patient may have pulmonary symptoms related to inhalation injury (freebasing) or chronic use (such as respiratory depression and PE).
- A hypermetabolic state results in weight loss, insomnia, fatigue.

DIAGNOSIS

- Same as for other opioids.

TREATMENT

- Cocaine overdose is cautiously treated with beta-blocking agents (propanolol), since the beta-blockers may result in unopposed alpha stimulation and worsening of BP.
- Alpha- and beta-blocking agents (esmolol, labetalol), ACE inhibitors, calcium channel blockers, and vasodilators may also be used.
- Ice lavage or dantrolene administered IV may be used to treat hyperthermia.

- Cocaine is metabolized to a less acute form in an alkaline medium. Whole bowel irrigation with PEG-ELS and sodium bicarbonate promotes rapid transit of cocaine into the small intestine, decreasing the risk of toxicity.
- Activated charcoal adsorbs cocaine well.
- Gastric lavage can be used if patient presents quickly after ingestion/use (body packets). Paper packets are rapidly broken down. Condom packets liberate less cocaine.

Hydrocarbons

(e.g., methane, propane, gasoline, kerosine, turpentine). Hydrocarbons vaporize at low temperatures. They enter the pulmonary tree easily.

SYMPTOMS

- Bronchospasm and PE resulting in aspiration pneumonitis.

DIAGNOSIS

- A hydrocarbon overdose is diagnosed by history and symptom presentation.

TREATMENT

- The patient must be lavaged with an ET in place because of the aspiration potential.
- Oxygen and mechanical ventilation are often needed.
- Activated charcoal poorly absorbs hydrocarbons.

Organophosphates

(e.g., commercial sprays, bug bombs, insect repellents, flea collars). Organophosphate exposure can occur through inhalation, ingestion, or the skin (3).

SYMPTOMS

- Organophosphates overstimulate the parasympathetic nervous system.
- An overdose produces SLUDGE syndrome (oversecretion) salivation, lacrimation, urination, defecation, GI manifestations, N/V, and emesis.
- Pinpoint pupils and muscle weakness occur.

DIAGNOSIS

- Diagnosis is by history and presence of symptoms.

TREATMENT

- Overdose/exposure is treated with IV atropine until pulmonary secretions dry.
- Pralidoxime chloride (Protopam) is administered as an IV drip of 2 g over 30 minutes. This medicine reactivates cholinesterase. It is most useful when administered

T

within 24 hours of exposure. Indications for use are muscle weakness and fasciculations. The dose is not based on heart rate or pupil size.

> **NURSING ALERT**
>
> The patient or family should not be given their removed clothing or any leather items. These articles absorb the pesticides for an indefinite period of time. Health care providers must avoid contact with patient secretions, since they may be contaminated.

Iron
SYMPTOMS
- Iron poisoning produces corrosive effects on the GI mucosa.
- Patients may vomit blood or have bloody stools.
- Hypovolemia may occur in children.
- Patients may not have any real ill effects for the first 6 to 8 hours.
- Patients may be inappropriately discharged from the ED after vomiting.
- Severe effects may occur later at home.
- An overdose produces anion gap acidosis and shock.

DIAGNOSIS
- Diagnosis is by abdominal radiographs and serum level.

TREATMENT
- Removed by using chelation therapy with deferoxamine.
- Approximately 100 mg of deferoxamine binds 8.5 mg of elemental iron.
- Deferoxamine is administered either IV (15 mg/kg/hr) or IM (90 mg/kg q 8 hr) until urine returns to yellow or serum iron level is normal.

Lead
SYMPTOMS
- Lethargy, decreased responsiveness, and confusion are symptoms of lead poisoning.
- Seizure activity may occur.

DIAGNOSIS
- Blood lead level >45 mcg/dl.

TREATMENT
- Lead poisoning is treated by administering a chelating agent, 2,3-DMSA. It is given orally. DMSA does not cause elimination of body stores of iron, copper, or zinc.

Anticholinergic and antihistamine drugs

These are over-the-counter drugs (e.g., sleeping pills, decongestants, antihistamines). Gypsum weed also has anticholinergic properties.

SYMPTOMS

- An overdose produces altered mental status (e.g., delirium, hallucinations), blurred and double vision, hyperreflexia, seizures, and coma.
- The patient may have dilated pupils that do not react to light because of paralysis of ciliary muscles.
- The patient is unable to sweat and may die from hyperthermia.
- Usually, an ileus and supraventricular tachycardia are present.

DIAGNOSIS

- Urine and serum toxicology screening detects these drugs.

TREATMENT

- An overdose is treated with physostigmine if the patient has tachycardia and cardiovascular instability.
- Gastric emptying and activated charcoal may be useful for several hours after ingestion as a result of slowed gastric motility.

Calcium channel and beta-blockers

(verapamil, nifedipine, diltiazem, Inderal)

These drugs decrease cardiac output and systemic vascular resistance. Individuals with preexisting pulmonary disease/asthma are at higher risk for serious complications as a result of the unopposed bronchoconstriction that occurs.

SYMPTOMS

- Bradycardia, blocks, respiratory depression, seizures, coma, and hypotension occur from an overdose of these agents.

DIAGNOSIS

- A serum drug level confirms the diagnosis.

TREATMENT

- Calcium and dopamine may be administered for calcium channel blocker overdose (9,12). The exact dose is individualized.
- Many of these agents are sustained release formulations. Patients who have taken the sustained release forms should be monitored overnight, since it may take 6 to 12 hours for effects to manifest.

T

- External pacing and pacemaker insertion may be required.
- An intraaortic balloon pump may be used to increase cardiac output.
- Atropine is administered for beta-blocker overdose.
- Glucagon is given to increase the availability of adenosine monophosphate that increases intracellular calcium. The increased calcium improves contractility and increases heart rate. A dose of 3 mg or 0.05 mg/kg to be given over 30 seconds followed by continuous infusion at 0.07 mg/kg/hr is administered.

Cardiac glycosides

(e.g., digoxin, foxglove)

SYMPTOMS

- Life-threatening dysrhythmias (e.g., bradydysrhythmias, conduction blocks, and multifocal premature ventricular contractions) and hyperkalemia may occur.

DIAGNOSIS

- Serum drug level confirms the overdose.

TREATMENT

- Emesis may enhance vagal tone and produce bradycardia. Activated charcoal may be used to absorb and to promote elimination.
- Digibind (digoxin-specific Fab antibody fragments) is used to counteract digoxin overdoses. These antibodies remove therapeutic, as well as toxic amounts, of the drug.
- Beware that the underlying condition that required digoxin use may be exacerbated (e.g., CHF).
- Electrolyte imbalances such as hyperkalemia and hypomagnesemia need to be corrected.

NURSING ALERT

Whatever antidote is ordered, make sure it is administered slowly. You do not want the patient to be totally alert, since the patient may become agitated. The medicine should be titrated. When the patient starts to sigh, stop. Try to keep the patient sleeping.

Table 20-2 summarizes common overdoses encountered in the ED.

TABLE 20-2   Common Antidotes in the ED Setting

Antidote	Common dosage	Use
Acetylcysteine	17 doses at 70 mg/kg or until acetaminophen level is 0	Acetaminophen overdose
2,3,-DMSA	30 mg/kg/day in 3 divided doses for 5 days followed by 20 mg/kg/day in 2 divided doses for 14 days*	Lead poisoning
Digoxin-specific Fab antibody fragments	Administered in equimolar dose to the digoxin load. 40 mg binds 0.6 mg of digoxin*	Cardiac glycoside overdose
Glucagon	3-5 mg up to 10 mg IVP, a continuous IV infusion may be used	Beta-blocker and calcium channel blocker overdose
Naloxone	2 mg IVP initially, can be repeated, a continuous IV infusion may be used	Opioid overdose
Flumazenil	0.2 mg IVP over 60 sec initially, if needed, 0.1 mg IVP over 60 sec can be repeated until a total dose of 1 mg is given	Benzodiazepines
Deferoxamine	1-2 g IM	Iron poisoning
Physostigmine	0.5-1 mg IVP over 60 sec	TCAs
Pralidoxime chloride	2 g IV infusion over 30 min	Organophosphates

*From Fine J, Goldfrank L: Update in medical toxicology, *Pediatr Emerg Med* 39:1031-1051, 1992.

T

NURSING SURVEILLANCE

1. Monitor responsiveness level.
2. Trend vital signs and oxygen saturation.
3. Monitor intake and output to assess fluid balance and effects of interventions.
4. Monitor for cardiac dysrhythmia.

EXPECTED PATIENT OUTCOMES

1. Level of responsiveness improves from time of arrival.
2. Mean arterial pressure is maintained between 70 and 105 mm Hg.
3. Airway remains patent without aspiration.
4. Drug absorption is inhibited.
5. ABGs trend toward normal limits.

DISCHARGE IMPLICATIONS

1. Check serum level before discharge if possible.
2. Teach family seizure precautions.
3. Teach family need for follow-up to rule out complications that may occur later.
4. Teach family about aspiration prevention, since the patient may vomit at home.
5. Beware of discharging a patient with a known overdose of acetaminophen or sustained release medications, since symptoms may occur later.

References

1. Clarke C: Drug overdose in teenagers, *Midwife Health Visitor and Community Nurse* 25:254-256, 1989.
2. Fine J, Goldfrank L: Update in medical toxicology, *Pediatr Emerg Med* 39:1031-1051, 1992.
3. Kirk M, Bowers L: Cluing in on the acutely poisoned patient, *JEMS* 16(5):64-78, 1991.
4. Palatnick W, Tenebein M: Activated charcoal in the treatment of drug overdose, *Drug Safety* 7:3-7, 1992.
5. Platt D: Pharmacokinetics of drug overdose, *Clin Lab Med* 10:261-269, 1990.
6. Pruchnicki S: Just say know: recognizing the dangers of commonplace drugs, *JEMS* 16(2):26-41, 1991.
7. Smith D, Leake L, Loflin J, Yearly D: Is admission after intravenous heroin overdose necessary? *Ann Emerg Med* 21:1326-1330, 1992.
8. Spiller H, Krenzelok E, Grande G, Safir E, Diamond J: A prospective evaluation of the effect of activated charcoal before oral N-acetylcysteine in acetaminophen overdose, *Ann Emerg Med* 23:519-523, 1994.

Specific Drugs

9. Boisvert S: A 27 year old woman with verapamil overdose, *J Emerg Nurs* 16:317-320, 1990.
10. House M: Cardiovascular effects of cocaine, *J Cardiovas Nurs* 6:1-11, 1992.

11. Johnson R, Steiner J: Tricyclic antidepressant overdose: a toxicologic emergency, *J Am Acad Physic Assist* 2(1):16-22, 1989.

12. Ramoska E, Spiller H, Winter M, Borys D: A one year evaluation of calcium channel blocker overdoses: toxicity and treatment, *Ann Emerg Med* 22:196-200, 1993.

13. Smilkstein M, Bronstein A, Linden C, Augenstein W, Kulig K, Rumack B: Acetaminophen overdose: a 48 hour intravenous *N*-acetylcysteine treatment protocol, *Ann Emerg Med* 20: 1058-1063, 1991.

Removal Techniques

14. Burkhart K, Wuerz R, Donovan J: Whole bowel irrigation as adjunctive treatment for sustained release theophylline overdose, *Ann Emerg Med* 21:1316-1320, 1992.

15. Votey S, Bayer M, Hoffman J: Flumazenil: a new benzodiazepine antagonist, *Ann Emerg Med* 20:181-188, 1991.

16. Weinbroum A, Halpern P, Geller E: The use of flumazenil in the management of acute drug poisoning: a review, *Intensive Care Med* 17:S32-38, 1991.

General Principles

17. Cuddy P, Hamburger S: Poisoning: responding to the crisis, *Physic Assist* 12:77-86, 1988.

18. ACEP: Clinical policy for the initial approach to patients presenting with toxic ingestion or dermal or inhalation exposure, *Ann Emerg Med* 25:570-585.

T

Chapter XXI

Trauma

Colleen Swartz
Steve Talbert

CLINICAL CONDITIONS
Chest Trauma
   Sentinel Injuries
   Blunt Cardiac Injury
   Cardiac Tamponade
   Aortic Transection
   Flail Chest
   Pneumothorax/Tension Pneumothorax
   Hemothorax/Tension Hemothorax
   Pulmonary Contusion
   Ruptured Diaphragm (Hemidiaphragm)
   Ruptured Bronchus/Trachea
Abdominal Trauma
Pelvic Fractures

TRIAGE ASSESSMENT

Although most trauma patients are transported to the ED by prehospital personnel, occasionally a patient may walk in or be brought to the ED by a friend or family member. It is essential that triage personnel recognize the potential severity of traumatic injury and escort the patient immediately to the treatment area where the initial assessment can occur. Care of the trauma patient begins with the primary assessment. This includes airway with cervical spine precautions, breathing, circulation, and a brief neurologic examination (deficit). Its purpose is to identify and correct any life-threatening conditions. Once the primary assessment is completed, the patient is completely exposed, covered to maintain body temperature, and a full set of vital signs is obtained. Finally, a thorough head-to-toe examination is done to identify all potential injuries. The box summarizes the trauma assessment and provides a simple acronym to help remember the proper sequence (2).

T

TRAUMA ASSESSMENT

Primary assessment

Airway with cervical spine precautions
Breathing
Circulation
Deficit (brief neurologic examination)

Secondary assessment

Expose (remove all clothing)/Evacuate (if necessary)
F (maintain body temperature)
Get full set of vital signs
Head-to-toe examination
Inspect the back

Primary Assessment
Airway with cervical spine precautions

1. Inspect for actual or potential obstruction:
   - Foreign body
   - Blood
   - Vomitus
   - Teeth
   - Tongue
   - Swelling
2. Listen and feel for air movement.

If the patient's airway is not patent, steps must be taken
   immediately to open it. Table 21-1 lists life-threatening
   airway problems, their signs and symptoms, and
   immediate interventions. A patent airway must be
   secured before proceeding with the primary assessment.

NURSING ALERT

A talking patient has a patent airway.

NURSING ALERT

Any blunt trauma patient and those experiencing penetrating
trauma above the nipple line must have their cervical spine
immobilized simultaneously with airway assessment.

TABLE 21-1 Life-Threatening Airway Problems

Problem	Signs and symptoms	Interventions
Airway obstruction (complete or partial)	• Dyspnea, labored respirations • Decreased or no air movement • Cyanosis • Presence of foreign body in airway • Trauma to face or neck	Airway opening maneuvers • Jaw thrust • Chin lift • Suction Airway adjuncts • Nasal airway • Oral airway • Endotracheal tube (ET) Surgical airway • Cricothyrotomy • Tracheostomy
Inhalation injury	• History of enclosed space fire, unconsciousness, or exposure to heavy smoke • Dyspnea • Wheezing, rhonchi, crackles • Hoarseness • Singed facial or nasal hairs • Carbonaceous sputum • Burns to face or neck	• Provide high-flow oxygen (100%) via nonrebreather mask or bag-valve device • Prepare for endotracheal intubation as soon as possible

Breathing

1. Inspect for rise and fall of chest.
   • Asymmetry may indicate a pneumothorax or hemothorax.
   • Paradoxical movement is present with a flail chest.
2. Inspect for open chest trauma.
   • Sucking chest wound may lead to a pneumothorax.
3. Inspect for work of breathing.
   • Increased work of breathing is a sign of potential breathing problems.

T

- Use of accessory muscles and nasal flaring are classic assessment findings.
4. Inspect and palpate for tracheal position.
   - The trachea will deviate away from a tension pneumothorax.
5. Auscultate lung fields for presence of breath sounds.
   - Unequal, diminished, or absent sounds may indicate a pneumothorax or hemothorax.

Initially, all trauma patients should receive 100% oxygen via nonrebreather mask or bag-valve device. Table 21-2 lists life-threatening breathing problems, their signs and symptoms, and immediate interventions.

NURSING ALERT

Tension pneumothorax is a clinical diagnosis. Treatment should not be delayed for confirmation by chest x-ray.

Circulation

1. Inspect for skin color.
   - Skin that is pale may indicate poor perfusion and shock.
2. Inspect for obvious external hemorrhage.
3. Palpate for pulse presence, rate, and quality.
   - Weak, thready, or absent pulses indicate poor perfusion and shock.
   - Tachycardia is the first and most sensitive sign of shock.
4. Palpate for skin temperature and moisture.
   - Skin that is cool and moist or diaphoretic indicates poor perfusion and shock.
5. Palpate for capillary refill.
   - Prolonged capillary refill time (>2 seconds) may indicate poor perfusion.

Initially, all trauma patients should receive two large bore intravenous (IV) lines with warm isotonic crystalloid solution infusing (Ringer's lactate or 0.9% NaCl). A large bore IV is a 14- or 16-gauge in adults and a 22-gauge or greater in pediatric patients (1). Table 21-3 lists life-threatening circulation problems, their signs and symptoms, and immediate interventions.

TABLE 21-2 Life-Threatening Breathing Problems

Problem	Signs and symptoms	Interventions
Tension pneumothorax (see the Nursing Alert box, p. 618)	• Dyspnea, labored respirations • Decreased or absent breath sounds on affected side • Unilateral chest rise and fall • Tracheal deviation away from affected side • Cyanosis • Jugular venous distention • Tachycardia and hypotension • History of chest trauma or mechanical ventilation	• Provide high-flow oxygen (100%) via nonrebreather mask or bag-valve device • Rapid chest decompression by needle thoracostomy on affected side • Chest tube placement on affected side
Pneumothorax	• Dyspnea, labored respirations • Decreased or absent breath sounds on affected side • May have unilateral chest rise and fall • May have visible wound to chest or back • History of chest trauma	• Provide high-flow oxygen (100%) via nonrebreather mask or bag-valve device • Chest tube placement on affected side • Place occlusive dressing over any open chest wound and secure on three sides with tape
Hemothorax	• Dyspnea, labored respirations • Decreased or absent breath sounds on affected side	• Provide high-flow oxygen (100%) via nonrebreather mask or bag-valve device • Chest tube placement on affected side

Continued.

TABLE 21-2 Life-Threatening Breathing Problems (cont'd)

Problem	Signs and symptoms	Interventions
	• May have unilateral chest rise and fall • Tachycardia and hypotension • May have visible wound to chest or back • History of chest trauma (usually penetrating)	• Consider autotransfusion (see Procedure 4)
Sucking chest wound	• Dyspnea, labored respirations • Visible, sucking wound to chest or back • Decreased or absent breath sounds on affected side	• Provide high-flow oxygen (100%) via nonrebreather mask or bag-valve device • Cover wound with occlusive dressing and secure on 3 sides with tape • Watch for signs of tension pneumothorax and remove dressing during exhalation if they are noted
Flail chest	• Dyspnea, labored respirations • Paradoxical chest wall movement • Chest pain • Tachycardia	• Provide high-flow oxygen (100%) via nonrebreather mask or bag-valve device • Prepare for intubation and mechanical ventilation
Full-thickness circumferential burn of thorax	• Dyspnea, labored respirations • Shallow respirations • Obvious circumferential burns to thorax	• Provide high-flow oxygen (100%) via nonrebreather mask or bag-valve device • Prepare for immediate escharotomy (see Chapter 3)

TABLE 21-3 Life-Threatening Circulation Problems

Problem	Signs and symptoms	Interventions
External hemorrhage	• Obvious bleeding site	• Direct pressure • Elevation (see box below)
Shock	• Tachycardia • Weak, thready pulses • Cool, pale, clammy skin • Tachypnea • Altered mental status • Delayed capillary refill • Oliguria or anuria	• Provide high-flow oxygen (100%) via nonrebreather mask or bag-valve device • Place two large bore IV lines with warm isotonic crystalloid solution infusing (Ringer's lactate or 0.9% NaCl) • Administer fluid bolus (2 L in adults or 20 cc/kg in children) • Prepare to administer blood

NURSING ALERT

Clamping bleeding vessels or placing a tourniquet are measures of last resort only.

Deficit (brief neurologic assessment)

The brief neurologic assessment consists of the best eye opening, best motor response, best verbal response, and pupil size and reactivity. The Glasgow coma scale score (GCS) combines the eye opening, motor response, and verbal response (Table 21-4).

1. Check for best eye opening.
   • Spontaneous to voice, to pain, or none.
2. Check for best motor response.
   • Oriented, confused, inappropriate words, incomprehensible sounds, or none.
3. Check for best verbal response.
   • Obeys commands, purposeful movement, withdraw, flexion, extension, or none.

T

TABLE 21-4 Glasgow Coma Scale

Clinical finding	Score	Clinical application
Best eye opening:		
Spontaneous	4	• Be sure to give the patient
Voice	3	the best score for
Pain	2	demonstrated eye opening
None	1	
Best motor response:		
Follows commands	6	• Localization should be tested
Purposeful to pain	5	and be present in both upper
Withdraws to pain	4	and lower extremities
Flexes to pain	3	• Be sure to give the patient
Extends to pain	2	the best score for
None	1	demonstrated motor
		response
Best verbal response:		
Oriented	5	• If the patient is intubated,
Confused	4	the score is "1" with a
Inappropriate words	3	notation of intubation
Incomprehensible		(e.g., "1T")
sounds	2	• Be sure to give the patient
None	1	the best score for verbal
		response

4. Check for pupil size and reactivity.
   • Fixed, dilated pupils are consistent with a closed-head injury.
   • Unilateral dilatation may indicate herniation.
   • Constricted pupils may indicate a drug overdose.

FOCUSED NURSING ASSESSMENT

Secondary Assessment

Once the primary assessment is complete and all life-threatening conditions are corrected, the secondary examination can be done. The secondary assessment involves a thorough head-to-toe examination and history of the events surrounding the injury.

Expose and evacuate

Expose the patient by removing all articles of clothing. If the patient is immobilized, it is usually necessary to cut off the clothes. Exposing the patient is necessary in order to rapidly identify all injuries. Evacuation may be necessary in order to match resources to patient needs.

Fahrenheit

The patient should not be left uncovered. Hypothermia in the trauma patient is common and has severe detrimental effects. Measures should be taken to preserve body heat and prevent hypothermia. These include warm blankets, special warming blankets, increasing the temperature of the resuscitation room, use of warming lights, and use of warm IV fluids. If continuous temperature monitoring is available (e.g., rectal probe or temperature-sensing indwelling urinary catheter), then it should be used to ensure the prevention of hypothermia.

Vital Signs

A full set of vital signs should be obtained as quickly as possible. These include heart rate, respiratory rate, blood pressure (BP), and a core body temperature.

Head-to-toe examination

The head-to-toe examination is a thorough and systematic assessment of the entire body. It includes auscultation, inspection, palpation, and percussion.

- *Head and neck:* The head should be inspected for obvious wounds (e.g., lacerations, contusions, abrasions, or burns), external hemorrhage, deformities, impaled objects, or drainage from the nose (rhinorrhea) or ears (otorrhea). It should be palpated for deformities, areas of tenderness, or subcutaneous air. Furthermore, the stability of the midface and alignment of the teeth should be assessed.

The neck should be assessed for any obvious wounds, external hemorrhage, or impaled objects. Presence or absence of jugular venous distention (JVD) should be noted. Tracheal position should be palpated. Any areas of tenderness should be noted. Auscultation of bruits over major vessels may indicate vascular injury.

T

NURSING ALERT

Alignment of the cervical spine must be maintained during assessment of the neck.

- *Chest:* The chest should be inspected for signs of obvious injury including the presence of a sucking chest wound, external hemorrhage, or impaled objects. Rise and fall of the chest wall should be observed for symmetry and equality. Palpate the chest wall for tenderness, crepitus, and presence of subcutaneous air. Finally, auscultate for depth, quality, and equality of breath sounds. Presence or absence of bowel sounds in the chest should be noted as well.

- *Abdomen:* Abdominal assessment begins by inspecting the abdomen for signs of obvious trauma, external hemorrhage, or impaled objects. Next, auscultate for bowel sounds in all quadrants. The abdomen should be palpated for areas of tenderness, firmness, and distention. Rigidness, distention, and pain are indicators of possible internal injury and ongoing hemorrhage.

- *Pelvis:* The pelvis should be inspected for signs of obvious trauma, external hemorrhage, or impaled objects. Next, it should be palpated for tenderness and stability. This is accomplished by pushing downward simultaneously on the anterior aspect of the iliac crests, followed by pushing inward simultaneously on the lateral aspect of the iliac crests. Finally, gentle pressure should be applied to the symphysis pubis. As a general rule, this assessment illicits pain or reveals instability if the pelvis is fractured.

- *Genitourinary:* The genitourinary and gynecologic assessment begins with inspection for signs of obvious trauma, external hemorrhage, impaled objects, blood at the urethral meatus, vaginal bleeding, or a scrotal hematoma. If blood is present at the urethral meatus, insertion of an indwelling urinary catheter should be postponed until the patency of the urethra is confirmed. All women should receive a vaginal examination to rule out any internal injuries.

- *Extremities:* Finally, the extremities should be assessed. Inspect for signs of obvious trauma, external hemorrhage, impaled objects, or deformities. Palpate each extremity for areas of tenderness or deformity, determine capillary refill time, and assess pulse presence and quality. Pulse quality should be compared bilaterally simultaneously for equality. Likewise, sensation should be checked for each extremity and compared bilaterally for equality. Lastly, range of motion may be checked unless contraindicated.

Inspect the back

> **NURSING ALERT**
>
> Cervical spine immobilization must be maintained while the patient is logrolled and the back assessed. Neurologic checks for movement and sensation of extremities should be performed before and immediately after the logroll.

The patient should be carefully logrolled onto either side. Inspect the back, buttocks, and dorsal side of lower extremities for signs of obvious trauma, external hemorrhage, or impaled objects. The spine should be palpated for areas of tenderness or deformity. Rectal tone should be determined and stool checked for presence of blood. The position of the prostate should also be established in all male trauma patients before insertion of an indwelling urinary catheter. When the back assessment is complete, the patient should be carefully rolled back into the supine position.

> **NURSING ALERT**
>
> Before performing the rectal examination, the practitioner should put on a new glove. This minimizes the risk of a false positive reading for rectal bleeding.

History

Another component of the secondary assessment is obtaining a rapid, focused history that provides important data for anticipating injuries and guiding patient care. This history includes *AMPLE A*llergies, *M*edications, *P*ast medical history, *L*ast oral intake, and *E*vents surrounding the traumatic event (e.g., mechanism of injury, seat belt or helmet use, type of weapon used, and loss of consciousness after the injury). The acronym AMPLE can serve as a reminder for the information needed. The history should include mechanism of injury, extent of injuries (based on prehospital assessment), vital signs in the field and interventions in the field (MIVI) (3).

T

Risk Factors
Age
Trauma is the leading cause of death during the first four decades of life. Although it is historically a disease of the young, trauma in the geriatric population is a growing problem. The mechanisms of injury differ for these age groups. Younger patients are frequently involved in motor vehicle crashes (driver, passenger, and pedestrian or bicyclist) or violence. The leading cause of injury in the geriatric population is falling.

Preexisting medical conditions
Certain medical conditions can predispose patients to injury. These diseases create one of several conditions that increase the risk of injury, such as altered level of consciousness, altered sensory input, or altered thought processes. Table 21-5 lists common chronic medical conditions and their mechanism for predisposing patients to traumatic injury.

Medications
As with preexisting medical conditions, certain medications can predispose patients to injury. Drugs that directly or indirectly alter the mental status are the prime contributors. Table 21-6 lists classes of medications and their mechanism for predisposing patients to traumatic injury.

Life Span Issues

NURSING ALERT

Assessment and intervention priorities are the same for all patients regardless of age.

Pediatric
GENERAL CONSIDERATIONS
1. Blunt trauma is the leading cause of injury, accounting for up to 80% of all pediatric trauma.
2. Deterioration of the child's clinical condition may be insidious—frequent systems reassessment is critical.
3. Children have higher metabolic rates and require increased amounts of oxygen and substrates.
4. The skeletal system is immature and flexible. It does provide protection for underlying structures.

TABLE 21-5 Common Medical Conditions that Increase Risk for Injury

Medical condition	Mechanism of increased risk	Etiology of increased risk
Diabetes mellitus	Altered level of consciousness	Hypoglycemia
		Hyperglycemia
Seizures	Altered level of consciousness	Hitting head or face
		Fracture extremity
		Fall into path of vehicle
Cardiovascular disease	Altered level of consciousness	Syncope
Peripheral vascular disease	Altered sensory input	Orthostatic hypotension
		Dysrhythmias
		Myocardial infarction
		Cerebral vascular accident
		Transient ischemic attack
		Neuropathies
Substance abuse	Altered level of consciousness	Altered judgement
	Altered sensory input	Altered reflexes
	Altered thought process	Unconsciousness
Psychiatric illness	Altered thought process	Depression
		Suicidal ideation
		Self-destructive behavior

T

TABLE 21-6 Common Medication Classes that Increase Risk of Injury

Medication class	Etiology of increased risk of injury
Antidiabetic	Hypoglycemia
Antiseizure	Depressed level of consciousness
Antihypertensives	Syncope
	Orthostatic hypotension
Antidysrhythmias	Hypotension
	Bradycardia
	Dysrhythmias
Antihistamines	CNS depression
Antineoplastics	Anemia
Antipsychotics	Extrapyramidal symptoms
	Hypotension
	Dysrhythmias
Barbiturates	CNS depression
Benzodiazepines	CNS depression
Diuretics	Hypovolemia
	Hypotension
	Electrolyte imbalances
Narcotics	CNS depression
Thyroid hormone	Thyroid storm

CNS, Central nervous system.

Consequently, a serious underlying injury may be present in the absence of fractures.

5. Children, especially young children, have immature or inadequate thermoregulation. Prevention of heat loss through the use of warmed fluids, blankets, and environment is critical.

6. Children have immature immune systems. Prevention of infection through the use of strict sterile technique is important.

7. Presence of the primary caregiver is important to help the child cope with the stress of a traumatic injury.

8. When assessing the child and intervening, keep the child's developmental level in mind.

Airway/Breathing

1. Children <12 months of age are obligatory nose breathers. Nasal passages must remain clear unless an artificial airway (e.g., endotracheal tube [ET]) is provided.

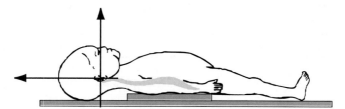

Figure 21-1 Proper spinal immobilization for children less than 8 years of age. (Adapted from Nypaver M, Treloar T: Cervical spine positioning, *Ann Emerg Med* 23:209, 1994.)

2. The trachea is shorter and more anterior in children. Intubation may be difficult.
3. Uncuffed ET use in smaller children necessitates frequent respiratory assessments to confirm placement. Securing these tubes is critical.
4. Provide high-flow oxygen (100%) via nonrebreather mask, bag-valve device, or mechanical ventilator.

CERVICAL SPINE
1. Children <8 years of age should have padding placed under their back and shoulders to alleviate flexion of the cervical spine. Figure 21-1 illustrates proper spinal immobilization for children.

CIRCULATION
1. Children compensate well for hypovolemia and clinical shock symptoms (especially hypotension) may be masked for a prolonged period of time.
2. Peripheral IV size selection should be as large as possible.
• Infant: 20 to 24 gauge
• Young child: 16 to 20 gauge
• Older child: 18 gauge or larger
3. Interosseous fluid and drug administration is an option if peripheral access cannot be obtained.
4. Fluid volume replacement is as follows:
• 20 ml/kg of isotonic crystalloid solution rapid IV push.
• If no response, repeat 20 ml/kg bolus of isotonic crystalloid solution IV push.
• If shock state persists, administer 10 ml/kg packed red blood cells IV push.
• Repeat blood administration as necessary.

T

NURSING ALERT

Hypothermia has severe detrimental effects on the pediatric trauma patient. All fluids should be warmed before administration if possible. Blood should be mixed with warm saline or given via blood warmer.

TABLE 21-7 Pediatric Glasgow Coma Scale (Children Ages 3 and Under)

Clinical finding		Score
Eye opening:		
Spontaneous		4
Reaction to speech		3
Reaction to pain		2
No response		1
Motor response:		
Spontaneous (obeys commands)		6
Localizes to pain		5
Withdraws to pain		4
Abnormal flexion to pain		3
Abnormal extension to pain		2
No response		1
Verbal response:		
Smiles, oriented to sound, follows objects, interacts		5
Crying	**Interacts**	
Consolable	Inappropriate	4
Inconsistently consolable	Moaning	3
Inconsolable	Irritable, restless	2
No response	No response	1

DEFICIT
1. When assessing mental status, keep the patient's development level in mind.
2. Table 21-7 is the pediatric GCS.

Geriatric

GENERAL CONSIDERATIONS
1. Hallmark of aging is a diminished ability to compensate (loss of physiologic reserve).
2. Mortality is higher in the geriatric population for every body region.

3. Mortality increases with age up to 85 years.
4. Falling is the leading cause of injury in the geriatric population.
5. Geriatric patients have an increased mortality from motor vehicle crashes and burns.
6. Physiologic changes are seen in every system and vary with lifestyle and preexisting medical conditions.
7. Response to medication can be altered with age because of altered body tissue (e.g., decreased lean body mass and increased adipose tissue), altered receptor response, altered absorption (e.g., decreased GI blood flow), or altered metabolism (e.g., decreased renal clearance).
8. Immune response is diminished. Careful attention to prevention of infection is important.
9. Thermoregulation, especially the ability to generate heat is also diminished. Steps to prevent hypothermia should be taken immediately. Core temperature should be continuously monitored if possible.
10. Medication use may further reduce the ability to compensate and/or mask clinical signs of shock. They may also impact on the effectiveness of interventions.

AIRWAY/BREATHING

1. There is a generalized reduction in pulmonary function.
2. Preexisting diseases (e.g., chronic obstructive pulmonary disease) may have a significant impact on compensatory mechanisms for shock.

CERVICAL SPINE

1. Arthritic changes may complicate assessment and immobilization.
2. Composition changes (e.g., osteoporosis) increase the likelihood of injury.

CIRCULATION

1. If arteriosclerosis or peripheral vascular disease are present, higher arterial pressures (hypertension) may be necessary to perfuse organs and extremities. "Normal" BPs may be present even though a state of inadequate tissue perfusion exists.
2. Fluids should be administered with caution. Do not withhold needed volume, but frequent reassessment of the cardiovascular and respiratory systems should be performed. Watch closely for signs of fluid overload.

T

3. Many geriatric patients are candidates for early invasive monitoring, and it should be used to guide resuscitation efforts if available.

DEFICIT

Cognitive skills may be slowed or diminished with increasing age and certain degenerative diseases (e.g., Alzheimer's and dementia). Make an early effort to determine a baseline neurologic status from reliable sources.

Obstetric

GENERAL CONSIDERATIONS

1. Motor vehicle crashes are the leading cause of maternal injury.
2. Intravascular fluid volume, cardiac output, minute ventilation, and oxygen consumption increase during pregnancy.
3. Normal WBC counts may be as high as 25,000.
4. Normal hematocrit and hemoglobin are decreased.
5. Gastric emptying and peristalsis are slowed.
6. Maternal concern may be focused on the well being of the fetus. Reassurance is important.

AIRWAY/BREATHING

Increased oxygen consumption requires an increase in oxygen delivery. Provide all pregnant trauma patients with high-flow oxygen.

CERVICAL SPINE

Fully immobilize the pregnant patient.

CIRCULATION

1. Increased plasma volume allows for maternal compensation, but harm may come to the fetus because of decreased oxygen and substrate supply.
2. Pregnant women may compensate for a prolonged period with only minimal clinical signs.
3. The supine position, especially in later gestation, causes the uterus to rest on the inferior vena cava, resulting in diminished venous return which, in turn, decreases cardiac output. The pregnant patient should be rolled slightly to the left side while immobilization is maintained.

INITIAL INTERVENTIONS

Once the primary and secondary assessments are complete and all life-threatening conditions are corrected, other initial interventions may be necessary.

1. Gastric distention poses two potential problems in the trauma patient. First, distention pushes a full stomach upward into the diaphragm decreasing pulmonary capacity and, consequently, gas exchange. Furthermore, gastric distention increases the risk of vomiting and aspiration. Decompression of the stomach should be accomplished via a nasogastric tube as early in the resuscitation as possible.

NURSING ALERT

If a basilar skull fracture is suspected, or if the midface is unstable, the gastric tube should be passed orally not nasally.

2. Bladder distention also poses a unique set of problems. Not only is it very uncomfortable for the patient, but it can increase anxiety, BP, and heart rate as well. An indwelling urinary catheter should be placed as early in the resuscitation as possible.

NURSING ALERT

Before an indwelling urinary catheter may be inserted, the meatus should be assessed for bleeding or signs of trauma. In males, assessment for a scrotal hematoma and prostate size and position must be done before catheter placement.

3. Other interventions include tetanus prophylaxis, dressing wounds, and immobilization of any known or suspected fractures.

4. Finally, the psychosocial interventions are an important part of the resuscitation. Trauma patients are under extreme stress and usually in a state of crisis. It is natural for them to mobilize usual coping mechanisms in order to adapt. However, normal coping mechanisms may be quickly overwhelmed by fear, pain, and loss of control. The nurse should facilitate the use of normal coping mechanisms, reduce anxiety and pain, and give the patient as much control as possible. Interventions such as informing the patient of procedures before they are done, maintaining eye contact, holding a hand, or taking time to listen can facilitate coping. Allowing a significant other to remain at or near the bedside may improve adaptation as well.

T

5. Significant others (e.g., family and friends) may also be experiencing feelings of anxiety, fear, anger, and guilt. Taking time to keep them informed of the patient's condition and prognosis is critical for their coping. Furthermore, allowing them to see the patient as quickly as possible and reassuring them that the trauma team truly cares about the patient also helps them deal with the crisis.

PRIORITY NURSING DIAGNOSES

Risk for altered tissue perfusion
Risk for pain
Risk for alteration in gas exchange

◆ **Altered tissue perfusion** related to hypoperfusion and shunting of blood.
   INTERVENTIONS
   • Initiate two large bore IVs for fluid resuscitation.
   • Administer warmed Ringer's lactate or 0.9% NaCl solution as indicated to maintain systolic BP ≥90 mm Hg and urine output 1 cc/kg/hr.
   • Apply pressure to external sources of bleeding.
   • Monitor for internal bleeding, abdominal rigidity, expanding hematomas, decreasing level of consciousness, diminishing breath sounds, dullness on lung percussion.
◆ **Pain** related to stimulation of nerve endings.
   INTERVENTIONS
   • Administer IM/IV nonsteroidal antiinflammatory agents per physician order.
   • Position of comfort postclearance for spinal fractures
   • Use of imagery
   • Use of distraction
   • Allow presence of support systems
◆ **Alteration in gas exchange** related to occluded or partially occluded airway, chest and lung injury, as well as hypoperfusion.
   INTERVENTIONS
   • Maintain patent airway, suction as necessary.
   • Administer high flow O_2 per mask or BVD and ET.
   • Monitor breath sounds, chest well excursion and movement.
   • Prepare for chest tube insertion if appropriate.

- Monitor ABGs, blood lactate levels, SaO_2 readings.

PRIORITY DIAGNOSTIC TESTS

During the initial resuscitation of the trauma patient, priority diagnostic tests should be individualized based on mechanism of injury and clinical findings. However, there are a number of laboratory tests, radiographic examinations, and special procedures that may be anticipated. Tables 21-8 to 21-10 list common diagnostic tests and special procedures, their clinical indications, and clinical implications.

COLLABORATIVE INTERVENTIONS

Although trauma may affect every body region and system, this chapter focuses on injuries to the chest, abdomen, and pelvis. Trauma to other regions are discussed in the appropriate chapters.

Clinical Conditions
Chest trauma
For patients admitted with chest injury, only 15% require thoracotomy for definitive management. Thus, 85% of patients with chest injury can be managed with general resuscitative techniques including ventilatory support, tube thoracostomy, or other interventions for management of chest injury.

Sentinel injuries
Some injury patterns are not particularly life threatening, in and of themselves, but should raise your suspicion of other potentially life-threatening injuries. These injuries are termed sentinel injuries and should prompt the emergency nurse to watch for the more life-threatening associated injuries. The sentinel injuries of particular importance are outlined in the box, p. 639.

Blunt cardiac injury
SYMPTOMS
- Anginal chest pain, dyspnea, hypoperfusion, hypotension may be present.
- Symptoms vary depending upon extent of contusion.
- The patient may present in frank left ventricular failure with crackles on auscultation, presence of S_3, and JVD.

TABLE 21-8 Common Laboratory Tests

Laboratory test	Clinical implications
Complete blood count (CBC)	• Hematocrit and hemoglobin may be normal or above normal despite acute hemorrhage. Normal values do not exclude hemorrhagic shock
Electrolytes	• Baseline data • Rule out electrolyte imbalance
Protime (PT) Prothrombin time (PTT)	• Baseline data • Rule out coagulopathies
Amylase	• Baseline data • Elevated value may indicate possible intraabdominal injury
Lipase	• Baseline data • Elevated value may indicate possible intraabdominal injury
Lactate	• Baseline data • Elevated level correlates with acute hemorrhage, shock, and increased anaerobic metabolism
Arterial blood gas (ABG)	• Assess ventilatory and respiratory status • Acidosis, especially in the presence of normal or decreased $PaCO_2$ level correlates with shock • Base deficit of −6 or greater correlates with acute hemorrhage and shock • Decreased PaO_2 and SaO_2 and an elevated $PaCO_2$ may indicate an airway or breathing emergency
Liver function tests (LFTs)	• Baseline data • Elevated values may indicate liver damage
Type and crossmatch	• Prepare for administration of blood and blood products

TABLE 21-9 Common Radiographic Examinations

Radiographic examination	Indication	Clinical implications
Chest x-ray	Chest trauma or pain Shortness of breath	• Anteroposterior examination with patient in supine position if immobilized. • Should be taken immediately upon arrival if possible. • Do not delay treatment of a suspected tension pneumothorax for a chest x-ray.
Pelvis x-ray	Blunt trauma Pelvic pain or instability Blood at urethral meatus	• Anteroposterior examination with patient in supine position.
Cervical spine x-ray	Blunt trauma Trauma above nipple line Neck tenderness Neurologic deficit	• Should be taken early in the resuscitation. • Cross-table lateral film usually obtained early in resuscitation. • Immobilization should be maintained until spine is radiographically and clinically cleared.
Thoracic and lumbar spine x-ray	Blunt trauma Back pain or trauma Neurologic deficit	• Patient should be logrolled until spine is cleared radiographically and clinically.
Extremity x-rays	Extremity trauma, deformity, or pain	• Suspected fractures should be immobilized before radiographs.
Head CT	Head trauma Loss of consciousness Focal neurologic findings Altered level of consciousness	• Transfer to a definitive care facility should not be delayed to obtain a head computerized tomography (CT).
Abdominal CT	Abdominal trauma or pain Altered level of consciousness Unreliable clinical examination	• Transfer to a definitive care facility should not be delayed to obtain an abdominal CT.

T

637

TABLE 21-10 Common Special Procedures

Procedure	Indication	Clinical implications
Angiography	Suspected vessel injury Cerebral blood flow study	• Be prepared to assess and intervene in the event of an anaphylactic reaction. • Insertion site must be watched closely for bleeding after procedure.
Ultrasound	Abdominal trauma Unable to perform diagnostic peritoneal lavage or abdominal CT	—
Diagnostic peritoneal lavage	Abdominal trauma or pain, especially in a hemodynamically unstable patient	• Gastric and bladder decompression must be done before performing a diagnostic peritoneal lavage. • This procedure does not evaluate the retroperitoneal space.
Transesophageal echocardiogram	Widened mediastinum Significant chest trauma	• Patient is usually rolled on side for procedure. • Patient may be sedated during procedure.

- A 12-lead ECG may reveal conduction/rhythm disturbances.
- PACs, PVCs, atrial fibrillation/flutter, ventricular tachycardia, and bundle branch block (especially right bundle branch block, since the right ventricle is situated to the right of the sternum, positioned anteriorly leaving

---

SENTINEL INJURY AND ASSOCIATED INJURY PATTERN

- First rib fracture: Heart/great vessel injury (subclavian vein and artery), CNS injury (head/neck)
- Scapula fracture: Brachial plexus, pulmonary contusion, great vessel, CNS injury
- Sternal fracture: Blunt cardiac injury, great vessel, pulmonary contusion
- Right lower rib fractures: Liver lacerations
- Left lower rib fractures: Spleen lacerations

---

it virtually unprotected with a high-energy impact) may occur.

DIAGNOSIS

- A 12-lead ECG and transthoracic or transesophageal imaging may be used for diagnosis.
- Some institutions utilize CPK and LDH with isoenzymes to evaluate blunt cardiac injury, however, these fail to detect one-third to one-half of patients who have actual myocardial damage detected via transthoracic imaging.
- Review your institutional blunt cardiac injury evaluation protocol.

TREATMENT

- Evaluate and intervene during primary assessment and evaluation of airway, breathing, and circulation.
- Oxygen should be applied and vigilant ECG monitoring should ensue with early recognition and treatment of dysrhythmias.
- Potential pump failure with large contusional patterns may occur, and interventions should be initiated accordingly to maximize contractility (addition of inotropes, maximizing filling pressures), reduce afterload (addition of vasodilators), and optimize preload (optimizing volume status via volume infusion or diuresis, infusion of vasoactives).
- Central venous pressures should be monitored closely to guide volume resuscitation.
- ICU or telemetry admission is likely and should be anticipated early during the patient's resuscitation.

T

Cardiac tamponade

Cardiac tamponade is actually an expression of injury (blunt or penetrating). Manifestation is denoted by a rapid accumulation of blood in the pericardial sac, resulting in restriction of myocardial pump motion, as well as, restriction of chamber filling. Diminished stroke volume occurs along with a noticeable increase in chamber pressures.

SYMPTOMS

- Anxiety, dyspnea, duskiness/cyanosis.
- Beck's triad: hypotension, muffled heart tones, JVD. Beck's triad manifests all three facets in only 35% to 65% of cases.
- Kussmaul's sign (a paradoxical rise in venous pressure with inspiration when breathing spontaneously) may occur when the patient inspires deeply.
- A progression of JVD occurs instead of the normal flattening of the jugular vein with deep inspiration.

DIAGNOSIS

- Because cardiac tamponade and tension pneumothorax present similarly, auscultation of breath sounds is crucial to diagnosis.
- The patient with cardiac tamponade will have adequate, equilateral breath sounds.
- The patient with a tension pneumothorax, tension hemothorax, or tension viscerothorax will not have clear, equal breath sounds.
- Transthoracic or transesophageal imaging should be anticipated if the patient's condition is amenable to further diagnostic evaluation.
- With acute deterioration, prepare for pericardiocentesis.

TREATMENT

- High-flow oxygen to maximize DO_2 (oxygen delivery).
- Prepare for pericardiocentesis. Have a basin available to evaluate the aspirated blood for coagulability and send a specimen to the lab to analyze hematocrit.
- Inherent to the procedure is the possibility of puncture of an uninjured chamber.
- Ongoing evaluation for recurrence of tamponade or creating an environment conducive to development of tamponade (by puncturing an uninjured chamber) must be considered and remain in the decision tree for ongoing assessment.

- Should the patient experience acute deterioration, prepare for open, resuscitative thoracotomy to decompress the pericardial effusion.
- Adequate technique and equipment is essential to the success of this procedure and should be done in centers where surgical backup is readily available (see Procedure 24).

Aortic transection

Eighty-five percent of patients with acute aortic transection expire before reaching the hospital. The 15% who live to make it to the hospital usually are experiencing aortic dissection. Remember, the vessel has three layers of tissue—the intima, the media, and the adventitia. With dissection the intimal and possibly the medial walls are torn. However, the adventitial layer is intact, containing a ballooning pseudoaneurysm or allowing for dissection down into the layers of the vessel. These patients are extremely fragile and must be diagnosed quickly and transferred where cardiothoracic services are immediately available. The usual site of injury is just distal to the subclavian artery at the ligamentum arteriosum that tethers the aorta posteriorly creating a focal point for the dissipation of the shear forces in blunt injury.

SYMPTOMS

- A conscious patient typically complains of intense and severe midscapular/low back pain possibly referring down into the pelvic area and lower extremities.
- Dyspnea, tachycardia, and anxiety are often evident.
- Pulse amplitude is often magnified in upper extremities and diminished in lower extremities.
- Acute coarctation syndrome may manifest itself (hypertension in upper extremities and hypotension in lower extremities).
- During auscultation, a harsh systolic parascapular murmur may be heard.
- Patients quite typically present with impressive variability in hemodynamic parameters, especially BP variability.
- Quite typically, patients' BPs may vary from 40 to 60 mm Hg diastolic to 150 to 170 mm Hg systolic. Such wide swings in hemodynamic parameters should encourage consideration of aortic dissection in the differential.

DIAGNOSIS

- Radiographic evaluation of the chest, specifically the mediastinum, with the following findings: Widened mediastinum, loss of aortic knob shadow (may be hazy or obscured), deviation of trachea to the right (if the patient is nasogastrically intubated, the nasogastric tube will also deviate to the right), left apical pleural cap, depressed/downward displacement of the left mainstem bronchus.

  Confirmation of the diagnosis of the aortic dissection has traditionally been done via aortography, however more studies are validating the role of transesophageal imaging for detection of acute aortic dissection. Transesophageal echo (TEE) circumvents the need for dye load, transport off site to special procedures, and arterial access. Nationally, aortography remains the gold standard for confirmation of diagnosis.

TREATMENT

- Hypervolemia should be avoided to minimize additional wall stress on the already stressed vessel.
- Intensive BP monitoring must be done to evaluate hypotension, as well as to treat hypertension as necessary, to avoid additional dissection of the aorta and possible rupture.
- Beta-blockers and other pharmacologics are given to reduce afterload thereby minimizing vessel wall stress and turbulent flow.
- A tube thoracostomy with autotransfusion may be performed for excessive blood loss.
- Resuscitative/open thoracotomy may be conducted to facilitate emergent surgical control of the aorta (see Procedure 14).
- Once the diagnosis is confirmed, anticipate hasty transport to the operating room with an armamentarium of blood products to minimize the potential for acute and excessive blood loss.

Flail chest/Multiple rib fractures

SYMPTOMS

- Crepitance over fracture sites may be palpated, pain is expressed by the patient, expression of concomitant tissue injury may be evident (e.g., pulmonary contusion, pneumothorax, hemothorax).

- Paradoxical chest wall movement with inspiration/expiration is indicative of a flail segment.
- The patient may also experience acute oxygen desaturation because of the contusional pattern that may create a shunt.

  The concept of shunt implies adequate perfusion to nonventilated alveoli. Some degree of physiologic shunt (2% to 5%) occurs in healthy individuals, however shunt resulting from pulmonary contusion, atelectasis, a right mainstem intubation, etc. may result in shunt as high as 40% to 50%. This obviously will tremendously affect gas exchange (both onloading oxygen to hemoglobin and offloading CO_2 for exhalation).

DIAGNOSIS

- Chest radiograph remains the hallmark in diagnosis of rib fractures and flail segment (two or more rib fractures at two or more adjacent sites).
- The diagnosis of flail chest can also be a clinical diagnosis without the necessity of a chest radiograph.
- Clinical evaluation of the chest wall movement may lead the clinician to the diagnosis of flail chest.

TREATMENT

- Tube thoracostomy is performed for pneumothoraces and hemothoraces.
- Intubation and positive pressure ventilation may be used for pulmonary contusion with flail segment.
- Pain management is critical in these patients in order to maximize respiratory effort/gaseous exchange and minimize atelectasis/pneumonia.
- Alternative methods for adequate pain management include analgesic IV administration, epidural anesthetic for pain management, traditional approaches to pain control, as well as other pain management techniques, such as imagery and therapeutic touch.
- Vigilant monitoring of oxygen saturation, respiratory effort, work of breathing, and CO_2 are critical in ongoing evaluation of respiratory function.
- An arterial line may be placed to facilitate serial ABG measurement and real-time BP monitoring.

Pneumothorax/Tension pneumothorax

A pneumothorax is manifested by the entry of air into the pleural space with loss of negative pressure resulting in partial or total collapse of the lung parenchyma on the affected side. A pneumothorax may progress to a tension pneumothorax if air continues to enter the pleural space with no mechanism for escape on exhalation. Pressure continues to rise within the thoracic cavity with collapse of lung parenchyma on the affected side. Unrelieved, the pressure shifts the heart, great vessels, and trachea and eventually collapses the contralateral lung. Detection and treatment of a tension pneumothorax should be conducted within the context of the primary assessment.

NURSING ALERT

You should be particularly concerned with the development of a pneumothorax/tension pneumothorax should the patient require intubation and positive pressure ventilation for the injuries sustained. Positive pressure ventilation can quickly convert a simple pneumothorax to a tension pneumothorax, thus a high index of suspicion must be maintained after intubation.

SYMPTOMS

- Dyspnea, tachypnea, hyperpnea, diminished or absent breath sounds ipsilateral, possibly diminished sounds bilateral if tension pneumothorax has progressed and is compressing contralateral lung parenchyma.
- Subcutaneous emphysema is possible with the development of a tension pneumothorax as is tracheal deviation away from the involved hemithorax.
- JVD may occur as can hypotension if severe compression of the thoracic mediastinal structures ensue.

DIAGNOSIS

- Clinical diagnosis is more than adequate. A radiograph is not and should not be necessary to make diagnosis.

TREATMENT

- Immediate decompression is indicated using needle or tube thoracostomy (see Procedure 7).
- Typically, a rush of air with either decompressive technique is heard and/or felt.
- An immediate improvement in the patient's condition and clinical appearance usually occurs within minutes after the decompression of a tension pneumothorax.

NURSING ALERT

REMEMBER: Once needle thoracostomy has been performed, a chest tube must follow to ensure adequate and ongoing, definitive chest management. The chest drainage system should be monitored closely for output and air leak (see Procedure 7).

Hemothorax/Tension hemothorax

The presence of blood in the pleural space represents a hemothorax. Each hemithorax can contain up to 2.5 liters of blood, thereby precipitating hemorrhagic shock with acute or ongoing blood loss.

SYMPTOMS

- Dyspnea, hyperpnea, dullness on percussion, oxygen desaturation, diminished or absent breath sounds on side of injury, possibly symptoms of shock state if blood loss is excessive.
- With tension hemothorax, the clinical presentation is same as tension pneumothorax, except the causative agent is blood instead of air.

DIAGNOSIS

- Usually detected via clinical examination.
- However, if the hemothorax is small (<250 ml), a chest radiograph may be necessary to definitively diagnose hemothorax.
- An anteroposterior film may not delineate the hemothorax if it is small, an upright chest may be necessary to allow the blood to collect and reveal itself radiographically.

TREATMENT

- Tube thoracostomy (see Procedure 7).
- Prepare for autotransfusion if the hemothorax is known to be or is suspected to be large (see Procedure 4).
- Monitor chest drainage closely.
- If the patient has >1000 cc out initially or evidences ongoing blood loss of >200 cc/hr for 3 to 4 hours, elective surgical thoracotomy may be pursued (in children, >5 ml/kg/hr).

Pulmonary contusion

Approximately 75% of patients with blunt chest trauma have some degree of underlying pulmonary contusion.

Signs and symptoms of the contusion may take as long as 48 hours to manifest themselves, especially in children. Again, a high index of suspicion is critical in evaluation and management of these patients. Initial lung hemorrhage occurs with interstitial and alveolar edema at the site of contusion with general inflammation developing. Ventilation/perfusion mismatching develops (shunt) resulting in systemic hypoxia and hypercapnea.

SYMPTOMS

- Surface ecchymosis over chest wall may be present, hyperpnea (without subsequent auscultation of breath sounds that would be expected with degree of hyperpnea).
- Diminished respiratory excursion, hemoptysis, and oxygen desaturation usually occur with pulmonary contusion.

DIAGNOSIS

- Chest radiograph initially may reveal contusional pattern, this may "fluff out" in 48 to 72 hours.

TREATMENT

- Supportive therapy is indicated as dictated by patient's condition.
- Intubation and positive pressure ventilation may be necessary to minimize shunting.
- Pain control is essential to maximize alveolar insufflation in the patient with pulmonary contusion.
- Vigilant monitoring of oxygen saturation is required.
- Judicious administration of IV fluids (crystalloid and colloid) so as not to exacerbate tissue edema should be the rule of thumb.
- Simultaneous independent lung ventilation (SILV) may be considered to minimize barotrauma sustained by the "good" lung. A double-lumen ET is necessary to achieve this but may be done in the ED.

Ruptured diaphragm (Hemidiaphragm)

Usually results from a rapid deceleration injury. Ruptured diaphragm is more common on the left than the right. This may be due to protection on the right by the liver or because of the pattern of the kinetic energy dissipated with certain types of injury. The diaphragm rupture allows herniation of the abdominal contents into the chest, compressing the lungs and possibly the mediastinum. Left untreated, a tension viscerothorax may result.

SYMPTOMS

- Dyspnea, Kerr's sign (sharp, relentless left shoulder pain as a result of irritation of the phrenic nerve), diminished breath sounds.
- Auscultation of bowel sounds in the thoracic cavity may occur with extreme case and severe herniation.
- Hamman's crunch may be appreciated with mediastinal emphysema. Hamman's crunch can best be characterized as a crunching sound heard best over the anterior chest wall at the apex. The crunching sound appreciated is synchronous with the cardiac cycle and can be auscultated in conditions leading to the presence of mediastinal air.

DIAGNOSIS

- Chest radiograph may reveal the herniation.
- Nasogastric intubation clarifies the diagnosis with the radiopaque nasogastric tube present in the thoracic cavity on radiograph.
- Diagnostic peritoneal lavage may be performed also to evaluate for additional intraabdominal injury.

NURSING ALERT

With ruptured diaphragm, when lavage fluid is instilled, a communication exists with the thoracic cavity. Monitor for lavage fluid drainage from the chest tube or a chest tube may need to be inserted if the fluid extravasates from the abdominal cavity to the thoracic cavity.

TREATMENT

- Nasogastric intubation and gastric decompression may lessen the effects of the herniation on chest structures.
- Inadvertent esophageal intubation and positive pressure ventilation is lethal as the herniated contents would then be insufflated, compounding the effects of the herniation.
- Prepare for immediate surgical intervention.

Ruptured bronchus/Trachea

The most common site of injury is at the distal trachea or proximal mainstem bronchus. This injury usually occurs as a result of compressive/shear forces or penetrating injury.

SYMPTOMS

- Respiratory distress, forceful coughing, subcutaneous emphysema, and hemoptysis are frequently present.
- With placement of tube thoracostomy, a persistent large air leak is usually present.

DIAGNOSIS

- Bronchoscopy, clinical examination.

TREATMENT

- Resuscitation initially per primary assessment.
- Tube thoracostomy is usually necessary to optimize ventilation.
- Again, monitor for persistent air leak and troubleshoot accordingly.
- The ET cuff must be distal to injury to maximize ventilation.
- Aggressive management and surgical intervention should be anticipated.

NURSING ALERT

With laryngeal injuries, the patient may often present with hoarseness, dysphagia, and the inability to tolerate the supine position as a result of a collapsing airway lumen with fracture. When the patient assumes the supine position, the usual airway lumen collapses on itself because of a fracture of the structure itself. Thus when patients are forced to lie supine, as we normally do to ensure adequate spinal immobilization, the false lumen achieved with a more upright position is collapsed and airway obstruction occurs. Laryngeal injuries are exceedingly difficult to manage and a position of comfort, maintaining immobilization should be the approach taken until management in a controlled environment can be achieved (e.g., the operating room).

Abdominal trauma

Unrecognized injuries to the abdomen present one of the major contributing factors to preventable mortality and morbidity for the trauma patient. As many as 20% of patients with acute hemoperitoneum have benign abdominal findings when first examined in the ED. The peritoneal cavity is a major reservoir for major occult blood loss (1).

A high index of suspicion must be maintained in patients
with suspected abdominal injury, especially related to
occult vascular and retroperitoneal injuries. Serial
abdominal examinations must be approached in a
systematic and meticulous fashion with thorough
documentation of findings and changes in findings. The
patient with peritoneal signs and/or signs of ongoing
blood loss must be approached with a vigorous/
aggressive posture in terms of discovery of injury and
appropriate management.

NURSING ALERT

The following is an outline for the approach to the abdominal
evaluation. It is not essential to identify a specific type of injury, but
it is most essential to determine that an abdominal injury exists.
The liver, spleen, and kidneys are the organs predominantly
involved after blunt injury. Essentially, you should be evaluating
the patient for blood loss following major solid organ injury (liver,
spleen, or kidney) or hollow viscus injury to the small or large
bowel. The initial systematic evaluation of the abdomen using
inspection, auscultation, percussion, and palpation are outlined
under Secondary Assessment. Refer to this section in the chapter
to review the initial approach to the abdominal examination.

DIAGNOSIS

- Definitive evaluation of abdominal injuries is conducted
  in different ways based on the philosophy and resources
  of the institution. Protocol for evaluation of blunt
  abdominal trauma should be developed and adhered to
  for cases presenting to your ED.
- Penetrating abdominal trauma is usually more
  straightforward in terms of evaluation.

NURSING ALERT

The diaphragm rises to the 4th intercostal space during exhalation and extends to the 6th or 7th intercostal space, midclavicular line on inspiration or the 8th or 9th intercostal
space, midaxillary line on inspiration. This must be a consideration, especially in evaluating penetrating thoracic/abdominal
trauma in that the adjacent cavity must also be closely evaluated to ascertain the extent of injury. With lower chest injuries,
abdominal injury must be entertained and with upper abdominal injuries, chest injuries must be suspected.

T

- Nasogastric intubation and urinary catheterization are both therapeutic and diagnostic.
- The nasogastric tube decompresses the stomach-removing gastric contents, reducing gastric volume and pressure thus reducing the risk of aspiration.
- The urinary catheter allows for bladder decompression and evaluation for hematuria. The catheter also allows for monitoring of urinary output that serves as a solid guide to the efficacy of fluid resuscitation.

NURSING ALERT

Inspection of the meatus and the rectal examination should be performed before insertion of the urinary catheter. Contraindications to urinary catheter placement such as blood at the meatus, inability to palpate the prostate, a high riding prostate, or boggy prostate may be discovered during the examination.

Laboratory screening

Laboratory screening should be conducted per the abdominal evaluation protocol for your facility. Baseline studies typically include CBC with differential, amylase, urinalysis, urine pregnancy test, and alcohol/drug determination.

Diagnostic studies

For evaluation of genitourinary trauma, see Chapter 12.

The two major mechanisms for definitive abdominal evaluation are diagnostic peritoneal lavage (DPL) and CT scanning of the abdomen. Determination of the approach taken is usually related to hemodynamic stability of the patient and the time available to determine the presence or absence of intraabdominal injury.

1. *DPL:* The DPL is usually conducted to evaluate those patients with hemodynamic instability. DPL is considered 98% sensitive for intraperitoneal bleeding. The only absolute contraindication for DPL is an existing indication for celiotomy. Relative contraindications include morbid obesity, previous abdominal operations, advanced cirrhosis, and preexisting coagulopathy. DPL may be approached with an open or closed (percutaneous) technique. Again, this is dictated by the general philosophy of the department of surgery.

NURSING ALERT

Before DPL, all patients should have nasogastric tube and urinary catheter in place. During DPL, a catheter is inserted and initially aspirated. If gross bloody aspirate is obtained, this is immediate indication for surgical intervention. If aspiration yields no blood, the patient should be lavaged with a liter of warmed isotonic fluid. Lavage fluid should then be sent to the lab. Microscopic evaluation leading to celiotomy are usually results of >100,000 RBCs or 500 WBCs for patients with blunt injury. A more sensitive indicator of bleeding (the presence of fewer RBCs) may be utilized as a surgical indicator for patients with penetrating injury (1).

2. *CT scan:* The CT scan is more specific, but less sensitive than DPL. Usually both IV and oral contrast are administered to heighten specificity of the examination. The CT scan provides information relative to specific organ injury and its extent and can also give information related to the pelvis and retroperitoneum. If the CT scan reveals free fluid, a DPL may be performed to evaluate the nature of the fluid.

NURSING ALERT

Be cautious regarding timing of administration of oral contrast to allow for a long enough dwell time to ensure an adequate study. Examination of the lower thoracic or upper lumbar vertebrae via plain films may be obscured or equivocal with the contrast dye.

The advantages of CT scanning vs. DPL must be weighed carefully in order to provide optimal care for the injured patient. Even patients with hemodynamic stability but with an impressive abdominal examination indicative of peritoneal signs may be candidates for DPL. Another consideration is the availability of resources in the facility and timing of marshalling those resources for the patient vs. transferring the patient to a higher level of care. These decisions must be made collaboratively with the attending physician, receiving physician, and attending nurse based on the patient's condition and facility that best matches needs of the patient with resources available.

Pelvic fractures

Pelvic fractures, especially those involving the posterior columns, can bleed vigorously, leading to exsanguination and formation of a retroperitoneal hematoma. The hematoma can become so enlarged as to extend from the pelvis into the lower anterior abdominal wall. To avoid the hematoma, the DPL may be done with an approach above the umbilicus to avoid a false positive finding for intraabdominal bleeding. (NOTE: Orthopedic consultation should be obtained quickly in these patients to facilitate definitive care of the pelvic fracture.)

The blood loss from the pelvic fracture should be addressed as with any source of blood loss precipitating a shock state. After alternative sources of blood loss have been ruled out, the pelvis should be stabilized (either by external fixation or possibly with a pneumatic antishock garment). This stabilization allows the retroperitoneal space to tamponade the bleeding and control ongoing blood loss.

In some instances (<10%), stabilization may not control blood loss from the fracture. Arteriography may be indicated to embolize ongoing arterial bleeding. Considerations must be given to the patients underlying renal function and physiologic condition before transport to arteriography. Management of the patient with ongoing blood loss from a pelvic fracture often requires very aggressive colloid resuscitation with attention to potential coagulopathy and hypothermia.

NURSING SURVEILLANCE

The ongoing assessment of the trauma patient is a repeated primary and secondary assessment. Airway patency, adequacy of breathing and circulation, and neurologic status should be reassessed as frequently as needed and anytime there is a change in the patient's condition. The secondary assessment may be more limited to identified injuries and known system involvement. Frequent reassessment should be done to rapidly identify any deterioration and, consequently, intervene appropriately.

EXPECTED PATIENT OUTCOMES

Expected patient outcomes vary widely from patient to
patient. Generally speaking, airway, breathing,
circulation, and neurologic status should be maintained
or improved. If spinal trauma is suspected or present,
then preservation of function is an expected outcome.
Preventing infection is important for patients with open
wounds or burns. Immobilizing fractures and
maintaining adequate peripheral tissue perfusion is
appropriate for patients with extremity injuries.

DISCHARGE IMPLICATIONS

Trauma patients present the clinician with a unique set of
challenges, both clinically and from a systems approach.
Although most patients suffering from injury are
admitted to the receiving hospital, a relatively small
percentage of injured patients require timely triage and
transfer to a higher level of care. Certain categories of
trauma patients require transfer to a higher level of care
based on the referring and receiving hospitals'
capabilities. One set of guidelines for consideration of
early transfer of patients is represented in the box, p.
654 and has been proposed by the American College of
Surgeons Committee on Trauma.

Specific issues arise with interhospital transfer to a higher
level of care. These issues include, but are not limited to,
the following:

1. Communications between the referring and receiving
   facilities, both written and verbal, physician and nursing.
2. Interhospital transfer forms.
3. Decisions regarding transport mode-ground vs.
   aeromedical evacuation and level of care of personnel
   attending the patient while in transit.
4. Matching the patient's needs with those offered by the
   receiving facility. An adequate match must occur
   between the patient's needs and those resources
   available at the receiving institution. This "match" must
   be done and the patient transferred in a timely fashion.
5. Optimal/maximal stabilization of the patient must occur
   before transport within the capabilities of the referring

T

institution. Often physicians from the receiving facility may offer guidance regarding stabilization and transport procedures.

Again, most injured patients can be adequately cared for by the initial receiving hospital. However, those patients requiring a higher level of care must be promptly recognized based on the limitations/capabilities of the receiving hospital, and appropriate transfer must ensue to the appropriate higher level of care.

HIGH-RISK CRITERIA FOR CONSIDERATION OF EARLY TRANSFER

(These guidelines are not intended to be hospital-specific.)

Central nervous system

Head injury
- Penetrating injury or open fracture (with or without cerebrospinal fluid leak)
- Depressed skull fracture
- Glasgow Coma Scale (GCS) <14 or GCS deterioration
- Lateralizing signs

Spinal cord injury
- Spinal column injury or major vertebral injury

Chest

Major chest wall injury
Wide mediastinum or other signs suggesting great vessel injury
Cardiac injury
Patients who may require prolonged ventilation

Pelvis

Unstable pelvic ring disruption
Unstable pelvic fracture with shock or other evidence of continuing hemorrhage
Open pelvic injury

Major extremity injuries

Fracture/dislocation with loss of distal pulses
Open long-bone fractures
Extremity ischemia

Multiple-system injury

Head injury combined with face, chest, abdominal, or pelvic
injury
Burns with associated injuries
Multiple long-bone fractures
Injury to more than two body regions

Comorbid factors

Age >55 years
Children
Cardiac or respiratory disease
Insulin-dependent diabetics, morbid obesity
Pregnancy
Immunosuppression

Secondary deterioration (late sequelae)

Mechanical ventilation required
Sepsis
Single or multiple organ system failure (deterioration in central nervous, cardiac, pulmonary, hepatic, renal, or coagulation systems)
Major tissue necrosis

References

1. American College of Surgeons, Committee of Trauma:
   Advanced trauma life support: course for physicians, Chicago, 1993,
   The College.
2. Emergency Nurses' Association: *Trauma nursing core course,*
   ed 3, Chicago, 1991, Award Printing Corp.
3. Emergency Nurses' Association: Trauma nursing core course,
   ed 4, Chicago, 1995 (in press).

T

Chapter XXII

The Unresponsive Patient

Steve Talbert

CLINICAL CONDITIONS
Alcohol
Electrolyte Abnormalities
Encephalopathy
Endocrine
Insulin
Intercranial Lesion
Overdose
Uremia
Trauma
Infection
Psychogenic
Seizure
Hypovolemic Shock
Cardiogenic Shock
Neurogenic Shock
Anaphylactic Shock
Hypoxia/Hypoxemia
Acid-Base Imbalance
Thermoregulation

TRIAGE ASSESSMENT

The unresponsive patient, regardless of etiology, constitutes a medical emergency and should be taken immediately to an appropriate treatment area. The initial triage assessment focuses on the airway, breathing, circulation, a brief neurologic examination, and critical history. It is followed by a detailed secondary assessment centered around the risk factors for unresponsiveness.

Airway and cervical spine

First, the patient's airway must be examined for patency (1,6). A method for checking patency is to apply a modified jaw-thrust maneuver, then observe the airway for any source of potential or actual obstruction, listen

657

for breath sounds, and feel for air movement. If compromised, the establishment of a stable, patent airway through the removal of any obstruction and/or the placement of an artificial airway is essential before continuing the assessment. Care must be taken to protect the cervical spine if the etiology of the patient's unresponsiveness is either unknown or known to be traumatic (1,6).

Breathing

Assessment of breathing includes the respiratory rate, depth, pattern, and work (12). Respiratory rates vary with age, anxiety, acid-base balance, and other physiologic and psychologic factors (4,12). Tachypnea or bradypnea, especially when prolonged, are signs of respiratory distress and/or metabolic problems (4). Assess respiration depth by auscultating lung sounds and inspecting chest rise and fall. Unequal chest rise and fall may indicate a pneumothorax. Paradoxical chest wall movement suggests a flail chest segment. Respirations that are continuously deep or shallow may be symptoms of an underlying respiratory or metabolic disorder. Diminished, absent, or abnormal breath sounds (e.g., wheezing, rales, or rhonchi) are symptoms of breathing problems that impair gas exchange and must be addressed. These conditions include pneumothorax or hemothorax, pulmonary edema (PE), and airway constriction. Respiratory patterns are also part of the breathing assessment. Abnormal respiratory patterns such as Biot's, Cheyne-Stokes, and Kussmaul's are classically associated with various medical conditions (Table 22-1) (10). Finally, work of breathing or respiratory effort should be assessed. Signs of increased work of breathing include nasal flaring, retractions, and use of accessory muscles. Initially, all unresponsive patients should receive 100% oxygen via an appropriate route (e.g., nonrebreather mask, bag-valve device, or ventilator) until deemed unnecessary by history and physical examination.

Circulation

Circulation or perfusion is assessed by noting pulse rate and quality, skin color, temperature, moisture, and capillary refill (1,2,10,12). The presence or absence of a pulse must be established quickly during the triage

TABLE 22-1 Respiratory Patterns and Associated Clinical Conditions

Respiratory pattern	Description	Associated clinical conditions
Biot's	Fast, deep inspirations interrupted by sudden periods of apnea	Increased intercranial pressure (late sign)
Cheyne-Stokes	Gradual rhythmic transition going from hyperventilation to apnea and then repeating the cycle over and over	Increased intercranial pressure Encephalopathy Overdose of narcotics, barbiturates, or hypnotics
Kussmaul's	Fast, deep respirations that may be labored	Metabolic acidosis Ketoacidosis Renal failure

assessment. Palpation for presence and quality of carotid, femoral, brachial, or radial pulses is the first step. Failure to palpate distal pulses in the absence of extremity trauma or the presence of weak, thready pulses are indicative of poor perfusion and hypotension. Other significant assessment findings consistent with poor perfusion are cool, pale or mottled and clammy skin. Capillary refill time may increase with aging and hypothermia (10). As a general rule, prolonged capillary refill time (>3 seconds) is associated with poor perfusion (1,6,9,12). If perfusion is compromised, steps should be taken to augment circulatory volume. Current recommendations are the placement of two large bore (e.g., 18-gauge or larger) IV lines and administration of an isotonic crystalloid solution (Ringer's lactate or 0.9% NaCl) (1). All unresponsive patients should have at least one IV line inserted during the initial assessment.

Deficit

The fourth step in the triage assessment is a brief neurologic examination consisting of pupil size and reactivity, best motor response, best verbal response, and best eye opening response (Table 22-2) (1,6,9,12). This

TABLE 22-2 Rapid Neurologic Assessment

A	Alert
V	Responds to verbal stimuli
P	Responds to painful stimuli
U	Unresponsive

Adapted from American College of Surgeons, Committee of Trauma: *Advanced trauma life support: course for physicians*, Chicago, 1993, First Impression.

TABLE 22-3 Neurologic Findings and Associated Clinical Conditions

Neurologic finding	Associated clinical condition
Dilated, nonreactive pupils Unilateral or bilateral	Increased intercranial pressure Overdose of barbiturates Anticholinergic drugs (e.g., atropine sulfate)
Constricted pupils	Overdose of narcotics Cholinergic activity
Sluggish pupil reactivity	Metabolic process (e.g., drug ingestion) Structural problem (e.g., closed-head injury)
Flaccid extremities	Spinal cord injury Closed-head injury
Spasticity of muscles	Seizure disorder Electrolyte imbalance
Abnormal flexion or extension of extremities	Closed-head injury Increased intercranial pressure
Unilateral flaccidity or weakness	Closed-head injury Intercranial lesion (bleed, mass, ischemia)

initial examination provides critical baseline data for later comparison. Table 22-3 lists some common neurologic findings and their associated clinical conditions.

Other interventions

Other early interventions include the administration of reversal agents such as naloxone HCl (Narcan) and flumazenil (Romazicon). Recently, the universal administration of $D_{50}W$ to the unresponsive patient has been questioned (13). If a bedside glucose level is readily available, it should be checked before administering $D_{50}W$.

History

Finally, a focused history should be obtained as quickly as possible. Since the unresponsive patient is unable to provide this information, it must be obtained from EMS personnel, family, friends, bystanders, or medic alert devices. Searching through pockets, wallets, purses, and bags may provide valuable information regarding medications, regular physicians, and preexisting medical conditions. Table 22-4 lists the questions asked during a focused history and their clinical application.

FOCUSED NURSING ASSESSMENT

Once the initial survey is complete and all life-threatening conditions are corrected, the nurse should begin a systematic, head-to-toe examination focusing on the risk factors associated with unresponsiveness. This secondary assessment should begin with exposing the patient, taking measures to maintain body temperature, and getting a complete set of vital signs including a rectal temperature.

Risk Factors

The mnemonic "AEIOU TIPS HAT" can be used to help remember risk factors leading to unresponsiveness (see the box, p. 663).

Life Span Issues

U

NURSING ALERT

Regardless of the patient's age, priorities of care always begin with airway, breathing, circulation, and deficit. The mnemonic "AEIOU TIPS HAT" is valid for patients of all ages.

TABLE 22-4 Patient History and Clinical Implications

Question	Clinical implication
Events surrounding the unresponsive episode	If traumatic, suspect closed-head injury or shock
	If ingestion, suspect overdose and alcohol
	Note any patient complaints before unresponsiveness occurred (chest pain, nausea, headache, etc.)
When the unresponsiveness occurred	If after trauma, suspect closed-head injury or shock
	If after medication (e.g., insulin), suspect adverse drug reaction or overdose
How unresponsiveness occurred	If a specific event caused the unresponsiveness (e.g., trauma), then it rapidly narrows the possible etiologies
Associated symptoms	Patient complaints such as dizziness, chest pain, shortness of breath, or headache may indicate a cardiovascular or neurologic etiology
	Symptoms like vomiting, diarrhea, or bleeding point toward hypovolemia
	Fever may indicate an infectious process
Regular medications	Insulin use may lead to hypoglycemia
	Diuretics may cause hypovolemia or electrolyte imbalances
	Patients on antihypertensives are prone to intercranial problems like CVA and bleeds
	Endocrine disorders may cause unresponsiveness
Past medical history	Renal failure may cause uremia
	Liver failure may cause encephalopathy
	Patients with a history of CVA, TIA, cerebral aneurysm, or hypertension are more prone to intercranial problems
	Patients with cardiovascular disease are prone to cardiogenic shock
	Immunocompromised patients are more susceptible to infections
Allergies	Exposure to a known antigen may result in anaphylaxis

RISK FACTORS FOR UNRESPONSIVENESS

A alcohol
E electrolytes, encephalopathy, endocrine
I insulin, intercranial lesion
O overdose
U uremia

T trauma
I infection
P psychogenic
S seizure, shock

H hypoxia
A acidosis, alkalosis
T thermoregulation

Pediatrics

1. Remember priorities of care are airway, breathing, circulation, and deficit.
2. Intraosseous infusion may be used in children if unable to obtain peripheral IV access.
3. Common etiologies of unresponsiveness include (2,13):
   * Infection
   * Trauma
   * Seizure
   * Overdose
4. Reye's syndrome must also be considered in children (13).
   * History of recent viral illness (e.g., cold or flu symptoms).
   * Progression from confusion and lethargy to unresponsiveness.
   * Abnormal liver enzyme studies.
   * May exhibit abnormal posturing or respiratory arrest.

Geriatrics

1. Remember priorities of care are airway, breathing, circulation, and deficit.
2. Common etiologies of unresponsiveness include (7):
   * Trauma
   * Overdose or medication interaction
   * Infection

U

- Endocrine
- Acidosis/alkalosis
- Intercranial lesion (cerebral vascular attack [CVA], subdural hematoma [SDH], mass)
- Hypoxia

Obstetric

1. Remember priorities of care are airway, breathing, circulation, and deficit.
2. Common causes of unresponsiveness include:
   - Infection (e.g., sepsis)
   - Shock (etiologies: ruptured uterus or abruptio placentae)
   - Overdose (suicide attempt or attention seeking behavior, takes available medication [iron pills are common])
   - Seizure
   - Endocrine
   - Trauma

INITIAL INTERVENTIONS

Immediate interventions involve the airway, breathing, circulation, and deficit. A patent airway should be established and maintained throughout the resuscitation. Breathing and ventilation should be supported through the administration of 100% oxygen. If the patient is breathing adequately, a nonrebreather mask may be applied. If, however, ventilation is inadequate or there are no spontaneous respirations, the patient should be ventilated via a bag-valve mask device. Circulation is supported through the establishment of two large bore IV lines (14 or 16 gauge in adults) with warm crystalloid solution (0.9% NaCl or Ringer's lactate). Deficit should be supported through proper positioning of the patient (e.g., do not occlude venous return from the head), special precautions (e.g., padded side rails), and repeated neurologic assessments to rapidly identify any changes.

PRIORITY NURSING DIAGNOSES

Risk for injury
Risk for altered cerebral perfusion

- **Risk for injury** related to etiology of unresponsiveness.
  INTERVENTIONS
  - Keep bed in low position with side rails up.
  - Maintain patent airway.

- Administer high flow oxygen (as stated above).
- Administer neuromuscular blocking agents and/or anticonvulsants per physician order.
◆ **Altered cerebral perfusion** related to etiology of unresponsiveness.
  INTERVENTIONS
  - Avoid increases in intracranial pressure.
  - Suction only as necessary.
  - Elevate head of bed.
  - Avoid hip flexion.
  - Avoid neck flexion.
  - IV fluids as keep-vein-open rates (30 cc/hr) unless hypovolemia coexists.

PRIORITY DIAGNOSTIC TESTS

As a general rule, diagnostic testing for the unresponsive patient may be referred to as the safety net approach, which provides screening for a multitude of potential etiologies in the shortest amount of time. The boxes list common diagnostic tests.

COLLABORATIVE INTERVENTIONS
Overview

Supportive measures for airway, breathing, circulation, and deficit should be continued until a specific etiology for unresponsiveness is known and the patient is stabilized. Once known, the underlying cause can be addressed.

Clinical Conditions
Alcohol
(See Chapter 20.)
SYMPTOMS
- Smelling ethanol on the breath of the unresponsive patient is a good indicator that alcohol may be involved.
- Other findings include an enlarged liver (hepatitis and cirrhosis), ascites, spider angiomas, and signs of malnutrition.
- Family, friends, or bystanders may also confirm ingestion of alcohol.

DIAGNOSIS
- Confirmation of alcohol toxicity is made through blood sample testing. It should be noted that the level of ethanol needed to induce unresponsiveness varies considerably.

U

COMMON LABORATORY DIAGNOSTIC TESTS

Complete blood count (CBC)
Electrolytes (Na, K, Cl, Ca, Mg, PO_4)
Blood urea nitrogen (BUN)
Creatinine
Glucose
Anion gap
Arterial blood gas (ABG)
Alcohols
Drug (toxicology) screen
Hepatic enzymes
Medication levels

COMMON RADIOGRAPHIC TESTS

Chest x-ray
Cervical spine x-ray
CT scan of head (without contrast first, then with contrast if needed)
Other radiographic tests as indicated by assessment and history

---

OTHER

ECG
Lumbar puncture

- Chronic drinkers may have high blood alcohol levels and still be conscious.

TREATMENT

- Initial treatment focuses on supporting airway, breathing, and circulation.
- Oxygen may be administered and IV fluids (usually isotonic crystalloid solutions) should be given to reverse dehydration and assist with clearing the alcohol from the body.

- It is common to administer thiamine, multivitamins, folic acid, and magnesium intravenously to reverse electrolyte imbalances and malnutrition.
- Many patients go home after their blood alcohol has returned to an acceptable level.
- Discharge teaching regarding alcohol abuse and detoxification facilities should be provided.

Electrolyte abnormalities

SYMPTOMS

- The symptoms associated with electrolyte imbalances are specific for the specific anion (negatively charged particle) or cation (positively charged particle) involved.
- The neurologic, cardiovascular, respiratory, and endocrine systems are the most common systems affected by electrolyte imbalances (10).

DIAGNOSIS

- Clinical signs and symptoms of an electrolyte imbalance are confirmed through blood sample testing.

TREATMENT

- Treatment revolves around correcting the imbalance through supplemental administration of the electrolyte (e.g., potassium chloride infusion) or measures to decrease the concentration of the electrolyte (e.g., dialysis).
- Support of airway, breathing, and circulation must be continued until the patient is stabilized.

Encephalopathy

SYMPTOMS

- Encephalopathy is usually associated with conditions causing hepatic or renal failure.
- When either of these systems fail, toxins (e.g., ammonia and urea) can build up in the blood causing neurotoxicity that is manifested by an altered level of consciousness (10).
- Unconscious persons with a history of cirrhosis, liver failure, renal failure, or alcohol abuse should heighten suspicion for an etiology of encephalopathy.

DIAGNOSIS

- Diagnosis is confirmed by laboratory values coupled with a history consistent with liver or renal failure.
- Elevations of the following tests are significant: BUN, creatinine, ammonia, and liver enzymes.

- It is also common to see an elevated potassium and phosphate level.

TREATMENT

- Until the underlying cause is resolved, airway, breathing, and circulation must be fully supported.
- Treatment is focused on removing the offending toxin(s) as quickly as possible.
- This may include the administration of lactulose for ammonia toxicity.
- The patient may also be a candidate for emergent dialysis.

Endocrine

(See Chapter 7.)

SYMPTOMS

- Endocrine etiologies for unresponsiveness typically involve one of the following glands: pancreas, thyroid, or adrenal (10).
- Symptoms associated with pancreatic problems (ketoacidosis) are tachycardia, Kussmaul's respirations, and a ketone odor to the breath.
- Symptoms associated with hyperthyroidism (thyroid storm) are tachycardia, hypertension, congestive heart failure, and extreme hyperthermia.
- Hypothyroidism (myxedema coma) is characterized by shock, hypothermia, generalized edema, and hypoventilation and is usually seen in people over age 50.
- Symptoms associated with acute adrenal crisis are shock, hypotension, and dehydration.

DIAGNOSIS

- Diagnosis of all endocrine disorders are made by combining history, clinical findings, and laboratory tests.
- Ketoacidosis is characterized by acidosis, excessive ketones, hyperglycemia, and hyperosmolarity.
- Thyroid storms may be associated with electrolyte imbalances and hypoglycemia.
- Myxedema coma can be differentiated by the presence of hyponatremia, hypoglycemia, and lactic acidosis.
- Hyponatremia and hypoglycemia are also found in acute adrenal crisis.

TREATMENT

- Treatment begins with support of airway, breathing, and circulation while correcting the underlying cause.

- Ketoacidosis is corrected with IV hydration and insulin.
- Thyroid storm is treated by cooling, IV hydration, and glucose. It is not uncommon for a beta-blocker to be administered to protect the cardiovascular system from the excess thyroxin. Glucocorticoids may also be necessary.
- Myxedema coma is usually managed by intubation, IV hydration, and hormone replacement.
- Acute adrenal crisis is treated with IV glucocorticoid therapy, saline infusion, and administration of glucose.

Insulin

(See Chapter 7.)

SYMPTOMS

- Clinical symptoms associated with insulin shock (hypoglycemia) are hypotension, diaphoresis, tachycardia, seizures, and pale, clammy skin.
- Usually, these patients are known diabetics who have missed meals, are experiencing an acute illness (e.g., infection), or have recently exercised.

DIAGNOSIS

- Diagnosis of insulin shock is confirmed by laboratory or bedside blood tests that demonstrate hypoglycemia.

TREATMENT

- Immediate treatment is support for airway, breathing, and circulation.
- In the presence of documented hypoglycemia, IV dextrose should be administered.
- Once consciousness has returned, the patient should be able to eat a meal before being discharged from the ED.
- Discharge teaching includes insulin/diet instructions, an explanation of the reason for hypoglycemia, and symptoms to watch for in the future with prevention strategies.
- Furthermore, patient compliance with medications, diet, and follow-up should be assessed.

Intercranial lesion (hemorrhage or mass)

(See Chapter 15.)

SYMPTOMS

- Regardless of the specific lesion, the unresponsive patient with an acute intercranial mass may present with a variety of symptoms.
- These include seizures, focal neurologic findings (e.g., hemiplegia), elevated mean arterial pressure, tachypnea, and bradycardia.

U

- The patient may also have obvious head trauma.
- Significant history includes recent trauma, previous intercranial lesion, known mass, old CVA or transient ischemic attack (TIA), history of a cerebral aneurysm, sudden onset of headache, or behavioral changes.

DIAGNOSIS

- Diagnosis of an intercranial lesion is usually confirmed by visualization of the lesion on CT scan or MRI.

TREATMENT

- Initial management of intercranial lesions are centered around maximizing cerebral perfusion.
- This begins by supporting the airway, breathing, and circulation.
- It is common to intubate and hyperventilate these patients.
- A neurosurgery or neurologic consult should be obtained as quickly as possible.

Overdose

(See Chapter 20.)

NOTE: Specific assessment findings vary with different agents.

SYMPTOMS

- Symptoms associated with overdoses vary depending on the agents ingested.
- Frequently, a description of the scene where the patient was found or a recent history by family or friends may be your best clues.
- Drugs, medications, or pill bottles at the scene could indicate an ingestion and should be brought to the ED.
- The patient may have a history of overdosing or suicide attempts in the past.
- A family member or friend may have witnessed the overdose.
- Some of the more common systems affected by overdoses are the cardiovascular system (tachycardia or bradycardia, hypertension or hypotension); the respiratory system (tachypnea or bradypnea); and the neurologic system (abnormal pupil size or reaction or seizures).

DIAGNOSIS

- The diagnosis of overdose is confirmed by results of a drug screen (blood or urine).

- A clinical diagnosis may also be supported by a response to reversal agents such as naloxone HCl (Narcan) and flumazenil (Romazicon).

TREATMENT

- Treatment begins with support of the airway, breathing, and circulation.
- Symptomatic support should be continued until the specific agent is identified.
- The Regional Poison Control Center is an excellent resource regarding treatment.

Uremia

SYMPTOMS

- Uremic patients are usually those with acute or chronic renal failure.
- Symptoms include edema, crackles (PE), hypertension, and seizures.
- The presence of dialysis access devices (e.g., shunts and central lines) may also be a clue.

DIAGNOSIS

- Laboratory values consistent with uremia are elevated BUN and creatinine, hyperkalemia, metabolic acidosis, and anemia.

TREATMENT

- Unless the patient is a known dialysis patient, initial management is usually conservative (e.g., diuretics).
- If conservative measures do not resolve the uremia, or if the patient normally undergoes dialysis, then hemodialysis is the treatment of choice.

Trauma

(See Chapter 21.)

NOTE: Three common causes for unresponsiveness associated with trauma are head injury, hypoxia, and shock.

SYMPTOMS

- Common signs and symptoms associated with trauma are tachycardia, tachypnea, signs of poor perfusion (e.g., weak pulses, clammy skin, diaphoresis), delayed capillary refill, and focal neurologic findings.
- These patients usually present with visible external trauma (e.g., ecchymosis, hematoma, lacerations, deformities, or edema) that provides clues to the etiology of their unresponsiveness.

U

DIAGNOSIS

- Diagnosis of a traumatic etiology is a combination of history, physical findings, and diagnostic testing.
- Common laboratory findings consistent with traumatic injury are acidosis, hypoxemia, hypercapnia, elevated base deficit, decreased hematocrit and hemoglobin, elevated lactic acid level, hematuria, hyperglycemia, and an elevated WBC count.
- Radiographic studies include x-rays of all suspected injury sites, CT scan, and possible angiography.
- Other diagnostic tools include diagnostic peritoneal lavage, ultrasound, and MRI.

TREATMENT

- Initial management focuses on supporting airway, breathing, circulation, and deficit.
- All traumatic injuries should be treated in the following order: life-threatening injuries first, limb-threatening injuries second, and finally all other injuries (1-3,6).

Infection (sepsis, CNS, respiratory)

(See Chapters 5,15,17.)

SYMPTOMS

- Symptoms vary with the severity of the infection, system(s) involved, and the individual response to the infectious process.
- General symptoms include tachycardia, tachypnea, and fever.
- Respiratory symptoms include abnormal breath sounds (e.g., wheezing, crackles, or rhonchi), diminished breath sounds, cough, and excessive respiratory secretions.
- Neurologic symptoms include seizures, focal neurologic findings, bulging fontanel, and nuchal rigidity.
- Systemic symptoms (sepsis) include hypotension, cool, mottled, clammy skin, petechiae and/or purpura, and weak, thready pulses.
- Patients with a history of immunosupression (e.g., AIDS or chemotherapy) and cancer patients are at higher risk for infections.

DIAGNOSIS

- Diagnosis is a combination of clinical symptoms and laboratory results.
- Blood test findings include elevated or decreased WBC, acidosis, hyperglycemia, hypoxemia, and hypercapnia.

- Gram stains may provide rapid identification of potential sources of infection.
- Positive cultures (respiratory, cerebral spinal fluid (CSF), blood, urine, or wound) are definitive diagnostic adjuncts, but may require several days for results.

TREATMENT

- Treatment begins with support of airway, breathing, circulation, and deficit.
- A high priority for the unresponsive patient with an infectious etiology is the rapid administration of broad-spectrum antibiotics.
- The use of isolation precautions should also be considered.

Psychogenic

NURSING ALERT

All psychiatric patients eventually die of an organic disease or process. Other life-threatening problems must be identified or ruled out in the presence of a psychiatric history and medication. Assessment findings vary widely from patient to patient.

SYMPTOMS

- Symptoms consistent with a psychiatric etiology vary widely. However, they are usually inconsistent with medical conditions or present conflicting symptoms.
- A psychiatric history and known psychiatric medication use should raise the index of suspicion for this etiology.
- However, it must be stressed again that other life-threatening causes for unresponsiveness must be ruled out.

DIAGNOSIS

- Psychiatric cause for unresponsiveness is a diagnosis of exclusion.
- After other medical and traumatic causes are ruled out, a psychiatric etiology should be considered.
- History of previous similar behavior, depression, and mental illness serve to strengthen the likelihood of a psychiatric cause.
- Drug levels for specific psychotropic medications may also be found.

U

TREATMENT

- As with other etiologies of unresponsiveness, treatment begins with supporting airway, breathing, circulation, and deficit until the underlying cause is determined.
- Treating the unresponsive psychiatric patient can be difficult and dangerous.
- The focus should be addressing the underlying cause and may require the intervention of specialists.
- Care must be taken to protect the patient, family members, and other health care workers from injury.

Seizure

(See Chapter 15.)

SYMPTOMS

- The unresponsive seizure patient may present actively seizing or postictal.
- Seizure activity could be localized (focal) or involve the entire body (generalized).
- The postictal patient may have reported witnessed seizure activity or a seizure history.
- Other associated symptoms found with the seizure patient are tachycardia and warm, flushed, moist skin.
- They may also be hyperthermic.
- Incontinence of both bladder and bowel are common as well.
- Identification of certain traumatic injuries such as lacerations to the tongue, mouth, or head and abrasions or fractures in the extremities, face, or skull may also suggest a seizure etiology.

DIAGNOSIS

- Diagnosis is usually confirmed by the physical findings, medical history, and witnessed seizure activity. However, the etiology may remain unknown until antiseizure drug levels are confirmed and the patient arouses enough to provide an adequate medical history.
- Other common laboratory findings include hyperglycemia and an elevated WBC count.

TREATMENT

- Treatment begins with support of the airway, breathing, circulation, and deficit.
- If the patient is actively seizing, antiseizure medication (e.g., diazepam or lorazepam) should be administered intravenously until the seizure has ceased (13).

- If postical, seizure precautions (e.g., padded side rails) should be instituted to protect the patient from further harm.
- In addition, airway breathing, circulation, and neurologic status should be carefully assessed and documented.
- Anticonvulsants may also be given if blood levels are subtherapeutic (13).
- Finally, discharge instructions should include education regarding medication regimen, follow-up instructions, and wound care.

Shock

NOTE: There are five shock states—hypovolemic, cardiogenic, neurogenic, anaphylactic, and septic. Sepsis is discussed under "Infection."

Hypovolemic shock

SYMPTOMS

- Hypovolemic shock is a condition brought about by intravascular fluid loss (internal or external) (11).
- A history of traumatic injury, vomiting, or diarrhea is significant and should raise suspicion for a hypovolemic etiology.
- Symptoms associated with hypovolemic shock are a manifestation of the body's compensatory mechanisms (e.g., catecholamine release) and inadequate tissue perfusion.
- Tachycardia, tachypnea, delayed capillary refill, narrowed pulse pressure, and pale, cool, clammy, diaphoretic skin are hallmark signs of catecholamine release.
- Inadequate tissue perfusion is manifested by the unresponsiveness, cyanosis, weak and thready peripheral pulses, and oliguria or anuria.
- Hypotension is associated with hypovolemia but it is a late sign (1,2,6,12).

DIAGNOSIS

- Diagnosis of hypovolemic shock is clinically based.
- If a history consistent with hypovolemia is present coupled with the physical correlates of catecholamine release and inadequate tissue perfusion, then the diagnosis is made.
- Obvious internal or external fluid loss (e.g., internal or external bleeding) serves to further confirm the diagnosis.

U

- Laboratory values seen in hypovolemia include normal, elevated, or decreased hematocrit and hemoglobin, acidosis, moderate or severe base deficit (e.g., ≥ -6), hyperglycemia, elevated WBC, and elevated lactate levels (5).

TREATMENT

- Treatment begins with support of airway, breathing, circulation, and deficit.
- The overall goal of managing shock is to maximize oxygen delivery to the tissues (8). This is accomplished through two primary mechanisms: (1) stopping the fluid loss and (2) replenishing the intravascular volume.
- Stopping the fluid loss is a combination of direct pressure (external loss) and surgical intervention (internal loss).
- Replenishing the intravascular volume begins with establishing two large bore IV lines and rapidly infusing warm isotonic crystalloid solution.
- Administration of blood and blood products should be considered.
- Patients with traumatic injuries require immediate surgical consult or transfer to the closest appropriate trauma center.

Cardiogenic shock

Cardiogenic shock has two primary causes—coronary (e.g., acute myocardial infarction [AMI]) and noncoronary (e.g., cardiomyopathy or valve disease). Regardless of the etiology, the underlying pathophysiology is impaired pumping ability of the left ventricle (11).

SYMPTOMS

- Cardiogenic shock is characterized by poor cardiac output and inadequate ventricular emptying.
- Symptoms include hypotension, delayed capillary refill, and pale, cool, moist skin.
- Other assessment findings include cyanosis and pulmonary edema (PE).
- If the origin of shock is coronary in nature, there may be ECG findings consistent with AMI.
- As cardiac output and, subsequently, tissue perfusion decrease, oliguria or anuria may also be noted.

DIAGNOSIS

- Diagnosing cardiogenic shock is a combination of history, physical findings, and other diagnostic tools.

- Twelve-lead or fifteen-lead ECG findings consistent with AMI, elevated cardiac enzymes, and coronary artery occlusion noted on catheterization confirm a coronary origin for cardiogenic shock.
- Other tests such as an echocardiogram and chest x-ray can confirm a noncoronary origin.

TREATMENT

- As with other forms of shock, treatment begins with support of airway, breathing, circulation, and deficit.
- Therapies specific for cardiogenic shock are directed at correcting the underlying cause and improving cardiac output. These include pharmacologic therapy to augment contractility (e.g., dobutamine) and mechanical adjuncts such as intraaortic balloon pumps or ventricular assist devices.
- If the etiology of the shock is coronary in nature, then thrombolytic therapy and angioplasty are probable interventions.
- Emergency cardiopulmonary bypass or extracorporeal membrane oxygenation (ECMO) are also possible modalities of treatment.
- Finally, both coronary and noncoronary causes may require surgical intervention.

Neurogenic shock

SYMPTOMS

- Neurogenic shock is caused by a blocked sympathetic response secondary to neuron damage (1).
- The underlying pathology is massive vasodilation resulting in a relative hypovolemia and poor venous return.
- Symptoms include warm, flushed skin, bradycardia, and hypotension.
- The patient may also exhibit oliguria or anuria.
- Motor and/or sensory deficits may also be present.

DIAGNOSIS

- Diagnosis of neurogenic shock is clinical in nature based on a history consistent with a spinal cord injury coupled with the above mentioned clinical findings.
- Confirmation of spinal cord injury is accomplished through the use of CT scan and MRI.

TREATMENT

- Treatment begins with support of airway, breathing, circulation, and deficit.

- A fluid challenge should be given initially to rule out a hypovolemic source and augment circulating volume.
- Vasoconstriction can be promoted through the use of vasopressors (e.g., dopamine).
- Frequently, the injured vertebrae are stabilized via a brace (e.g., halo), surgery, or traction.
- The use of high-dose methylprednisolone is also currently being used in an effort to decrease spinal cord edema and minimize secondary cellular damage (3).

Anaphylactic shock
SYMPTOMS
- Anaphylactic shock is a life-threatening situation caused by an antigen-antibody reaction in which chemical mediators (e.g., histamine and kinins) are released in great quantity and exhibit systemic effects (10).
- Tachycardia, tachypnea, respiratory distress, wheezing, hypotension, and cyanosis are classic symptoms.

DIAGNOSIS
- As with other forms of shock, anaphylaxis is a clinical diagnosis.
- History of a known antigen exposure is a critical piece of history.
- In addition, there is an elevated white count, especially eosinophils.

TREATMENT
- As with the other forms of shock, treatment begins with support of airway, breathing, circulation, and deficit.
- Interventions specific to anaphylaxis include removing the offending antigen if possible and administration of specific pharmacologic agents that inhibit chemical mediator activity and the detrimental effects of the acute inflammatory response.
- These drugs include epinephrine, antihistamines, steroids, and bronchodilators.

Hypoxia/Hypoxemia
(See Chapter 17.)
SYMPTOMS
- Hypoxia and the resultant hypoxemia can manifest itself in a variety of ways. The underlying cause is usually related to inadequate gas exchange at the alveolar capillary membrane or decreased minute ventilation.
- Patients may present with a respiratory rate ranging from apnea or agonal respirations to tachypnea.

- Auscultation of the lungs may reveal adventitious sounds such as stridor, wheezing, crackles, or rhonchi.
- Breath sounds may be diminished or absent unilaterally or bilaterally.
- Heart rate may also vary from asystole to tachycardia and almost any electrophysiologic rhythm may be seen on ECG (10).
- Inspection of the airway may reveal a complete or partial obstruction.
- Inspection of the chest wall may reveal a mechanical defect (e.g., flail chest segment) or a structural deformity (e.g., sucking chest wound).
- Cyanosis may also be noted.

DIAGNOSIS

- Diagnosis of hypoxia and hypoxemia is confirmed through ABG analysis that confirms a decreased PaO_2 and SaO_2.
- Other findings may include hypercapnia and acidosis.
- The patient may have a known exposure to toxins like smoke, chemicals, or vapors.

TREATMENT

- Treatment is targeted at correcting the underlying problem and resolving the hypoxia and hypoxemia.
- It begins with ensuring a patent airway through the use of manual manipulation (e.g., jaw thrust or chin lift), clearing techniques (e.g., suctioning), and airway adjuncts (e.g., oral and nasal airway or endotracheal tube).
- Once an airway has been secured, the patient should be given 100% oxygen via nonrebreather mask, bag-valve mask, or ventilator.
- Any life-threatening breathing problems (e.g., tension pneumothorax) should be corrected immediately before moving on to support of the circulation.
- Serial blood gas analysis and ongoing respiratory assessments should also be performed to evaluate the effectiveness of any interventions.

Acid-base imbalance

(See Chapter 11.)

SYMPTOMS

- Conditions leading to acid-base imbalance are either respiratory or metabolic in nature.
- Regardless of the etiology, the underlying pathology is an excess of either acid or base. The resulting symptoms may vary widely.

- Respiratory acidosis is associated with poor gas exchange that results in hypercapnia.
- The patient usually presents with partial or complete airway obstruction in either the upper or lower airways or has a history of inadequate minute ventilation.
- In contrast, respiratory alkalosis is associated with hypocapnia usually resulting from hyperventilation.
- Metabolic acid-base imbalances are caused by inadequate tissue perfusion (shock and lactic acidosis), renal failure, and drug ingestion.
- Symptoms associated with acid-base imbalance are usually associated with the cardiovascular, respiratory, and neurologic systems (10).
- Cardiovascular manifestations include dysrhythmias.
- Respiratory symptoms range from tachypnea to apnea.
- Neurologic manifestations are altered level of consciousness, seizures, and hyperreflexia.

DIAGNOSIS

- Diagnosis of acid-base imbalance is seen through blood analysis.
- A pH >7.45 is classified as alkalosis.
  A pH <7.35 is classified as acidosis.
- The determination of a respiratory or metabolic etiology may be established through blood gas analysis.
- Other laboratory findings associated with acid-base imbalance include alterations of the following: bicarbonate, potassium, and urine ammonia levels.

TREATMENT

- Again, treatment begins with support of airway, breathing, circulation, and deficit.
- Therapy must then be targeted at correcting the underlying cause and resolving the acid-base imbalance through the use of ventilation techniques and administration of buffer solutions.

Thermoregulation

(See Chapter 8.)

SYMPTOMS

- The patient who is unresponsive secondary to thermoregulation issues suffers from either extreme hyperthermia or hypothermia (10,12). Symptoms are different for each condition.
- Early hyperthermia is characterized by hot and dry skin and hypertension.

- Late hyperthermia is characterized by cool skin, hypotension, dysrhythmias, and seizures.
- In either case the core body temperature exceeds 40° C (104° F).
- Hypothermia is associated with a core body temperature <35° C (95° F).
- The skin is cool or cold to touch.
- Cardiac manifestations include hypotension, dysrhythmias, and weak, thready pulses.
- Bradypnea and dilated pupils are also common findings.

DIAGNOSIS

- Diagnosis of hypothermia or hyperthermia is confirmed through core body temperature readings and clinical findings.
- Electrolyte imbalances, hyperglycemia, and an elevated WBC may also be present.

TREATMENT

- Treatment begins with support of airway, breathing, circulation, and deficit.
- If the patient is hyperthermic, interventions include the provision of a cool environment, IV hydration, and possibly active cooling by special blanket or water.
- The treatment for hypothermia is to rewarm the patient safely. Techniques include warm, humidified air, warming blanket, heat lamps, and blankets.
- If hypothermia is severe enough, warm fluid may be circulated into the peritoneal cavity or passed through a nasogastric tube.

NURSING SURVEILLANCE

In general, ongoing surveillance of the unresponsive patient is a continuation of the primary assessment combined with the safety net approach to diagnosis. Regardless of etiology, every unresponsive patient should have their airway, breathing, circulation, and deficit reassessed on a regular basis with appropriate assessment findings documented. Furthermore, if a significant change is noted in the patient's condition, the primary assessment should be repeated noting any changes from the initial assessment.

Components of Primary Assessment

1. Airway patency and cervical spine control.
2. Effectiveness of breathing and ventilation.
3. Adequacy of perfusion.
4. Mental status and neurologic checks.
5. Exposure of all body surface areas including extremities and back.
6. Vital signs including core body temperature.

Focused Assessments

Each specific etiology for unresponsiveness lists characteristic assessment and diagnostic findings. Once an etiology has been determined, those specific parameters should be reassessed for any improvement or worsening of the patient's condition.

EXPECTED PATIENT OUTCOMES

1. Airway remains patent.
2. Breathing and ventilation are effective.
3. Circulation and perfusion are adequate.
4. Mental status improves or remains the same.
5. Known underlying etiologies are corrected.

DISCHARGE IMPLICATIONS

Very few unresponsive patients are discharged home from the ED. Exceptions may include alcohol overdose, chronic seizure patients, hypoglycemic patients who are holding down PO food, and psychiatric patients. Furthermore, patients should have a safe environment to which they may go upon leaving the ED. When discharged, it must be stressed to these individuals the reason for their unresponsiveness. Timely follow-up with a primary care provider or clinic is essential.

References

1. American College of Surgeons, Committee of Trauma: *Advanced trauma life support: course for physicians,* Chicago, 1993, First Impression.
2. Aoki BY, McCloskey K, editors: *Evaluation, stabilization, and transport of the critically ill child,* St. Louis, 1992, Mosby.
3. Bracken MB, Shepard MJ, Collins WF, et al: Randomized, controlled trial of methylprednisolone or naloxone in the treatment of acute spinal cord injury, *N Engl J Med* 322: 1045-11, 1990.

4. Charnow JA, editor: *Professional guide to signs and symptoms,* Springhouse, Pa, 1993, Springhouse Corp.
5. Davis JW, Mackersie RC, Holbrook TL, and Hoyt DB: Base deficit as an indicator of significant abdominal injury, *Ann Emerg Med* 20:842-4, 1991.
6. Emergency Nurses' Association: *Trauma nursing core course,* ed 3, Chicago, 1991, Award Printing Corp.
7. Fadem JJ, Rosenberg SJ: Geriatric neurology: five acute problems, *Emerg Med* 62-78, September 30, 1992.
8. Fiddian-Green RG, Haglund U, Gutierrez G, and Shoemaker WC: Goals for the resuscitation of shock, *Crit Care Med* 21: S25-S31, 1993.
9. Lee G, editor: *Flight nursing: principles and practice,* St. Louis, 1991, Mosby.
10. Porth CM, editor: *Pathophysiology: concepts of altered health states,* ed 3, Philadelphia, 1990, JB Lippincott.
11. Rice V: Shock—a clinical syndrome: an update, (Entire Issue) New York, 1991, Cahners Publishing Co.
12. Sheehy SB, editor: *Emergency nursing: principles and practice,* ed 3, St. Louis, 1992, Mosby.
13. Wagner MB: Neurologic emergencies in the young: parts 1 and 2, *Emerg Med,* 204-24, June 15, 1992.

U

Procedures

Ace Wrap Application

Betty Gaudet Nolan

DESCRIPTION

An ace wrap is an elastic bandage that is available in sizes ranging from 2, 3, 4, and 6 inches in width. An ace wrap can provide or assist with support, pressure, and immobilization.

INDICATIONS

1. Support the injured area and decrease swelling in soft tissue and/or ligamentous injuries of the extremities.
2. Anchor dressings.
3. Secure and maintain pressure dressings to stop or decrease bleeding.
4. Secure splints for the purpose of immobilization.

EQUIPMENT

- Ace wrap (elastic bandage)
- Tape or pins/clips
- Dressings as indicated
- Splints as indicated
- 3 to 6 inch wide ace wrap for lower extremities
- 2 to 4 inch wide ace wrap for upper extremities

INITIAL NURSING ACTIONS

1. Assess distal pulses, skin color, temperature, capillary refill, sensation, and amount of edema to extremity before applying the ace wrap.
2. When applying the wrap, start at the distal portion of the extremity. Anchor the wrap by circling around the extremity twice.
3. Unroll the bandage and gently stretch the bandage as you wrap the body part. Overlap each layer of the bandage. Avoid wrinkling.
4. Avoid pressure over the antecubital and popliteal space.
5. Use a figure-eight wrap on joints.

A. Wrist or hand application
1. Anchor the bandage on hand first, then cross over the wrist. Cross back and forth in a figure-eight maneuver until part is adequately covered.

B. Elbow application
1. Anchor the bandage below the elbow, then cross under the antecubital space, and wrap above the elbow. Cross back and forth in a figure-eight maneuver until part is adequately covered.

C. Knee application
1. Anchor the bandage below the knee, cross over the knee diagonally, and wrap above the knee. Cross back and forth over the knee in a figure-eight maneuver until part is adequately covered. Avoid pressure on the popliteal space because of the vasculature in the area.

D. Ankle application
1. Anchor the bandage around the foot. Cross over the top of the foot and around the back of the ankle, and bring back over foot and under the arch. Cross back and forth in a figure-eight maneuver until the foot (not toes) and ankle are adequately covered (Figure P1-1).

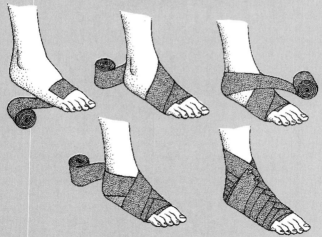

Figure P1-1 Figure-eight ace bandage application to ankle.

NURSING ALERT

The ace wrap bandage should be loose enough to insert one finger under the bandage comfortably. Check distal pulses, color, temperature, sensation, and capillary refill of the distal digits.

PATIENT CARE MANAGEMENT

1. Elevate the extremity and apply ice or cold packs as directed to prevent and decrease swelling.
2. If appropriate, instruct the patient to remove and reapply the bandage if too loose, too tight, or for bathing.
3. Teach the patient how to correctly apply the ace wrap.
4. Teach the patient how to assess for a tight ace wrap. Instruct the patient to check for changes in sensation, temperature, swelling, and color to distal digits. If present, the patient should remove or loosen bandage and elevate the extremity. If no improvement, call physician immediately.

Bibliography

Ace Wrap

Proehl JA: *Adult emergency nursing procedures,* Boston, 1993.
National Safety Council: *First aid essentials,* Boston, 1989, Jones and Bartlett.

Arterial Blood Gas

Janet Rodgers

DESCRIPTION

Arterial blood gases (ABGs) are obtained by direct aspiration of blood from an artery. This may be done by aspiration of blood from an indwelling arterial line or by percutaneous arterial puncture. This procedure focuses on percutaneous arterial puncture.

INDICATIONS

ABGs are useful in the evaluation of oxygenation, ventilation and perfusion, and acid-base disturbances. Often ABGs are obtained to document a baseline for future reference.

EQUIPMENT

- Povidone-iodine swab
- Alcohol swab
- 2 × 2 gauze pads
- Gloves
- Heparinized syringe (usually available in a prepackaged kit): 1 ml for pediatrics, 3 ml for adults
- 25-gauge, ⅜ inch needle
- 20-22 gauge, 1½ inch needle (for deeper arteries)
- Butterfly catheter
- Adhesive tape
- Specimen label
- Container of ice

INITIAL NURSING ACTIONS

1. Explain the procedure to the patient.
2. Select the arterial puncture site. Any accessible artery may be used; however, the radial, brachial, and femoral arteries are the most commonly used sites. Hospital policy may dictate sites from which arterial samples may

be taken. In choosing a site for arterial puncture, the following four factors are considered:

- The site must be easily accessible.
- The pulse must be easily palpable.
- The artery must be easily compressible.
- There should be no associated injuries or alterations in skin integrity that would increase the risk of circulatory compromise or infection.

In the absence of palpable peripheral pulses, the femoral artery is the recommended site for arterial puncture. The location of the femoral artery may be estimated by drawing an imaginary line between the anterior-superior iliac spine and the symphysis pubis. Midpoint of that line over the inguinal area should be the femoral artery.

Before selection of the radial artery as the puncture site, the Allen's test must be performed to evaluate collateral circulation to the hand. The Allen's test is performed by asking the patient to make a fist and compressing the ulnar and radial arteries with your fingers. After a few seconds, ask the patient to open their hand. The hand should appear pale and blanched. Now release the ulnar artery and observe the palm or hand for flushing. Rapid flushing indicates good collateral circulation. If the hand remains blanched, collateral circulation may be compromised and another site should be selected.

3. Cleanse the area with povidone-iodine and allow to dry.
4. Wipe off area with an alcohol swab. Povidone-iodine leaves a sticky residue on the skin and may interfere with subtle finger movements.
5. Palpate the pulse with the middle and index finger or the index finger only of the nondominant hand. Arterial puncture may then be performed by insertion of the needle between the two fingers or by insertion of the needle just proximal to the index finger.
6. The angle of insertion varies depending on the site selected. For a radial artery puncture, the syringe should be held at a 45-degree angle with the bevel of the needle turned upward. Brachial artery puncture may be performed at a 45- to 60-degree angle. Femoral artery puncture should be performed at a 90-degree angle.
7. Slowly insert the needle over the point of maximal pulsation. Observe closely for the appearance of blood within the needle hub. Arterial pressure should be sufficient to fill the syringe without manual aspiration.

However, in patients with decreased peripheral perfusion or hypotension, gentle aspiration may be necessary. The amount of blood required for ABG analysis may vary between institutions, however, 0.5 to 1.0 ml is usually sufficient.

8. During insertion the needle may inadvertently puncture both sides of the artery resulting in a small flash of blood into the needle hub but no further flow into the syringe. If this occurs, slowly withdraw the needle until blood return is noted. If no blood return occurs, and the pulse remains palpable, withdraw the needle until the bevel is visible and redirect it toward the point of maximal pulsation.

9. Loss of arterial pulsation during puncture attempts may indicate arterial spasm or hematoma formation. If this occurs, withdraw the needle, apply manual pressure for 5 to 10 minutes, and select another site.

10. After the arterial blood sample is obtained, withdraw the needle and apply manual pressure for 5 to 10 minutes.

11. Remove air bubbles from the specimen and cap the syringe as soon as possible. Air can be removed from the specimen by holding the syringe upright, tapping the sides of the syringe to direct air bubbles upward, and expelling the air by gently pushing upward on the plunger.

12. Apply a dressing to the site.

13. Label the specimen. Be sure to include the patient's temperature and the type and concentration of supplemental oxygen.

14. Place the specimen in a sealed container and then place on ice. Ziplock bags work very well. Place one bag inside another. Put the labeled specimen in the inner bag and seal it. Pour ice into the outer bag around the specimen and seal it. Pushing the specimen into a prefilled ice container may result in inadvertent expulsion of the syringe contents.

NURSING ALERT

All arterial puncture sites require manual pressure for a minimum of 5 minutes. Larger, higher pressure arteries such as the femoral artery may require 10 minutes of manual pressure to establish hemostasis. Clotting times vary depending on the presence of preexisting diseases that alter clotting factors, medical and surgical interventions that deplete clotting factors, reduction of clotting factors resulting from hemorrhage and multiple blood transfusions, and the use of anticoagulants. The length of application of manual pressure should be increased accordingly. Patients receiving IV thrombolytics require the application of manual pressure followed by a pressure dressing.

NURSING ALERT

To obtain accurate blood gas results, wait 30 minutes after suctioning, respiratory treatments, and ventilator and oxygen concentration changes.

PATIENT CARE MANAGEMENT

1. Assess the puncture site for bleeding after manual pressure is released.
2. If alert and oriented, instruct the patient to notify you if bloody drainage is noted on or around the dressing or if visible bruising occurs around the puncture site.
3. If the patient is disoriented or unconscious, frequently assess the site for bleeding and hematoma formation for approximately 30 minutes.
4. Assess the circulatory status distal to the puncture site by evaluating skin color and temperature, capillary refill, and distal pulses.
5. Document the arterial puncture site on the nursing record.

Bibliography

Knighton D, Locksley RM, Mills J: Emergency procedures. In Saunders CE and Ho MT, editors: *Current emergency diagnosis and treatment*, Norwalk, Conn, 1992, Appleton & Lange.

American Heart Association: *Textbook of cardiac life support*, 1994, Dallas, The Association.

Arterial Line Monitoring

Patricia Brisky

DESCRIPTION

Arterial pressure lines enable the nurse to continuously monitor a patient's blood pressure and draw frequent arterial blood specimens.

INDICATIONS

1. Significant respiratory compromise
2. Diabetic ketoacidosis
3. Shock
4. Adult respiratory distress syndrome (ARDS)
5. Titration of vasopressor agents
6. To determine the mean arterial pressure and cerebral perfusion pressure in patients with a ventricular catheter device

EQUIPMENT

- 500 cc IV bag of normal saline (flush solution)
- 500 cc pressure bag
- 20-gauge, 1½ or 2 inch angiocath
- Antiseptic solution
- Tincture of benzoin
- 4-0 nylon sutures
- Lidocaine 1%, 10 cc vial
- Needles and syringes of different sizes
- Sterile towels
- Sterile scissors
- Sterile needle-holder
- Sterile gauze
- Sterile gown
- Sterile gloves
- Male Luer-Lok cap
- Pressure tubing with flush device, transducer, stopcock, and extension set
- Central or deepline dressing kit, or tegaderm

- Armboard
- Monitor with hemodynamic capabilities
- Transducer cable

INITIAL NURSING ACTIONS

1. Explain procedure to patient.
2. Gather equipment.
3. Determine from physician which site is to be cannulated. Either the radial, brachial, or femoral artery may be selected. The radial artery is commonly used because it usually has good collateral circulation and is easily accessible. If the radial artery is to be used, perform the Allen's test (see Procedure 2).
4. Position the extremity properly. The hand should be supinated and the wrist slightly hyperextended. The hand can be taped to an armboard with a small gauze roll under the wrist to maintain this position.
5. Prepare flush solution. Heparin (500 to 1000 U of a 1:1000 heparin solution) may be added to the 500 cc bag of normal saline depending on your hospital's protocols.
6. Attach flush solution to the pressure tubing. If not fully assembled, connect the transducer to the pressure tubing proximal to the flush device. Attach a stopcock to the end of the pressure tubing and add a pressure extension set.
7. Place flush solution into the pressure bag and hang on an IV pole.
8. Clear all air from the pressure tubing and transducer by opening the roller clamp and activating the flush device according to the manufacturer's directions.
9. Pump the pressure bag to 300 mm Hg and clamp to maintain the pressure.
10. Connect the transducer to the transducer cable. Attach the cable to the monitor.
11. Place the transducer at the level of the catheter tip (1).
12. Turn the stopcock off to the patient side. Open the transducer to air and zero the system. The exact mechanism used to zero the system depends on the manufacturer. Once zeroed, close the system to air. Zeroing the system negates other pressure influences.
13. When the physician has cannulated the artery, firmly attach the pressure tubing to the catheter.

14. Activate the flush device to clear the line and catheter of any blood.
15. Once the catheter is sutured in place by the physician, clean the site with antiseptic solution. Apply benzoin around the area. Place a sterile gauze over the site. Tape securely.

PATIENT CARE MANAGEMENT

1. Apply pressure to the site for 10 to 15 minutes if the catheter accidentally falls out.
2. Monitor the color, temperature, sensation, and movement of the area distal to the catheter. Complications can include hematoma formation, intraluminal clotting, arterial spasm, thrombosis, and nerve injury.
3. Withdraw blood for arterial blood gas (ABG) analysis and other laboratory tests as ordered by the physician and based on the patient's clinical condition.
   * Attach a 5 cc syringe to the stopcock port closest to the catheter.
   * Turn the stopcock off to the monitor and on to the patient. Withdraw 3 to 5 cc of blood to clear the line of heparinized solution and blood. Turn the stopcock off to the port and discard the syringe.
   * Coagulation studies are usually drawn last to ensure use of a nonheparinized specimen.
   * Attach another syringe to obtain needed blood specimens. Use a heparinized syringe to obtain blood for an ABG. Turn the stopcock off to the monitor and on to the patient. Withdraw the necessary blood. Turn the stopcock on to the monitor and patient (off to the port). Remove the syringe.
   * Flush the line to the patient. Turn the stopcock off to the patient and flush the access port. Turn stopcock on to the patient and monitor. Recap the stopcock port with a Luer-Lok cap.
4. Dampening of the waveform may be caused by air in the tubing or transducer, clot formation, and kinking of the catheter.
5. Rezero the transducer every 4 to 8 hours and each time the patient is repositioned.

References

1. Hudak C, Gallo B: *Critical care nursing–a holistic approach,* Philadelphia, 1994, JB Lippincott.

Bibliography

Kidd, PS: Nursing care of the patient with altered tissue perfusion. In Kidd PS, Wagner KD, editors: *High acuity nursing,* Norwalk, Conn, 1992, Appleton and Lange.

Kitt S: Arterial line insertion and monitoring. In Proehl JA, editor: *Adult emergency nursing procedures,* Boston, 1993, Jones and Bartlett.

Lanros N: *Assessment and intervention in emergency nursing;* Norwalk, Conn, 1988, Appleton and Lange.

Thelan L: *Textbook of critical care nursing,* St Louis, 1990, Mosby.

Autotransfusion

Patty Sturt

DESCRIPTION

Autotransfusion is used for the collection and reinfusion of autologous blood. Benefits of autotransfusion include the immediate availability of blood and the diminished incidence of tranfusion reactions. Shed blood collected from post-traumatic patients should be tranfused or discarded within 4 to 6 hours from the time collection begins. Autotransfusion of >25% of estimated blood volume has been associated with a reduction in platelets, fibrinogen, and clotting factors. For this reason, the amount of blood autotransfused should not exceed 2000 ml (2). Hyperkalemia may result from red blood cell destruction from mechanical forces during collection and reinfusion.

INDICATIONS

Massive hemothorax (see Chapter 21)

CONTRAINDICATIONS

- Suspected thoracoabdominal injury. The risk of sepsis is significant when blood contaminated with gastric or intestinal contents is autotransfused. Thoracoabdominal communication may occur from injuries that disrupt or tear the diaphragm.
- Pulmonary or systemic infections
- Coagulopathies
- Malignant neoplasms
- Blood from injuries more than 4 hours old should not be autotransfused.

ATRIUM SYSTEM*

Equipment

- Atrium 2050 blood recovery system

---

*Atrium 2050 blood recovery system instruction sheet, Hudson, NH, 1994, Atrium Medical Corp.

- Atrium ATS blood recovery bag
- Y-type blood administration set with 500 to 1000 ml bag of normal saline (NS)
- Microaggregate blood filter
- Alcohol swab
- Citrate phosphate dextrose (CPD) solution (if ordered by physician)
- 60 ml syringe
- 18-gauge needle

Initial Nursing Actions

1. Prepare 2050 blood recovery chest drainage unit and assist physician with chest tube insertion (see Procedure 7). Flush Y-type blood administration set with NS.

2. Cleanse collection chamber anticoagulant injection site with an alcohol swab.

3. With an 18-gauge needle and syringe, add the CPD directly to the ATS collection chamber through the anticoagulant injection site located on top of the drain. CPD can be added at the discretion of a physician at a control dosage of 14 ml CPD per 100 ml of collected blood (1).

4. Remove ATS blood recovery bag from the sterile wrap. Place a label on the bag to include the patient's name, identification number, date, and time of collection.

5. Close ATS blood bag clamp and the ATS access line clamp on the drainage system.

6. Remove the access line cap and insert the ATS blood recovery bag spike into the chest drainage access line using a firm twisting motion. Maintain aseptic technique (Figure P4-1).

7. Once connected, open the blood bag clamp and the access line clamp.

8. For optimal blood transfer results, hold the ATS blood recovery bag 2 to 4 inches below the chest drain.

9. To activate the blood transfer, bend bottom of ATS blood bag upward where indicated. The ATS bag will begin to fill and expand as blood enters from the chest drain (Figure P4-2).

10. Once full, displace any residual air into the chest drain by gently squeezing the ATS blood bag.

11. Once blood evacuation is complete, close the access line clamp and blood bag clamp.

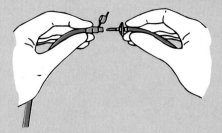

Figure P4-1   Insertion of ATS blood recovery bag spike into the chest drainage access line.

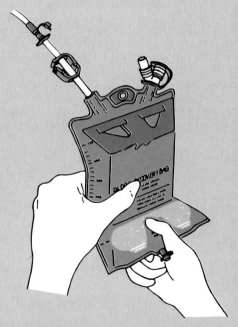

Figure P4-2   Activation of blood transfer by bending bottom of ATS blood bag upward.

12. Remove the bag spike from the access line and place the spike into the ATS bag spike holder.

13. Replace the access line cap and place the access line in the holder located on top of the chest drain.

14. A microaggregate (microemboli) filter must be used for each new ATS bag. Remove the blood filter cap and spike the microaggregate filter into the blood bag. Spike the Y-type blood administration set (the Y portion not connected to NS) into the microaggregate filter.

15. Prime blood filter by gently squeezing the blood bag before opening the air vent. Filling the microaggregate filter with NS before squeezing the bag may facilitate the flow of blood through the filter.

16. Open the air vent if the blood is to infuse by gravity. Leave the air vent closed if the blood bag is squeezed by hand or placed on a pressure infuser. Maximum ATS blood bag infusion pressure is 150 mm Hg.

17. When the infusion is complete, close the air vent (if open) by replacing the tethered vent plug. Remove the microaggregate blood filter from the blood bag and replace the tethered cap on the blood filter port. Turn on the Y portion of the blood administration set leading to the NS. Infuse the NS as needed for volume replacement and to maintain a patent line for further blood administration.

THORA-KLEX SYSTEM[†]

Equipment
- Thora-Klex autotransfusion kit 7756
- Thora-Klex chest drainage unit
- Y-type blood administration set with 500 to 1000 ml bag of NS
- Microaggregate blood filter
- Citrate phosphate dextrose (CPD)
- 60 ml syringe
- 18-gauge needle

Initial Nursing Actions
A. Preparing the autotransfusion unit

[†]*Thora-Klex autotransfusion quick reference guide*, Cranston, RI, 1990, CR Bard.

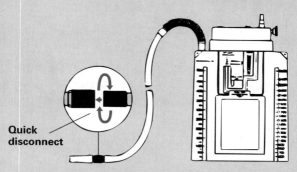

Figure P4-3 Location of Quick Disconnect on the Thora-Klex Chest drainage unit.

1. Prepare Thora-Klex chest drainage system as per manufacturer's instructions. Assist physician with chest tube insertion.
2. Connect the chest tube to the Thora-Klex chest drainage unit.
3. Remove the protective seal from the quick disconnect locking connector located midway on the patient tube of the Thora-Klex chest drainage unit.
4. Separate connector by twisting the quick disconnect locking connector counterclockwise and pulling apart. Clamp or pinch the chest tube to present outflow of blood (Figure P4-3).
5. Using aseptic technique, remove the red cover from the filter of the autotransfusion unit and insert the corresponding red-color-coded quick disconnect locking connector of the patient tube to the filter. The connector is locked into place by twisting clockwise. Insert and lock blue-color-coded connector into bottlecap (Figure P4-4).
6. Release the clamp from the patient's chest tube.
7. The Thora-Klex unit should be positioned below the patient's chest and in an upright position.
8. Place the Thora-Klex unit on suction. The wall or machine suction should be between 80 and 120 mm Hg. The suction control on the chest drainage unit is usually set to -20 cm H_2O.

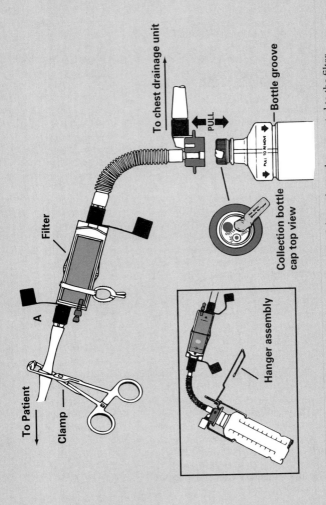

To Patient

Clamp

Filter

A

To chest drainage unit

PULL

Collection bottle
cap top view

Bottle groove

PULL TO REMOVE

Hanger assembly

Figure P4-4 Red-color-coded quick disconnect locking connector (A) of the patient tube connected to the filter.

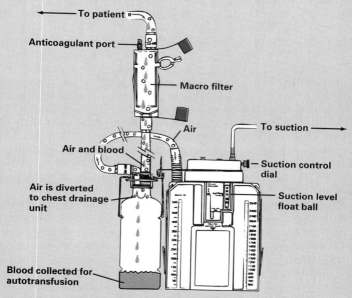

Figure P4-5 Fluid flow into the drainage collection bottle for autotransfusion. Anticoagulant may be added at the anticoagulant port of the filter.

9. Inject CPD or anticoagulant (as ordered by physician) through the anticoagulant port on the filter. The ratio of CPD to blood is 1:7 (2). Add the anticoagulant by inserting a needle through the latex injection port of the filter housing (Figure P4-5).

B. Steps for Reinfusion

1. Disconnect the Thora-Klex chest drainage unit from suction.
2. Clamp the patient tube above the filter.
3. Separate patient tube from the filter connector by rotating quick disconnect locking connector counterclockwise and pulling apart.
4. Similarly, separate Thora-Klex chest drainage patient tube at the bottle cap by rotating locking connector counterclockwise.

5. Join the patient tubes together at the quick disconnect locking connector.
6. Release clamp from the patient tube.
7. Reconnect to suction.
8. Remove the spike adapter package from side of bottle.
9. Remove the bottle from hanger.
10. Grasp the bottle cap and pull away from the bottle, exposing the rubber stopper.
11. Discard the bottle cap and filter.
12. Attach primed (flushed) Y-type blood administration set to microaggregate blood filter (attach to the portion of the Y not connected to NS).
13. Using aseptic technique, remove the IV spike adapter from the package and insert it onto the spike of the microaggregate blood filter.
14. Remove the red protective cap from the adapter and insert the adapter firmly into the port of rubber stopper marked "FLUID."
15. Remove protective seal from air vent on bottle stopper.
16. Invert bottle and hang from an IV pole using the hanger loop. Place a label on the bottle to include the patient's name, identification number, date, and time of infusion (Figure P4-6).
17. Infuse blood using gravity.
18. When the autologous blood has infused, turn off the Y clamp leading to the blood bottle. Turn on the Y clamp leading to the NS to maintain a patent IV line for further blood and fluid administration.

PLEUR-EVAC SYSTEM‡

Equipment
- Pleur-evac chest drainage unit
- Pleur-evac A-1500 autotransfusion replacement bag
- Y-type blood administration set with 500 to 1000 cc bag of NS
- Microaggregate blood filter
- Citrate phosphate dextrose (CPD) or heparin
- 60 ml syringe
- 18-gauge needle

---

‡*Pleur-evac autotransfusion replacement bag instruction sheet*, Fall River, Mass, 1992, DeKnatel.

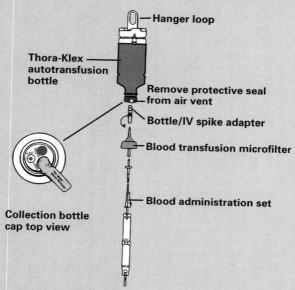

Figure P4-6 Preparation for gravity infusion.

Initial Nursing Actions

1. Prepare Pleur-evac chest drainage unit per manufacturer's instructions. Assist physician with chest tube insertion.
2. Unwrap the A-1500 replacement bag. Close the two clamps on top of the replacement bag (Figure P4-7).
3. Close the clamp on the Pleur-evac patient tubing and milk blood from the tubing into the Pleur-evac.
4. Disconnect red and blue connectors on the patient tubing.
5. Remove the red protective cap from the collection tubing on the autotransfusion bag and connect to the patient chest drainage tubing using red connectors.
6. Remove the blue protective cap from the tubing on the A-1500 autotransfusion bag and connect to the 6 inch Pleur-evac tube using blue connectors.
7. Open all clamps. Make sure connections are tight.
8. Anticoagulants may be used at the discretion of the physician. Add anticoagulant into the collection bag

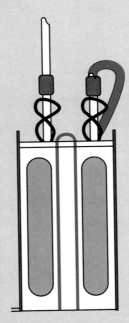

Figure P4-7 A-1500 Autotransfusion bag.

through the injection site in the autotransfusion system connector.

9. Attach the bag to the Pleur-evac using the foot hook and hanger on side of unit (Figure P4-8).

10. After blood is collected, close the clamp on the patient tubing and on top of the autotransfusion bag.

11. Disconnect all red and blue connectors.

12. Attach red and blue connectors on top of the autotransfusion bag.

13. Securely attach red and blue connectors joining the patient tube (red) to the 6 inch Pleur-evac tube (blue).

14. Open clamp on patient tube. Patient drainage is collected in the Pleur-evac.

15. Remove the autotransfusion bag from hanger on side of unit.

16. Invert the bag so the spike port points upward. Place a label on the bag to include the patient's name, identification number, date and time of infusion.

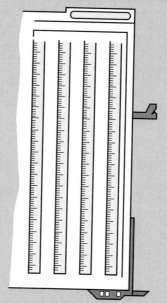

Figure P4-8 Attach the A-1500 Autotransfusion bag to the Pleur-evac using foot hook and ATS hanger on side of unit.

17. Remove the protective cap and insert microaggregate filter into the spike port.
18. Attach one end of the Y-blood administration set to the microaggregate blood filter. The other end of the Y is connected to a bag of NS. Prime the microaggregate filter and blood set with NS. Turn off Y portion leading to NS.
19. Invert the autotransfusion bag and suspend from an IV pole using the plastic strap. Turn on Y portion leading to autotransfusion bag.

PATIENT CARE MANAGEMENT (FOR ALL AUTOTRANSFUSION SYSTEMS)

1. Use a new microaggregate filter for each new autotransfusion bag or bottle.
2. Monitor the patient for coagulopathies and air embolism.
3. Prepare the patient for surgery as indicated (see Chapter 21).

References

1. *Atrium 2050 blood recovery system instruction sheet,* Hudson, NH, 1994, Atrium Medical Corp.
2. Kitt S: (1993) Autotransfusion using the Thora-Klex system. In Proehl JA, editor: *Adult emergency nursing procedures,* Boston, 1993, Jones and Bartlett.

Burn Dressing

Julia Fultz

DESCRIPTION

Burn dressings are applied to:
1. Provide an optimal environment for healing.
2. Help prevent infection.
3. Absorb exudate.
4. Assist in debridement of burned tissue.
5. Protect uninjured skin from excretions and secretions.

There are two types of burn dressings, open and closed. Open dressings are used on areas that would be hard to dress such as the head, neck, or perineum. An antibacterial cream is applied to the wound. After the cream is applied, the wound may be covered with a layer of fine mesh gauze. Leaving the wound without a dressing diminishes the proliferation of bacteria because of the decreased moisture. Closed dressings involve placing a layer of antibacterial cream or a nonstick layer of gauze over the wound and covering it with a bulky dressing. Closed dressings are most frequently used with patients treated on an outpatient basis, ambulatory patients, those who must work specifically with their hands, children, and burns in areas that will be covered with clothing.

INDICATIONS

Burn injuries that interrupt skin integrity

EQUIPMENT

- Pain medication
- Sterile gloves, hats, masks, gowns, eye protection
- Tongue blades
- Mild soap or antiseptic solution
- 4 × 4 gauze sponges
- Semielastic coarse mesh gauze such as Kerlex
- Nonadherent porous mesh gauze saturated with a water soluble lubricant

- Antibacterial agent
- 35 cc syringe attached to an 18-gauge IV catheter (needle removed) for irrigation
- Sterile saline solution with a sterile basin
- Sterile, curved scissors
- Sterile forceps
- Good light source

INITIAL NURSING ACTIONS

1. Administer pain medication in enough time before procedure, so effective analgesia is obtained.
2. Don sterile hats, gowns, masks, eye protection during irrigation of burn (to prevent splash back into eyes), and sterile gloves before initiation of care.
3. Fill sterile basin with sterile saline. Using the 35 cc syringe and the 18-gauge catheter, irrigate the burn to remove gross debris.
4. Gently cleanse the burned area with mild soap or antiseptic solution and rinse again with sterile saline.
5. If permitted by your institution's nursing policies and procedures, remove any loose skin, debris, blisters (broken, tense, or infected) using sterile forceps and scissors. If not permitted, notify the physician to perform the debridement.
6. If the patient is to be transferred to a burn unit within 1 to 2 hours, burns can be cleansed with saline and a mild soap or antiseptic solution, grossly debrided, and wrapped in sterile sheets or dry dressings for the transfer.
7. Cotton-tipped applicators dipped in sterile saline can be used to gently remove loose skin from lips, around eyes, ears, and nose. Do not vigorously debride the eyelids as the skin is very thin. Cotton-tipped applicators should only be used on the outer ear, never in the ear canal.
8. Apply neomycin or bacitracin ointment to burns of the face and do not cover area.
9. If ordered, apply antibacterial cream using a sterile tongue blade, or a sterile gloved hand. (If using a jar of antibacterial cream, do not dip the tongue blade or gloved hand back into the jar after it has come into contact with the wound. Contamination of the cream will occur.)

10. Dress the wound. (Dressings are usually not applied to the head, neck, and perineum because of difficulty securing them.)

   a. Describe procedure to patient. (If the patient is to be discharged home and expected to do dressing changes, explain each step as it is done.)

   b. Apply mesh gauze that contains a water soluble lubricant to prevent sticking if no antibacterial cream is used.

   c. Cover mesh gauze or antibacterial cream with a bulky dressing such as 4 × 4 gauze sponges about ½ inch thick to absorb drainage.

   d. Secure bulky dressing with semielastic mesh gauze (e.g., Kerlex), wrapping extremities distal to proximal.

   e. Hands must be wrapped in a functional position. (Fingers slightly flexed with the thumb abducted away from the palm with a roll of gauze such as Kling or Kerlex in the patient's palm to support the position.)

   f. Wrap fingers and toes individually to allow for range of motion. Leave tips of fingers and toes exposed to evaluate circulation.

COMPLICATIONS

1. Infection
2. Diminished perfusion distal to a circumferential dressing

PATIENT CARE MANAGEMENT

1. Check circulation distal to any circumferential dressing.
2. Administer tetanus toxoid as ordered.
3. Elevate extremity to minimize swelling.
4. If patient is to be discharged, teaching regarding dressing changes and signs of infection must be reinforced, and written instructions must be given to the patient. If wound is infected, ensure patient receives a prescription for antibiotics. Plans for follow-up care (with a private physician or with the emergency department) must be made before discharging the patient.

EXAMPLE OF DISCHARGE INSTRUCTIONS

1. How to change your dressing:
   - Assemble your supplies and keep the area around the supplies clean.
   - Wash your hands, do not touch anything (hair, face, clothes, pets) other than the dressing supplies.
   - Remove old dressing (if the dressing sticks to the burn, soak it off with cool, clean water).
   - Clean the burn with soap and water, then pat dry with a clean, dry cloth such as a wash cloth or dish towel.
   - Look for one or more of these signs and symptoms of infection:
     a. Increased redness around the burn
     b. Swelling
     c. Red streaks extending away from the burn
     d. Pus
     e. Elevated temperature
     f. Increased pain
   - Apply a thin layer of the antibacterial cream and cover with a gauze dressing as was done in the hospital.
2. If you think your burn has become infected, call your private physician or the ED.
3. Take your pain medicine as prescribed.
4. Elevate the extremity for 24 hours if possible.
5. It is very important for you to have your burn checked in about 24 hours. Please comply with the follow-up directions given to you before leaving the ED.
   Follow-up directions:
   _____
   _____
   _____
6. If you have any questions, call your private physician or the ED at _____ .

Central Venous Pressure Measurement

Patty Sturt

DESCRIPTION

Central venous pressure (CVP) monitoring refers to the measurement of pressure within the right atrium. Right atrial pressure is synonymous with CVP. The CVP can provide an estimate of the volume status of the right heart. The normal range is 3 to 10 cm H_2O.

INDICATIONS

1. Alteration in fluid volume status. A low CVP often occurs in hypovolemic patients. An elevated CVP occurs in cases of fluid overload or retention.
2. To guide fluid replacement in hypovolemia.
3. To assess the effectiveness of diuretic administration.
4. To assess right heart function. The CVP may be increased in right-sided heart failure.

NURSING ALERT

The CVP is not a reliable indicator of left ventricular failure. Left ventricular failure increases filling pressure of the left side of the heart. Eventually this increased pressure results in the backup of blood into the pulmonary vasculature. Pulmonary edema is present by the time the CVP becomes elevated.

EQUIPMENT

1. For catheter placement:
   - Single-, double-, or triple-lumen infusion catheter
   - 1% lidocaine
   - 5 and 10 cc syringes and different size needles for injection of lidocaine
   - Antiseptic skin solution such as povidone-iodine solution

- Sterile towels
- Needle introducer
- 10 to 20 cc syringe
- Guidewire

NOTE: These are available in commercially prepackaged kits often referred to as CVP kits or venous pressure trays.

2. For CVP monitoring:
   - CVP water manometer with three-way stopcock
   - Extension tubing
   - IV fluid and administration set
   - Indelible marker

INITIAL NURSING ACTIONS

1. Attach stopcock to end of manometer. Attach extension tubing to one port and IV administration set to the other port. Turn stopcock off to the manometer, and flush entire length of tubing with IV solution.
2. Explain the procedure to the patient and obtain informed consent.
3. Prep the catheter insertion site with antiseptic solution.
4. Position patient supine and in slight Trendelenburg position (if patient will tolerate this).
5. After injecting with local anesthetic and draping the area, the physician usually inserts the infusion catheter into the subclavian or internal jugular vein. A needle is inserted, then a guidewire is placed through the needle. The needle is removed and a catheter is placed over the guidewire. The guidewire is removed and the catheter is sutured in place. The catheter tip is usually placed into the superior vena cava just above the right atrium.

NURSING ALERT

Monitor for arrhythmias during catheter insertion. Inform physician immediately if this occurs.

6. Obtain an order for a chest x-ray to confirm accurate placement.
7. Connect end of extension tubing to the catheter.
8. Adjust IV rate as prescribed by physician.

9. For CVP measurement, the patient should be supine or the head of bed can be elevated 30 to 45 degrees.
10. Position the zero mark of the water manometer at the phlebostatic axis. This is located at the junction of the midaxillary line and 4th intercostal space. This point approximates the level of the atria.
11. Mark the point with an indelible marker. This site becomes the zero reference point—the location to be used for all subsequent readings.
12. Turn the stopcock off to the patient (catheter) and open to the IV solution and manometer. Allow IV solution to slowly fill the manometer to the 25 cm level. Do not let fluid overflow from the top of the manometer.
13. Turn the stopcock off to the IV solution and open to the patient (catheter) and manometer. The fluid level will fall and fluctuate with respirations.
14. Take the reading when the fluid level stabilizes. The CVP reading should be taken at the end of expiration. The measurement should be recorded at the lowest point of the water meniscus.
15. Turn the stopcock off to the manometer and on to the patient (catheter) and IV solution.
16. Infuse IV solution through the central venous line as prescribed.
17. Document CVP reading.

PATIENT CARE MANAGEMENT

1. Note the trend of the CVP readings.
2. Instruct patient to report any tubing disconnections.

Bibliography

Gray MC, Littleton AD: Central venous pressure measurement via manometer. In Proehl JA, editor: *Adult emergency nursing procedures,* Boston, 1993, Jones and Bartlett.

Hogsten P: Hemodynamic monitoring. In Kidd PS, Wagner KD, editors: *High acuity nursing,* Norwalk, Conn, 1992, Appleton and Lange.

Sudarth DS: *Lippincott manual of nursing practice,* Philadelphia, 1991, JB Lippincott.

Thelan L, Davie JK, Urden LD, Lough ME: *Cardiovascular diagnostic procedures,* Philadelphia, 1994, Mosby.

Chest Tubes

Patty Sturt

DESCRIPTION

Chest tubes are used to remove air and/or fluid from the pleural cavity, to restore normal negative intrapleural pressure, and to achieve full reexpansion of a lung.

INDICATIONS

1. Hemothorax
2. Pneumothorax
3. Empyema
4. Large pleural effusion

EQUIPMENT

- Povidone-iodine solution
- 4 × 4 gauze sponges
- Local anesthetic
- Needles of various sizes
- 5 and 10 ml syringes
- Sterile gloves
- Sterile drapes
- Scalpels
- Large clamps/hemostats
- Suture material
- Needle-holders
- Occlusive gauze
- 3 to 4 inch tape
- Chest drainage systems
- Chest tube of appropriate size as follows:

Age	Chest tube sizes
Newborn	12-18 Fr
6 months	14-20 Fr
1 year	14-24 Fr

Age	Chest tube sizes
3 years	16-28 Fr
5 years	20-32 Fr
8 years	24-32 Fr
12 years	28-36 Fr
Adults	28-40 Fr

Smaller sizes can be used for removal of air and larger sizes for removal of fluid. Anticipate the need for a 36 to 40 Fr tube in an adult trauma patient.

INITIAL NURSING ACTIONS

1. Assemble chest drainage system. Fill water seal and suction control chambers as specified by instructions with the system.
2. If patient is on a cardiac monitor, move electrodes on involved side of chest to shoulder and lateral-posterior chest wall.
3. Monitor patient throughout procedure. Provide verbal support and comfort measures.
4. The 4th intercostal space in the midaxillary line is often used as the insertion site. The physician cleanses the area with a povidone-iodine solution. The area is draped and locally infiltrated with an anesthetic solution. An incision is made with a scalpel along the rib. A curved clamp is inserted into the incision. A small tunnel is formed by separating the clamp. The clamp is closed and then placed further into the thoracic cage through the intercostal muscles and parietal pleura. The clamp is opened and closed again to enlarge the puncture site. At this point, the physician removes the clamp and inserts a gloved finger into the pleural space to ensure a clear passage for the chest tube. The chest tube is inserted into the opening with a curved clamp. The tube is sutured in place.
5. After insertion, connect the chest tube to the tubing from the collection chamber. Connect tubing from suction control chamber to the suction source.
6. After the chest tube is sutured in place, apply a dressing with occlusive gauze, 4 × 4 sponges, and 3 to 4 inch tape.
7. Wrap tubing connections with adhesive tape to ensure they are airtight.

8. Coil extra tubing from the drainage system, and place it flat on the bed.
9. Secure an x-ray to confirm correct tube placement.

PATIENT CARE MANAGEMENT

1. Assess and trend patient's vital signs, skin color, and breath sounds.
2. Monitor for blood/fluid in the collection chamber. Mark the level of drainage hourly on the drainage system. Notify physician if drainage is >100 ml/hour.
3. Observe for fluctuation ("tidaling") of the fluid level in the water seal chamber. The fluid level rises when the patient inhales and drops when the patient exhales. If the patient is on a ventilator, the opposite occurs. The fluid level drops on inspiration (because intrapleural pressure becomes more positive) and rises on expiration. Fluctuation indicates patency of the system. Lack of fluctuation may be indicative of an obstruction or kink in the system.
4. Milk tubing by gently kneading a small piece of tubing between your fingers if blood clots or tissue obstruct the tubing.
5. Do not clamp the chest tube. Clamping may lead to an accumulation of air in the pleural space and result in a tension pneumothorax.
6. If the patient is to be transported, or if suction is not being used, leave the suction tubing connector open to air. Do not clamp it off.
7. If the chest tube is accidentally pulled out, cover the site with a dressing taped on three sides. Immediately notify the physician.

NURSING ALERT

It may be difficult to assess tidaling and breath sounds when suction is in use. Suction may be turned off. The purpose of the suction control chamber is to facilitate the removal of air and fluid. The water seal remains intact when suction is not in use.

Bibliography

Simons RS, Brenner BE: *Emergency procedures and techniques,* Baltimore, MD, 1994, William and Wilkins.
Sudarth DS: *Lippincott manual of nursing practice,* ed 5, Philadelphia, 1991, JB Lippincott.

Conscious Sedation

Patty Sturt

DESCRIPTION

IV conscious sedation (IVCS) is produced by the administration of pharmacologic agents. A patient under conscious sedation has a depressed level of consciousness but retains the ability to independently and continuously maintain a patent airway and respond appropriately to physical stimulation and/or verbal command. The objectives of IVCS include the following:
1. Alteration of mood
2. Maintenance of consciousness
3. Cooperative patient
4. Increased pain threshold
5. Stable vital signs
6. Amnesia dependent on medications

INDICATIONS

IVCS may be used in ED patients requiring the following:
1. Closed manipulation/reduction of dislocations and/or fractures
2. Suction curettage
3. Extensive laceration repairs
4. Incision and drainage
5. Foreign body removal
6. Endoscopic procedures
7. Diagnostic procedures

CONTRAINDICATIONS

IVCS should be used cautiously in patients that have a history of recent alcohol ingestion. Alcohol can compound the actions of many of the medications used for IVCS. Other contraindications can include the following:
1. Pregnancy
2. Thyroid, adrenal, or renal dysfunction

3. Patients on MAO inhibitors (MAOIs) or tricyclic antidepressants (TCAs)
4. Respiratory failure

EQUIPMENT

- IV fluid, tubing, and catheter
- IVCS medications and their antidotes (see Table P8-1)
- Pulse oximeter
- Code cart with airway equipment, bag-valve-mask device, resuscitation drugs, and a monitor/defibrillator
- Oxygen and oxygen delivery devices such as nasal cannula and nonrebreather mask
- Suction
- Automatic blood pressure (BP) device or BP cuff and stethoscope

INITIAL NURSING ACTIONS

1. Obtain a history and baseline assessment data to include the following:
   - Current medications and drug allergies
   - Medical/surgical history
   - History of substance abuse
   - Physical parameters such as vital signs, level of consciousness, skin color, temperature, oxygen saturation, and an Aldrete score (Table P8-2)
   - Planned method of transport home
   - Food or fluid intake within the past 8 hours
2. Establish IV access. Use an 18-gauge or greater, if there is the possibility of significant blood loss.
3. Place the patient on a pulse oximeter.
4. Administer and titrate the medications (see the box, p. 724) based on the attending physician's order and the individual's response. The desired effects of conscious sedation include the following:
   - Relaxed and cooperative patient
   - Diminished verbal communication
   - Initiation of slurred speech
   - Arousable sleep

PATIENT CARE MANAGEMENT

1. A patent IV must be continuously maintained during the procedure.

TABLE P8-2 Discharge Guidelines Using the Aldrete Scoring System

Physical parameters	Score
Activity	
Voluntary movement of all limbs to command	2
Voluntary movement of two extremities to command	1
Unable to move	0
Respiration	
Breathe deeply and cough	2
Dyspnea, hypoventilation	1
Apneic	0
Circulation	
BP 20% of preanesthetic level	2
BP 20%-50% of preanesthetic level	1
BP 50% of preanesthetic level	0
Consciousness	
Fully awake	2
Arousable	1
Unresponsive	0
Color	
Pink	2
Pale, blotch	1
Cyanotic	0

2. The RN managing the care of the patient receiving IVCS should not leave the patient unattended.
3. Oxygen saturation must be continuously monitored during the procedure. Supplemental oxygen should be given if there is a drop in the oxygen saturation from the patient's baseline.
      Oxygen Saturation Levels as follows:
      Normal reading: 95% to 100%
      Mild hypoxemia: 89% to 94.5%
      Severe hypoxemia: <75%

COMMONLY ADMINISTERED MEDICATIONS FOR IVCS

Benzodiazpines

Midazolam (Versed)
Diazepam (Valium)
Lorazepam (Ativan)

Antagonists

Naloxone (Narcan)
Flumazenil (Romazicon)

Narcotics

Meperidine (Demerol)
Morphine
Sublimaze (Fentanyl)

4. Anticipate the need to administer oxygen in any patient with a baseline SpO_2 equal to or <90.
5. The BP, heart rate, respiratory rate, and pulse oximeter values should be obtained and recorded every 5 to 15 minutes during the procedure.
6. Anticipate the need to continuously monitor cardiac rhythm and rate on patients with a history of cardiac or respiratory disease.
7. Vital signs and an Aldrete score should be evaluated and documented at least every 15 minutes until the patient's values return to baseline. The Aldrete score provides objective, measurable information regarding the degree of sedation. Other sedation scoring systems are available.
8. Before discharge from the ED, the patient and significant others should receive verbal and written instructions to include signs and symptoms of complications, restrictions on diet and activity, and a follow-up appointment as needed. Documentation should reflect that the patient and significant others received, verbalized, and understood the instructions.
9. Never allow the patient to drive self home.

Bibliography

Association of Operating Room Nurses: Position statement on the role of the RN in the management of patients receiving IV conscious sedation for short-term therapeutic, diagnostic, or surgical procedures, *AORN* 51:1513, 1991.

Association of Operating Room Nurses: Recommended practices on the patient receiving IV conscious sedation, *Standards and recommended practices,* Denver, 1993, The Association.

Kidwell JA: Nursing care for the patient receiving conscious sedation during gastrointestinal endoscopic procedures, *Gastroenterol Nurs* 13:136-137, 1991.

Levy L, Pandit S: Is midazolam a dangerous drug? *J Post Anesth Nurs* 3:40-43, 1991.

Murphy E: OR nursing law: monitoring IV conscious sedation, the legal scope of practice, *AORN* 57:512-514, 1993.

Skidmore-Roth L: *Nursing drug reference,* St Louis, 1994, Mosby.

TABLE P8-1 Drug Summary

Drug	Dose/Route	Special considerations	Half-life
Flumazenil (Romazicon) benzodiazepine antagonist	0.2 mg. May be repeated at 1 min intervals until desired level of consciousness is achieved or a total dose of 1 mg has been given. IV over 15 sec.	Used to reverse the effects of benzodiazepines in adults. Not recommended for use in children. Some side effects include nausea/vomiting, headache, dizziness, sweating, and flushing.	41-79 min
Meperidine (Demerol) narcotic	Initial dose of 10-25 mg. IV over 30 sec–2 min into an infusing IV. May repeat every 10-15 min.	Monitor the patient for weakness, nausea/vomiting, respiratory depression, and hypotension.	3-4 hr
Lorazepam (Ativan) benzodiazepine	1-2 mg or 0.05 mg/kg. 2 mg IV over 1 min.	Potentiates narcotics, MAOIs, and TCAs. Effective in 15-20 min.	14 hr
Diazepam (Valium) benzodiazepine	2.5-5 mg. Slow IV push over 1 min. Repeat every 5-10 min. Onset is within 1-5 min.	Monitor patient for hypotension and respiratory depression.	20-50 hr
Midazolam (Versed) benzodiazepine	0.5 to 2.5 mg. IV push over 2 min into an infusing IV line.	Do not give to patients on MAOIs or TCAs.	1.2-12.3 hr

Drug	Dose	Notes	Duration
Morphine narcotic	Initial dose of 2-5 mg. Slow IV push over 5 min into an infusing IV line.	Reduced doses should be used in those with renal or hepatic dysfunctions.	2.5-3 hr
Sublimaze (Fentanyl) narcotic	2 mcg/kg. 0.1 mg over 1-2 min.	Respiratory depressant effects outlast analgesics effect; 80 times more potent than morphine. Usually used under the direct observation of an anesthesiologist.	2.5-4 hr
Naloxone (Narcan) narcotic antagonist	0.1 to 0.2 mg. IV at 2-3 min intervals into an infusing IV line.	Antagonist for narcotic-induced hypotension and respiratory depression.	1 hr

Crutch Walking

Lee Garner

DESCRIPTION

Crutches may be needed in emergency department (ED) patients to facilitate unilateral, non–weight-bearing ambulation. The most frequently used crutches are the underarm or axillary crutches with hand bars (1).

INDICATIONS

Lower extremity injuries such as sprains, contusions, or fractures.

EQUIPMENT

Adjustable crutches with axilla pads, hand bar pads, and crutch tips.

INITIAL NURSING ACTIONS

A. Measuring for crutches
1. Place axilla pads, hand bar pads, and crutch tips on the crutches.
2. Have patient stand and bear weight on nonaffected extremity. Place crutches 2.5 to 5 cm (1 to 2 inches) or 2 to 3 finger breadths below axilla. Adjust crutches so they extend 5 cm (2 inches) in front of and 15 cm (6 inches) to the side of the feet. Crutches can be adjusted by removing the screws in the lower portion and shortening or lengthening the inner lower piece. Replace the screws and bolts and tighten firmly.
3. With the patient standing upright and erect, adjust the hand bars to the point where there is approximately 30 degree elbow flexion. The hand grips can be adjusted by removing the screws and sliding the hand grips to the appropriate level. Slide screws back into the crutches. Replace the bolts and tighten firmly. The patient's arms should never be straight (Figure P9-1).

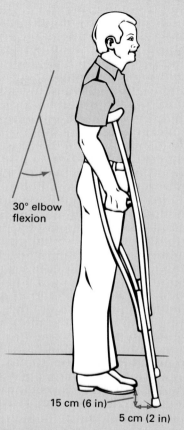

30° elbow flexion

15 cm (6 in)

5 cm (2 in)

Figure P9-1 The standing position to measure the correct length of crutches. (From Kozier B, et al: *Fundamentals of nursing,* ed 4, 1991, Addison-Wesley.)

B. Ambulating with crutches
   1. Place weight on palms of the hands and not the axilla.

NURSING ALERT

Continual pressure on the axilla can injure the radial nerve, resulting in weakness to the forearm, wrist, and hand.

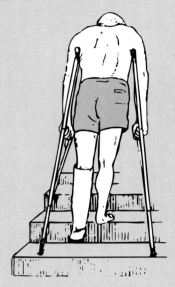

Figure P9-2 When climbing stairs the client places weight on the crutches while first moving the unaffected leg onto a step. (From Barber J, Stokes L, Billings D: *Adult and child care*, ed 2, St Louis, 1977, Mosby.)

2. Use the proper standing position called the tripod position. In this position, the crutch tips are placed about 5 cm (2 inches) in front of the feet and out laterally about 15 cm (6 inches). This creates a wide and stable base of support.
3. Look forward (not at the feet) and advance crutches and affected leg forward at the same time.
4. Move the unaffected leg forward and through to a position slightly ahead of the crutches (2).

C. Going up stairs (Figure P9-2)
   1. Assume the tripod position at the bottom of the stairs.
   2. While balancing weight on the hands, move the unaffected leg onto the step.
   3. Shift body weight to the unaffected leg and move affected leg and crutches up onto the step. Keep the affected leg slightly bent during this move.

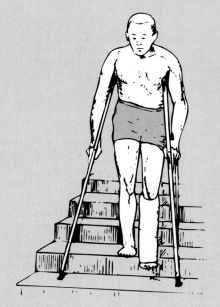

Figure P9-3 When descending stairs the client first moves the crutches and affected leg down to the next step. (From Barber J, Stokes L, Billings D: *Adult and child care*, ed 2, St Louis, 1977, Mosby.)

D. Going down stairs (Figure P9-3)
   1. Shift body weight to the unaffected leg. Move the crutches and affected leg onto the step. Keep the affected leg slightly in front of the body during the move.
   2. Transfer body weight to crutches and move unaffected leg to that step. When moving unaffected leg to the step, land on the heel and not the toes.

NURSING ALERT

A simple way to remind patients of these steps is the "good" (unaffected leg) goes up first toward heaven when traveling up stairs. Thus the bad (affected) leg goes down first when moving down the stairs.

E. Sitting on chair or bed
   1. Slowly turn around and back up until the back of the unaffected leg touches the chair or bed.
   2. Transfer both crutches to the hand on the same side as the affected leg. Hold onto the crutches with the hand bars. Grasp arm of the chair with the other hand.
   3. Hold affected leg slightly forward, and slowly lower self into a sitting position.
F. Getting out of chair or bed
   1. Move forward to the edge of the chair or bed.
   2. Grasp the crutches by the hand bars in the hand on the affected side. Grasp the arm of the chair by the hand on the unaffected side.
   3. Push self up.
   4. Assume tripod position before moving.

PATIENT CARE MANAGEMENT

Instruct patient to:
1. Remove loose rugs and small objects on the floor at home.
2. Stay off wet or waxed floors, ice, and grass. These can be slick.
3. Wipe off wet crutch tips.
4. Avoid escalators.
5. Wear sturdy, low-heeled shoes.
6. Avoid alcohol or medications that may impair balance, perception, and judgment.

References

1. Kozier E, Erb G, Olivier R: *Fundamentals of nursing: concepts, process, and practice,* Redwood City, Calif, 1991, Addison-Wesley.
2. Swimm DM: Measuring for crutches/teaching crutch walking. In Proehl JA, editor: *Adult emergency nursing procedures,* Boston, 1993, Jones and Bartlett.

Defibrillation

Darlene Welsh
George P Glessner III

Defibrillation is the treatment of choice for ventricular fibrillation and pulseless ventricular tachycardia. Until recently, this procedure has been performed only in settings equipped for advanced cardiac life support with the use of complex defibrillators. With the advent of automated external defibrillators(AEDs), defibrillation can now be executed in a variety of settings by emergency cardiac care providers and eventually laypersons. The emergency nurse will be dealing with the prehospital use of AEDs more frequently and therefore must have an understanding of their use and integration into the emergency department (ED) resuscitation of the cardiac arrest patient. AEDs are classified as "fully" automatic or "semiautomatic." Fully automatic AEDs require no intervention beyond application and initial activation of the device. Semiautomatic AEDs require the operator to initiate the "analyze" feature of the device and then press the appropriate button to deliver the shocks after being advised to do so by the AED. Both devices are considered safe and effective (1). The semiautomatic AEDs applied in the prehospital setting can be used to continue defibrillation in the ED while other definitive cardiac care measures such as intubation, IV cannulation, and initial resuscitation drug administration are instituted. It is important for the ED nurse to be competent with defibrillation, since the survival of the patient with serious cardiac complications often depends on the successful completion of this procedure.

DESCRIPTION

Defibrillation can be accomplished by delivering nonsynchronized electrical energy (joules) to the myocardium in order to depolarize the pacemaker cells. With successful defibrillation, a brief period of asystole is followed by an

effective cardiac rhythm eliminating ventricular fibrillation
or pulseless ventricular tachycardia.

INDICATIONS

1. Ventricular fibrillation
2. Pulseless ventricular tachycardia

EQUIPMENT

- Automatic external defibrillator or standard defibrillator
  with cardiac monitor
- ECG electrodes
- Conductive gel, two gel pads, or two self-adhesive
  disposable defibrillator electrodes (DDE)

INITIAL NURSING ACTIONS

Defibrillation with Standard Defibrillator

1. Turn on the ECG monitor. Hook the patient up to the
   ECG monitor in lead II, while someone else performs
   CPR. Turn on continuous ECG recorder. Confirm
   ventricular fibrillation/pulseless tachycardia.
2. Apply conductive gel to defibrillator paddles. Gel pads
   designed specifically for defibrillation can be substituted
   for the defibrillator gel. Do not use ECG gel. Some
   institutions use pregelled, self-adhesive disposable
   defibrillator electrodes in place of paddles for repeated
   defibrillation (1). Many defibrillators have the capacity
   for cardiac monitoring through the defibrillator paddles,
   omitting the need for ECG electrodes.
3. Charge the defibrillator to 200 joules. Make sure the
   defibrillator is in the "unsynchronized" mode.
4. Place the paddles on the chest wall for defibrillation or
   to monitor without ECG cables. The sternal or posterior
   paddle is placed on the right upper sternum below the
   clavicle (right atrial area). The apex or anterior paddle is
   placed near and lateral to the left nipple at the
   midaxillary line (apex). See Figure P10-1 for standard
   paddle placement. Infants weighing <10 kg require 4.5
   cm pediatric paddles. Children weighing over 10 kg,
   approximately 1 year of age, can be defibrillated with 8
   to 10 cm paddles (3,4). Adults require 13 cm paddles
   (5). Paddle placement in children is similar to adults,
   with one paddle over the right side of the upper chest

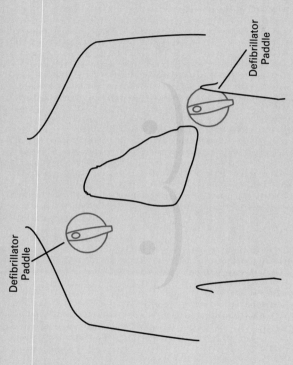

Figure P10-1 Recommended anterior-apex position for defibrillation. The anterior electrode should be to the right of the upper sternum below the clavicle. The apex electrode should be placed to the left of the nipple with the center of the electrode in the midaxillary line. (From American Heart Association, *Textbook of advanced cardiac life support*, 1994, Dallas, The Association.)

and the other over the apex of the heart to the left of the nipple.

5. Press the paddles on the chest wall with approximately 25 lb of pressure.

6. Determine that everyone in the room is not in contact with the patient or equipment touching the patient. Verify verbally that all rescuers are not in contact by stating, "All clear" before delivering the shock. This reminds everyone to check their status and move to a safe location.

7. Deliver the electrical current by simultaneously pressing the appropriate buttons. Defibrillators vary, therefore, it is recommended that nurses seek appropriate training for equipment used in their clinical area.

8. For adults, three consecutive shocks are delivered at 200, 200 to 300, and 360 joules if resolution of ventricular fibrillation/tachycardia does not occur after each attempt (2). Remember to confirm ventricular fibrillation/tachycardia by cardiac monitor before each countershock. It is important to deliver the initial three consecutive shocks with little time in between in order to increase the probability of successful defibrillation. Therefore, CPR between the three consecutive shocks is not recommended. Pediatric patients require 2 joules/kg initially, followed by successive shocks of 4 joules/kg.

NURSING ALERT

Do not defibrillate over nitroglycerine patches or permanent pacemaker pulse generators. Avoid pulse generators by placing one paddle opposite the insertion site below the clavicle and the other lateral to the sternum at least 5 inches from the pulse generator. See Figure P10-2 for alternate paddle placement (5). Do not allow gel to form a path between paddles. Burn injury to the patient could occur under these circumstances.

9. If the patient does not convert to a pulse generating rhythm after the third attempt, initiate ACLS.

PATIENT CARE MANAGEMENT

1. Continue CPR if delays in defibrillation occur. Do not perform CPR between the three initial consecutive shocks.

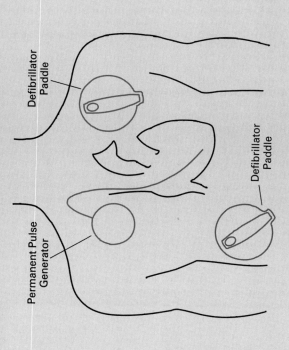

Figure P10-2 Alternate paddle placement for synchronized cardioversion and defibrillation in the patient with a permanent pulse generator. (From Boggs R, Wooldridge-King M: *AACN procedure manual for critical care*, ed 3, Philadelphia, 1993, WB Saunders.)

2. Continue monitoring and assessing cardiopulmonary status after defibrillation.

3. Other interventions before and after defibrillation may include airway and ventilation management by intubation or cricothyrotomy, IV medication administration, and in some instances, endotracheal medication instillation if rapid IV access cannot be achieved.

4. Routine care of the defibrillation equipment includes inspection of the equipment every shift. Determine that ECG paper, monitoring electrodes, and defibrillator gel or pads are available. Examine the cables, connectors, paddles, and defibrillator for damage. Test the adequacy of the battery power supply and the ECG display by turning on the equipment and charging the paddles. For most models, the paddles can be safely discharged into the equipment. Clean the equipment and restock supplies after each use.

Defibrillation with AED

1. Turn power on.
2. Attach the device and "hands off" defibrillation pads to the patient.
3. Initiate analysis of the rhythm if not "fully" automatic.
4. Deliver the shock if needed (if not fully automatic).
5. If the device is already in place and can be used to continue defibrillation in the ED, skip steps 1 through 4 as they have already been done and continue defibrillation without delay by using the "manual" feature of the AED.

NURSING ALERT

Some models of AEDs lack a rhythm interpretation monitor and should be removed immediately and a standard defibrillator used upon arrival at the ED (1).

References

1. American Heart Association: Defibrillation, *Textbook of advanced cardiac life support,* Dallas, 1994, The Association, 1-22.
2. American Heart Association Emergency Cardiac Care Committee and Subcommittee: Adult advanced cardiac life support part 3, *JAMA* 268(16):2199-2241, 1992.

3. American Heart Association Emergency Cardiac Care
   Committee and Subcommittee: Pediatric advanced life
   support part 6, *JAMA* 268(16):2262-2275, 1992.
4. Suddaby EC, Rider SL: Defibrillation and cardioversion in
   children, *Pediatr Nurs* 17(5):477-481, 1991.
5. Walker CB: Precordial shock. In Boggs RL, Wooldridge-King
   MW, editors: *AACN procedure manual for critical care,*
   Philadelphia, 1993, WB Saunders.

Bibliography

Johnston JB: Defibrillation in the emergency care setting: present
and future shock, *Emerg Nurs Reports* 3(3):1-8, 1988.
Smith M: Rules for joules, *JEMS* 17(2):13, 1992.
Stewart JA: Defibrillation training for general unit nurses, *J Emer
Nurs* 18(6):519-524, 1992.

Diagnostic Peritoneal Lavage

Patty Sturt
Barbara Blake

DESCRIPTION

Diagnostic peritoneal lavage (DPL) is a procedure used to detect intraabdominal bleeding or viscus perforation after abdominal trauma. The accuracy of peritoneal lavage is approximately 95% to 98%. It is less useful in children than in adults. An abdominal CT scan is commonly used in children to assess internal abdominal injury (1). DPL is neither organ or injury specific. It is also unable to detect retroperitoneal bleeding. DPL can be performed using either the percutaneous or open (operative) approach. The open approach allows direct visualization of the peritoneum when the catheter is inserted. Thus inadvertent insertion of the catheter into the preperitoneal space is less likely to occur.

INDICATIONS

1. Blunt Trauma
   - Unreliable examination because of altered level of consciousness, central nervous system or spinal cord injury, and/or alcohol or drug intoxication
   - Unexplained history of hypotension in the field or ED (4)
   - Major thoracic or multisystem injuries
   - Multiple trauma patient requiring general anesthetic for nonabdominal surgical procedures
2. Penetrating Trauma
   - Gunshot or stab wound with questionable peritoneal penetration. Depending on the size and shape of the instrument used, stab wounds at or below the nipple line may involve the abdominal/peritoneal cavity.
   - Multiple stab wounds to lower chest and/or abdomen

CONTRAINDICATIONS

1. Previous intraabdominal surgery (relative contraindication)
2. Multiple previous abdominal surgeries increase the risk of adhesions. Adhesions may cause the intestines to adhere to the abdominal wall. Intestinal perforation may occur when the catheter is introduced.
3. Pregnancy >12 weeks of gestation (relative contraindication) (5)
4. Definite abdominal penetration. Gunshot wounds to the abdomen require surgical exploration.
5. Patient is hemodynamically unstable and immediate abdominal surgery is indicated based on the physical examination (see Chapter 21).
6. Radiographic evidence of free air in the abdomen

EQUIPMENT

- Gastric tube
- Urinary catheter
- Antiseptic solution (povidone-iodine solution commonly used)
- Sterile gloves
- Mask
- Gown
- Razor
- 5, 10, and 20 cc syringes
- Needles of various sizes
- Sterile drapes (four sterile towels are usually used)
- Gauze sponge
- Local anesthetic (1% lidocaine with or without epinephrine is frequently used)
- Peritoneal lavage catheter and introducing stylet (commercially available in preassembled kits)
- 1000 ml warmed (36.6 to 37.7°C) normal saline (NS) or Ringer's lactate solution (3)
- IV tubing: maxidrip solution set
- Needle-holder and straight scissors
- Suture material (4-0 nylon on a cutting needle for the percutaneous approach. Suture material for open procedure depends on the physician's preference.)
- For open technique: Two Allis or Kocher clamps, one Kelly clamp, and two small right angle retractors

- Blood collection tubes and sterile specimen container
- Antibiotic ointment
- Small dressing for covering catheter entrance site. (NOTE: Preassembled kits containing much of this equipment are available.)

INITIAL NURSING ACTIONS

1. If at all possible, diagnostic abdominal x-rays should be taken before performing DPL. The procedure may produce artifacts on the x-rays such as intraperitoneal air.
2. Explain procedure to the conscious patient.
3. Insert an indwelling urinary catheter before the procedure.

NURSING ALERT

This is extremely important, since a full bladder may be punctured during the advancement of the catheter toward the pelvis.

4. Pass a nasogastric or orogastric tube to decompress the stomach and prevent stomach perforation during peritoneal catheter insertion.
5. Spike the IV bag with the maxidrip IV tubing set. Flush IV tubing. Keep end of tubing capped and sterile.
6. Place the patient in a supine position. Provide verbal support in the conscious patient.
7. The nurse or physician should shave the abdomen at and around the insertion site if necessary.
8. The nurse or physician should prep the abdomen with antiseptic solution from the umbilicus and to the symphysis pubis.
   NOTE: At this point the physician drapes the abdomen and injects the area with lidocaine. A small transverse incision through the skin and fascia may be performed to allow easy passage of the catheter and stylet (percutaneous approach). In the open approach, an incision is made and Kelly clamps are used to dissect through the fascia until the parietal peritoneum is exposed. In adults, the usual site for catheter insertion is midline and 2 to 3 cm below the umbilicus or one-third of the distance between the umbilicus and symphysis pubis. In young children an infraumbilical or

supraumbilical approach may be used. The catheter is directed through the peritoneum toward the pelvis. Once the catheter is in place, a 10 or 20 cc syringe is attached to aspirate peritoneal fluid. If more than 5 to 10 ml of blood or any gastric/bowel contents are aspirated, the lavage is considered positive, and it is not necessary to infuse the NS or Ringer's lactate into the peritoneal space.

9. If no blood or gastric contents are aspirated, attach the IV tubing to the catheter. Open the IV tubing clamp and infuse 1 liter. For children, infuse 15 to 20 cc/kg. The physician may gently massage the abdomen to distribute the fluid.

10. When the infusion is complete, lower the IV bag and allow the fluid to return by gravity. As much of the fluid as possible should be removed from the peritoneal cavity. A reasonable return is 75% to 80% of the fluid instilled (3). If the patient's condition permits, turning the patient may facilitate removal of the fluid.

11. Laboratory specimens of the peritoneal fluid should be obtained as ordered by the physician. Commonly ordered laboratory tests include red blood cell count (RBC), white blood cell count (WBC), hematocrit (Hct), bilirubin, amylase, alkaline phosphatase, SGOT, culture and sensitivity, and gram stain. The fluid should be placed in a sterile specimen container or the same laboratory tubes that would be used if the tests were being performed on blood.

   The following findings (based on 1000 ml infused) are associated with a positive lavage:
   - RBC >100,000/mm^3 in blunt trauma
   - RBC >10,000/mm^3 in penetrating trauma
   - WBC >500/mm^3
   - Hct >2% within the first hour after trauma
   - Amylase >200 somogyi units
   - Presence of bile, bacteria, or fecal material (indicates viscus injury) (2).

   NOTE: The ability to read newspaper print through the fluid in the IV bag is not a reliable indicator of a negative lavage.

12. Once the catheter is removed, and the wound is sutured (if applicable), place a thin layer of antibiotic ointment and a sterile dressing over the site.

PATIENT CARE MANAGEMENT

1. Monitor for bleeding or signs of infection at the site.
2. Continue to assess abdomen for pain, distention, rigidity, and tenderness.
3. Prepare the patient for surgery as indicated.

References

1. Clemence B: Procedures involving the gastrointestinal and genitourinary systems. In Bernardo LM, Bove M, editors: *Pediatric emergency nursing procedures,* Boston, 1993, Jones and Bartlett.
2. Emergency Nurses' Association: *Trauma nurse core course,* Chicago, 1991, The Association.
3. Knighton D, Locksley RM, Mills J: Emergency procedures. In Saunders CF, Ho MT, editors: *Current emergency diagnosis and treatment,* Norwalk, Conn, 1992, Appleton and Lange.
4. Marx JA: Abdominal trauma. In Barkin RM, Rosen P, editors: *Emergency pediatrics,* St Louis, 1990, Mosby.
5. Proehl, JA: Peritoneal lavage. In Proehl JA, editor: *Adult emergency nursing procedures,* Boston, 1993, Jones and Bartlett.

Diarrhea

Mary Phillips

DESCRIPTION

Diarrhea is a frequently encountered complaint in the emergency department (ED) among adults and children. It is defined as an increase in frequency, fluid content, and volume of stool. There are many causes of diarrhea including viral infections such as rotaviruses, bacterial infections such as *Shigella* and *Salmonella*, and parasitic invasion such as *Giardia lamblia*. Other noninfectious causes include immune deficiencies, hepatic and pancreatic disorders, and use of antibiotics. If persistent, diarrhea can lead to dehydration, shock, and subsequent electrolyte imbalances, as well as breakdown in skin integrity. When caring for the patient with diarrhea, the nurse will be concerned with identifying the cause, treating dehydration and electrolyte imbalances if they exist, and relieving discomfort.

INITIAL NURSING ACTIONS

1. Triage assessment and history
   * General appearance and level of consciousness
   * Symptoms and their duration
   * Diet and oral intake
   * Number and appearance of stools
   * Estimated urine output
   * Recent exposure to illness
   * Presence of fever
   * Age of patient
   * Preexisting medical conditions
   * Present medications
   * Vital signs including temperature, pulse, blood pressure, and respirations
   * Weight (in pediatric patients)
2. Determine the degree of dehydration. Table P12-1 is a helpful guide to use with children.
   * Similar guidelines (excluding fontanels) can be used for adults.

TABLE P12-1 Degrees of Dehydration Including Signs and Symptoms

Percentage of loss of body weight	Mild 5%	Moderate 10%	Severe 15%
Signs and symptoms			
Mucous membranes and lips	Dry	Very dry, cracked	Parched
Skin turgor	Normal	Slightly decreased	Tenting
Anterior fontanel	Normal	Sunken	Sunken
Eyeballs	Normal	Sunken	Sunken
Tearing	Normal	Decreased	Absent
Heart rate	Normal or slightly increased	Increased	Increased
Respirations	Normal or slightly increased	Increased	Increased
Blood pressure	Normal	Normal	Decreased
Skin perfusion	Normal, pale	Mottled, cool	Slow capillary refill time, cold, cyanotic

From Emergency Nurses' Association: *Emergency nursing pediatric core course manual*, Park Ridge, Ill, 1993, The Association.

- Orthostatic vital signs in adults (these are not an accurate indicator of fluid volume status in children).
- Laboratory data such as electrolytes, BUN, creatinine, glucose, and urinalysis.

3. Determine the cause of diarrhea.
   - It may be necessary to collect a stool sample for culture, WBC, ova, and parasite testing.
   - Other diagnostic procedures such as x-rays including an abdominal series may be indicated.
   - Laboratory data such as CBC with differential, blood cultures, liver function studies, amylase, and ABG may be useful.

OTHER NURSING ACTIONS

1. Use antidiarrheal agents if appropriate (these are not routinely used in children because of side effects such as lethargy, nausea and vomiting, and possible respiratory depression).
2. The method of fluid replacement depends on the severity of dehydration and the patient's ability to retain fluids (see the box below and on p. 746).

PATIENT CARE MANAGEMENT

Infants and Children

1. Instruct parent to give clear liquids for 24 hours. If breastfeeding, clear liquids may be used in addition to breast milk.
2. Avoid juices such as apple juice as this may worsen diarrhea.
3. If the infant's diet is solely formula, advance to half-strength formula the second day and full-strength formula the third day if stool output decreases.

ORAL REHYDRATION FOR MILD DEHYDRATION

Infants (≤1 year old)

Give clear liquids such as Pedialyte, half-strength "flattened or defizzed" clear soda (no caffeine), or half strength Jell-O water offered in frequent small amounts (½ oz every 10-20 min).

Children (>1 year old)

Give clear liquids such as half-strength "flattened or defizzed" clear, decaffeinated soda, half-strength Jell-O water, or Popsicles offered in frequent small amounts (½ oz-1 oz every 10-20 min).

Adults

Give clear liquids such as ice chips, "flattened or defizzed" decaffeinated clear soda, Jell-O, or Gatorade in frequent small amounts.

IV FLUID REHYDRATION FOR MODERATE-TO-SEVERE DEHYDRATION

Infants and children

1. Establish a patent airway and deliver supplemental oxygen as necessary.
2. Establish two large bore IV lines using 22-gauge or larger IV catheter, if possible.
3. Administer 20 cc/kg bolus of warmed normal saline or Ringer's lactate solution. Repeat crystalloid bolus as needed.
4. Strict fluid intake and output monitoring.
5. Frequent monitoring of vital signs, pulses, and perfusion.

Adult

1. Establish a patent airway and deliver supplemental oxygen as needed.
2. Establish two large bore IV lines using 18-gauge or larger IV catheters.
3. The amount of fluid replacement depends on the amount of fluid loss. In the geriatric patient, or patients with heart disease, rehydration should be done cautiously. In some cases, it may be necessary to place a central venous line to monitor central venous pressure (see Procedure 6). Normal saline or Ringer's lactate solutions are most often used for IV rehydration.
4. Strict fluid intake and output monitoring.
5. Frequent monitoring of vital signs, pulses, and perfusion.

4. If the infant or child eats baby food, advance to applesauce, bananas, and rice cereal mixed with water (in addition to clear liquids) on the second day.
5. If stool output decreases, advance to rice cereal mixed with formula, and full-strength formula on the third day.
6. Instruct parent on proper dosage and administration of medications if prescribed.
7. Instruct parent to change diapers frequently keeping diaper area clean and dry to prevent skin rash and breakdown.
8. Instruct parent on signs and symptoms of dehydration:
   - Decreased number of wet diapers
   - Sunken anterior fontanel (soft spot)

- Decreased or absent tears with crying
- Lethargy

NOTE: Advise parent to seek health care immediately if these symptoms occur.

9. Advise follow-up with pediatrician or pediatric nurse practitioner.

Adults

1. Instruct patient to continue clear liquids for 24 hours.
2. Instruct patient to advance to bland diet on second day if stool output decreases.
3. Advance to regular diet on third day if stool output remains decreased. Avoid milk products, spicy or greasy foods for 4 to 5 days.
4. Instruct patient on proper dosage and administration of medications if prescribed.
5. Advise follow-up with private physician or clinic.

Bibliography

Barkin R, Rosen P, editors: *Emerg pediatrics, ed 3*, St Louis, 1990, Mosby.

Emergency Nurses' Association: *Emergency nursing pediatric core course manual*, Park Ridge, Ill, 1993, The Association.

Ear Irrigation

Mark Parshall

INDICATIONS

Ear irrigation is commonly ordered for removal of cerumen impaction or a foreign body from the external auditory canal. On occasion, both ear canals may be impacted.

CONTRAINDICATIONS

Contraindications include ruptured tympanic membrane (TM) myringotomy tubes and Ménière's disease. Irrigation should not be performed if the patient is experiencing vertigo. If the patient develops vertigo or nystagmus during the procedure, it should be discontinued and the physician should be notified.

EQUIPMENT

- Metal piston syringe or dental irrigation device (e.g., Water-Pik)
- 30 or 60 cc Luer-Lok syringe
- 16 or 18 gauge teflon angiocath sheath or a hub and clipped tubing from a butterfly (A metal needle should never be used.)
- Warm water or saline (body temperature)
- Two basins: one for irrigant and one for runoff
- Otoscope
- Cerumenolytic drops (docusate sodium (1) Debrox, or Cerumenex)
- Towels and a gown to drape patient's clothing
- Examination gloves

INITIAL NURSING ACTIONS

1. Explain the procedure to the patient. Ask the patient to report any discomfort, vertigo, or nausea.
2. Examine both ears with an otoscope, even if only one is impacted, as this will establish a baseline for subsequent inspection.

3. If a cerumenolytic agent is being used, it should be instilled at least 10 minutes before irrigating.
4. The irrigation tip should not be advanced beyond the cartilaginous portion of the ear canal. In an adult, the pinna may be pulled upward and backward (in a small child, downward and backward), to straighten the ear canal.
5. The direction of the irrigation should be toward the anterosuperior aspect of the ear canal, not at the TM (e.g., at the 1 o'clock position in the left ear and the 11 o'clock position in the right ear) (2). Irrigation can be continued until the impaction is relieved or the patient reports discomfort.
6. If a Water-Pik is used, great care must be taken to assure that the pressure is not excessive and remains constant. For this reason, the author's preference is a manual technique.

PATIENT CARE MANAGEMENT

1. At times a large plug will be irrigated free. If a cerumenolytic agent was used before irrigation, the impaction may tend to break up in small pieces as irrigation progresses.
2. The ear canal should be examined otoscopically at frequent intervals during the irrigation. The ear should be examined again at the conclusion of the procedure.
3. If irrigation is successful, patients generally report a marked improvement in hearing and relief from the feeling of fullness in the ear.
4. There is often some degree of redness of the ear canal after irrigation. There may even be a small amount of superficial bleeding, which should stop spontaneously. At times the physician may decide to treat the inflammatory reaction as an external otitis. Frequently, it resolves spontaneously within a day or two without treatment.
5. Assuming the TM is intact, some sources recommend instillation of a few drops of isopropyl alcohol or other drying agent (e.g., VoSol Otic Solution or Domeboro Otic) following irrigation (2).
6. Recommendation of cerumenolytic agents to prevent recurrence is at the discretion of the physician. Docusate sodium liquid, 1% solution (Colace liquid, 1%) and

Debrox are available over the counter; Cerumenex is available by prescription only.

References

1. Chen DA, Caparosa RJ: A nonprescription cerumenolytic, *Am J Otol* 12:475, 1991.
2. Zivic RC, King S: Cerumen impaction management for clients of all ages, *Nurs Pract* 18(3):33, 1993.

Bibliography

Reich JJ, Turbiak TW: Otic emergencies, *Top Emerg Med* 6 (3):19, 1984.

Votey S, Dudley JP: Emergency ear nose and throat procedures, *Emerg Med Clin North Am* 7:117, 1989.

Emergency Thoracotomy

Theresa M. Glessner

DESCRIPTION

Open thoracotomy is an emergent procedure during which the chest is opened surgically in order to correct exsanguinating hemorrhage or cardiac arrest from an unknown cause after blunt or penetrating trauma.

INDICATIONS

Cardiopulmonary arrest in the patient who has had signs of life (pulse, blood pressure, cardiac electrical activity, respiratory effort, or motor function of any type) just before or after arrival in the ED—the patient may have suffered blunt or penetrating trauma to the chest or abdomen.

CONTRAINDICATIONS

This procedure is NOT indicated in those patients who have not had signs of life since the time of the traumatic injury and/or it has been >15 minutes since the injury.

EQUIPMENT

- Povidone-iodine solution
- 4 × 4 sponges
- Sterile gowns, gloves, masks, hats, and shoe covers
- Open chest tray to include some or all of the following:
  - Finchietto-Buford rib spreader with two large blades and two small (pediatric) blades
  - Tuffier rib spreader
  - 2 9½-inch DeBakey aneurysm clamps
  - 1 medium Satinsky clamp
  - 6 Vanderbilt clamps
  - 2 8-inch Sarot needle-holders
  - Curved Mayo scissors
  - 2 Metz scissors
  - 8 large towel clamps

- 1 straight Liston bone cutter
- 1 Lebsche sternal chisel
- 1 mallet
- 2 9-inch DeBakey forceps
- 2 5½-inch tissue forceps
- 4 sterile towel packs (6 each)
- Sterile teflon sheet (6 × 6 felt)
- 4 packs lap sponges
- 2 2-0 silk suture
- Dacron tape
- 4 4-0 prolene suture
- 10 2-0 ticron suture
- No. 21 scalpel
- 3-0 prolene suture
- ¼-inch pledget
- ⅜-inch pledget
- 6 3-0 prolene suture with strung ¼-inch pledget
- Small Satinsky clamp
- 2 9½-inch sponge forceps
- 2 8-inch Allis clamps
- 2 8-inch Gemini clamps (right angle forceps)
- 2 6-inch Gemini clamps
- 2 8-inch standard needle-holders
- 2 7-inch Sarot needle-holders
- 2 Duval lung clamps
- 8-inch curved Metz scissors
- 6 ¾-inch straight Mayo scissors
- 6 curved Kelly clamps
- Large Allison lung retractor
- Small Allison lung retractor
- Medium Richardson retractor
- Small Richardson retractor
- 2 9½-inch DeBakey forceps
- 2 7¾-inch DeBakey forceps
- 2 vessel clude neuromedics
- No. 10 scalpel
- No. 11 scalpel
- Sterile Foley catheter

INITIAL NURSING ACTIONS

1. Assist the surgeon in donning his or her sterile gown, gloves, mask, and cap. Assist in preparing the patient for

the procedure—prep the patient with 4 × 4's and povidone-iodine solution and sterilely drape the patient's thorax for the procedure.

2. Assure that the sterile thoracotomy tray is opened sterilely and awaiting the surgeon when he/she is ready to perform the procedure.

   Physician Actions

   - After the patient is prepped and draped, the physician makes a skin incision with the scalpel, then either the sternal chisel and mallet are used to make a mediastinal opening or the fascia is cut away and the rib spreaders are utilized to gain access to the heart.
   - Occasionally, a rib will have to be cut away for better visualization using the bone cutter.

3. Prepare yourself or an assistant sterilely in order to perform the duties of a scrub nurse—to hand the surgeon the instruments as needed. Another nurse will have to monitor the patient's vital signs and continually assess the patient during the procedure.

   Physician Actions

   - The physician will be looking for the source of bleeding.
   - He/she will need lap sponges and 4 × 4's to dry the area, and when the source of bleeding is found, he will need a variety of clamps and suture to close the bleeder.

4. Cardiopulmonary resuscitation will have to be stopped during the time that the incision is made but will be continued internally after the chest is opened. The incision is a left thoracotomy incision made at the 4th or 5th intercostal space and can be extended to the right. Occasionally, the incision is a mediastinal approach, but it is much easier to spread the ribs than to saw the sternum.

5. The patient's airway must be secured by endotracheal intubation before initiation of this procedure because there is less access to the head, making bag-valve-mask ventilation very difficult.

6. Be prepared to do internal defibrillation—be sure that the defibrillator is in working order. Have the surgeon hand the end of the cable that attaches to the defibrillator to someone, so it can be properly attached to the defibrillator and ready when the chest is open.

Physician Actions
- The internal defibrillator paddles are placed one on either ventricle, and the maximum amount of joules that can be delivered internally is 20.

7. Be ready to perform internal cardiac massage and internal defibrillation as ordered by the physician.

8. The patient must be on a cardiac monitor throughout this procedure.

9. If the surgeon is successful in resuscitating the patient, be ready to proceed to the operating room for further evaluation of the patient's injuries.

10. The surgeon may place a Foley catheter in the heart for tamponade of bleeding if there is a visible hole in the heart or aorta, or it may be placed for fluid resuscitation if the heart is flat—without any circulating volume. Warm IV fluids must be given through this catheter.

Physician Actions
- If the patient is successfully resuscitated, the physician will sterilely drape the patient and proceed to the operating room; he/she will not close the chest in the emergency department.

PATIENT CARE MANAGEMENT

1. Continuously assess and trend the patient's vital signs, noting any return of pulse, blood pressure, or cardiac electrical activity.

2. Monitor the continuing fluid resuscitation that will be ongoing during this procedure.

3. Note the amount of joules utilized with each internal defibrillation attempt (up to 20 joules).

4. Note any change in the patient's condition during this procedure. This may give the surgeon data to diagnose a specific problem that can be corrected.

5. The patient may need to be transported to the operating room while internal cardiac massage is ongoing. If this occurs, try to maintain sterility as much as possible. Cover the patient with a sterile sheet if possible.

6. If the patient has an indwelling Foley catheter in the heart to tamponade bleeding or for fluid resuscitation, be sure that the balloon is inflated and that it does not get dislodged during the procedure or during transport.

POTENTIAL COMPLICATIONS

The most common complication of this procedure is death. Other complications include further injury to the thorax, exsanguination, and further myocardial and pleural injury.

Bibliography

Alexander RH, Proctor HJ: *Advanced trauma life support course for physicians,* ed 5, Chicago, 1993, First Impression.

Neff J, Kidd PS: *Trauma nursing: the art and science,* St Louis, 1993, Mosby.

Vasquez M, Lazear SE, Larson E: *Critical care nursing,* ed 2, Philadelphia, 1992, WB Saunders.

Endotracheal Tube Insertion

George P. Glessner III

Endotracheal intubation can be accomplished orally with the use of a laryngoscope on patients of all ages or nasally (without the use of a laryngoscope) on adult and adolescent patients. Endotracheal intubation is used for definitive airway control in the injured and ill patient. The intubated patient may be unconscious and apneic or conscious with impaired breathing capabilities. Endotracheal intubation may require the use of induction and/or neuromuscular blockade (NMB) agents. Different patient situations may require modifications of the basic principles of endotracheal intubation presented in this section.

DESCRIPTION

Endotracheal intubation requires the use of an endotracheal tube (ET) (3). The ET is a hollow, flexible, clear tube with an opening at both ends (Figure P15-1) (2).

The distal end has an additional opening on the side referred to as the Murphy's eye that allows air passage if the larger opening distal to it becomes clogged. The proximal end has a standard 15 mm adapter that connects to ventilatory devices. ETs vary in size from 2 to 9 mm. The size correlates to the interior diameter of the tube. All ETs have centimeter markings on the sides at the proximal end. These markings allow quick visual identification of the distance of the tube in the trachea. Adult and pediatric ETs have some important differences.

Adult ETs have a cuff on the outside of the distal end that is connected by a small hollow tube to a pilot balloon and an inflation port with a one-way valve on the proximal end. This port allows air to be injected into the low pressure, high volume cuff via the use of a syringe. The pilot balloon inflates when air is in the cuff allowing the health care provider to determine if the cuff is inflated. The cuff is designed to fill the void space in the adult trachea past the

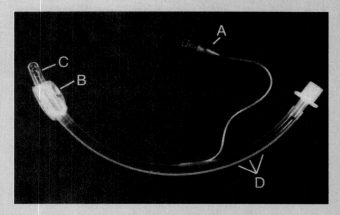

Figure P15-1 Endotracheal tube. **A,** Pilot balloon; **B,** cuff; **C,** Murphy's eye; and **D,** centimeter markings of tube length from tip. (From Dailey R, Simon B, Young G: *The airway: emergency management,* St Louis, 1992, Mosby.)

vocal cords and thus help to protect the patient from aspiration. The pediatric ET does not have a cuff.

The trachea of the pediatric patient is less rigid than the adult's and narrows past the vocal cords. This allows a "seal" to be created when a properly sized ET is passed through the vocal cords and into the narrow portion of the pediatric trachea. A pediatric uncuffed ET has black rings around the distal aspect of the tube where a cuff would have been. Adult and pediatric endotracheal intubation is usually accomplished orally with direct visualization of the glottic opening and vocal cords with a laryngoscope.

The laryngoscope is a two-piece instrument consisting of a handle and blade. The blade is either straight or curved and varies in length from size zero for neonates and infants to size four for large adults. Laryngoscopes are battery operated and have a source of light in the distal end of the blade that facilitates visualization of the glottic opening. A laryngoscope is not used for nasal-tracheal intubation.

Nasal-tracheal intubation is performed on spontaneously breathing adolescent or adult patients who require definitive airway control with a less invasive method or no head

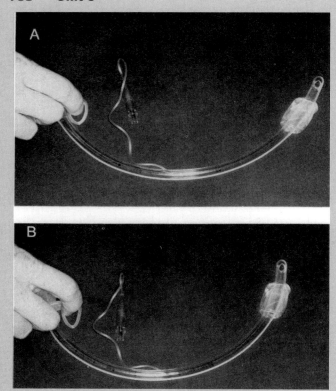

Figure P15-2 Endotrol tube. **A,** Relaxed position. **B,** Trigger pulled. Note increased angulation to direct tip of tube anteriorly. (From Dailey R, Simon B, Young G: *The airway; emergency management,* St Louis, 1992, Mosby.)

movement because of a possible spinal injury. Nasaltracheal intubation is a blind intubation. The ET is passed through the nasal passage, past the pharynx and vocal cords, and into the trachea without direct visualization. The use of a flex-tip ET such as the Endotrol (Figure P15-2) (2) may help with the procedure. With an Endotrol the tip of the ET can be flexed with the use of a pull ring at the proximal end attached to a monofilament line that runs the length of the ET through the wall and is anchored to the end.

If a flex-tip ET is not being used to perform nasal-tracheal intubation, flexing the ET into a circle, inserting the distal tip into the proximal end, and placing it on ice while the patient is being prepared for intubation may help. The increased flex in the ET assists the intubator in passing the tip of the ET through the cords similar to flexing the tip of the Endotrol. The cooling of the tube helps maintain this flexed shape longer.

INDICATIONS

Oral-Tracheal Intubation

1. Establishment, maintenance, or protection of the airway
2. Enhancement of the physiologic aspects of breathing, oxygenation, and ventilation
3. Intubation requiring a larger tube than one that can be advanced through the nasal passage

CONTRAINDICATIONS

There are no absolute contraindications for oral-tracheal intubation in patients who need definitive airway control. There are some relative contraindications when oral-tracheal intubation may be very difficult or could worsen or complicate an existing condition.

1. Anticipated surgical access through the mouth
2. Major maxillofacial fractures or trauma
3. Significant bleeding in the supraglottic area
4. Potential unstable cervical spine injuries
5. Epiglottitis
6. Miscellaneous (rheumatoid arthritis, ankylosing spondylitis) (1)

INDICATIONS

Nasal-Tracheal Intubation

1. Dyspneic patients whose condition could worsen or who cannot tolerate the supine position (e.g., COPD, asthma, pulmonary edema).
2. Oral cavity not sufficiently accessible to permit oral-tracheal intubation.
   * Wired jaws
   * Anatomic problems (e.g., small mouth, temporomandibular joint ankylosis)
   * Trismus (e.g., tetanus, intraoral infections)

- Actively seizing
- Obstructing lesions of the anterior oropharynx (e.g., tumors, Ludwig's angina, lingual swelling/hematoma, dental abscesses)

3. Inability to attain proper sniffing position.
   - Suspected/proven unstable cervical spine injury
   - Decerebrate rigidity
   - Tetanus
   - Severe degeneration joint disease (DJD) or rheumatoid arthritis of the cervical spine
4. Comatose, breathing patients (e.g., sedative overdose, cerebrovascular accidents, head injury).
5. When NMB agents are contraindicated (e.g., hyperkalemia secondary to burns or renal failure (2).

EQUIPMENT

- Suction equipment set up and functioning
  1. Proper devices to suction the oral pharynx (e.g., rigid tonsillar-tip suction device)
  2. Suction catheters properly sized for the ET being used
- Oxygen source
- Bag-valve device and a proper fitting mask
- Two properly sized ETs (Table P15-1)
- 10 cc syringe

TABLE P15-1 Properly Sized Endotracheal Tubes

Age	Average weight (lbs/kg)	ET size	Blade size
Premature	3/1.5	2.5, 3.0	0
Term	7.5/3.5	3.5	0
6 mo	15/7	3.5	0 or 1
1 yr	22/10	4.0	1
3 yr	33/15	4.5	1 or 2
6 yr	44/20	5.5	2
8 yr	55/30	6.0	2
11 yr	77/35	6.5	2 or 3
14 yr	99/45	7.0	3
Adult females	120 lbs and up	7.0-8.0	3
Adult males	160 lbs and up	8.0-9.0	3 or 4

- Laryngoscope handle with two different sized blades, curved and straight
- Properly sized stylet
- Anesthetic and lubricating water soluble topical agents
- Towel
- Protective eye wear, mask, and gloves
- Stethoscope
- Pulse oximeter (optional)
- End-tidal CO_2 monitor/detector (optional)
- NMB agents (optional)
- Sedation and or induction agents (optional)
- Surgical cricothyrotomy kit
  —May be needed if the patient cannot successfully be intubated

INITIAL NURSING ACTIONS

General Endotracheal Intubation

1. Discuss the procedure thoroughly with the conscious patient.
2. Preoxygenate the patient with 100% O_2 via bag-valve-mask device for 2 to 5 minutes.
3. Start an IV access line (if not already done).
4. Assure proper noninvasive monitors are in place (e.g., ECG, blood pressure, pulse oximeter, and end-tidal CO_2).
5. Gather all the needed equipment and personnel.
6. Check the laryngoscope and blades to ensure that batteries and light source are functional.
7. Prepare the ETs while keeping the distal two-thirds sterile.
   A. Check the patency of the ET cuff and balloon.
   B. Insert a malleable stylet (oral intubation) into the ET making sure that it does not extend past the distal end of the tube.
      1. Bend the ET and stylet to create a gentle curve in the tube with a sharp upward turn of the distal end at an approximate 30-degree angle (oral intubation).
   C. Lubricate the distal aspect of the ET with Xylocaine jelly or another water soluble lubricant.
8. Ensure that universal precautions are being maintained (protective eye wear, mask, and gloves).
9. Place the patient in the proper position.

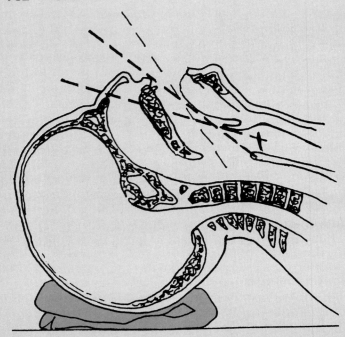

Figure P15-3 Intubating or "sniffing" position. Note approximation of three critical axes. (From Dailey R, Simon B, Young G. *The airway: emergency management*, St Louis, 1992, Mosby.)

A. Sniffing position with head resting on a folded towel (Figure P15-3) (2).
B. If there is a possibility of a cervical spine injury, the patient is kept in neutral alignment with manual immobilization being maintained.

Oral-Tracheal Intubation

1. Visualize the glottic opening and vocal cords.
   A. With the left hand, insert the blade of the laryngoscope into the right side of the mouth and sweep the tongue to the left.
   B. Lift the lower jaw and displace it up and forward at a 30 to 45 degree angle with the laryngoscope
      1. Keep the blade away from and off of the teeth.

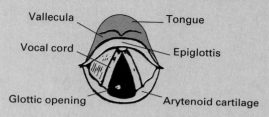

Figure P15-4 Anatomic structures seen during direct laryngoscopy.

2. Do not pull back on the handle, instead push it forward and up with a lifting motion.

  C. Visualize the glottic opening and the vocal cords (Figure P15-4) (1).

2. With the right hand, insert the ET into the mouth and through the glottic opening and vocal cords.

  A. Advance the ET until the cuff completely disappears through the vocal cords or one or more of the black rings on the distal end of the pediatric uncuffed ET passes through the vocal cords.

  B. Grasp the ET at the mouth with the left hand after setting down the laryngoscope and carefully pull out the stylet.

3. Inflate the cuff with a 10 cc syringe.

  A. Use only enough air to stop exhaled air from leaking around the cuff.

4. Check placement of the ET.

  A. Auscultate breath sounds over the anterior and lateral aspect of the chest.

    1. Breath sounds should be present and equal bilaterally.

  B. Look for fogging of the ET.

  C. Watch for equal bilateral rise and fall of the chest.

  D. Auscultate the epigastrium.

    1. Breath sounds may be faintly heard, but they should be less audible than those heard over the anterior chest

      a. Stomach bubbling should not be heard (coarse basilar rales may mimic air bubbling in the stomach)

E. Assess the patient for signs of improved oxygenation and ventilation
   1. Improved skin color and/or capillary refill
   2. Improved pulse oximetry readings (this may take several minutes)
   3. Positive detection of end-tidal CO_2 by a colormetric CO_2 detector or a measurable reading of CO_2 on a continuous end-tidal CO_2 monitor
F. Feel for adequate compliance of the lungs while ventilating the patient.
5. Note the cm marking at the lips or teeth and document.
6. Secure the ET with a commercial ET-holding device or adhesive tape.
   A. Secure the ET in place making sure that the ET cannot be moved by activity such as suctioning and ventilating.
   B. Secure the ET in place with adhesive tape
      1. Have someone manually secure the ET with their hand
      2. Clean and dry the surface of the face
      3. Apply mastisol or other adhesive to the skin surface of both cheeks beside the mouth
      4. With 1-inch adhesive tape, secure the ET by wrapping the middle portion of a 6-inch strip of tape around the ET at the level of the teeth and secure the other portions of tape to the previously prepared skin surface.
   C. Follow the manufacturer's directions for commercially prepared ET holders.
7. Insert a nasogastric or orogastric tube and attach it to suction in order to evacuate and deflate the stomach.
8. If endotracheal intubation cannot be accomplished within 15 to 20 seconds, stop and reoxygenate and hyperventilate the patient for 2 to 5 minutes and then reattempt intubation.

Nasal-Tracheal Intubation

1. Prepare the nares and nasal passage with 2% Xylocaine jelly or a water soluble lubricant.
   • A nasal pharyngeal airway may be placed and then removed to evenly spread the topical agents.
2. Gently introduce the distal end of the ET into the nares, and advance it through the nasal passage into the posterior oropharynx.

- A slight gentle twisting motion may help.
- If passage on one side cannot be accomplished, try the opposite side.

3. Advance the ET until it reaches the glottis.
   - This usually causes the patient with an intact gag reflex to cough.

4. Advance the ET through the glottic opening.
   - Listen with your ear for breath sounds through the proximal end of the ET.
   - Gently but quickly advance the ET 5 to 6 cm through the glottic opening when the patient inhales.

5. Confirm tube placement same as for oral intubation.

6. Secure the ET with a commercial-holding device or adhesive tape.
   - Secure the ET in place making sure that the tube cannot be moved by activity such as suctioning and ventilating.
   - Follow the manufacturer's directions for commercially prepared ET holders.

7. Insert a nasogastric or orogastric tube and attach it to suction in order to evacuate and deflate the stomach.

8. If endotracheal intubation cannot be accomplished within 15 to 20 seconds, stop and reoxygenate and hyperventilate the patient for 2 to 5 minutes and then reattempt intubation.

PATIENT CARE MANAGEMENT

1. Suction the oral pharynx and ET as needed.
   - Neither the ET cuff or the narrowing of the pediatric trachea seals well enough to completely protect the patient from aspiration. Suctioning of the oral pharynx is still required.

2. Assess and reassess the patient's ventilation, oxygenation, and perfusion status.

3. Assess for impairment of oxygenation, sometimes associated with the intubated patient.
   - Pneumothorax or tension pneumothorax
   - Dislodgement of the ET
   - Inadvertent advancement of the ET into the right mainstem bronchus
   - Clogged ET
   - Air leaks around the ET associated with a ruptured or leaking ET cuff

4. Be prepared to intervene if intubation efforts are unsuccessful.
   - Continue to assist ventilation and hyperventilate the patient with 100% O_2.
   - Prepare and set up for surgical cricothyrotomy if intubation is unsuccessful.

References

1. American Heart Association: *Textbook of advanced cardiac life support*, Dallas, 1994, The Association.
2. Dailey R, Simon B, Young G, and Stewart R: *The airway: emergency management*, St Louis, 1992, Mosby.
3. Jablonski S: *Dictionary of medical acronyms and abbreviations*, Philadelphia, 1987, Hanley & Belfus.

Eye Irrigation

Mark Parshall

INDICATIONS

1. Decontamination of chemical injuries
2. Cleansing debris (e.g., dust) from the eyes

CONTRAINDICATIONS

Open or impaled globe

EQUIPMENT

- Eye shower (if available)
- Ophthalmic topical anesthetic drops
- pH test strips (if acid or alkali exposure)
- 1 to 2 liters of normal saline (NS) or Ringer's lactate per eye
- Standard drip IV tubing (e.g., 10 to 15 gtt/ml)
- Hairwash tray or sink, or chux to divert runoff
- Irrigating lens (Morgan Lens) (optional)
- Lid retractors (optional)
- Towels/gloves

INITIAL NURSING ACTIONS

1. Explain procedure to patient.
2. Instill topical anesthetic as prescribed by physician.

Eye Shower

If an eye shower is available, instruct the patient to place his/her face in the middle of the two streams so that water is flushing over the eyes and lids. Instruct the patient to blink eyes in the streams and look in all directions with eyes open. Continue for at least 15 minutes.

Manual Irrigation

1. Position the patient to catch runoff and drape clothing with chux or towels to keep from getting wet. Topically anesthetize the eye(s).

2. Gently retract the lids with nondominant hand. If the lids are swollen, an assistant may be necessary. A Desmarres lid retractor, or a retractor fashioned from a paper clip may be used if permitted by institutional policy and the nurse is comfortable in their use (1).

3. Begin the flow of irrigant through the IV tubing, holding the distal end of the tubing in the dominant hand. The irrigant should be free flowing, not dripping. The rate can be adjusted to patient comfort.

4. Direct the flow in all directions on the anterior globe. The lower conjunctival fornix can be exposed by gentle traction on the lower lid. The palpebral conjunctiva of the upper lid can be exposed by a retractor, by gentle traction, or by eversion over an applicator swab.

5. In general, a liter of irrigant to each eye that needs irrigation is sufficient, except in the case of corrosives (strong acids, alkali), for which the amount of irrigant needed depends on the conjunctival pH (see Chapter 10).

Irrigation Via an Irrigating Contact Lens (Morgan Lens)

1. Explain the equipment to patient and instill topical anesthetic. Position and drape the patient.

2. Attach IV tubing to the extension on the irrigating lens.

3. Run a small amount of irrigant over the ocular surface of the lens to lubricate.

4. Ask the patient to look down, grasp the extension tubing of the lens, and slip the lens under the upper lid (it should go into the upper fornix without resistance).

5. Ask the patient to look up. With your free hand, gently retract the lower lid until the lower lid is outside the margin of the lens. Release the lid so that it covers the lower part of the lens.

6. Open the flow clamp and adjust rate to patient comfort. Irrigate 1 to 2 liters/eye.

7. To remove the lens, ask the patient to look up. Retract the lower lid gently, the lens will pop off the ocular surface. Ask the patient to look down and slide the lens out from under the upper lid.

PATIENT CARE MANAGEMENT

1. An eye shower achieves much higher volumes at relatively lower pressure than other methods. If there is

not one in the ED, often there is one in the hospital laboratory. It may be followed by use of an irrigating lens or manual irrigation.

2. Apart from the eye shower, other methods of irrigation are safest if the patient is supine.

3. There are Y-connectors for the Morgan Lens so that the nurse can irrigate both eyes simultaneously from one bag of irrigant and one infusion set. When using the Y-connector, the volume of irrigant should be doubled (e.g., a minimum of 2 liters should be used if 1 liter/eye is desired). Independent setups can also be used for each eye if needed.

4. Most patients tolerate the Morgan Lens very well, but a few do not. The nurse should remain with the patient or close at hand in case the patient becomes restless or frightened.

5. The Morgan Lens comes with a very clear package insert in each lens packet. It is a good idea to post one wherever eye irrigation is regularly performed in the ED.

References

1. Smallwood M: Eye irrigation. In Proehl JA, editor: *Adult emergency nursing procedures,* Boston, 1993, Jones and Bartlett.

Fever Care

Mary Phillips

DESCRIPTION

Fever is one of the most common chief complaints of patients presenting to the emergency department (ED). Fever is not a disease but rather a nonspecific symptom of an underlying infectious or inflammatory process (1). Other factors that contribute to a rise in body temperature include excessive clothing, physical exertion, and increased environmental temperature. Fever results when there is a rise in the core body temperature following a resetting of the body's thermostat that is regulated by the hypothalamus. In general, for the appropriately dressed patient at rest, a rectal (core) temperature of $\geq100.4°F$ ($38°C$) in children and $\geq99.6°F$ ($37°C$) in adults is considered a fever. Remembering that fever is a symptom, nursing care will focus on identification of its cause and relief of associated discomfort.

INITIAL NURSING ACTIONS

1. Triage assessment and history
   - General appearance and level of consciousness
   - Symptoms and their duration
   - Vital signs including temperature, pulse, respirations, and blood pressure
   - Diet and oral intake history
   - Presence of rash
   - Estimated urine output
   - Recent exposure to illness
   - Immunization status in children
   - Preexisting medical conditions
   - Current medications and allergies
   - Time and amount of last antipyretic
   - Activity level
   - Weight of patient

NURSING ALERT

Immunocompromised patients with a fever, such as those on chemotherapy or with acquired immunodeficiency syndrome (AIDS), should be considered emergent and quickly escorted to a private treatment area.

2. Determine the cause of the fever.
   - Anticipate septic work-up including laboratory data such as CBC with differential, electrolytes, glucose, and blood cultures. A septic work-up is indicated in febrile infants <3 months old and febrile immunocompromised patients.
   - Anticipate urine culture and urinalysis.
   - Anticipate lumbar puncture to obtain cerebrospinal fluid for culture and analysis.
   - Anticipate cultures from any potential focal site (e.g., wounds, central lines).
   - Anticipate sputum cultures.
   - Anticipate need for chest radiography.
   - Explain all diagnostic procedures to patient.

OTHER NURSING ACTIONS

1. Administer antibiotics as ordered (dosage is based on weight in children).
2. Administer antipyretics for fever and pain reduction (see box).
3. Encourage increased oral intake (clear liquids may be better tolerated).
4. Administer IV fluids if patient's condition warrants (e.g., severe dehydration, inability to manage oral fluids).
5. Implement other fever reduction efforts as follows:
   - Remove excess clothing
   - Sponge bathing with tepid water if fever exceeds 104°F (40°C)
   - Prevent shivering as this may increase body temperature

PATIENT CARE MANAGEMENT

Children

1. Instruct parent on proper dosage and administration of antipyretic. A dosage chart is helpful (Table P17-1).

ACETAMINOPHEN AND IBUPROFEN DOSING

Children

Acetaminophen	15 mg/kg
Pediatric ibuprofen	10 mg/kg

Adult

Acetaminophen	650-1000 mg
Ibuprofen	400-800 mg

---

2. Discourage use of aspirin because of its association with Reye's syndrome.
3. Instruct on proper dosage and administration of antibiotics if prescribed. Emphasize importance of completing antibiotic therapy.
4. Inform parent that sponge baths can be used as an aid in fever reduction for fever ≥104°F (40°C). Use tepid water sponge on head, axilla, and groin.
5. Emphasize prevention of shivering, since this increases body temperature.
6. Discourage use of alcohol baths because of the potential for alcohol toxicity.
7. Instruct parent on proper technique for taking rectal temperature (if applicable).
8. Encourage increased intake of oral fluids to prevent dehydration (clear liquids such as "flattened" or "defizzed" decaffeinated clear soda may be better tolerated).
9. Give follow-up instructions including correct procedure for obtaining culture results.
10. Give guidelines regarding signs and symptoms that would require a child to be reevaluated such as persistent fever that does not respond to antipyretics or antibiotics, decreased level of consciousness, development of petechiae or purpuric rash, seizure activity, and dehydration.
11. Encourage rest and use of cool, comfortable attire.
12. Instruct to follow-up with private physician or clinic.

TABLE P17-1 Proper Dosage and Administration of Acetaminophen

Age	Weight (lbs)	Mg	Drops (ml)	Elixir (tsp)	Chewable tablets	Adult tablets
0-3 mo	6-11	40	0.4	¼	—	—
4-11 mo	12-17	80	0.8	½	—	—
12-23 mo	18-23	120	1.2	¾	1½	—
2-3 yr	24-35	160	1.6	1	2	—
4-5 yr	36-47	240	—	1½	3	—
6-8 yr	48-59	320	—	2	4	1
9-10 yr	60-71	400	—	3	6	1
11 yr	72-95	480	—	—	—	1½

12 years and older may take two regular adult tablets (640 mg total).

Adults

1. Instruct on proper dosage and administration of antipyretics and antibiotics.
2. Emphasize need to complete antibiotic therapy.
3. Encourage increased oral intake to prevent dehydration.
4. Encourage rest and use of cool, comfortable attire.
5. Instruct to follow-up with private physician or clinic as appropriate.

References

1. Emergency Nurses' Association: *Emergency nurse pediatric course,* Park Ridge, Ill, 1993, The Association, 200.

Gastric Lavage

Kim Sparks

DESCRIPTION

Gastric intubation is a very common procedure performed in the emergency department (ED). Gastric intubation involves the insertion of a tube, through either the nose or mouth, into the stomach for gastric evacuation or lavage.

INDICATIONS

1. Empty gastric contents and suppress vomiting caused by an ileus or mechanical obstruction.
2. Remove toxic substances.
3. Prevent gastric dilatation and aspiration in patients with major trauma.
4. Instill radiopaque contrast.
5. Perform therapeutic or diagnostic gastric lavage. Lavage facilitates removal of blood and clots in patients with upper gastrointestinal bleeding.

CONTRAINDICATIONS

1. Insertion of a gastric tube in patients that have ingested a caustic substance (e.g., acid, lye) may cause further esophageal damage.
2. A gastric tube should not be inserted nasally in patients with massive facial trauma or a basilar skull fracture. In such cases, the tube shall be inserted orally.

EQUIPMENT

- Gastric tube: Gastric tubes are also known as Levin, Salem-sump, Ewald, or Levacuator tubes. The Salem-sump tube has a vent lumen that allows for controlled suction force at the drainage eyes. The sump tube is also less likely to be sucked against the stomach wall.

NURSING ALERT

The size and type of tube used depends on the reason for placement. In adult patients with active upper gastrointestinal bleeding, a large bore tube (32 to 36 Fr) should be inserted through the mouth.

- Water soluble lubricant
- 60 ml piston or catheter tip syringe
- Emesis basin
- Tape
- Stethoscope
- Suction equipment
- Gloves
- Normal saline (NS)

INITIAL NURSING ACTIONS

1. Explain procedure to patient.
2. If alert, place the patient in a higher Fowler's position.

NURSING ALERT

Maintain spinal immobilization in trauma patients. Have suction readily available. Be prepared to logroll patient if vomiting occurs.

Nasogastric Placement

- Measure distance of insertion by placing the tip of the tube at the patient's nose and following the length of the tubing to the ear and then from the ear to the xiphoid process. Mark the tubing at this point.
- Examine the nose and select the largest nare.
- Lubricate the end of the tube with water soluble lubricant. Occasionally lidocaine jelly is used to lubricate the tube and anesthetize the nasal tract.
- Insert the tube into the nostril at a 60 to 90 degree angle to the plane of the face.
- Once the tube is in the oropharynx, have the patient flex the head forward and swallow several times. If possible, have the patient swallow a few sips of water through a straw. Advance the tube (while the patient swallows) to the previously marked point.

NURSING ALERT

If the tube slips into the trachea, violent coughing will ensue. Withdraw the tube into the oropharynx and try again to advance the tube into the esophagus and stomach.

Orogastric Placement

- If alert, place the patient in a high Fowler's position. If lavage is to be performed, place the patient on the left side in slight Trendelenburg position to promote return of lavage fluid and to prevent aspiration.
- Measure the distance of insertion by placing the tip of the tube at the lips. Follow the length of the tubing to the angle of the jaw and then from the jaw to the xiphoid process. Mark the tubing at that point.
- If the patient is uncooperative, place a bite block in the mouth to prevent the patient from biting the tube.
- Lubricate the tip of the tube and pass it gently over the tongue aiming down and back towards the pharynx.
- Flex the patient's head forward and advance the tube when the patient swallows.

NURSING ALERT

Do not flex the head if there is the possibility of a cervical spine injury.

3. Verify proper placement by aspirating gastric contents and by injecting 20 to 30 cc of air (with piston or catheter tip syringe) into the tube while listening over the stomach with a stethoscope.
4. Secure the tube with tape or a gastric tube holder. Do not tape to the forehead as this places pressure on the nares.

PATIENT CARE MANAGEMENT

1. Connect the tube to suction as prescribed by the physician.
2. Lavage may be needed in patients with upper gastrointestinal bleeding or ingestion of toxic substance.
   - Pour NS solution into a container. The use of iced saline is controversial. Some clinicians prefer using

room temperature tap water on the grounds that it breaks up clots better and it does not lower core body temperature as much.

- Instill 60 to 500 ml (the actual volume is controversial) of fluid by a piston or catheter tip syringe. Gently withdraw the fluid with the syringe and discard into a measured basin.
- Continue the lavage until the fluid returns clear or an endoscopy is performed. Prepackaged gastric lavage kits, that can be connected to suction, are commercially available.

3. Consider providing the patient with anesthetic throat lozenges or spray to relieve throat discomfort from the tube.

Bibliography

Bitterman RA: Upper gastrointestinal hemorrhage, *Emerg Med*, 77-86, October 30, 1989.

Gervin AS, Gostout CJ, and Zinner MJ: Upper GI bleeding: treatment options, *Patient Care*, 59-77, January 30, 1991.

Knighton D, Locksley RM, Mills J: Emergency procedures. In Saunders CE, Ho MT, editors: *Current emergency diagnosis and treatment*, Norwalk, Conn, 1992, Appleton & Lange.

Novotny-Dinsdale V: Gastric lavage for gastrointestinal bleeding. In Proehl JA, editor: *Adult emergency nursing procedures,* Boston, 1993, Jones & Bartlett.

Qureshi WA, Netchvolodoff CV: Acute bleeding from peptic ulcers, *Postgrad Med* 93(4):167-176, 1993.

Simon RR, Brenner BE: *Emergency procedures and techniques,* Baltimore, 1994, Williams & Wilkins.

Swimm D: Insertion of nasogastric and orogastric tubes. In Proehl JA, editor: *Adult emergency nursing procedures,* Boston, 1993, Jones & Bartlett.

Wardell TL: Assessing and managing a gastric ulcer, *Nurs 91,* 34-41, March 1994.

Head Injury

Lisa Creech

DESCRIPTION

Patients sustaining mild head injuries will often be discharged from the emergency department (ED). Discharge teaching is imperative, and the nurse must ensure that the patient and family understand signs and symptoms that warrant immediate return to the ED. Proper education may assist patients and family members in assessing the need for return to the hospital.

INDICATIONS

Generally, patients who have no loss of consciousness, or a loss of consciousness lasting <5 minutes will be discharged from the hospital. Discharge instructions should include both monitoring for symptoms of a worsening head injury and symptoms associated with post concussion syndrome.

INITIAL NURSING ACTIONS

The patient and family should be alerted to signs and symptoms that warrant return to the hospital. Instruct the patient and family that it will be necessary for a responsible person to remain with the patient for the first 24 hours following the injury, in order to observe and monitor for the following:

- Obvious pupillary changes (one large, one small)
- Blurred vision
- Vomiting
- Severe headache
- Slurred speech
- Gait or balance disturbance
- Noticeable new weakness of either arm or leg
- Unusual behavior
- Confusion
- Severe lethargy or unusual drowsiness (3)

The patient should be awakened every 2 hours, or as determined by the physician, to ensure that he or she is arousable to a normal state of alertness (1).

> **NURSING ALERT**
>
> Patients and families should be instructed to call or return to the ED immediately if any of the above are noted. In addition, alcohol and other sedative medication should be avoided for 24 hours. Activity levels should be kept to a minimum for 48 hours. Acetaminophen and ibuprofen are acceptable measures for pain control unless contraindicated.

PATIENT CARE MANAGEMENT

Post concussion syndrome is a generalized term used to describe a specific group of symptoms following a head injury. These symptoms may persist for weeks to months. It has been estimated that nearly 50% of all patients sustaining mild head injuries will develop some degree of post concussion syndrome (2). Complaints vary among individuals, but those most commonly noted include headache, mood changes, and forgetfulness. Because treatment is palliative, families must understand the need for follow-up care after discharge from the ED.

References
1. Bartkowski H: Head trauma. In Saunders C, Ho M, editors: *Current emergency diagnosis and treatment*, 1992, Lange.
2. Evans RW: The post concussion syndrome and the sequalae of mild head injury, *The neurology of trauma*, vol 10, 1992, WB Saunders.
3. Leahy NM: *Quick reference to neurologic critical care nursing*, 1990, Aspen.

Intracranial Pressure Monitoring

Patty Sturt

Intracranial pressure (ICP) monitoring provides continuous data regarding the pressure exerted within the cranial vault. Direct measurement of ICP is best achieved by use of an intraventricular catheter placed into the lateral ventricle. The intraventricular catheter also allows withdrawal of cerebrospinal fluid (CSF) to control ICP. The normal ICP is 0 to 15 mm Hg. In addition, it is possible to calculate the cerebral perfusion pressure (CPP) if the ICP is known. The CPP is an indirect measurement of cerebral blood flow and is calculated by subtracting the ICP from the mean arterial pressure. Normal is considered 60 to 100 mm Hg. Monitoring the ICP may provide evidence of intracranial hypertension before serious signs and symptoms exhibit thus permitting earlier intervention. ICP monitoring is based on the concept of converting fluid pressure (CSF) into electrical current and displaying it on a monitor.

INDICATIONS

The decision for which patients should be monitored for ICP varies among physicians (4). Patients with certain pathophysiologic conditions may be considered candidates for ICP monitoring. These pathophysiologic conditions include the following:
1. Head injury
2. Intracerebral hematoma
3. Subarachnoid hemorrhage
4. Space-occupying lesions
5. Central nervous system infections
6. Toxic or metabolic encephalopathies
7. Cerebral edema
8. Hydrocephalus
9. Ischemic/hypoxic insults

A depressed level of consciousness with a Glasgow Coma Scale (GCS) score ≤8 in any of the above conditions is a commonly used indicator for ICP monitoring.

ICP monitoring may also be indicated in patients that are clinically difficult to assess because of paralytic agents.

CONTRAINDICATIONS

1. Coagulation abnormalities
2. Generalized cerebral edema resulting in small compressed ventricles

INTRAVENTRICULAR CATHETER SETUP, INSERTION, AND MONITORING

Description

The intraventricular catheter is most commonly placed into the anterior horn of the lateral ventricle of the nondominant hemisphere. The right hemisphere is considered the nondominant hemisphere in most humans. The catheter is inserted through a burr hole for the purposes of:

1. Monitoring intracranial pressure
2. Removal of CSF for culture and laboratory specimens
3. Removal of CSF to control and reduce ICP
   The catheter is inserted by a neurosurgeon.

Equipment

- Razor
- Betadine scrub brush or container of sponges with povidone-iodine solution
- Lidocaine with or without epinephrine for injection
- 5 to 10 cc syringe and different size needles for injection
- IV pole attached to the bed
- Pressure module and monitor
- Stopcock
- Transducer
- 12 inch pressure tubing
- One bottle of nonbacteriostatic normal saline (NS)
- 10 cc syringe with 18-gauge needle for drawing up NS
- Luer-Lok
- Betadine ointment, sterile eye patch, and 3 inch tape for dressing over insertion site
- Intraventricular catheter and external drainage collection system

ICP insertion tray includes the following:

- Iodine cup
- Twist drill

- Needle-holder
- Sharp, blunt scissors
- Knife handle and scalpel
- 4 × 4 sponges
- 16-gauge and 18-gauge ventricular needles
- 10 cc syringe

INITIAL NURSING ACTIONS

1. Fill a 10 ml syringe with sterile nonbacteriostatic NS for injection.
2. Attach open end of transducer to side port of stopcock.
3. Attach 12 inch pressure tubing to the other side port of the stopcock.
4. Attach 10 cc syringe of NS to the vertical port of the stopcock.
5. Turn stopcock off to the transducer and flush the pressure tubing.
6. Turn stopcock off to the pressure tubing and flush the transducer. Turn stopcock on to transducer and tubing.
7. Remove the syringe and place Luer-Lok on the open end of the stopcock.

NURSING ALERT

Aseptic technique should be used when assembling and flushing the system. Never use a transducer with a flush system.

8. Attach transducer to the pressure cable. The pressure cable should be connected to a pressure module on the monitor.
9. Tape the transducer to a towel roll to maintain the position of the transducer at the correct level.
10. Elevate the head of bed. The neck should be kept in a neutral position. Place a protective barrier under the head.
11. The physician will shave the hair around the insertion site and prep the area with a betadine brush or sponges soaked with povidone-iodine solution. The physician should wear a mask and sterile gloves. Depending on the patient's condition and the urgency of the situation, lidocaine may be injected to anesthetize the insertion site. Using a twist drill, a burr hole is made

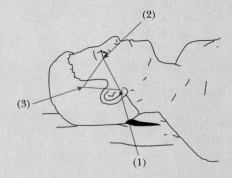

Figure P20-1 Location of foramen of Monro for transducer placement. Map an imaginary equilateral triangle from (1) the external auditory meatus, to (2) the outer canthus of the eye, to (3) behind the hairline. Point 3 is the location of the foramen of Monro. (From Stillwell S: *Mosby's critical care nursing reference,* 1992, Mosby.)

anterior to the coronal suture. A catheter over a guidewire is inserted aiming at the inner canthus of the eye. The guidewire is withdrawn. Using aseptic technique, the end of the external drainage collection system is connected to the catheter via a port or valve. Attach the pressure tubing from the transducer to the other end of the port. The distal end of the catheter is sutured to the scalp.

12. Record the opening pressure.
13. Maintain the transducer at the level of the foramen of Monro (Figure P20-1).
14. Place betadine ointment (as directed by the physician) over the insertion site. Cover the site with a sterile eye patch or gauze and tape in place.
15. Using the cord provided, suspend the external drainage collection system from the IV pole attached to the bed. The drip chamber is usually placed 10 to 20 cm above the level of the foramen of Monro.
16. CSF should be drained intermittently or continuously, as prescribed. With intermittent drainage, the system is turned on to drainage when the ICP reaches a certain level. The physician usually orders drainage of CSF when the ICP is 20 mm Hg or greater.

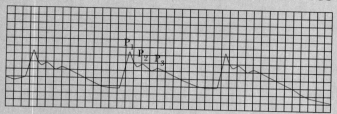

P20-2 ICP waveform. (From Stillwell S: *Mosby's critical care nursing reference,* 1992, Mosby.)

17. The system should be turned off to drainage when an ICP reading is obtained for documentation (3). Pressure vented toward the collection system and away from the transducer may cause an artificially low ICP.

PATIENT CARE MANAGEMENT

1. Avoid kinks in the drainage system.
2. Evaluate and document the clarity, color, and amount of CSF drainage.
3. Notify the physician if there is no CSF drainage in the presence of intracranial hypertension.
4. Ensure integrity of the system to prevent the entrance of air and infection.
5. Zero the transducer every shift, after position changes, or when there is a sudden change in the ICP reading or waveform.
6. Prophylactic antibiotics may be ordered by the physician to prevent brain infection.
7. Monitor the waveform on the monitor. The waveform consists of at least three peaks (Figure P20-2). As ICP increases, P_2 becomes elevated. If P_2 is higher than P_1, suspect decreased compliance.
8. Notify the physician if abnormal waveforms are noted. A-waves (plateau waves) are seen with sudden transient elevations of 50 to 100 mm Hg that last 5 to 20 minutes. B-waves (sawtooth waves) are seen with increases in ICP of up to 50 mm Hg and occur every 30 seconds to 2 minutes. B-waves indicate an unstable ICP (1).

TABLE P20-1 Checklist For ICP Monitoring

Problem	Action
No waveform	Check power to monitor and to trace
	Check gain setting
	Check all connections
	Check for air bubbles in system
High pressure reading	Check transducer level placement
	Check calibration and rezero
	Evaluate patient:
	Check airway
	Check ventilator settings
	Check ABGs for hypoxemia, hypercarbia
	Check head of bed (15-30 degrees)
	Check position of head (do not rotate head)
	Check extremities (limit flexion in lower extremities and hips)
	Check excessive muscle activity (administer muscle relaxants, paralyzing agents as ordered)
	Check abdominal distention
	Check noxious stimuli and remove
	Check temperature
	Check PAP, CO, SvO_2, BP
	Check electrolytes
Low pressure reading	Check transducer level placement (Figure P20-1)
	Check for otorrhea and rhinorrhea
	Check for dislodged catheter—notify physician
	Check if 15-20 mm Hg positive pressure exists (with use of external ventriculostomy)

9. See Table P20-1 for possible problems that can occur with ICP monitoring and the appropriate nursing actions.

CAMINO ICP SYSTEM SETUP, INSERTION, AND MONITORING

Description

The Camino catheter contains a miniature transducer located at the distal end of a fiberoptic catheter to sense ICP. A fluid-filled external transducer system is not used, since the transducer is placed directly into the brain parenchyma.

Equipment

- Sterile gloves
- Camino OLM intracranial kit. This kit contains the following: sterile transducer-tipped pressure monitoring catheter, Camino bolt, compression cap, drill bit, stylet, Allen wrench, zero adjustment tool, and strain relief sheath (Figure P20-3)
- Camino disposable twist drill procedure kit. This kit contains the hand drill, scalp retractor, needle-holder, Metzenbaum scissors, 18-gauge spinal needle, forceps, scalpel with handle, NS ampules, 1% lidocaine, sponges, medicine cups, betadine swabs, syringes, and various size needles
- Camino V420 direct pressure monitor with power cord and pole mount (2)
- Pole stand

INITIAL NURSING ACTIONS

1. After the insertion site is chosen by the physician, the area is shaved and prepped in a sterile fashion with betadine solution. The area is then draped with sterile towels. The physician injects the area with lidocaine and makes an incision to the bone with the scalpel. The drill bit is secured to the hand drill and a twist drill hole is made through the skull. The hole is irrigated with NS and an 18-gauge spinal needle is used to open the dura. The Camino bolt is screwed into the skull. The stylet is inserted through the dura to clear the passage for the Camino catheter. The Camino Bolt is then irrigated with nonbacteriostatic sterile saline.

2. The catheter is removed from the sterile package. Firmly attach the transducer connector to the preamp connector (Figure P20-4).

3. If the Camino 420 display does not read zero after a short system self-check, use the tool from the catheter kit to turn the zero adjustment on the bottom side of the transducer connector until the Camino 420 display reads zero. Once this is accomplished, it is not necessary to zero the system again (Figure P20-5).

4. The physician inserts the Camino catheter into the bolt. A waveform should appear if the V420 is connected to a bedside monitor. The compression cap on the bolt is turned to lock the catheter in place. The physician then

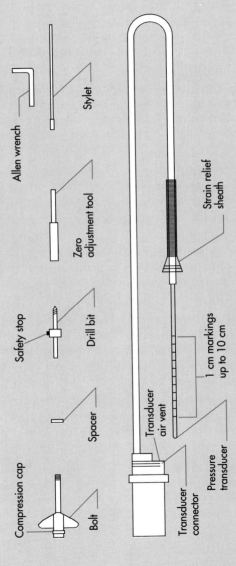

P20-3 Camino OLM intracranial kit. Courtesy Camino Laboratories.

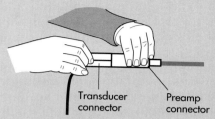

P20-4 Connection of transducer connector and preamp connector. Courtesy Camino Laboratories.

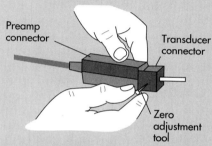

P20-5 Technique for zeroing transducer. Courtesy Camino Laboratories.

slides the strain release sheath (on the catheter) down onto the compression cap.
5. Do not attach anything to the transducer air vent. The vent must remain open for proper operation.
6. After the catheter has been inserted into the patient, select the appropriate scale on the monitor by repeatedly pressing the SCALE button on the V420 front panel (2).

PATIENT CARE MANAGEMENT

1. If the V420 is connected to an external bedside monitor, the CAL STEP button may be used to calibrate or balance the bedside monitor.
   - Press the CAL STEP button repeatedly until zero is displayed on the V420.
   - While keeping the button depressed to maintain zero, simultaneously zero the bedside monitor.
   - Release the CAL STEP button. The CAL STEP does not affect the transducer calibration.

2. The V420 can be connected to a 427 recorder as follows:
   - Connect the V420 interface cable to the V420 monitor accessory receptacle.
   - Insert the V420 power cable into the V420 power cord receptacle.
   - Insert the power cord into its receptacle on the back of the 427 recorder. Then insert the plug into a grounded outlet.
   - Turn on the power by moving the circuit breaker switch to its "up" position.
   - To record waveforms, press the 25 mm/sec button. The recording will continue until the STOP button is pressed (2).

3. Monitor the waveforms as described under patient care management with intraventricular catheters.

References

1. Barker E: Avoiding increased intracranial pressure. *Nursing '90,* May 64Q-64RR, 1990.
2. Camino user information guide, Camino Laboratories, San Diego, Calif.
3. McQuillan KA: Intracranial pressure monitoring technical imperatives, *AACN Clinical Issues* 2(4):624-636, 1991.
4. Richmond TS: Intracranial pressure monitoring, *AACN Clinical Issues* 4(1):148-160, 1993.

Intraosseous Infusion

George P. Glessner III

DESCRIPTION

Intraosseous infusion is used for fluid and medication administration in infants and children 8 years of age or less when attempts at venous access have been unsuccessful. There is minimal risk of complications if the procedure is performed properly and appropriately. Colloids, crystalloids, and medications that can be administered intravenously can be administered intraosseously. The proximal tibia is the usual sight for intraosseous cannulation. The distal femur of an infant can also be used. Intraosseous access is a temporary measure and should be replaced with venous access as soon as possible (1).

INDICATIONS

1. The indications for intraosseous cannulation and infusion are the same as for venous cannulation (see Chapter 11).
2. Intraosseous cannulation is indicated in an emergency after unsuccessful attempts have been made to establish venous access.

CONTRAINDICATIONS

1. Anyone older than 8 years of age
2. When the intraosseous site is in an extremity with a recent or possible acute fracture
3. Bone disorders
4. When using marrow-toxic drugs

EQUIPMENT

- Appropriate IV administration set and IV fluid
- Spinal needles with stylets, bone marrow needles, or standard 16 or 18 gauge hypodermic needles (hypodermic needles sometimes bend or break)

INITIAL NURSING ACTIONS

1. Assemble all the necessary equipment.
2. Prepare the patient and the site with povidone-iodine solution. The usual site is 2 to 3 cm or two finger breadths below the tibial tuberosity.
3. Insert the needle that has been attached to a syringe into the anterior-medial aspect of the leg perpendicularly or pointed slightly inferiorly to avoid the epiphyseal plate (Figure P21-1, *B*).
4. Advance the needle until reaching the bone. With firm pressure and control, advance the needle through the bone and into the bone marrow cavity. This is evidenced by feeling the "pop" of the needle entering the bone marrow cavity.
5. Confirm placement of the intraosseous cannula by withdrawing bone marrow with the attached syringe.
6. Attach the appropriate IV administration set and fluid.
7. Secure both the leg and the intraosseous cannula in order to prevent dislodgement (Figure P21-1, *A*).

PATIENT CARE MANAGEMENT

1. Assess the intraosseous sight frequently for signs of infiltration to assure patency.
2. Prepare for and anticipate the need to gain venous access as soon as the patient's condition has stabilized or resuscitation is complete. This minimizes the chance of developing osteomyelitis.
3. Assist with gaining venous access by means of a saphenous vein cutdown or central venous cannulation.
4. If the intraosseous needle becomes clogged with bone marrow and will not clear, replace the needle with a similar needle passed through the same hole in the bone.
5. Assess for development of infection and administer antibiotics when ordered.
6. Be prepared to secure the leg to prevent excessive movement causing dislodgement.
   * Secure the leg to a padded IV board or padded full leg splint.

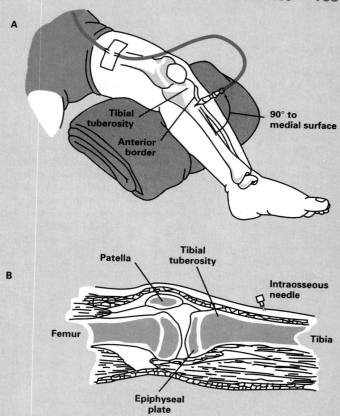

Figure P21-1 A, Intraosseous infusion technique. **B,** Insertion.
(**A** Redrawn from Chameides L, editor: *Pediatric advanced life support,*
Dallas, 1988, American Heart Association. **B** from Barkin RM,
Rosen P: *Emergency pediatrics: a guide to ambulatory care,* ed 3, St Louis,
1990, Mosby.)

References

1. American Heart Association, American Academy of Pediatrics:
   Textbook of pediatric life support, 1988, Dallas, The Association.

Lumbar Puncture

Barbara Blake

DESCRIPTION

Lumbar puncture (LP) involves insertion of a hollow needle with a stylet into the subarachnoid space between the L3 and L4 or L4 and L5 vertebrae to obtain cerebrospinal fluid (CSF) for diagnostic purposes.

INDICATIONS

In the ED setting, an LP may be performed to:

1. Obtain CSF for microscopic examination and/or culture and sensitivity. This may be necessary in cases where meningitis or encephalitis is suspected (see Chapter 15).
2. Determine the presence of blood in the CSF. Blood in the CSF is suggestive of subarachnoid hemorrhage.
3. Measure CSF pressure.
4. Instill blood, medications (such as antibiotics), or radiopaque contrast material into the subarachnoid space.

CONTRAINDICATIONS

1. Local infection of the lumbar area
2. Suspected spinal cord mass lesion
3. Anticoagulant therapy
4. Signs of increased intracranial pressure from a suspected intracranial mass (brain abscess, lesion, tumor, or posterior fossa lesion). In these cases, a CT scan should be performed before the LP, since fluid drainage may cause herniation (see Chapter 15).

EQUIPMENT

Prepackaged sterile disposable LP trays are commercially available. If the tray is not available, gather the following:

- Sterile gloves
- 1% lidocaine (some physicians prefer 1% lidocaine with epinephrine)

- Antiseptic solution such as povidone-iodine solution
- Sterile towels or drapes
- Sterile gauze sponges
- Four sterile collection tubes
- 3 to 5 ml syringe
- 22 or 25 gauge needle, 1½ inch in length for lidocaine infiltration
- Pressure manometer with a three-way stopcock
- Spinal needles with stylet
  Adults: 20 to 22 gauge, 3 to 3½ inch
  <1 year: 22-gauge, 1½ inch
  >1 year: 22-gauge, 2½ inch
- Small adhesive dressing for puncture site
- Stool or chair for physician to sit on during procedure

INITIAL NURSING ACTIONS

1. Explain procedure to the patient.
2. Obtain informed consent. Written consent can be obtained in accordance with the hospital policies.
3. Position the patient. Proper positioning is necessary to perform an LP.
   - *Lying position:* Assist patient to the lateral decubitus position with the shoulders and pelvis perpendicular to the stretcher. Instruct the patient to curl his back by drawing the knees up to the abdomen and flexing the neck forward. Place a small pillow under the head to keep the spine in the horizontal position. Assist the patient in maintaining this position during the procedure by placing your hands and/or arms behind the neck and knees (Figure P22-1).
   - *Sitting or upright position:* Assist patients to a sitting position on side of examination table. Have patient curl his/her back by placing head and arms over a padded bedside table. For an infant, place in an upright position with thighs flexing up to the abdomen and the neck flexed forward. Stabilize the infant against your upper torso and immobilize the extremities with your hands (Figure P22-2).

NURSING ALERT

Avoid hyperflexion of neck in infants as this may lead to airway obstruction. Observe for signs of respiratory distress.

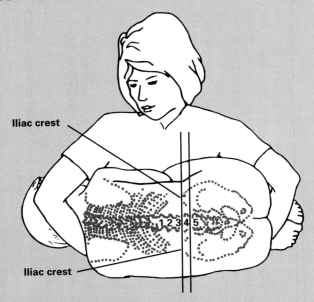

Figure P22-1 Position for lumbar puncture. The desired sites are the interspaces between L3 and L4, or L4 and L5.

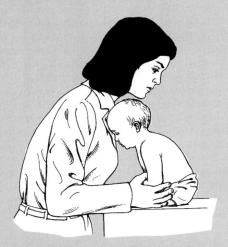

Figure P22-2 Position for lumbar puncture of an infant.

4. Once the patient is positioned correctly, the physician will proceed as follows:
   - Cleanse the skin with antiseptic solution.
   - Place a sterile drape under the patient and across the back.
   - Inject the area with 1% lidocaine.
   - Insert and slowly advance the needle until the subarachnoid space is entered (will feel a "pop").
   - Remove the stylet to observe for flow of CSF.
   - Attach stopcock and manometer to the needle to measure opening CSF pressure. Normal pressure is between 70 and 180 mm H_2O. Have patient slowly relax legs and neck to prevent falsely elevated readings (the nurse may need to assist the patient to a relaxed position).
   - Remove manometer and collect CSF in the four collection tubes.
     Tube no. 1 is usually for culture and sensitivity, gram stain, and red cell count.
     Tube no. 2 is for protein and glucose determinations.
     Tube no. 3 is for cytology.
     Tube no. 4 is for cell count.
   - Reinsert stylet and remove the needle.
5. The nurse or physician will place a small adhesive dressing over the puncture site.
6. Cleanse antiseptic solution from the back.
7. Send specimens to the laboratory for studies ordered by the physician.

PATIENT CARE MANAGEMENT

1. Document the patient's reaction to the procedure, specimen disposition, and appearance of the CSF. For example, was the CSF clear, cloudy, or blood tinged?
2. Instruct the patient to lie prone for at least 2 hours or per physician's instructions to decrease the chance of a spinal headache.
3. A lumbar puncture or spinal headache may occur afterwards from CSF leakage. A blood patch (injection of autologous blood into the epidural space) may be required.

Bibliography

Barkin R, Rosen P: *Emergency pediatrics*, St Louis, 1990, Mosby.

Knighton D, Locksley RM, Mills J: Emergency procedures. In Saunders CE, Ho MT, editors: *Current emergency diagnosis and treatment,* East Norwalk, Conn, 1992, Appleton and Lange.

Lang S: Procedures involving the neurologic system. In Bernardo LM, Bove M, editors: *Pediatric emergency nursing procedures,* Boston, 1993, Jones and Bartlett.

Leahy NM: *Neurologic critical care nursing,* Rockville, Md, 1990, Aspen.

Neff JA: Lumbar puncture. In Proehl JA, editor: *Adult emergency nursing procedures,* Boston, 1993, Jones and Bartlett.

Medicolegal Evidence

Patty Sturt

DESCRIPTION

Forensic laboratories have been established to serve a vital need in the criminal justice system. Their purpose is to scientifically analyze physical evidence from possible criminal activities in the event of a trial. However, analysis of the evidence is only possible when the evidence has been collected and preserved in the correct manner. Emergency department (ED) nurses play a vital role in the collection and preservation of evidence from patients.

Physical evidence deals with material objects and can include hair, fibers, blood, body secretions, glass, bullets, or almost anything that can be collected or deposited. Physical evidence is helpful in proving that a crime has been committed.

INDICATIONS

Indications for the collection and preservation of medicolegal evidence may include cases involving suspected suicide, homicide, physical assault, sexual assault (see Sexual Assault Evidence Collection, Procedure 26), and driving under the influence of alcohol or illegal drugs.

INITIAL NURSING ACTIONS

1. Medicolegal evidence should be collected and preserved, keeping in mind specific state laws and following the hospital's policies and guidelines.
2. ALWAYS maintain the chain of evidence. The chain of evidence is simply documentation of who has possession of the evidence at all times. Transfer of evidence from one health care professional to another should be documented. This documentation should include the person that received the evidence and the time. In most cases, the evidence is handed over to a police or law enforcement officer. The law enforcement officer

should sign that he/she received the evidence and the time. This chain of evidence can be kept on the patient's medical record (chart) or a chain of evidence form. Evidence may be rendered invalid in court if the chain of evidence is not maintained and recorded.

3. If the evidence is placed in a lock box or refrigerator, document the name of the individual who placed the evidence in the lock box and the time.

4. The following principles should be followed with the collection and preservation of clothing:

- Articles of clothing may provide useful information regarding gun powder residue and the type of gun used in patients with bullet wounds. Do not cut or rip though bullet holes when cutting clothing for removal. Allow the garment to air dry (if wet) before packaging. Place paper or cardboard over and under the bullet hole and fold the garment over twice. Place in a paper bag. Do not use plastic bags.

- Stains on clothing (such as semen, blood, grass, or soil) may provide crucial evidence. Blood stains may help to identify the suspected assailant. Make sure that all stains are dry. If the stain is wet, it must be air dried. Package each item of clothing separately to avoid contamination. Do not use plastic bags, since plastic holds in moisture thus permitting bacterial and fungal growth. Avoid unnecessary handling of garment with stains.

- A law enforcement officer may request clothing for analysis of fibers. Fibers on clothing may be microscopically examined for the type, dye content, or weave content. This may be useful evidence if the fibers found match the fibers of the suspected assailant's clothing or fibers at the scene of the crime from carpet or other objects.

NURSING ALERT

Each bag of clothing collected for evidence should be labeled with the patient's name, hospital identification number, date, time, and the name of the person collecting the clothing for evidence.

5. A bullet can be examined in a forensic laboratory to determine whether it was fired from a specific firearm by comparing striated marks with the aid of a microscope. For the collection and preservation of bullets, wrap each one in clean soft tissue paper and place in a rigid container such as a sterile specimen cup. Place a label on the container to include the patient's name, hospital identification number, date, time of collection, and the name of the person collecting the bullet.

6. Many guns have gaps around the firing chamber through which residue can escape and coat the hand which fired it. The first priority of the nurse is always resuscitation of the patient. When possible, paper bags placed over the hands may prevent removal of gunshot residue. Many state forensic laboratories provide gunshot residue kits for law enforcement officers to obtain the residue for analysis. This may provide useful information in suspected suicide cases.

7. Occasionally, syringes and other drug paraphernalia may be found on a patient. Generally, if you cannot see residue in the syringe or paraphernalia, there is not enough to identify the substance. The needle should be capped or taped and placed in a rigid container. Always mark the container with "Contains Syringes" in bold lettering.

8. The following principles should be followed with the collection of blood for alcohol or drug identification and levels for medicolegal purposes:
   - Follow the hospital policy regarding the collection of blood for medicolegal purposes. Many state forensic laboratories have specific kits for the collection of blood.
   - Utilize nonalcohol swabs when prepping the skin for obtaining blood.
   - Label each blood tube with patient's name, hospital identification number, date, time, and name of the person collecting the specimen.

PATIENT CARE MANAGEMENT

Never leave evidence in an area of the ED where it can be tampered with by patients or visitors.

Bibliography

Huber DJ, Stokes JL: *Physical evidence handbook*, Kentucky State Police, Forensic laboratories section, 1994, Frankfort, KY.

Pericardiocentesis

Janet Rodgers

DESCRIPTION

A pericardiocentesis is performed by placing a needle and/or catheter into the pericardial space and aspirating fluid and/or blood from the pericardial sac. Decreasing the amount of fluid that has accumulated within the pericardial sac may allow for improved filling of the heart and increased contractility.

INDICATIONS

1. Cardiac tamponade
2. Aspiration of fluid for cytology and microbiology evaluation
3. Increasing pericardial effusion

EQUIPMENT

- Cardiac monitor
- Resuscitation medications and equipment
- Povidone-iodine solution
- Local anesthetic (lidocaine 1% without epinephrine)
- Needles of various sizes
- 10 ml syringe
- Sterile 4 × 4 gauze pads
- Razors
- Sterile gowns, gloves, and drape
- Masks and hair covers
- Sterile specimen containers
- Three-way stopcock
- 60 ml syringe
- Suture material
- Hemostat
- Sterile IV tubing
- Sterile drainage collector
- Catheter adapter
- 1 inch tape

- Occlusive dressing
- Alligator clamps, sterile
- ECG machine
- Pericardiocentesis needle (may be a spinal needle, a through-the-needle or an over-the-needle type catheter per physician's preference)

INITIAL NURSING ACTIONS

1. Position the patient with the head of bed elevated approximately 30 degrees. May use reverse Trendelenburg position.
2. Explain procedure to the patient.
3. Place patient on a cardiac monitor.
4. Establish a large bore peripheral IV for fluid, blood, or medication administration as ordered.
5. Monitor the patient throughout the procedure. Observe closely for changes in cardiac rhythm, dysrythmias, and elevation of the PR and ST segment from baseline. These changes indicate that the catheter/needle is in contact with the epicardium.
   Conduction of electrical activity from the epicardium through the pericardiocentesis needle, signaling contact with the epicardium, is most accurately assessed by attaching a sterile alligator clamp to the needle and connecting it to the V lead on an ECG. If time allows, this is recommended.
6. After insertion, if a catheter is left in place, attach it to the collection device using the sterile IV tubing and a catheter adapter. Secure all connections with tape. Place a Luer-Lok cap over the stopcock opening. Occasionally in critical situations, the physician may secure and clamp the catheter by using a hemostat to clamp the catheter to the chest wall.
7. Cover the insertion site with an occlusive dressing after the catheter has been secured or after it has been removed.
8. Coil extra tubing from the collection system and place it on the bed.

NURSING ALERT

If CPR is in progress, continue chest compressions until needle insertion is initiated.

NURSING ALERT

Isolated pericardial effusion fluid will not rapidly clot, whereas, blood inadvertently aspirated from within the cardiac chambers will rapidly clot. Remember that clotting times may vary greatly depending on the presence of preexisting diseases that alter clotting factors, medical and surgical interventions that reduce clotting factors, hemorrhage, and the use of anticoagulants.

Traumatic cardiac tamponade may result from rapid hemorrhage into the pericardial space. The blood may clot within the pericardial sac making aspiration impossible or may clot rapidly after aspiration.

PATIENT CARE MANAGEMENT

1. Assess vital signs, peripheral perfusion, heart sounds, and cardiac rhythm every 15 minutes for 1 hour, then advance according to the patient's condition. If invasive monitoring has been initiated, such as a pulmonary artery catheter or central venous catheter, these pressures should also be assessed. Notify the physician if symptoms of pericardial tamponade reoccur.
2. Monitor and record blood/fluid drainage within the collection system every 15 minutes for one hour, then hourly.
3. If clots develop within the collection tubing, gently squeeze the tubing between your fingers and advance the clot into the collection chamber.

Bibliography

Emergency procedures, Springhouse, Pa, 1993, Springhouse Corp.
Lippincott manual nursing practice, Philadelphia, 1991, JB Lippincott.
Textbook of advanced cardiac life support, 1994, Dallas, American Heart Association.

Pulmonary Arterial Catheter

Theresa M. Glessner

DESCRIPTION

Pulmonary arterial (PA) catheters are IV catheters inserted through a large central vein (femoral, internal jugular, or subclavian) into the right side of the heart with the tip of the catheter extending into the PA. The purpose of this catheter is to directly measure pressures in the right side of the heart, indirectly measure pressures in the left side of the heart, and measure cardiac output utilizing the thermodilution method.

INDICATIONS

1. Monitoring of fluid status
2. Right or left heart failure
3. Shock states
4. Titration of vasoactive drugs

CONTRAINDICATIONS

Any bleeding disorder or coagulation disorder would be a reason to consider the risk vs. the benefit of this procedure. There are no absolute contraindications to this procedure.

EQUIPMENT

- PA catheter (Figure P25-1)
- Introducer kit
- Local anesthetic
- Gloves
- Povidone-iodine solution
- Transducer setup with pressure bag—need two transducers or a cardiac bridge to monitor CVP readings
- Monitor with pressure capability and appropriate cables
- Cardiac output monitor with appropriate cable and cardiac output setup—includes IV solution, tubing, and 10 cc syringe
- 4 × 4 gauze

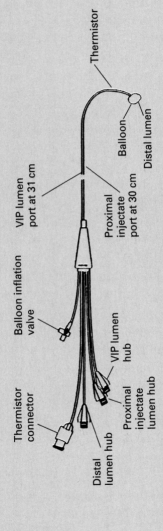

Figure P25-1 Swan-Ganz Venous Infusion Port (VIP) Thermodilution Catheter.

- Sterile normal saline for flushing ports and syringes and needles

INITIAL NURSING ACTIONS

1. Assure that this procedure is thoroughly explained to the patient and/or family before initiation and that informed consent has been obtained.
2. Assemble the transducer and flush system, then completely flush through the system eliminating all air bubbles. Assure that the pressure bag is inflated to 300 mm Hg.
3. Assemble the cardiac output measurement system and flush through this system. Assure that the computation constant for the cardiac output computer is appropriate for the size of the catheter used and the temperature of the diluent.
4. Assure that all the monitoring equipment is functional and zero the transducer(s) at the phlebostatic axis (4th or 5th intercostal space, midaxillary line) remembering to turn the stopcock off to the patient side and open to air (atmosphere).
5. Assure that the patient's ECG is being continuously monitored for ventricular arrhythmias (ventricular tachycardia, PVCs, and ventricular fibrillation can occur during insertion through the right ventricle), and remain with the patient throughout the procedure providing verbal support and comfort measures.
6. Before insertion of the catheter, assure that the catheter is flushed. Utilize the flush system for the PA port and the CVP port (either separately or bridged) to flush these ports respectively. Utilize a 10 cc syringe of saline to flush the infusion port. Also, ensure patency of the balloon by inflating it and allowing it to passively deflate.

Physician Actions

- Initially the physician palpates the area where the catheter is placed to locate the landmarks for insertion such as the sternal notch and the clavicle.
- The physician, after donning a mask, sterile gloves, a sterile gown and a cap, preps and sterilely drapes the area where the catheter will be placed.
- The area is anesthetized with a local anesthetic such as 1% lidocaine.
- The physician then attempts to locate the blood vessel with a large needle and syringe. Once there is blood return, the syringe is removed and a wire is

threaded through the needle. The needle is then removed and a large catheter is threaded over the wire. The physician may need to lacerate the skin in order to pass the large catheter into the vessel.

- The physician is now ready to float the PA catheter through the introducer (which was just inserted). The PA catheter must have the sterile sleeve placed over it before being placed into the patient.
- When the physician has the catheter advanced approximately 10 to 15 cm, the balloon needs to be inflated by the nurse (or whomever is helping).
- Once the catheter is floated to a wedge position, the physician will ask for the balloon to be deflated.

7. During insertion of the catheter, monitor the ECG for dysrhythmias especially while passing through the right ventricle because irritation of the ventricle can cause ventricular arrhythmias—ventricular tachycardia, PVCs, and ventricular fibrillation.

8. After insertion of the catheter, obtain a stat portable chest x-ray to verify line placement and to rule out a pneumothorax caused by insertion of the introducer.
   - When the physician is satisfied with the catheter placement, it is sutured in place and dressed sterilely.

9. Continuously monitor the PA pressure (and the central venous pressure if the ports are monitored with separate transducers).

10. Record all hemodynamic parameters—CVP, PAP, PCWP, CO/CI, SVR, and other parameters per unit protocol.

11. After the catheter is sutured in place, apply a sterile, deep-line dressing utilizing strict aseptic technique. Secure the catheter to the patient with tape in order to avoid catheter dislodgement from the weight of the catheter or accidental pulling on the catheter.

PATIENT CARE MANAGEMENT

1. Assess and trend patient's vital signs and hemodynamic parameters, and note improvement or deterioration.

2. Record all hemodynamic parameters every hour or per unit protocol, and notify physician of any significant changes in the patient's condition.

3. Assure that transducer(s) are zeroed to atmosphere at least every shift or per unit protocol.

4. Monitor insertion site for infection and change dressing every 72 hours or per unit protocol.

5. Monitor PA waveform for signs of catheter migration. If the catheter floats in (distally), the waveform changes to a permanent wedge waveform. If the catheter floats out (proximally), the waveform shows a right ventricular tracing (Figure P25-2). Notify the physician if either occurs, both are dangerous conditions.

6. Continuously monitor the patient's ECG. Ventricular arrhythmias may indicate catheter migration into the right ventricle. This can be corrected by the physician floating the catheter back into the pulmonary artery.

7. Change pressure tubing, including bridge systems and Luer-Loks, every 72 hours or per unit protocol utilizing strict aseptic technique including gloves and a mask. Assure that all stopcocks have sterile Luer-Loks on each unused port.

8. If blood specimens are being withdrawn through the PA catheter system, assure that the system is thoroughly flushed after each blood draw to prevent clot formation in the catheter.

9. Assure that the system pressure bag is always inflated to 300 mm Hg in order to prevent clot formation and to assure a crisp waveform at all times.

10. Assure that the balloon passively deflates after each wedge reading. If it does not, attempt to manually deflate the balloon with the syringe. If the normal resistance is not felt when inflating the balloon, and the balloon does not passively deflate, the balloon is probably ruptured and should not be reinflated at any time until the catheter is replaced.

11. If utilizing an SVO_2 or oximetrix PA catheter (Figure P25-3), assure the following:

   • The SVO_2 monitor and cable are available and functional.

   • The optical connector is attached to the cable and monitor and is calibrated before removing the catheter from the package.

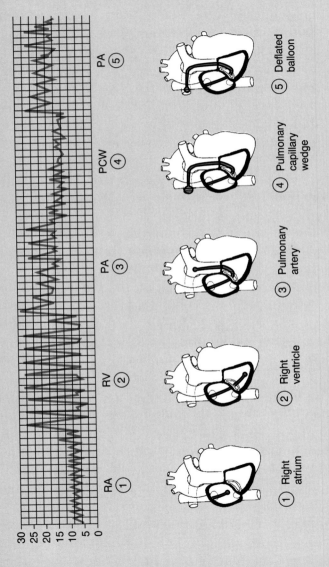

Figure P25-2 PA waveforms: RA, RV, PA, wedge.

① Right atrium ② Right ventricle ③ Pulmonary artery ④ Pulmonary capillary wedge ⑤ Deflated balloon

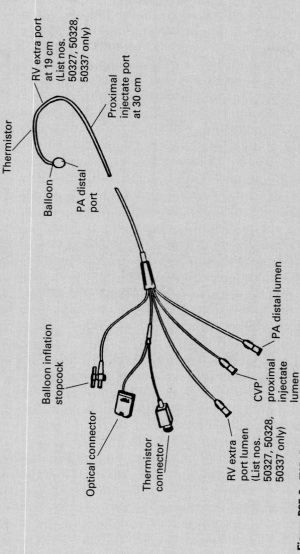

Thermistor

RV extra port
at 19 cm
(List nos.
50327, 50328,
50337 only)

Proximal
injectate port
at 30 cm

Balloon

PA distal
port

Balloon inflation
stopcock

Optical connector

Thermistor
connector

RV extra
port lumen
(List nos.
50327, 50328,
50337 only)

CVP
proximal
injectate
lumen

PA distal lumen

Figure P25-3 SVO₂ PA catheter.

TABLE P25-1 Troubleshooting

Problem	Cause	Solution
Bleed back	Loose connections	Check connections
	Open stopcock	Check system
	Crack in transducer or connection	
Dampened waveform	Air bubbles	Check connections
	Clot	Flush system
	Loose connections	Check system
No waveform	Transducer not properly connected to monitor	Check system
False readings	Transducer not properly zeroed or not at the phlebostatic axis	Zero transducer always zero at the phlebostatic axis

- The SVO$_2$ system is calibrated utilizing the in vivo method every 24 hours or per unit protocol.

POTENTIAL COMPLICATIONS

1. Pneumothorax from deep-line insertion
2. Bleeding at the site
3. A life-threatening arrhythmia
4. Puncture of a great vessel or the heart with the catheter
5. Poor catheter placement
6. Balloon breakage during insertion
7. For troubleshooting problems, see Table P25-1.

Bibliography

Horvath, PT, editor: *Care of the adult cardiac surgery patient,* New York, 1984, John Wiley and Sons.

Lamb JI, Carlson VR, editors: *Handbook of cardiovascular nursing,* Philadelphia, 1986, JB Lippincott.

Neff JA, Kidd PS: *Trauma nursing: the art and science,* St Louis, 1993, Mosby.

Vazquez M, Lazear SE, Larson EL: *Critical care nursing,* ed 2, Philadelphia, 1992, WB Saunders.

Sexual Assault Evidence Collection

Patty Sturt

DESCRIPTION

Rape and sexual assault are crimes that remain prevalent in our society. Emergency department (ED) nurses need to be aware of their role in the care of these patients. The primary role of the nurse includes (1) minimizing further physical and psychologic trauma of the victim and (2) collecting and preserving medicolegal evidence for potential use in the legal system.

INDICATIONS

Patients that present to the ED reporting they have been raped or sexually assaulted.

CONTRAINDICATIONS

The chances of finding physical evidence decrease in direct proportion to the length of time which has elapsed between the assault and examination. Generally, if the assault took place more than 48 hours before the examination, it is unlikely that trace evidence will still be present on the patient. However, evidence may still be gathered by documenting any findings obtained during the examination such as lacerations, bruises, bite marks, and statements about the assault. In addition, counseling on prophylaxis for sexually transmitted diseases (STDs) and community support services should be provided.

EQUIPMENT

- Speculum: Have different sizes available. If vaginal trauma is present, a small speculum may be needed to prevent additional discomfort.
- Sexual assault evidence collection kit. If this is not available, obtain the following:
  - Paper bags (for clothing)

- Comb
- 8 to 12 packaged cotton-tipped applicators
- Microscopic slide with slide cover and container
- Two blood tubes with an anticoagulant
- Several envelopes and ziplock bags
- Labels with the patient's name, hospital identification number, date, time of evidence collection, and specimen (evidence collected)
- *Chlamydia* and gonorrhea cultures
- Personal care items such as toothbrush, tooth paste, and soap for the patient's use after the sexual assault examination.

INITIAL NURSING ACTIONS

1. Some sexual assault victims may suffer life-threatening injuries. Always assess and treat any life-threatening injuries first.
2. Place the patient in a private area away from other patients and visitors. Never allow a sexual assault victim to wait in the lobby.
3. Approach the patient in a nonjudgmental manner, conveying empathy and concern. Sexual assault victims do experience psychologic trauma, although the effects of this trauma may be more difficult to recognize than the physical trauma. Each person has his or her own way of coping with sudden stress. Victims can appear to be calm, indifferent, submissive, jocular, angry, withdrawn, or even uncooperative and hostile toward those who are trying to help. All of these responses are within the range of anticipated reactions. These patients should be treated with special consideration to help alleviate the psychologic trauma associated with sexual assault.
4. Explain the plan of care, which includes identifying injuries, collecting medicolegal evidence, STD and pregnancy prophylaxis, and support service referrals.
5. If the patient does not have a friend or family member present, ask if there is someone he/she would like to call. Offer to call the rape crisis center that serves the area. Many rape crisis centers will send a counselor to the ED.

NURSING ALERT

Every effort should be made to have one primary nurse assigned to the patient. Sexual assault victims often experience shame, guilt, and fear. The patient is more likely to express his/her concerns and cooperate with the examination if a rapport is established with one nurse.

6. Obtain consent for treatment in the ED and for collection of medicolegal evidence. If adult victims are reluctant to sign a consent form for the collection of evidence, they should be assured that evidence will NOT obligate them to pursue prosecution of their case.

7. Notify police per hospital policy and state laws. Sexual assault victims should be gently encouraged to report and/or cooperate in the police investigation. However, they may refuse to do so out of fear, embarrassment, or other reasons.

8. Follow the hospital policy regarding the collection of sexual assault medicolegal evidence. In some institutions the nurse can collect the appropriate clothing, saliva swabs, and hair and blood specimens.

9. Have the patient undress and put on a hospital gown while standing on a sheet or pad. Hair, grass, fibers, or other evidence may fall from the clothing while the patient undresses. Carefully fold the pad (or sheet) and place in a paper bag with a label or in the sexual assault evidence collection kit. Collect the panties and place in a small paper bag. Seal the bag with tape. Attach a patient label to the outside of the bag.
Rationale: The panties can be analyzed for seminal fluid, spermatozoa, or foreign debris.

10. Other pieces of clothing should be collected if they are damaged or torn or if there are stains such as blood or semen. Each piece of clothing collected should be air dried (if wet) and placed in a separate paper bag. Attach a patient label to each bag.

NURSING ALERT

Plastic bags should not be used, since they hold on to moisture that can deteriorate evidence.

11. Obtain four saliva swabs. Place all four in the patient's mouth and instruct the patient to saturate them with saliva. The patient should not have anything to eat, drink, or smoke for a minimum of 15 minutes before obtaining the saliva swabs. Allow the swabs to air dry. Place the swabs in an envelope. Tape the envelope and label.
    Rationale: The saliva swabs are used to determine if the patient secretes properties of his/her blood groups (secretor status).

12. Have the patient pull at least fifteen head hairs from different locations on the scalp. Place in a ziplock bag and label.
    Rationale: Hair may have been transferred from the suspect to the victim. Hair can be analyzed using a comparison microscope. It is best to use pulled hair as the roots can also be analyzed for comparison purposes.

13. Place the pad provided in the evidence kit or a paper towel under the patient's perineal area. Thoroughly comb the pubic hair with downward strokes. Place the comb on the paper and gently fold the paper to retain the comb and any evidence. Place in an envelope, tape the envelope, and label.

14. Pull (or have the victim pull) at least fifteen pubic hairs from different locations. Place in a ziplock bag. Seal the bag and label.
    Rationale: The pulled pubic hairs are used for comparison with hairs found at the crime scene or on the assailant's body.

15. Obtain 1 to 2 tubes of blood for medicolegal purposes. Many crime laboratories prefer blood tubes with an anticoagulant. Place a patient label on each tube.
    Rationale: The purpose of this is to determine the victim's blood groups. Blood groups include ABO type and properties or groupings of certain proteins. This may be useful in identifying the victim's blood if found on the suspect or the crime scene. Determining the victim's blood groups makes it possible to determine if the victim secretes properties of his/her blood groups in body secretions such as saliva. Other blood should be obtained at this time if ordered by the physician. Blood/urine screens for toxicology should be

performed if the victim states that he/she was drugged by the assailant and/or the victim's medical condition appears to warrant toxicology screening for optimal patient care. For patients at risk for pregnancy, a urine or blood test should be done to rule out preexisting pregnancy.

16. Assist the physician with collection of evidence during the pelvic examination. Four vaginal swabs should be collected. Use one of these swabs to prepare a smear on the slide. Allow the vaginal swabs to air dry. Place them in an envelope. Tape the envelope and label. Place the vaginal smear in a slide holder, tape it closed, and label. These should be collected if vaginal assault occurred. The slide should not be fixed or stained. Write "vaginal" on the frosted end of the slide.
    Rationale: The vaginal swabs and smear are analyzed for spermatozoa and blood groups. If the assailant is a secretor, properties of his blood may be found in the vaginal swabs. The alleged assailant (if known) will have blood drawn to test for his blood groups. If there is a match between the swabs and his blood groups, it can serve as medicolegal evidence in court.

17. Four anal swabs should be collected if anal assault occurred.

18. Four buccal swabs should be collected if oral-genital assault occurred. Swab along the buccal area and gum line.

PATIENT CARE MANAGEMENT

1. The physician and/or nurse should document the patient's description of the assault. This should include any oral, vaginal, or rectal penetration.

2. Document and describe any bruises, lacerations, bite marks, or other signs of trauma. Body diagrams are very useful in describing the location and type of injury.

3. The patient's last menstrual period and contraceptive history should be recorded.

4. Administer antibiotics for STD prophylaxis as ordered by the physician.

5. Treatment for prevention of pregnancy should be discussed with the patient. Ovral, two tablets orally and repeated in 12 hours may be prescribed. This should be given only if a urine or blood pregnancy test is negative.

Inform the patient that nausea and vomiting may occur. Small frequent meals may decrease the nausea.

6. Refer the patient to a rape crisis center or sexual assault counselor for counseling.
7. Refer the patient to a gynecology clinic for follow-up STD and pregnancy testing and possible HIV testing. HIV testing of sexual assault victims in the ED is controversial. Emergency departments do not routinely provide confidential individual HIV counseling. For this reason the patient can be referred to a clinic or office that performs the test and provides counseling.
8. Provide clean clothing for the patient. Assist the patient in finding transportation home.
9. Maintain the chain of evidence at all times. If at all possible, one nurse should assist with the evidence collection and maintain possession of the evidence until it is signed over to a law enforcement officer.

Bibliography

1. Evidence collection handbook, Frankfort, KY, 1994, Kentucky State Police, Forensic Laboratories.
2. State sexual assault protocol, Frankfort, KY, 1987, Office of the Attorney General, Victims Advocacy Commission.

Splint Application

Betty Gaudet Nolan
Patty Sturt

DESCRIPTION

Splinting is a technique used to immobilize or stabilize an injured extremity. Immobilization decreases pain, swelling, muscle spasm, bleeding into the tissue, and the risk of fat emboli. Immobilization can also prevent a closed fracture from converting to an open fracture.

INDICATIONS

Splinting is indicated anytime there is trauma to an extremity with evidence of deformity, angulation, crepitus, edema, ecchymosis, significant pain, open soft-tissue injury, an impaled object, or neurovascular compromise (1).

EQUIPMENT

Splinting material that is appropriate for the injury. The following are four general categories of splints:
- Soft-nonrigid splints: Pillows, cravats, clavicle straps, sling and swathe, cervical collars (Figure P27–1).
- Hard-rigid and semirigid splints: Aluminum, wooden boards, molded plastic, plaster, fiberglass, cervical collars.
- Pneumatic-inflatable splints: Air splints and pneumatic antishock garments (PASG).
- Traction splints: Hare, Sager, and Thomas splints.
- Other equipment may include tape, padding material, and elastic bandages (ace wraps).

INITIAL NURSING ACTIONS

1. Explain the procedure to the patient.
2. Prepare the patient for splinting by removing clothing over the injury site, dressing any open wounds, removing jewelry, and completing a baseline neurovascular assessment (distal and proximal pulses, color,

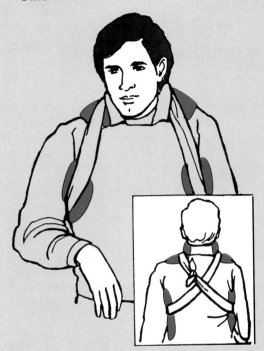

Figure P27–1 Posterior and anterior view of clavicle strap with a cravat.

    temperature, movement, sensation, and capillary refill of the digits).
3. Splint the joint in the position found unless the distal pulse is diminished or absent. When there is no palpable pulse present, apply sustained and gentle traction along the long axis of the extremity, distal to the injury until the pulse can be palpated (1).
4. Use padding over bony prominences. For nonjoints, immobilize the injured area along with the joint above and below the site.
5. Splints should not be tight enough to be constrictive.
6. Check the neurovascular status with each application or removal of splint or repositioning of extremity.

PREASSEMBLED PLASTER SPLINTS

Certain splinting can be done with preassembled plaster splints with incorporated padding such as those made by Orthopedic Casting Laboratory (OCL). They come in 2, 3, 4, and 6 inch widths.

General Preparation Steps for OCL Splinting Material

1. Prepare OCL splint with template (a cutting guide for different splints). Wear goggles to prevent plaster from getting into eyes.
2. Immerse in cool water.
3. Squeeze and remove excess water.
4. Stretch and smooth out on a towel.
5. Apply foam side to skin and wrap.

Application of Common Splints
Posterior short leg splint (ankle)

1. Measure (from toes to below the knee) and cut a 4 or 6 inch wide roll (Figure P27-2, *A*). (Figures P27-2, *A* to *D* show application of posterior short leg splint.)

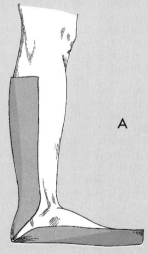

A

Figure P27-2 *A* to **D**, application of posterior short leg splint.

Continued.

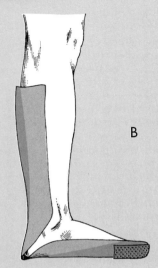

B

Figure P27-2 Cont'd.

2. Place the foot in a 90-degree angle to the leg.
3. Apply the roll posteriorly, folding back plaster at the toes (Figure P27-2, *B*).
4. Tuck in fold at heel area. Secure with elastic bandage (Figure P27-2, *C*).
5. Flare back plaster below knee, secure with elastic bandage, and position and hold foot at 90-degree angle to leg until plaster is set (Figure P27-2, *D*) (3).

Volar cock-up splint
1. Measure from base of fingers to below the elbow and cut a 3 or 4 inch wide roll.
2. Apply and secure roll to volar side (inner aspect) of arm and palm, positioning the wrist in a 15 to 30 degree dorsiflexion (Figure P27-3).

Ulnar gutter (boxer) splint
1. Use template to cut a 3 or 4 inch roll measuring from fingertips to just below the elbow.
2. Fold to form desired gutter, place flap in palm of hand (Figure P27-4).
3. Pad between buddied fingers. Position the hand with the fingers in "position of function" at a 50-degree flexion at the metacarpophalangeal joint and 15 to 20 degree

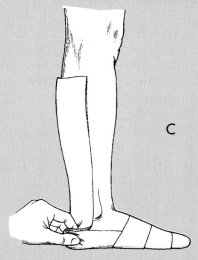

C

Figure P27-2 Cont'd.

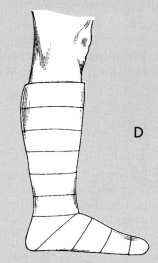

D

Figure P27-2 Cont'd.

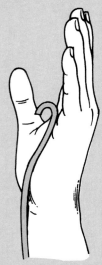

Figure P27-3   Application of Volar cock-up splint.

flexion at the interphalangeal joint with wrist in neutral position (4).

Sugar tong splint

1. Forearm: Measure from knuckles over the flexed elbow and around back to the hand at the midpalmar crease.
2. Humerus: Measure from the acromion process down the humerus, around elbow, and up to the axilla.
3. Using a 3 or 4 inch wide roll, apply the splint with the elbow at 90-degree flexion and secure with elastic bandage (Figure P27-5) (3).

PATIENT CARE MANAGEMENT

1. Instruct the patient to keep the splint clean and dry.
2. Plaster requires 12 to 24 hours to dry. Prevent impression of the plaster during this time or it may become misaligned and pressure sores may develop.
3. If plaster gets wet, it will crumble and not harden again.
4. Look for changes in fingers or toes—coolness, dusky color, swelling, or decrease in sensation.
5. Report pain that increases and does not respond to pain medication.

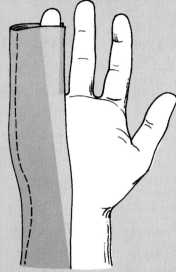

Figure P27-4 Placement of Ulnar gutter splint to form desired gutter.

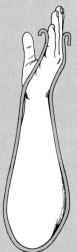

Figure P27-5 Application of Sugar tong splint.

6. Elevate limb to decrease swelling and pain, apply cold packs as directed.
7. Do not put sharp objects inside the splint for scratching.
8. Instruct on crutch walking as needed (see Procedure 9).

Traction Splints

DESCRIPTION

Traction splints are designed to reduce muscle spasms of the injured limb. Traction consists of pull parallel to the long axis of the fractured extremity and opposite to the pull of the major muscles in the area around the fracture site.

INDICATIONS

Traction splints are used to align and stabilize a midshaft femur or proximal tibial fracture.

CONTRAINDICATIONS

Traction splints should not be used for fractures of the distal fibula, distal tibia, ankle, foot, or upper extremity.

EQUIPMENT

There are various types of traction splints currently available including the Thomas half ring, Hare traction, and Sager traction splint.

INITIAL NURSING ACTIONS

1. Remove any constrictive clothing or jewelry.
2. Assess pedal pulses, skin color and temperature, capillary refill, sensation, and movement in the foot of the injured leg.
3. Generally, two clinicians, and optimally three, are needed to apply a traction splint. The first clinician applies manual traction by holding the lower leg and pulling with both hands. Manual traction must be maintained until the splint is in place.

Hare Traction Splint

1. Check Hare traction splint for any missing parts (Figure P27-6).

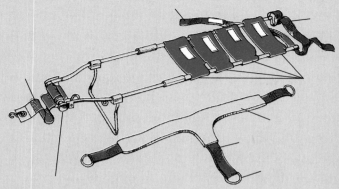

Figure P27-6 Hare traction equipment.

2. Adjust the length of the splint utilizing the patient's uninjured leg. Placing the padded ischial strap or padded ring next to the patient's iliac crest, extend the distal end of the splint by loosening the sleeve-locking device. The end of the splint should be approximately 10 inches past the heel of the foot (Figures P27-7 and P27-8).

3. Tighten the sleeve-locking device.

4. Open all support straps (those that support the thigh and lower leg) or tie cravats with overhand knots spaced evenly throughout the splint.

5. With manual traction still being applied, slide the splint under the affected extremity until the padded ischial strap or ring is against the ischial tuberosity.

6. Pad the groin area with gauze or other suitable material. Secure the ischial strap.

7. Place the ankle hitch under the heel of the foot and cross the side straps over the top of the foot.

8. Pull the release ring on the traction ratchet and release the traction strap. Connect the D rings of the ankle hitch to the S hook of the traction strap.

9. Apply mechanical traction by turning the ratchet knob until splint equals manual traction (2).

10. Extend the heel stand into place to elevate the leg.

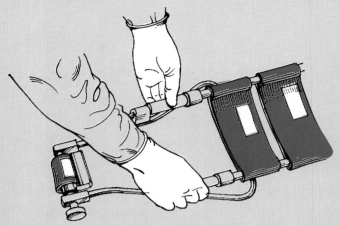

Figure P27-7 Adjusting length of splint with sleeve-locking device.

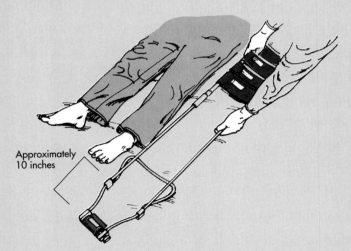

Approximately
10 inches

Figure P27-8 Extending Hare traction splint 10 inches past foot.

11. Secure the Velcro straps or cravats; two above and two below the knee. Do not place straps over the suspected fracture site (Figure P27-9).

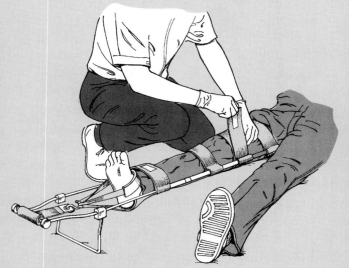

Figure P27-9 Application of strap.

12. Assess the pedal pulses, skin color and temperature, capillary refill, sensation, and movement in the foot of the splinted extremity.

Sager Traction Splint

1. Place the splint medial to the injured extremity with the padded bar resting against perineum (Figure P27-10).
2. Adjust the length until the wheel of the pulley is level with the heel of the patient.
3. Secure the thigh strap.
4. Wrap the ankle harness snugly above the ankle and secure under the heel.
5. Shorten the loop of the ankle harness by threading the strap through the D buckle.
6. Release the lock on the splint and pull the shaft out until the desired amount of traction tension is noted on the marking of the pulley wheel. The amount of traction should equal approximately 10% of the patient's body weight.

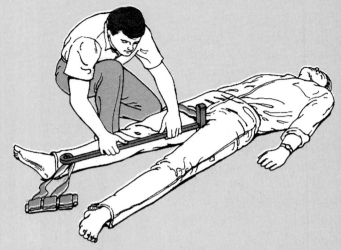

Figure P27-10 Sager traction splint to medial aspect of injured leg.

7. Secure straps at thigh, knee, and lower leg.
8. Strap ankle and feet together to prevent rotation of the injured extremity (Figure P27-11).
9. Reassess pedal pulses, skin color, temperature, capillary refill, sensation, and movement in the foot of the injured extremity (2).

PATIENT CARE MANAGEMENT

1. Continue to monitor the neurovascular status of the injured extremity at frequent intervals.
2. Maintain traction until definite stabilization, such as insertion of a Steinmann pin, is initiated.
3. If pedal pulses are absent, or there are other significant changes in the neurovascular status, inform the physician. The amount of traction may need to be slightly decreased or increased.

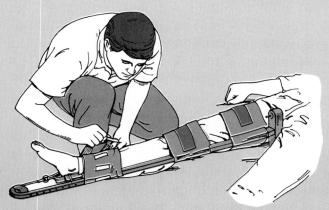

Figure P27-11 Application of straps.

References

1. Emergency Nurses Association, *Trauma nurse core course*, Chicago, 1991, The Association.
2. Grant HD, Murray RH, Bergeron JD: *Emergency care*, Englewood Cliffs, NJ, 1990, Prentice Hall.
3. OCL splinting manual, Eudora, KS, 1992, M-PACT Management Cooperation.
4. Proehl JA: *Adult emergency nursing procedures*, Boston, 1993, Jones & Bartlett.

Suture/Staple Removal

Betty Gaudet Nolan

DESCRIPTION (SUTURE REMOVAL)

Suture removal of nonabsorbable sutures is performed on a wound that shows signs of healing with no gaps in the skin integrity.

INDICATIONS

The amount of time stitches stay in place is dependent on several factors such as the laceration, type of wound closure, age and health of the patient, and presence of infection (see box).

TIMING OF SUTURE REMOVAL	
Location	**Time (Days)**
Eyelid	3
Cheek	3-5
Nose, forehead, neck	5
Ear, scalp	5-7
Trunk	7-10
Arms and legs	7-10
Hands and feet	7-14
Joints	10-14

The above timeframes are general guidelines. Modifications of these recommendations should be tailored to individual needs. Older patients or patients with a chronic illness may have delayed healing times. Leaving sutures in too long increases the risk of abscess and scar formation. Premature removal of sutures may result in wound disruption and delayed healing.

EQUIPMENT

- Suture removal kit (forceps, scissors, 4 × 4 gauze)
- Normal saline or an antiseptic solution
- Dressings as needed

INITIAL NURSING ACTIONS

1. Explain the procedure to the patient.
2. Gently clean the suture line with normal saline—use hydrogen peroxide if there is dried blood.
3. With forceps, grasp the suture knot and gently pull upwards.
4. Cut the stitch as close to the skin as possible and pull the stitch out. Avoid pulling the outside suture through the skin to decrease contamination of the underlying tissue.
5. Document the number of stitches removed.
6. When removing continuous sutures, cut the stitches on one side of the suture line and remove them through the opposite side.
7. Clean the site as before. Apply a small dressing if there is any bleeding or per physician order.

PATIENT CARE MANAGEMENT

1. Instruct the patient to watch for signs and symptoms of infection such as redness, swelling, pus, red streaks, increased pain or tenderness, or unexplained fever.
2. Remind patient to keep wound clean until completely healed and not to pick at crusts or scabs—they will fall off naturally.

DESCRIPTION (STAPLE REMOVAL)

Staple removal is performed on a wound that shows signs of healing with no gaps in the skin integrity.

INDICATIONS

The amount of time staples stay in place is dependent on the part of the body affected: head and neck, 3 to 5 days; chest and abdomen, 5 to 7 days; lower extremities, 7 to 10 days.

EQUIPMENT

- Staple removal kit (staple extractor, gauze)
- Normal saline or an antiseptic solution
- Dressings as needed

INITIAL NURSING ACTIONS

1. Gently clean the staple line with normal saline—use hydrogen peroxide if dried blood is present.
2. Place the nose of the extractor device beneath the center of the staple.
3. Squeeze down with the thumbs to lift the edges of the staple up until it is reformed.
4. When the extractor is fully closed and the staple reformed, lift the extractor from the skin.

PATIENT CARE MANAGEMENT

1. Instruct the patient to watch for signs and symptoms of infection such as redness, swelling, pus, red streaks, increased pain or tenderness, or unexplained fever.
2. Remind patient to keep wound clean until completely healed and not to pick at crusts or scabs—they will fall off naturally.

Bibliography

Kitt S: Staple removal. In Proehl JA, editor: *Adult emergency nursing procedures,* Norwalk, Conn, 1993, Appleton and Lange.

Kitt S: Suture removal. In Proehl JA, editor: *Adult emergency nursing procedures,* Norwalk, Conn, 1993, Appleton & Lange.

TAC Application

Michele Nypaver

DESCRIPTION

TAC is a topical anesthetic solution utilized for repair of small lacerations. It is beneficial in that, if used correctly, it avoids the need for injectable anesthetics. Effective topical anesthesia for laceration repair decreases pain, enhances patient cooperation and trust, and often results in a more pleasant experience for the child. The efficacy of TAC is dependent on proper application technique.

INDICATIONS

Repair of small lacerations (usually <5 cm), especially in children. TAC is less effective on the trunk or extremities than on the face or scalp.

CONTRAINDICATIONS

1. TAC should **never** be applied to:
   * Wounds involving the nose, ears, penis, digits, or eyelids because of the vasoconstrictive properties of the epinephrine and cocaine.
   * Mucous membranes, burns, or large abrasions. Rapid absorption from these areas increases the risk for systemic toxicity.
2. Known hypersensitivity to tetracaine, epinephrine, or cocaine.
3. Known or suspected coronary artery disease (relative contraindication).
4. Previous seizure disorders (relative contraindication).
5. Agitated child in which inadvertent mucous membrane application might occur.

MEDICATION

TAC is a mixture of tetracaine, Adrenalin, and cocaine. A commonly used concentration of the agents includes:

Tetracaine: 0.25%
Adrenaline: 1:4000
Cocaine: 5.9%
The dose can vary from 2 to 5 ml or 0.09 ml/kg.

EQUIPMENT

- Cotton swab
- Cotton-tipped applicators
- Gauze

INITIAL NURSING ACTIONS

1. Explain procedure to the child and caregiver.
2. TAC should be applied to the inner margins of the wound cavity. This can be achieved by either dripping TAC solution directly into the wound cavity until filled or by directly placing a TAC-soaked cottonball or cotton-tipped applicator into the wound.
3. The remainder of the TAC solution can then be placed on gauze and placed firmly and directly over the wound (perhaps with the cottonball or Q-tip beneath the gauze) for 10 to 15 minutes.
4. After 10 minutes, observe the area for blanching (whitening) of the skin around the wound; this indicates adequate anesthesia has been achieved. If this is not evident, the gauze may be reapplied for 5 more minutes.
5. If adequate anesthesia has not been achieved, injectable lidocaine may be used as an adjunct.

NURSING ALERT

Most failures of TAC are due to an inadequate amount of TAC applied, not using firm pressure to apply TAC, or not applying TAC in the appropriate amount of time before the procedure is done.

PATIENT CARE MANAGEMENT

TAC inadvertently dripped into the eyes of patients has caused pupillary dilatation and conjunctivitis. **TAC used inappropriately on mucosal surface wounds (lip lacerations, buccal mucosal lacerations) has resulted in death secondary to cocaine absorption.**

Bibliography

Altieri, MF, MD, Greene A MD, Hawk WH MD, et al: Comparison of topical tetracaine, adrenaline, and cocaine anesthesia with lidocaine infiltration for repair of lacerations in children, *Ann Emerg Med* 19:63-67, 1990.

Bragdon R MS, RPh, Crabbe LH MD, Ernst AA MD et al: Comparison of tetracaine, adrenaline, and cocaine with cocaine alone for topical anesthesia, *Ann Emerg Med* 19:51-54, 1990.

Grant SAD, MD, Hoffman RS, MD: Use of tetracaine, epinephrine, and cocaine as a topical anesthetic in the emergency department, *Ann Emerg Med* 21:987-997, 1990.

Thoracentesis/Paracentesis

Mary Rose Bauer

DESCRIPTION (THORACENTESIS)

Thoracentesis is a procedure used to evacuate air and/or fluid and to obtain sterile fluid specimens from the pleural space. This procedure can be performed at the bedside using sterile technique.

INDICATIONS

1. Accumulation of fluid (pleural effusion) because of an inflammatory or infectious process
   - Removal of fluid from the pleural cavity may be done for therapeutic or diagnostic purposes.
2. Accumulation of air (pneumothorax) because of chest trauma or trauma of the visceral pleura
   - Removal of air will facilitate lung expansion. However, tube thoracostomy is the treatment of choice.

CONTRAINDICATIONS

1. Respiratory status that is compromised because of certain conditions such as ruptured diaphragm or emphysema. These patients have a higher incidence of a pneumothorax secondary to lung perforation (1).
2. Coagulopathy should be corrected before this procedure, unless there is severe respiratory failure (2).
3. Pleural adhesions increase the risk of perforation of the lung (1).

EQUIPMENT

- Sterile drapes
- Antiseptic solution (povidone-iodine solution commonly used)
- Needles, several sizes, for aspiration (may use 18 or 20 gauge spinal needles, or 16-gauge, 3 inch needle) or through-the-needle catheters. Through-the-needle catheters are preferable in patients that must remain in the supine position.

- 60 cc and 10 cc syringes
- 25-gauge, ⅝-inch and 22-gauge, 1½-inch needles
- Local anesthetic (1% lidocaine usually used)
- Mask
- Sterile gloves
- Three-way stopcock
- 4 × 4 gauze sponges
- Three sterile specimen tubes
- Drainage tube and 500 cc vacuum bottle or collection bag. (If this is unavailable, you may substitute with IV tubing and a 500 cc bag of normal saline. Spike and drain the bag of fluid, then invert, maintaining sterility and connect the sterile tubing to the three-way stopcock for drainage collection.)
- Puncture site bandage
  NOTE: Preassembled kits containing much of this equipment are available in many settings.

INITIAL NURSING ACTION

1. Diagnostic x-rays are generally taken before procedure to determine the highest level of the effusion.
2. Explain procedure to patient.
3. Ideally patient should be placed in seated position, leaning slightly forward, with back to person performing procedure. This can be accomplished by having patient lean forward over a padded bedside table or the back of a chair. If patient must be supine, lateral approach may be used. For this approach, the affected side should face the person performing the procedure with the arm extended above the head for accessibility of site.
4. Prepare site using antiseptic solution. For the removal of pleural fluid, the insertion site is the midscapular or posterior axillary line at a level below the top of the fluid (1). Use 2nd intercostal space, midclavicular line for pneumothorax.
5. Instruct patient to refrain from coughing throughout procedure.
   NOTE: At this point the physician drapes the patient with sterile towels exposing the site of insertion. When the physician inserts the needle, and there is a return of fluid, the nurse connects the tubing, (maintaining sterility), to the stopcock and fastens securely.

6. Provide verbal support and comfort measures during procedure.

7. Sterility should be maintained throughout procedure and sterile connection should not be broken to ensure specimen is not contaminated. Record amount, appearance, and consistency of all fluid obtained during procedure.

8. Following procedure, apply pressure to site to prevent bleeding. Apply a small dressing to puncture site. Obtain a chest x-ray.

9. All specimens should be appropriately labeled and sent to the laboratory for analysis as ordered by physician. Some of the commonly ordered tests are gram stain, culture and sensitivity, cell count, cytology, pH, specific gravity, acid-fast staining, lactic dehydrogenase and total protein.

PATIENT CARE MANAGEMENT

1. Monitor vital signs every 15 minutes for 1 hour, every 30 minutes for 2 hours, and then every hour following until patient is stable.

2. Monitor for signs and symptoms of complications such as pneumothorax, hemothorax, pulmonary edema, hypoxia, respiratory distress, and later, infection. Symptoms may include dizziness, increased respirations, uncontrollable cough, tightness in chest, frothy blood-tinged sputum, tachycardia, and shortness of breath.

3. Continue to assess for any pain, tenderness, redness, or drainage from the site.

DESCRIPTION (PARACENTESIS)

Paracentesis is a procedure used to remove fluid from the peritoneal space using a large bore needle and closed drainage system. It may be performed to obtain specimens used in the diagnosis of certain conditions or as a preparation for other procedures.

INDICATIONS

1. Accumulation of fluid or pressure in the abdominal cavity because of trauma or disease process
   - Aspiration of fluid in the peritoneal space for analysis and culture

- Drainage of fluid to relieve intraabdominal pressure
2. Preparation for other procedures such as peritoneal dialysis or surgery

CONTRAINDICATIONS

1. Coagulopathy or thrombocytopenia should be corrected before this procedure to avoid predispostion to bleeding.
2. Severe bowel distension
   - Placement of nasogastric tube and/or rectal tube may be required for decompression before procedure.
3. Previous abdominal surgery

EQUIPMENT

See equipment list for Thoracentesis on pp. 857, 858.

INITIAL NURSING ACTIONS

1. Explain procedure to patient.
2. Bladder must be emptied before procedure either by voiding or placement of a catheter.
3. Raise head of bed to a 45-degree angle (if tolerated). Allow at least 10 minutes for fluid to pool in the abdominal cavity.
4. Prepare the insertion site by cleansing the abdomen between the umbilicus and the symphysis pubis, including both lower quadrants, with antiseptic solution. NOTE: At this point the physician drapes the patient with sterile drapes, exposing the site of insertion. Attach collection device to tubing and three-way stopcock. After insertion of catheter and aspiration with syringe, connect the stopcock and tubing to the catheter.
5. Be sure to record amount, color, and consistency of all drainage.
6. Continue to assess vital signs during procedure.
7. Apply pressure to site for approximately 5 minutes, then place a small sterile dressing to puncture site following procedure.
8. Label all specimens appropriately and send to laboratory for testing per physician request.

PATIENT CARE MANAGEMENT

1. Monitor for pain or discomfort. Provide comfort measures.

2. Monitor vital signs every 30 minutes for 2 hours, then every hour until stable.
3. Check dressing for signs of leakage, bleeding, tenderness, swelling, or redness.

References

1. Gray MJ, Littleton AD: Thoracentesis. In Proehl JA, editor: *Adult emergency nursing procedures*, Boston, 1993, Jones & Bartlett.
2. Knighton D, Locksley RM, Mills J: Emergency procedures. In Saunder CE, Ho MT, editors: *Current emergency diagnosis and treatment*, Norwalk, Conn, 1992, Appleton & Lange.

Vascular Access Devices

Patty Sturt

In recent years there have been major advances in vascular access devices (VADs). These devices are placed in patients requiring frequent, prolonged, or repeated administration of fluids or drugs such as chemotherapy, antibiotics, or hyperalimentation. Emergency nurses may encounter patients with various VADs including peripherally inserted central catheters (PICCs), central venous tunneled catheters (CVTCs), and implanted ports. Blood products can be administered through these devices.

PICCS

Description
Available in sizes ranging from 23 to 16 gauge. Length varies from 3 to 24 inches. These catheters are inserted into the antecubital region with the tip resting at the superior vena cava or another major vessel. These catheters can remain in place for several weeks to months.

INITIAL NURSING ACTIONS

1. **Obtaining blood:** It may be difficult to obtain blood from a PICC with a very small lumen because the catheter tends to collapse on aspiration. Flushing the catheter with 5 to 10 ml of normal saline before aspirating makes it easier to obtain blood from PICCs with larger lumens. When obtaining blood, discard the first 3 ml. Pull back on the syringe plunger gently and slowly for best results. Correct catheter placement can be confirmed by a chest x-ray.
2. **Flushing:** Flush the line after you infuse any agent. The flush should consist of 5 to 10 ml of normal saline or 2 to 3 ml of normal saline followed by 1 ml of heparin solution (100 U/ml). When flushing always use at least a 5 ml syringe. Smaller syringes generate higher pressures that can result in catheter rupture.

3. **Infusing fluids/medications:** Avoid excessive pressure when infusing fluids or IV push medications. Excessive pressure may tear the catheter. Never forcefully inject through a PICC. To start an infusion, connect a 1 inch or shorter needle to the IV tubing and insert needle into PICC latex port.

4. **Dressing:** Keep a transparent occlusive dressing over the entrance site.

CVTCs

Description

These are also referred to as long-term indwelling catheters or right atrial catheters. Two examples of such catheters include the Hickman catheter (Figure P31-1) and the Groshong catheter (Figure P31-2). The catheter tip is placed in the superior vena cava proximal to the right atrium. The catheter is tunneled under the skin and exits at the 4th to 5th intercostal space onto the chest.

INITIAL NURSING ACTIONS

Hickman

1. **Obtaining blood:** Stop infusions for 1 minute before obtaining blood. Prep injection cap with antiseptic swab. Insert 20 gauge, 1 inch needle into the injection cap. Open clamp, slowly withdraw 5 ml of blood, and waste. Use another syringe and needle to obtain needed blood.

2. **Flushing:** Cleanse injection cap with antiseptic swab. Irrigate the catheter with 10 ml normal saline between drug infusions and after drawing blood. Flush with 2.5 to 3 ml of heparin solution after using the catheter and once a day to keep the catheter patent. One hundred U/ml of heparin solution is commonly used for adults. Other heparin concentrations (10 to 1000 U/ml) (amount of solution is adjusted as appropriate for dosage) may be used depending on the patient's medical condition and laboratory values. If more than one lumen is present, flush each lumen. Inject heparin slowly. Withdraw needle from injection cap as last 0.5 cc of solution is infused. Close each clamp.

3. **Infusing fluids:** For continuous IV fluid administration, remove the male adapter (injection cap) from the hub

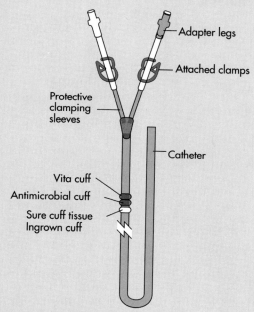

Figure P31-1   Hickman Dual-Lumen Catheter.

of the catheter and connect IV tubing. Unclamp catheter and start IV infusion.

4. **Dressing:** Transparent occlusive dressing.

Groshong

1. **Obtaining blood:** Same as the Hickman catheter except the Groshong catheter will not have a clamp because of the closed distal tip. A small slit near the tip stays closed under normal conditions, which prevents backflow of blood. Often helpful to pull back plunger 0.5 ml, pause for 2 second count, then slowly withdraw blood.

2. **Flushing:** Cleanse injection cap with antiseptic swab. Flush with 20 ml of normal saline after drawing blood. Flush with 5 ml of normal saline each week (no heparin). Withdraw needle while injecting last 0.5 ml of saline.

3. **Infusing fluids:** Same as Hickman except there is no catheter clamp.

4. **Dressings:** Same as Hickman.

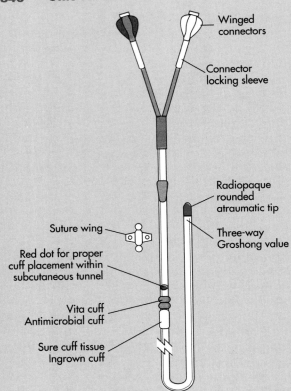

Figure P31-2 Groshong Dual-Lumen Catheter.

IMPLANTABLE PORTS

Description

Examples include Port-A-Cath Mediport, and Bard Implanted Ports. Consists of a catheter attached to a stainless steel, plastic, or titanium chamber that contains a self-sealing silicone diaphragm (Figure P31-3). The catheter is completely internal with the skin acting as a protective covering. The catheter's tip is placed in the superior vena cava. The port usually lies near the 2nd and 4th rib subcutaneously.

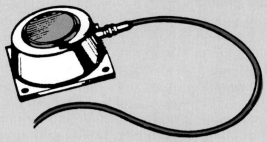

Figure P31-3 Implantable Port.

NURSING ALERT

Manufacturers of metal ports recommend that the port not be exposed to the magnetic field in magnetic resonance imaging (MRI).

INITIAL NURSING ACTIONS (ACCESSING THE PORT)

1. Open sterile gloves and use glove package as sterile field. Place following on the sterile field:
   - Alcohol and povidone-iodine swabs
   - 90-degree noncoring VAD needle (Huber, Lifeport)
   - Tegaderm dressing
   - 20 gauge, 1 inch needle
   - Eye patches
   - Male Luer-Lok with injectable diaphragm
   - 10 ml syringe
   - Extension tubing

NURSING ALERT

The VAD needles vary in size from 22 to 19 gauge and ⅝ to 1 inch in length. Use the larger size if the patient requires blood products.

2. Put on sterile gloves.
3. Cleanse skin over the injection port with 1 to 3 alcohol swabs using circular motions with each swab.
4. Cleanse same area with povidone-iodine swabs. Let dry for 1 minute and then wipe area with one alcohol swab.

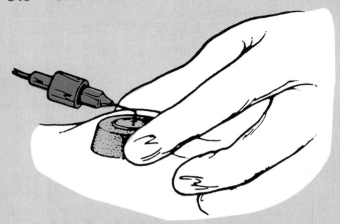

Figure P31-4 Accessing the port.

5. Connect Male Luer-Lok to extension tubing.
6. Connect extension tubing to 90-degree VAD needle (some needles come with attached extension sets).
7. Draw up 5 to 7 ml of normal saline. Remove air bubbles.
8. Insert needle of syringe into Luer-Lok and flush extension tubing and VAD needle.
9. Feel injection site (port) with one hand.
10. Place thumb on one side of the port and index finger on the other to stabilize the port.
11. With other hand, hold needle perpendicular to the skin. Firmly insert needle through the skin into the port until it touches the bottom of the chamber. Do not rock or move needle from side to side during insertion (Figure P31-4).
12. Unclamp extension tubing.
13. Gently pull back on plunger of syringe until you see blood. If there is no blood return with aspiration, have patient raise arms, cough, or turn sideways. If unable to achieve blood return, remove needle and try again with a new needle.
14. Push the normal saline into the injection site.
15. Clamp extension set. Place one eye patch under and one above the 90-degree VAD needle. Cover with an occlusive dressing such as Tegaderm.

NURSING ALERT

If the patient is to have long-term IV fluids or blood products, connect the IV tubing directly to the extension tubing. If the patient is to receive IV fluids and be discharged from the ED, the IV tubing can be connected to the Luer-Lok by a needle. Contact patient's physician, hospice, or home health nurse (if appropriate) to determine if the VAD needle and extension tubing should stay in place for IV fluids or medication while the patient is home.

16. **Starting an infusion:** Connect primed IV tubing into extension tubing. Unclamp extension tubing. Start infusion.
17. **Disconnecting an infusion:** Draw up 10 ml of normal saline and 5 ml of heparinized solution (100 U/ml for adults and 10 U/ml for children). Clamp extension tubing. Remove IV tubing. Inject normal saline and then heparinized solution into male Luer-Lok. Clamp the extension set while flushing the last 0.5 ml of solution.
18. **Obtaining blood:** Unclamp extension set. Withdraw 3 to 5 ml of blood from Luer-Lok and discard. With another syringe and needle, obtain needed blood. Flush with 5 ml of normal saline and continue infusion. If no infusion, inject 10 to 20 ml of normal saline. Administer heparinized solution as when discontinuing infusion.
19. **Removing VAD needle:** Remove dressing. Cleanse end of Luer-Lok with povidone-iodine swab. Insert a needle with a 5 ml syringe with heparinized solution into Luer-Lok. Stabilize port with thumb and index finger. Push in solution. Begin pulling the needle out while pushing in the last 0.5 ml.
20. **Flushing requirements:** When not accessed, the port should be flushed every 4 weeks with 5 ml of heparinized (100 U/ml for adults, 10 U/ml for children) solution.

Wound Care

Chris Lindsey
Kim Short

INDICATIONS

A. Treatment of wound may begin at triage.
   1. Be familiar with patient's medical history and allergies, including tetanus status (see Reference Guide 8).
   2. Bleeding may need to be controlled by direct pressure or pressure bandage and/or elevation.
   3. Inform patient of wound care procedure.
   4. Using clean technique, gently cleanse the wound with normal saline. Apply a normal–saline-soaked dressing to wound, and secure with a dry dressing.
   5. Apply ice to the area if edema is present. Instruct the patient to elevate the affected area at or above the level of the heart.

Ice packs should never be placed directly onto the skin because of possibility of skin damage related to the cold contact. Always provide a protective barrier between ice pack and skin.

   6. Instruct patient to inform triage nurse of active bleeding.

B. Simple wound care is used to clean abrasions, superficial lacerations, minor puncture wounds, and minor bites.
   1. Rinse the area thoroughly with normal saline.
   2. Allow the area to air dry or gently dry with gauze.
   3. Apply thin layer of triple antibiotic ointment. Ointment may be applied with a sterile tongue blade.
   4. Apply a dry sterile dressing to the area as needed.
   5. Discharge patient home with wound care instructions.

C. Wound care procedure for deep lacerations, deep puncture wounds or avulsions vary depending on

severity and length of time since injury. All wounds
need to be cleansed following simple wound care
procedure. In addition, deep irrigation, exploration,
and closure of wounds may be done in the emergency
department (ED) or operating room. Use the following
procedure if performed in the ED:

1. Be familiar with patient's medical history, allergies,
   and tetanus status.
2. Continue to monitor wound for active bleeding and
   control as needed.
3. Inform patient of wound care procedure.
4. Organize supplies as in simple wound care. Include a
   catheter-tipped 60-cc syringe, a 20- or 60-cc syringe,
   18-gauge IV catheter, and anesthetic supplies as
   needed.
5. Administer appropriate analgesics and anesthetics:
   a. If IV conscious sedation is used, monitor patient
      according to IV conscious sedation (see
      Procedure 8).
   b. If TAC is used, follow facility's potocol (see
      Procedure 29). Never apply TAC to mucosal surface.
6. Gently cleanse the area with cleansing agent of
   choice using 4 × 4 sponges (Table P32-1).
7. Normal saline is usually the preferred irrigating
   solution because of its nontoxicity and cost. A 35 cc
   syringe with 19-gauge needle provides high pressure
   irrigation when held 1 to 2 inches from the wound
   (1). Caution should be used when irrigating with a
   needle. An 18-gauge IV catheter with the needle
   removed can be safely used for irrigation.
8. Allow wound to dry.
9. Prepare for wound closure as indicated in the
   following guidelines: (see Table P32-1 for wound
   closures).
   a. Wounds <8 hours old may be closed by suturing or
      steri-strips.
   b. Facial wounds have a 12-hour window for suturing.
   c. Wounds >8 to 12 hours old may be considered
      contaminated, have a higher infection risk, and
      may be left open to heal by secondary intention.
      (Hand wounds are those with the highest risk for
      infection).

10. When cleansing and closure are completed, apply a thin layer of triple antibiotic ointment with sterile tongue blade.
11. Apply dry, sterile dressing when indicated. Light pressure may be needed to decrease edema related to inflammatory response and contusions and to control bleeding.

References

1. Edlich R, Rodeheaver G, Morgan R, Berman D, Thacker J: Principles of emergency wound management, *Ann Emerg Med* 17:1284-1302, 1988.

TABLE P32-1 Antiseptic Solutions

Agents	Antimicrobial activity	Mechanics of action	Tissue toxicity	Indications and contraindications
Povidone-iodine solution (iodine complexes) (Betadine)	Available as a 10% solution with polyvinyl-pyrrolidine (povidone) containing 1% free iodine with broad rapid-onset antimicrobial activity	Potent germicide in low concentrations	Will decrease PMN migration and life span at concentration >1% May cause systemic toxicity at higher concentrations; questionable toxicity at 1% concentration	Probably a safe and effective wound cleanser at a 1% concentration 10% solution is effective to prepare the skin about the wound
Povidone-iodine surgical scrub	Same as the solution	Same	Toxic to open wounds	Best as a hand cleanser; never use in open wounds
Nonionic detergents (Pluronic F-68, Shur-Clens)	Ethylene oxide is 80% of its molecular weight It has no antimicrobial activity	Wound cleanser	No toxicity to open wounds, eyes, or intravenous solutions	It appears to be an effective, safe wound cleanser
Hydrogen peroxide	3% solution in water has brief germicidal activity	Oxidizing agent that denatures protein	Toxic to open wound	Should not be used on wounds after the initial cleaning; may be used to clean intact skin

Continued.

853

TABLE P32-1 Antiseptic Solutions (cont'd)

Agents	Antimicrobial activity	Mechanics of action	Tissue toxicity	Indications and contraindications
Hexachlorophene (pHisoHex) (polychlorinated bisphenol)	Bacteriostatic (2% to 5%) Greater activity against gram-positive organisms	Interruption of bacterial electron transport and disruption of membrane-bound enzymes	Little skin toxicity; the scrub form is damaging to open wound	Never use scrub solution in open wounds Very good preoperative hand preparation
Alcohols	Low-potency antimicrobial most effective as a 70% ethyl and 70% isoproyl alcohol solution	Denatures protein	Will kill irreversibly and function as a fixative	No role in routine care
Phenols	Bacteriostatic >2% Bactericidal >1% Fungicidal 1.3%	Denatures protein	Extensive tissue necrosis and systemic toxicity	Never use >2% aqueous phenol or >4% phenol plus glycerol

From Simon R: Principles of wound management. In Rosen P, Barkin RM, Braen GR, et al editors: *Emergency medicine: concepts and clinical practice,* ed 3, vol I, St. Louis, 1992, Mosby.